# CLINICAL HYPERTENSION

Fifth Edition

# CLINICAL HYPERTENSION

## Fifth Edition

## Norman M. Kaplan, M.D.

*Professor of Medicine*
*Department of Internal Medicine*
*University of Texas Southwestern Medical School*
*Dallas, Texas*

WITH A CHAPTER BY

## Ellin Lieberman, M.D.

*Professor of Pediatrics*
*University of Southern California*
*School of Medicine*
*Los Angeles, California*

*Editorial Consultant*
*William W. Neal, M.D.*
*Veterans Administration Medical Center*
*Dallas, Texas*

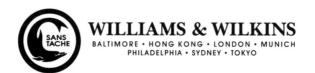

**WILLIAMS & WILKINS**
BALTIMORE · HONG KONG · LONDON · MUNICH
PHILADELPHIA · SYDNEY · TOKYO

*Editor:* Michael G. Fisher
*Associate Editor:* Carol Eckhart
*Copy Editor:* Susan Vaupel
*Designer:* Norman W. Och
*Illustration Planner:* Ray Lowman
*Production Coordinator:* Charles E. Zeller

Copyright © 1990
Williams & Wilkins
428 East Preston Street
Baltimore, Maryland 21202, USA

Accurate indications, adverse reactions, and dosage schedules for drugs are provided in this book, but it is possible that they may change. The reader is urged to review the package information data of the manufacturers of the medications mentioned.

*Printed in the United States of America*

First Edition 1973

**Library of Congress Cataloging in Publication Data**

Kaplan, Norman M., 1931–
    Clinical hypertension / Norman M. Kaplan, with a chapter by Ellin Lieberman. — 5th ed.
        p.    cm.
    Includes bibliographical references.
    ISBN 0-683-04522-9
    1. Hypertension.  I. Title.
    [DNLM: 1. Hypertension.   WG 340 K17c]
RC685.H8K35   1990
616.1′32—dc20
DNLM/DLC
for Library of Congress                                                      89-24802
                                                                                   CPI

                                                                    92  93  94
                                                        3   4   5   6   7   8   9  10

*To those such as:*

Goldblatt and Grollman,
Folkow and Pickering,
Braun-Menéndez and Page,
Tobian and Laragh,
Chesley and Freis,
and the many others,

*whose work has made it possible for me to*
*put together what I hope will be a useful book*
*on clinical hypertension.*

# Preface

Almost 20 years ago, in putting together the first edition of *Clinical Hypertension*, I wrote, ''There is a need for a clinically oriented, up-to-date book on hypertension that focuses all of the significant advances made during the last ten years into a practical, rational approach toward the management of patients. I hope this book will serve that need.'' The favorable reception accorded the first four editions indicates that this book has met at least part of this need.

It has only been a little over four years since the fourth edition, but the increase in research and clinical work in the field demands a frequent update. Once again, almost every page has been revised, using the same general aims:

- Give most attention to the most common problems. Primary (essential) hypertension takes up almost half of the book.
- Cover every form of hypertension. References are provided for forms of hypertension that are mentioned only briefly.
- Include the latest data, even if available only in abstract form.
- Provide enough pathophysiology to base clinical judgment on sound reason.
- Be objective and clearly identify biases. Although my views may be counter to those of others, I have tried to give reasonable attention to those with whom I disagree.

Once again I am pleased that Dr. Ellin Lieberman, Head of Pediatric Nephrology at the Children's Hospital of Los Angeles, has contributed a chapter on hypertension in children and adolescents. Many others have helped. Portions of the text have been reviewed by colleagues at the Medical School, including Drs. Hong Tjoa, Robert Boldrick, and William Henrich. I am particularly indebted to Dr. William Neal for the many hours spent in proofing and organizing the content. I have been fortunate in being in an academic setting wherein such endeavors are nurtured, much to the credit of our former chief, Dr. Donald Seldin. I have been greatly helped by my secretaries, Susan Beaubien and Sharon Washington. And lastly, the forbearance of Audrey, my wife, can only be acknowledged by the promise that I will not do it again—at least for another four years.

The time and energy required to write a medical book almost single-handedly have made the endeavor increasingly rare and perhaps foolhardy. But I believe the reader benefits from having a single overall perspective, systematically presented, with little redundancy but considerable cross-reference. To divide the task between multiple coauthors may provide greater depth in certain areas but almost certainly will leave some areas uncovered and others rehashed unevenly.

As I went through this revision, I was amazed at the tremendous amount of new information published over the past four years. Some is repetitious and minor; multiple journals about hypertension are now being published whereas no journals on hypertension existed when the first edition of this book was written. A considerable amount of significant new information is included in this book, hopefully presented in a manner that enables the reader to grasp its significance and place it in perspective. The task of keeping up with all of clinical hypertension is almost beyond one person's ability; I hope that my attempt will prove both interesting and informative for those who care for the millions of people with hypertension, our most common disease.

# Contents

# 1 Hypertension in the Population at Large

Hypertension, in the United States, is now the leading indication for both office visits to physicians (National Center for Health Statistics—McLemore and DeLozier, 1987) and the use of prescription drugs (National Center for Health Statistics—Koch and Knapp, 1987). These leading positions reflect the tremendous increase in the number of people with hypertension who have been identified and brought under active treatment over the past 25 years. This increase has occurred throughout the world but probably nowhere to the degree as in the United States where, in 1985, 85% of adults had their blood pressure taken and two-thirds of all of those found to have an elevated blood pressure at least twice were currently taking antihypertensive medication (National Center for Health Statistics—Schoenborn, 1988).

Nonetheless, for many, here and elsewhere, the risks of unrecognized and untreated hypertension persist. High blood pressure is a major risk factor for premature death and disability because of the large number of people afflicted and the consequences of uncontrolled hypertension. The main burden of illness associated with hypertension arises not from the relatively few with severe disease but from the masses of people with pressures that are only minimally elevated (MacMahon et al, in press).

On the other hand, there are risks of therapy, some of which have only surfaced in the last few years as more and more of the larger population of patients with mild hypertension have been given antihypertensive drug therapy. In the rush to identify and treat all with high blood pressure, there is a need for caution not to falsely label and inappropriately treat many millions of people.

In this first chapter, the overall problems of hypertension for the population at large will be considered. I will attempt to define the disease, quantitate its prevalence and risks, classify types, and describe the current status of detection and control. The next chapter will consider the individual patient, covering the measurement of the blood pressure, the management of its variability, and guidelines for evaluation of the types, consequences, and risks of hypertension.

## CONCEPTUAL DEFINITION OF HYPERTENSION

Although it has been more than 100 years since Mahomed clearly differentiated hypertension from Bright's renal disease, authorities still debate the level of blood pressure to be considered abnormal. Sir George Pickering for many years challenged the wisdom of that debate and decried the search for an arbitrary dividing line between normal and high blood pressure. In 1972 he restated his argument that "there is no dividing line. The relationship between arterial pressure and mortality is quantitative; the higher the pressure, the worse the prognosis." He saw "arterial pressure as a quantity and the consequence numerically related to the size of that quantity" (Pickering, 1972).

However, as Pickering realized, physicians feel more secure in dealing with precise criteria, even if they are basically arbitrary. To consider

1

a blood pressure of 138/88 as normal and one of 140/90 as high is obviously arbitrary, but medical practice requires the setting of criteria. Those criteria are required in order to decide upon the need for workup and therapy. They should be established on some rational basis, and that basis must include the risks of disability and death that are associated with various levels of blood pressure as well as the ability to reduce those risks by lowering the blood pressure. As stated by Rose (1980): "The operational definition of hypertension is the level at which the benefits . . . of action exceed those of inaction."

Even this definition should be broadened, since action, i.e., making the diagnosis of hypertension at any level of blood pressure, involves risks and costs as well as benefits, and inaction may provide benefits (Table 1.1). Therefore, I have proposed that the conceptual definition of hypertension be "that level of blood pressure at which the benefits (minus the risks and costs) of action exceed the risks and costs (minus the benefits) of inaction" (Kaplan, 1983).

Most of the elements of this conceptual definition are fairly obvious, although some—such as interference with life style and risks from biochemical side effects of therapy—may not be obvious and will be analyzed further in this and later chapters. Let us turn first to the issue of the risks of premature cardiovascular disease, since they have been widely taken as the prime, if not the only, basis for deciding the level of blood pressure that is to be called abnormal.

**Table 1.1. Factors Involved in the Conceptual Definition of Hypertension**

|  | Action | Inaction |
|---|---|---|
| Benefits | Reduce strokes, heart failure, renal damage<br>Decrease mortality from heart attacks (?)<br>Prevent progression of hypertension<br>Diagnose other family members | Maintain nonpatient role<br>Less interference with life style |
| Risk/cost | Assume role of patient<br>Interfere with life style<br>Add risks from biochemical side effects of therapy<br>Add costs of health care | Increase risk of premature cardiovascular disease<br>Fail to diagnose other family members |

## Risks of Inaction: The Risks of Elevated Blood Pressure

The risks of elevated blood pressure have been determined largely from large scale epidemiological surveys. A meta-analysis has been performed on all available major prospective observational studies relating blood pressure levels to the development of stroke and coronary heart disease (CHD) (MacMahon et al, 1990). These nine studies involved almost 420,000 people followed for 6 to 25 years among whom 599 fatal strokes and 4260 CHD deaths were recorded (Table 1.2). In this analysis, the associations were examined for diastolic blood pressure (DBP), which has been the usual index.

The overall results demonstrate "direct, continuous and apparently independent associations" with "no evidence of any 'threshold' level of DBP below which lower levels of DBP were not associated with lower risks of stroke and CHD" (Fig. 1.1).

MacMahon et al have taken account of the common practice in all of these studies to measure DBP on only one occasion, which leads to a substantial underestimation of the true association of the usual or long-term average DBP with disease. This arises because there is a strong tendency for both lower and higher readings to regress toward the middle on repeated readings. Since there are relatively few events associated with the lower readings and a much greater number associated with the higher readings, this "regression dilution bias" makes it appear that the risk is greater with higher readings than in fact exist over the longer term. Since most events occur in people whose first reading is higher than subsequent readings, it appears that the events develop at higher DBP than at the significantly lower levels actually present over the longer term. By applying a correction based upon the three sets of readings over 4 years in the Framingham study to all nine sets of data, MacMahon et al come up with estimates of risk that are about 60% greater than those previously published using uncorrected data. They estimate that a persistently higher DBP of 5.0 mm Hg is associated with at least a 34% increase in stroke risk and at least a 21% increase in CHD risk. Parenthetically, as will be noted in Chapter 5, a 5.8-mm Hg difference in DBP was the average difference noted in the major clinical trials of the treatment of hypertension between those who were given active drug therapy and those who were given placebo. The therapy-induced fall in

**Table 1.2.  Study Populations, Follow-up Durations, and Number of Events Provided in Nine Prospective Observational Studies[a]**

| | Number of Subjects | Age Range at Baseline | % Male | Follow-up Duration (Years) after DBP Measurement | Number of Events | |
|---|---|---|---|---|---|---|
| | | | | | Stroke (Fatal/Not) | CHD (Fatal/Not) |
| MRFIT Screenees (Neaton et al, 1984) | 350,977 | 35–57 | 100 | 6 | 230/– | 2,125/– |
| Chicago Heart Association (Stamler et al, 1975) | 22,777 | 35–64 | 52 | 12 | 81/– | 545/– |
| Whitehall (Reid et al, 1976) | 16,372 | 40–64 | 100 | 10 | 78/– | 557/– |
| Puerto Rico (Garcia-Palmieri and Costas, 1986) | 8,155 | 45–64 | 100 | 6 | –/– | 82/158 |
| Honolulu (Kagan et al, 1974) | 7,317 | 45–68 | 100 | 12 | 80/164 | 151/223 |
| LRC Prevalence (Lipid Research Clinics, 1980) | 4,674 | 25–84 | 65 | 9 | –/– | 65/– |
| Framingham (Dawber, 1980) | 4,641 | 40–69 | 44 | 6[b] | 22/80 | 116/215 |
| Western Electric (Dyer et al, 1977) | 2,025 | 40–59 | 100 | 25 | 46/– | 341/– |
| People's Gas (Dyer, 1975) | 1,402 | 40–59 | 100 | 25 | 62/– | 279/– |
| All studies | 418,340 | 25–84 | 96 | 10 | 599/244 | 4,260/596 |

[a]From MacMahon S, Peto R, Cutler J, et al: *Lancet*, 1990.
[b]The data from Framingham are based on 6-year follow-up among subjects who at survey 3 (1953–56) and among subjects who at survey 6 (about 6 years later) did not have a history of myocardial infarction or stroke. Some subjects contribute to both periods.

DBP provided the full 34% decrease in stroke risk predicted by the estimate of MacMahon et al but less than half of the 21% decrease in the predicted CHD risk.

## Other Epidemiological Data

Data from other populations than those included in Table 1.2 have shown similar relations between blood pressure and both morbidity and mortality from cardiovascular diseases. These include actuarial data of 4.5 million people followed for up to 20 years after application for life insurance (Society of Actuaries, 1980) and surveys of black and white women in Evans County, Georgia (Johnson et al, 1986); young Canadian pilots (Rabkin et al, 1978); the general population in South Wales (Miall, 1982); and middle-aged men in diverse locations, including 7735 in 24 towns in England, Wales, and Scotland (Shaper et al, 1988); 39,207 in Norway (Tverdal, 1987); and 1712 living in rural Italy (Farchi et al, 1987).

One discrepant report came from a 13-year follow-up of 1917 40- to 69-year-old Swedish men and women wherein overall mortality had a U-shaped association with blood pressure (Lindholm et al, 1986). The authors ascribe the higher mortality in the 20% with the lowest pressures to the coexistence of chronic debilitating disease.

## Gender and Risk

Women tolerate hypertension better than men: Morbidity and mortality rates from any level of hypertension are higher in men (Levy and Kannel, 1988). It takes higher pressures to hurt women, but when their pressures are high, they suffer. This is clearly demonstrated in the Framingham Study (Fig. 1.2) and in the actuarial data. Nonetheless, the lower rates of cardiovascular disease at all levels of either systolic or diastolic blood pressure among women aged 35 to 64 and even more strikingly among those aged 65 to 94 followed for 30 years in the Framingham study suggest that somewhat higher levels could be used to define hypertension among women.

## Race and Risk

Blacks tend to have higher levels of blood pressure than nonblacks and suffer more overall mortality at all levels (Fig. 1.3) (Neaton et al, 1984). The data in Figure 1.3 were obtained during the 5-year Multiple Risk Factor Intervention Trial (MRFIT) involving over 23,000 black men and 325,000 white men. When these men were followed for an additional 5 years, an interesting racial difference was confirmed: Black men with DBP above 90 had lower mortality rates than white men from coronary heart disease (relative risk of 0.84) but higher mor-

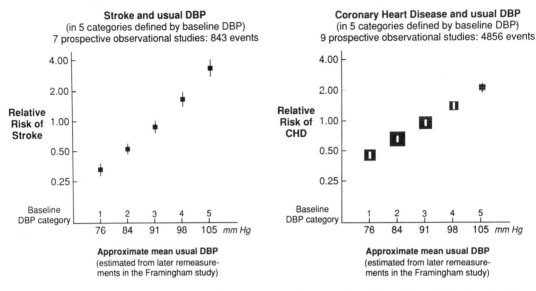

**Figure 1.1.** The relative risks of stroke and of coronary heart disease, estimated from the combined results of the prospective observational studies, for each of five categories of diastolic blood pressure. (Estimates of the usual DBP in each baseline DBP catagory are taken from mean DBP values 4 years postbaseline in the Framingham study). The *solid squares* represent disease risks in each category relative to risk in the whole study population; the sizes of the squares are proportional to the number of events in each DBP category, and 95% confidence intervals for the estimates of relative risk are denoted by *vertical lines*. (From MacMahon S, Peto R, Cutler J, et al: *Lancet*, 335:765, 1990).

tality from cerebrovascular disease (relative risk of 2.0) (Neaton et al, 1989). However, black men and women in Minneapolis-St. Paul have been found to have a higher rate of both coronary heart disease and stroke mortality than whites (Sprafka et al, 1988).

The greater risk of hypertension among blacks suggests that more attention be paid to even lower levels of hypertension among them, but there seems little reason to use different criteria for the diagnosis of hypertension in blacks than in whites.

Other races differ in their relative risk from hypertension in both the frequency and type of cardiovascular complications. These in turn may largely reflect differences in diet and life style (Stamler and Liu, 1983).

### Age and Risk: The Elderly

The number of people over age 65 is rapidly increasing: In 50 years, one of every five people in the United States will be over 65 (Kirkendall and Hammond, 1980). Blood pressure, particularly the systolic, tends to increase progressively with age (Fig. 1.4), and the elderly with hypertension have a greater risk of dying from cardiovascular disease although it may be a weaker predictor of mortality in the elderly than in the younger population (Ekbom et al, 1988).

Unfortunately, almost nothing is now known about the ability to reduce this risk by reduction of the blood pressure, but a proper study is now in progress (Perry et al, 1989).

*Diastolic Elevations.* With advancing age, diastolic blood pressures above 95 mm Hg are associated with a progressively increased risk of cardiovascular events (Vokonas et al, 1988). Data from the Veterans Administration Cooperative Study (1972) portray the danger: Among men with diastolic pressures between 90 and 114 mm Hg, 62.8% of those 60 years or older developed a major cardiovascular complication during an average 5 years on placebo.

*Isolated Systolic Elevations.* With increasing age, the prevalence of an isolated elevation in systolic blood pressure, defined as a diastolic below 90 and a systolic above 160 mm Hg, progressively rises so that it is present in about one-fourth of people over age 65 (Wilking et al, 1988). Over a 30-year interval, systolic elevations were more of a determinant of risk than were diastolic in the Framingham study (Vokonas et al, 1988). The risks involve both stroke and heart attack: Those with isolated systolic hypertension had 3 to 4 times more strokes (Kannel et al, 1981) and considerably more myocardial infarctions (Kannel, 1989) (Fig. 1.5) than did those without it.

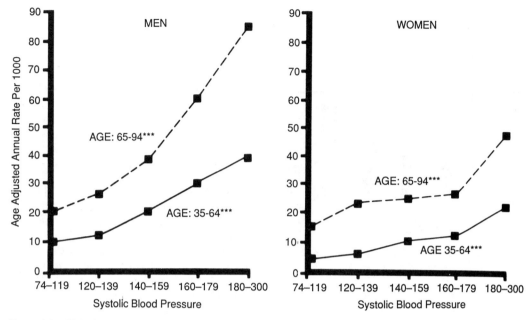

**Figure 1.2.** Risk of cardiovascular disease by age, sex, and level of systolic blood pressure, from a 30-year follow-up in the Framingham Study. ***, p < 0.001 (Wald statistic for logistic regression analysis. (From Vokonas PS, Kannel WB, Cupples LA: *J Hypertension* 6(Suppl 1):S3, 1988.)

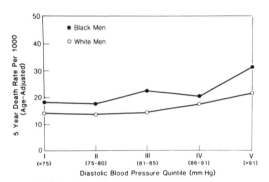

**Figure 1.3.** Five-year age-adjusted total mortality rate per 1,000 by diastolic blood levels among the 23,490 black men and the 325,384 white men screened in the Multiple Risk Factor Intervention Trial. (From Neaton JD, Kuller LH, Wentworth D, et al: *Am Heart J* 108:759, 1984.)

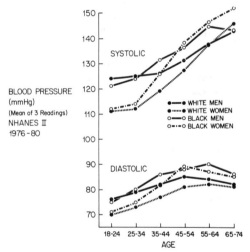

**Figure 1.4.** The mean systolic and diastolic blood pressures for white and black men and women in various age groups in the 1976 to 80 National Health and Nutrition Examination Survey. (From Rowland M, Roberts J: NCHS Advance Data, No. 84, Vital and Health Statistics of the National Center for Health Statistics, October 8, 1982.)

## Old Versus Very Old

As people become very old, into their 70s and 80s, hypertension becomes less and less of a risk factor, presumably because those most susceptible to the cardiovascular risks of hypertension will already have died. In fact, unlike what has been seen in people below age 65, 2-year mortality rates were found to be *lower* in those aged 85 or more with high blood pressure (Mattila et al, 1988). Similar data have been reported in a 10-year follow-up of 2270 people over age 65 (Langer et al, 1989). It may be that those who survive to a very old age despite elevated blood pressure simply are immune to the adverse effects of hypertension or that low blood pressure in the very old is simply a marker

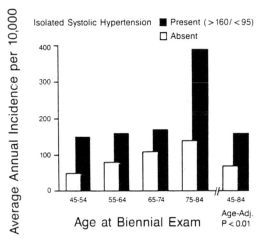

**Figure 1.5.** Risk of myocardial infarction with isolated systolic hypertension (>160/<95 mm Hg). Framingham Study, 24-year follow-up. Men 45 to 84 years of age. (From Kannel WB: Risk factors in hypertension. *J Cardiovasc Pharmacol* 13(Suppl 1):S4-S10, 1989.)

of an impending cardiovascular event. This latter possibility is supported by the increased mortality seen in two groups of untreated elderly patients with the lowest levels of systolic pressure, producing a J-curve for cardiovascular events (Coope et al, 1988; Staessen et al, 1988).

Regardless of the explanation, the data suggest that people over age 75 with mildly elevated blood pressure may not require treatment. As will be noted further in Chapter 5, treatment of hypertensive patients over age 80 has not been found to reduce their risk for cardiovascular events (Amery et al, 1986).

Nonetheless, hypertension remains a risk for the overall population over age 65. In two such groups followed for 9 and 10 years, respectively, high blood pressure had predictive value for all cause mortality in one (Barrett-Connor et al, 1984) and cardiovascular morbidity in the other (Agner, 1983).

### Systolic Versus Diastolic

As noted, the presence of isolated systolic hypertension is clearly a marker for cardiovascular disease (CVD) in the elderly, not surprising since such systolic hypertension is in itself a reflection of rigid, atherosclerotic arteries. However, as noted in both the Framingham and the Whitehall studies, systolic elevations are more a determinant of cardiovascular risk than are diastolic over the entire adult age range. The high pressures generated during systole put an immediate, direct burden on the heart and vas-

culature, so that all forms of CVD are logically more frequent with elevated systolic pressures (Birkenhäger and de Leeuw, 1988). Systolic pulse waves create turbulence and perturbations of flow and pressure that damage the endothelium, leading to atherosclerotic plaque formation. In the hypertensive aorta, progressive structural rigidity impedes left ventricular ejection, which is only manifest during systole, so that systolic pressure is easily seen to be more of a threat to left ventricular function than is diastolic pressure.

As evidence for this, in the untreated half of the large Medical Research Council (1988) and the smaller European Working Party (Amery et al, 1986) trials of therapy, the systolic pressure was more closely correlated with the risk of heart attack than was the diastolic (Medical Research Council Working Party, 1988). Clearly, as much attention must be given to the systolic pressure as to the diastolic in considering the risks of hypertension.

### Relative Versus Absolute Risk

In most of the data presented to this point, the risks related to elevated blood pressure have been presented in relation to those found with lower levels of blood pressure, in a relative manner. This way of looking at risk tends to exaggerate its degree.

For example, the Pooling Project data (Pooling Project Research Group, 1978) show a 52% increase in the relative risk for coronary disease over an 8.6-year interval for white men with initial DBP in the 80- to 87-mm Hg range, as compared with that for those with DBP below 80 (Table 1.3). The 52% increase is derived by taking the rate per 1000 persons of actual coronary events in the two groups, 100.6 versus 66.0, and dividing the difference (34.6) by the rate for those with the lower DBP (66.0). This increase in relative risk of 52%, then, reflects a 3.5% increase in absolute risk, i.e., 34.6 per 1000. The importance of this greater risk with higher pressure should not be ignored if one uses the smaller change in absolute risk numbers rather than the larger change in relative risk numbers, but caution is needed in applying epidemiological statistics to individual patients.

Fortunately, the Framingham data provide an easy way to assess the actual risk for every patient above age 35. As we shall see in the next chapter, that risk is unevenly distributed and closely related to the number and extent of concomitant risk factors.

**Table 1.3. Risk (8.6-Year) for Major Coronary Events in 7054 White Men by Diastolic Blood Pressure at Entry[a]**

| Diastolic BP at Entry[b] | Adjusted Rate of Major Coronary Events per 1000 | Relative Risk | Absolute Excess Risk Per 1000 |
|---|---|---|---|
| Below 80 (Quintiles 1 and 2) | 66.0 | 1.0 | |
| 80–87 (Quintile 3) | 100.6 | 1.52 | 34.6 |
| 88–95 (Quintile 4) | 109.4 | 1.66 | 43.4 |
| Above 95 (Quintile 5) | 143.3 | 2.17 | 77.3 |

[a]Data reprinted with permission from The Pooling Project Research Group: Relationship of blood pressure, serum cholesterol, smoking habit, relative weight, and electrocardiogram abnormalities to incidence of major coronary events: Final Report of the Pooling Project. *J Chronic Dis* 31:201, 1978 and by permission of the American Heart Association, Inc.
[b]The blood pressure ranges varied slightly for various 5-year age groups: 40 to 44, 45 to 49, etc.

For now, the problem seems well defined: For the population at large, risk clearly increases with every increment in blood pressure, and levels of blood pressure that are accompanied by significantly increased risks should be called "high." However, for individual patients, the absolute risk from slightly elevated blood pressure may be quite small. Therefore, more than just the level of blood pressure should be used in the determination of risk and, even more importantly, in the decision to diagnose the person as hypertensive and to begin treatment.

## Benefits of Action: Reducing Cardiovascular Disease

Let us now turn to the second major factor listed in Table 1.1 as being involved in a conceptual definition of hypertension, the level at which it is possible to show benefit from the use of available means of lowering the blood pressure. Inclusion of this factor is predicated on the assumption that it is of no benefit—and, as we shall see, is potentially harmful—to label a person as hypertensive if nothing is to be done to lower the blood pressure.

### Natural Versus Induced Blood Pressure

Before proceeding, one caveat is in order. As we have noted, the lower the blood pressure, the less cardiovascular disease seen in the general population that is not on antihypertensive therapy. However, that fact cannot be used as evidence in support of the benefits of therapy. A blood pressure that is naturally low may offer a degree of protection that is not provided by a similarly low blood pressure resulting from antihypertensive therapy.

The available evidence supports that view: Patients under antihypertensive drug treatment do continue to have a higher morbidity and mortality rate than untreated people with similar levels of blood pressure. This has been shown in analyses of populations in England (Bulpitt, 1982), Australia (Doyle, 1982), Hawaii (Yano et al, 1983), Framingham (Kannel et al, 1985), and Scotland (Isles et al, 1986). Recall, too, the data of MacMahon et al (1989) (Fig. 1.1) that predict a much greater fall in CHD risk than has been seen with the degree of blood pressure reduction achieved in the major clinical trials of the treatment of hypertension. As these investigators point out, the therapeutic trials have been much shorter in duration than the observational studies, and the rather sudden changes in blood pressure induced by treatment may not reflect the effect of natural changes in pressure. More will be said about this issue in Chapter 5, but it should be noted that the gap may be narrowing with better therapy (Waal-Manning et al, 1988).

For now, let us consider two of these studies. The data from Hawaii involved a 10-year follow-up of 7610 Japanese men, aged 45 to 68 at baseline. Those who were receiving antihypertensive therapy at baseline had a higher mortality from cardiovascular diseases overall, coronary heart disease, and stroke, as compared with untreated men whose blood pressures were comparable (Fig. 1.6). The authors conclude that "after adjustment of age, blood pressure, and nine other risk factors in multivariate logistic analysis, antihypertensive medication remained significant as a risk factor for CVD, CHD, and stroke (Yano et al, 1983).

The Framingham data report a greater than 2-fold increased risk of sudden death over 30 years among people receiving antihypertensive drug treatment, and this escalated risk was not accounted for by higher pressure or by any other known predisposing factor for sudden death (Kannel et al, 1988).

These disquieting data should not be taken as evidence against the use of antihypertensive drug therapy. They do not, in any way, deny that protection against cardiovascular complications can be achieved by successful reduction of the blood pressure with drugs. They simply indicate that the protection provided may only be partial, perhaps because of only partial reduction of the blood pressure; perhaps because of dangers in-

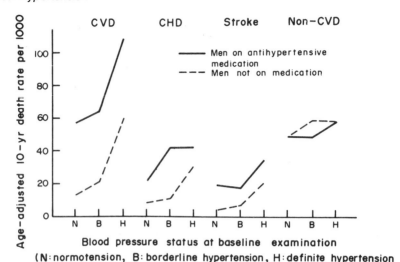

**Figure 1.6.** Age-adjusted 10-year mortality rates according to baseline blood pressure status and use of antihypertensive medication. (Reprinted with permission from Yano K, McGee D, Reed DM: *J Chron Dis* 36:569, copyright 1983, Pergamon Press PLC.)

herent in the use of some drugs; perhaps because of irreversible damage already done by the hypertension; perhaps because of underlying features, either causal or coincidental to the hypertension (Hansson, 1988). Whatever their explanation, these data do document a difference between natural and induced levels of blood pressure.

### Rationale for Reduction of Elevated Blood Pressure

Despite these disquieting data, there is considerable evidence, experimental, epidemiological, and clinical, for benefits from reduction of elevated blood pressure (Table 1.4). Only the last point, the reduction of cardiovascular disease, can be quantitated in a manner that will provide evidence as to the level of blood pressure wherein benefit can be shown from the use

**Table 1.4. Rationale for the Reduction of Elevated Blood Pressure**

1. The frequency of cardiovascular disease and death is directly related to the height of the blood pressure.
2. The blood pressure rises most in those whose pressures are already high.
3. In humans, vascular damage is less where the blood pressure is lower: beneath a coarctation, beyond a renovascular stenosis, and in the pulmonary circulation.
4. Experimentally, lowering the blood pressure protects the vascular system.
5. Antihypertensive therapy reduces cardiovascular disease and death.

of available means to lower the blood pressure. That level can be used as part of the operational definition of hypertension.

Over the past 20 years, there have been controlled therapeutic trials that have included patients with diastolic blood pressure levels as low as 90 or 95 mm Hg. Detailed analyses of these trials will be provided in Chapter 5. For now, it is enough to say that there is disagreement as to whether they have shown protection against cardiovascular disease for patients with DBP below 95 or even 100 mm Hg. On the one hand, some believe the data validate the need for drug therapy for those with DBP above 90 mm Hg (Gifford et al, 1983). On the other hand, some believe they do not validate the need for drug therapy, even for those with DBP as high as 104 mm Hg (Råstam et al, 1986a; Oliver, 1987).

The differences are highlighted in recent reports of four expert committees: The Report of the British Hypertension Society Working Party (1989) and the Canadian Hypertension Society Consensus Conference (Myers et al, 1989) recommend that antihypertensive treatment should be initiated with diastolic pressure consistently above 100 mm Hg for 3 to 4 months; the World Health Organization and International Society of Hypertension (1989) recommend treatment for diastolic pressures above 95 mm Hg; the fourth Joint National Committee on Detection, Evaluation, and Treatment of High Blood Pressure (1988) recommends treatment for those with a persistently elevated diastolic blood pressure above 94 mm Hg and for those with DBP from 90 to 94 who are otherwise at high risk.

As a compromise—and likely as the consensus—a diastolic pressure of 95 mm Hg seems to be the level wherein therapy has been shown to provide protection. That level may then be used in the operational definition of hypertension.

As a separate but related issue, the protection shown in the various therapeutic trials has been against stroke, heart failure, and renal damage. Little if any protection has been shown against the major cardiovascular risk from hypertension, coronary disease, an issue that will be discussed further in Chapter 5.

### Prevention of Progression of Hypertension

One of the other benefits of action listed in Table 1.1 is to prevent progression of hypertension. The evidence for that benefit is strong, as shown in the results of the four therapeutic trials that followed half of their patients while they were on placebo (Table 1.5). From 10 to 17% of these patients had progression of hypertension beyond their respective thresholds, whereas fewer than 1% of the treated half did so.

### Additional Risks and Costs of Action

The decision to label and treat a person for hypertension at any given level of blood pressure entails assumption of the role of a patient, interferences with life style, risks from biochemical side effects of therapy, and financial costs (Table 1.1). As will be emphasized in the next chapter, the diagnosis should not be based on one or only a few readings. In a survey of 6258 adults in two Canadian cities, more people—14.3%—were found to have been falsely labeled as hypertensive as the number—11.4%—

who were found to have hypertension (Birkett et al, 1986). The fact that 85% of United States adults had a blood pressure taken in 1985 (National Center for Health Statistics—Schoenborn, 1988) is then a mixed blessing: It may help identify many who are in need but it may lead to considerable mischief in overdiagnosis and unnecessary treatment.

### Assumption of the Role of a Patient

The mere labeling of a person as "hypertensive" may provoke ill effects. This should come as no surprise considering the common lay name for hypertension—"the silent killer." After review of the literature on the effects of labeling, these conclusions were made (Macdonald et al, 1984):

—Labeling by itself, without treatment, may be harmful.
—Absenteeism from work because of illness and psychological distress is increased more among aware hypertensives than among either normotensives or unaware hypertensives.
—People who are labeled but who receive appropriate counseling and care and who are compliant with therapy usually do not have increased absenteeism or psychological distress.

These findings were reiterated in a subsequent review by Lefebvre et al (1988) who addressed the issue of labeling in large-scale screening programs. Clearly, labeling can lead to increased absenteeism (Rudd et al, 1987) but, with proper debriefing and counseling, the psychological burdens can be mitigated. Nonetheless, the consequences of labeling may be insidious: The average yearly income of 230 hypertensive Canadian steelworkers, 5 years after they were identified, was an average of $1093 less than

**Table 1.5. Progression of Hypertension in Placebo-Controlled Trials of the Treatment of Hypertension**

| | Veterans Administration | United States Public Health Service[a] | Australian | Oslo[b] | Medical Research Council |
|---|---|---|---|---|---|
| No. of patients | 380 | 389 | 3427 | 785 | 17354 |
| Initial level of DBP (mm Hg) | 90–114 | 90–115 | 95–109 | 90–109 | 95–109 |
| Threshold level of DBP (mm Hg) | 125 | 130 | 110 | 110 | 110 |
| Progression beyond threshold: no. of patients (%) | | | | | |
| On placebo | 20 (10%) | 24 (12%) | 198 (12%) | 65 (17%) | 1011 (11.7%) |
| On treatment | 0 | 0 | 4 (0.2%) | 1 (0.3%) | 76 (0.9%) |

[a]Smith WM: *Circ Res* 40(Suppl 1):I-98, 1977.
[b]Helgeland A: *Am J Med* 69:752, 1980.

for a matched group of normotensives despite similar incomes in the year before screening (Johnston et al, 1984). Awareness of the presence of hypertension is followed by increases in various bothersome psychological characteristics, e.g., neuroticism, anxiety, anger, and hostility (Irvine et al, 1989).

### Interferences with the Quality of Life

One-third of the 3844 patients who were begun on antihypertensive medications for the Hypertension Detection and Follow-up Program developed side effects, about one-third of which resulted in discontinuation of their drug treatment (Curb et al, 1988). These side effects were recognized by detailed surveillance procedures.

In ordinary practice, neither physicians nor patients may be so aware of side effects that, nonetheless, may impair the quality of life of those who take drugs. A survey was performed on 75 consecutive patients from an English group practice who had hypertension controlled by the usual antihypertensive drugs, including diuretics, beta-blockers, and methyldopa (Jachuck et al, 1982). A series of questions about the quality of life was asked of the patients, their physicians, and their closest relatives (Table 1.6). Most of the patients responded that they were improved or no different after therapy, and all of the physicians stated that the patients were improved. However, 99% of the patient's closest relatives said the patients were worse after therapy. The symptoms that they described in the patients included loss of memory (33%), more irritability (45%), depression (46%), more hypochondria (55%), and decreased sexual interest (64%).

This study, though small in scope and uncontrolled, suggests that the treatment of hypertension may often interfere with patients' enjoyment of life in ways of which neither they nor their physicians are aware. Beyond these effects of drugs, the various nonpharmacological therapies that are often advocated may interfere further. Though none should suffer from

**Table 1.6. Estimates of the Effects of Antihypertensive Therapy on Quality of Life[a]**

| | Physician (%) | Patient (%) | Relatives (%) |
|---|---|---|---|
| Improvement | 100 | 48 | 1 |
| No change | | 43 | |
| Worse | | 9 | 99 |

[a]Data from Jachuck SJ, Brierley H, Jachuck S, et al: *J Royal Coll Gen Practitioners* 32:103, 1982.

a moderate reduction in calories and sodium intake, these restrictions may be perceived as unpleasant intrusions.

### Risks from Biochemical Side Effects of Therapy

These biochemical risks are less likely to be perceived by the patient than the interferences with life style, but they may actually be hazardous. A great deal more about them will be considered in Chapters 6 and 7. For now, mention will be made of only two: diuretic-induced hypokalemia that develops in about one-third of patients (Kaplan, 1984) and elevations in serum cholesterol or triglycerides that may accompany the use of either diuretics or beta-blockers (Weinberger, 1985).

### Overview of Risks and Benefits

We have now examined some of the issues involved in determining the level of blood pressure that poses enough risks to mandate the diagnosis of hypertension and to call for the use of appropriate therapy, despite the potential risks that such therapy entails. Another analysis of the issue of risk factor intervention by Dr. Allan S. Brett (1984) clearly defines the problem:

Risk factor intervention is usually undertaken in the hope of long-term gain in survival or quality of life. Unfortunately, there are sometimes trade-offs (such as inconvenience, expense, or side effects) and something immediate must be sacrificed. This tension between benefits and liabilities is not necessarily resolved by appealing to statements of medical fact, and it is highlighted by the fact that many persons at risk are asymptomatic. Particularly when proposing drug therapy, the physician cannot make an asymptomatic person feel any better, but might make him feel worse, since most drugs have some incidence of adverse effects. But how should side effects be quantitated on a balance sheet of net drug benefit? If a successful antihypertensive drug causes impotence in a patient, how many months or years of potentially increased survival make the side effect acceptable? There is obviously no dogmatic answer; accordingly, global statements such as "all patients with asymptomatic mild hypertension should be treated" are inappropriate, even if treatment were clearly shown to lower morbidity or mortality rates.

The example of mild hypertension may be further developed. It is widely acknowledged that, with successively higher blood pressure levels, the risk of complications increases gradually rather than abruptly. Therefore, the reasons to intervene should be viewed as gradually more compelling as blood pressure rises, rather than suddenly compelling at a specific level such as 90 mm Hg. Guttmacher et al (1981) argue persuasively that selection of a cutoff for critically elevated blood pressure reflects a value judgment about the point at which a risk is thought to be serious enough to warrant treatment. Each decision must be individualized, depending on the patient's aversion to risk, perception of the intrusiveness of medical care in his life, tolerance for discomfort or untoward drug effects, etc. When the medical data base contains considerable uncertainty, as it does for mild hypertension, the risk-benefit calculation is even more difficult. (From Brett AS: *Am J Med* 76:557, 1984.)

## OPERATIONAL DEFINITIONS OF HYPERTENSION

Now that the issues of risk and benefit have been examined, operational definitions of hypertension can be offered.

### WHO Criteria

In 1978, an expert committee of the World Health Organization (WHO Expert Committee Report, 1978) considered the evidence and recommended these criteria:

—Normotension: systolic ≤ 140 and diastolic ≤ 90 mm Hg;
—Borderline: systolic 141 to 159 and diastolic 91 to 94 mm Hg;
—Hypertension: systolic ≥ 160 and/or diastolic ≥ 95 mm Hg.

Since then, the increasing awareness of increased risk with blood pressures in the "borderline" category (Fig. 1.1) has caused a reassessment of these criteria (Working Group, 1985).

### Fourth Joint National Committee (JNC-4) Criteria

On the basis of these data, the fourth Joint National Committee on the Detection, Evaluation, and Treatment of High Blood Pressure (1988) recommended that hypertension be diagnosed, in people aged 18 years or older, at a DBP of 90 or above, regardless of the level of SBP, and that DBP between 85 and 89 be called "high normal" (Table 1.7). Notice the separation of hypertension into three degrees—mild, moderate, and severe—by level of DBP.

The JNC-4 report states that "Hypertension should not be diagnosed on the basis of a single measurement. Initial elevated readings should be confirmed on at least two subsequent visits, with average DBP levels of 90 mm Hg or greater or SBP levels of 140 mm Hg or greater required for diagnosis."

**Table 1.7. Fourth Joint National Committee Classification of BP[a]**

| Range (mm Hg) | Category[b] |
|---|---|
| Diastolic | |
| <85 | Normal BP |
| 85–89 | High normal BP |
| 90–104 | Mild hypertension |
| 105–114 | Moderate hypertension |
| ≥115 | Severe hypertension |
| Systolic (when DBP <90) | |
| <140 | Normal BP |
| 140–159 | Borderline isolated systolic hypertension |
| ≥160 | Isolated systolic hypertension |

[a]Classification based on the average of two or more readings on two or more occasions.
[b]A classification of borderline isolated systolic hypertension (systolic BP, 140 to 159 mm Hg) or isolated systolic hypertension (systolic BP ≥160 mm Hg) takes precedence over a classification of high normal BP (diastolic BP, 85 to 89 mm Hg) when both occur in the same person. A classification of high normal BP (diastolic BP, 85 to 89 mm Hg) takes precedence over a classification of normal BP (systolic BP <140 mm Hg) when both occur in the same person.

### Systolic Hypertension in the Elderly

In view of the recognized risks of isolated systolic elevations (Fig. 1.5), the report of JNC-4 recommends that, in the presence of a DBP below 90, systolic levels of 160 or higher be classified as "isolated systolic hypertension," and that in the presence of SBP between 140 and 159 they be called "borderline isolated systolic hypertension."

### Children

For children, JNC-4 utilizes the Report of the Second Task Force on Blood Pressure Control in Children (Task Force, 1987) to identify "*significant hypertension* as blood pressure persistently equal to or greater than the 95th percentile for age and *severe hypertension* as blood pressure persistently equal to or greater than the 99th percentile for age." This will be covered in Chapter 16 and the levels of elevated blood pressure at various ages are given in Table 16.7.

### Operational Definition Based on Risk and Benefit

Considering all of the factors shown in Table 1.1, I believe that the definition for hypertension in adults, *based upon the average of multiple readings*, should be those listed in Table 1.7 from the JNC-4 report.

In using these DBP levels to make the diagnosis, three caveats should be considered:

—Systolic levels likely should be used alongside the diastolic and not just in those people with DBP below 90 mm Hg.

—The levels for women probably should be set a bit higher, likely 150/95, since their risk is less than for men.

—The acceptance of these levels for the diagnosis of hypertension does not automatically mean that drug treatment should be given to all whose levels are elevated.

From what is now known, drug treatment should probably be given to most with DBP above 95 and virtually to all with DBP above 100 and to most with SBP above 160 mm Hg. However, among people prone to stroke, e.g., blacks in the United States, Japanese and Chinese, therapy might be started at lower levels since reducing the pressure below 90 mm Hg has been shown to protect against stroke. Among diabetics who are known to be susceptible to nephropathy, treatment at considerably lower levels than 95 mm Hg may be found to be protective. Among people at high risk for CHD because of other factors, therapy at DBP below 95 may turn out to useful even though it has not been shown among mostly lower risk individuals. Hopefully, with newer agents that will avoid some of the problems of those used in the clinical trials now completed, therapy will be found to offer the protection against CHD predicted for a fall in pressure from the observational studies.

My belief has changed somewhat through the years. Although I accept the advice of George Pickering that the risks are directly proportional to the level of blood pressure and that there is no critical hypertensive level, I have felt that there was no reason to label a person as hypertensive unless active, i.e., drug, therapy were indicated. Now I am willing to utilize lower levels of blood pressure as indicative of the diagnosis for two main reasons: First, those whose readings are not as high as to mandate drug therapy may achieve a reduction in risk by making changes in their life-style and the diagnosis of hypertension may motivate the physician and the patient to make these changes; second, the impressive protection shown against stroke by reduction of even mild degrees of hypertension is in itself a justification of diagnosing such patients as hypertensive while giving hope that they will be protected against CHD and the other cardiovascular sequelae by currently available therapies.

These criteria will obviously identify a larger number of people as hypertensive than would the WHO and other previously used criteria that took 160/95 as the dividing line. Since this chapter addresses the population at large, let us now consider how the use of the lower levels of blood pressure to define hypertension influences the prevalence of the diagnosis and the estimates of the overall risks in the population.

## PREVALENCE OF HYPERTENSION

Perhaps the best sources of data for the United States population are the National Center for Health Statistics National Health and Nutrition Examination Surveys (NHANES), first performed in 1960 to 1962, again in 1971 to 1974, and in 1976 to 1980 (Table 1.8). We will focus on the results of the latter survey in which a representative sample of the American population, a total of 16,204 people from ages 6 to 74, was examined.

### NHANES Surveys

The prevalence of hypertension—defined in these surveys as a systolic level of 160 mm Hg or higher or a diastolic of 95 mm Hg or higher, or as taking antihypertensive medications—is shown to have increased, mainly by growth of the population, from about 22 million to over 30 million people from ages 25 to 74. The percentages of these people aware of their hypertension, on medication, and well controlled all have risen from the levels of 1960 to 1962 to the levels of 1976 to 1980 (Fig. 1.7). (The percentages in Fig. 1.7 are based upon data that also include persons aged 18 to 24 and other groups not included in the NHANES survey, so they differ somewhat from those in Table 1.8.)

Even more striking percentages of people in areas of high health awareness and medical coverage, such as around the Mayo Clinic, have been identified, treated and well controlled (Phillips et al, 1988).

Further analysis of the NHANES data for the entire United States, however, reveals that despite the improvements in the recognition and treatment of hypertension, the mean diastolic blood pressure of white men in the United States has *increased* from its 1960 to 1962 levels to those of 1976 to 1980, whereas the DBP of other groups has changed little. Mean systolic pressures have fallen for all four groups and this is responsible for the overall decrease in the prevalence rates for hypertension that have been almost exclusively noted among those over age 50.

As we examine these data, remember that they are the average of three blood pressures—

**Table 1.8. Findings of Three Hypertension Surveys Using Data from Persons 25 to 74 Years of Age**

| | National Health Survey (1960–1962) | National Health and Nutrition Examination Survey I (1971–1975) | National Health and Nutrition Examination Survey II (1976–1980) |
|---|---|---|---|
| No. of people examined | 6,672 | 17,796 | 16,204 |
| % with BP ≥160/95 | 20.3 | 22.1 | 22.0 |
| % of hypertensives aware of diagnosis | 49 | 64 | 73 |
| % of hypertensives being treated | 31 | 34 | 56 |
| % of hypertensives under control | 16 | 20 | 34 |
| References | Roberts and Maurer (1977) | Roberts and Maurer (1977) | Rowland and Roberts (1982) |

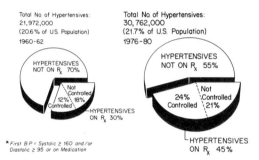

\* First B.P. = Systolic ≥ 160 and/or Diastolic ≥ 95 or on Medication

**Figure 1.7.** The total number of hypertensive people in the United States aged 18 to 74, estimated from the National Health and Nutrition Examination Surveys of 1960 to 1962 to 1980 and the percentages of those not on therapy, on therapy not controlled, and on therapy controlled.

two sitting, one lying—taken at one examination. In a survey of 2737 Canadians, the prevalence of hypertension was overestimated by 30% when the diagnosis was based on data from only one visit compared with three visits (Birkett et al, 1987).

## Effects of Lower Criteria on Prevalence

Supposedly in keeping with the recommendations of JNC-4 (shown in Table 1.7) the NHANES-II data have been reanalyzed, defining hypertension as a blood pressure of 140 mm Hg or higher for the systolic and 90 mm Hg or higher for the diastolic (Subcommittee on Definition and Prevalence of the 1984 Joint National Committee on Detection, Evaluation, and Treatment of High Blood Pressure, 1985). I believe this reanalysis is inappropriate, since JNC-4 clearly states that the diagnosis of hypertension be based on at least three sets of readings and there is a fall in blood pressure from definitely high to distinctly normal in as many as one-third of patients at a second examination. Nonetheless, the reanalysis has been justified as an appropriate way to identify the total number of

people at risk. The report of the reanalysis concludes that "58 million Americans are estimated to be at increased risk of morbidity and premature mortality associated with high blood pressure, warranting some type of therapy or systematic monitoring" (Subcommittee on Definition and Prevalence of the 1984 Joint National Committee on Detection, Evaluation, and Treatment of High Blood Pressure, 1985).

In addition to lowering the level of blood pressure used to define hypertension, the reanalysis attempted to include those populations excluded in the NHANES-II survey— institutionalized, military, elderly over age 74, and young persons aged 6 to 17. The data for the elderly were based upon a survey of 5566 people 75 years and older performed by the Systolic Hypertension in the Elderly Program (SHEP), which found that 75% of these people had hypertension, again defined as a blood pressure higher than 140 mm Hg systolic or 90 diastolic.

When the data for these additional groups are added to those obtained in NHANES-II and are applied to the 1983 United States Census data, the total estimated prevalence of hypertension in the United States population is seen to be over 57 million people, rather than the 30 million based upon a blood pressure level of 160 mm Hg systolic or 95 mm Hg diastolic (Table 1.9). The newer prevalence rates continue to show a higher percentage of men and blacks to be hypertensive (Fig. 1.8).

### Implications of the New Criteria

*On the Prevalence of Hypertension.* When the prevalence estimates using the lower levels of pressure to define hypertension were applied to the NHANES-II survey findings, a rather striking realignment of the proportions of hypertensive people aware, treated, and controlled was noted. Though this can be used as an ar-

**Table 1.9. Prevalence Estimate of Hypertension[a] for the Total United States Population in 1983[b]**

| Population Groups | Prevalence |
|---|---|
| Adult (ages 18 through 74 years; civilian, noninstitutionalized) | 46,035,000 |
| Institutionalized (ages 18 through 74 years) | 471,000 |
| Military | 312,000 |
| Elderly (75 years and above) | 8,170,000[c] |
| Young (6 through 17 years) | 2,724,000 |
| Total | 57,712,000[d] |

[a]Hypertension defined as systolic of 140 mm Hg or higher, or diastolic of 90 mm Hg or higher, or use of antihypertensive medication.
[b]Data from Subcommittee on Definition and Prevalence of the 1984 JNC, 1985.
[c]Derived by applying SHEP pilot study rates to 1983 United States Census data.
[d]Excludes children under 6 years of age and hypertensives who controlled their blood pressure without medications.

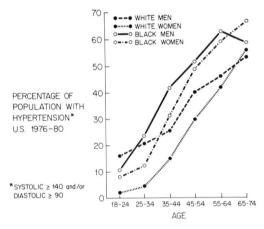

**Figure 1.8.** The prevalence of hypertension among white and black men and women in the United States, defined as systolic of 140 and/or diastolic of 90 or higher. (From Rowland M, Roberts J: NCHS Advance Data, Vital and Health Statistics of the National Center for Health Statistics, No. 84, October 8, 1982. Washington, D.C., United States Department of Health and Human Services.)

gument that effort must be intensified to identify and treat many millions more people, the realignment should be recognized for what it is—not a demonstration of less adequate management of hypertension but simply a redrawing of the criteria. When the same criteria are used, a definite improvement in the management of hypertension in the United States from the 1960 to 1962 levels to the 1976 to 1980 levels is obvious (Table 1.8).

*On the Prevalence of Isolated Systolic Hypertension.* Another consequence of the new criteria is the striking increase in the number of elderly people with isolated systolic hypertension (Fig. 1.9). Though the majority of these are "borderline," i.e., systolic levels of 140 to 159 mm Hg, 30% of people aged 65 to 74 have isolated systolic hypertension (Fig 1.9), and even more of those over age 74 have it. Remember that in the elderly, as in the younger in the Framingham population, systolic levels are more closely predictive of cardiovascular complications than are diastolic levels (Rutan et al, 1988).

## Differences Among Racial Groups

The preceding has referred to the overall population within the United States. Within that population, different racial groups may have different prevalence rates. Moreover, populations in other countries may show prevalence rates different from those of the United States population.

### Blacks

As noted in Figure 1.8, blacks in the United States have more hypertension than whites and, as noted in Figure 1.3, they suffer more morbidity and mortality from it (Anderson et al, 1989). Fortunately, the 1976 to 1980 NHANES-II data showed a significant decrease in the prevalence of hypertension among black adults as compared with that in the 1960-62 NHES I Survey (Dannenberg et al, 1987).

A higher prevalence of hypertension has been noted in blacks than in whites in Brazil (Ribeiro and Ribeiro, 1986) and parts of Africa (Akinkugbe, 1987) so that the association may be widespread. Possible underlying causes for this higher prevalence of hypertension in blacks will be covered near the end of Chapter 3, after considering the various pathogenetic mechanisms for hypertension. The higher prevalence and greater morbidity of hypertension in blacks may reflect three factors: (1) an earlier onset, (2) a more rapid progression, or (3) less adequate control.

In regard to earlier onset, although most surveys find that the average blood pressures of black and white young children are similar (Morrison et al, 1980), during adolescence blacks experience a greater increase in average blood pressure and in the prevalence of hypertension that they maintain throughout adult life (Liebman et al, 1986). Moreover, blacks tend to have a lesser fall in nocturnal blood pressure than do whites with similar daytime pressure levels (Murphy et al, 1988).

In regard to more rapid progression of hypertension, black hypertensives have more strokes (Gillum, 1988) and renal damage (Shulman,

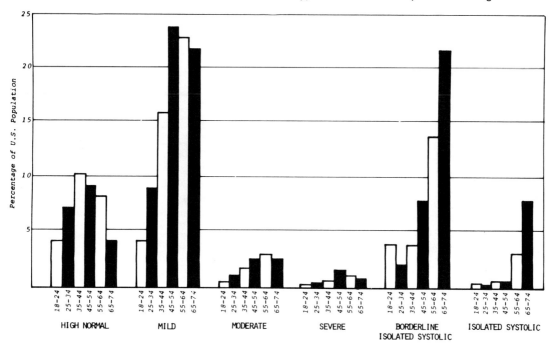

**Figure 1.9.** The percentages of the United States population in various age groups from 18 to 74 years with various types of hypertension, based upon the National Health and Nutrition Examination Survey (NHANES-II), 1976 to 1980. (From the Subcommittee on Definition and Prevalence of the 1984 Joint National Committee: Hypertension prevalence and the status of awareness, treatment and control in the Unites States: Final report of the Subcommittee on Definition and Prevalence of the 1984 Joint National Committee. *Hypertension* 7:457, 1985, and by permission of the American Heart Association, Inc.)

1987) and about the same or a slightly lower susceptibility to coronary heart disease (CHD) (Neaton et al, 1989).

In regard to the lesser degree of control of hypertension in blacks, this is well documented in the United States (Sprafka et al, 1988). This likely reflects various barriers, mainly socio-economic, to the delivery of health care to blacks (Blendon et al, 1989). When these barriers have been removed, blacks achieve marked reduction in mortality from both coronary disease and stroke (Folsom et al, 1987).

Interestingly, blacks with homozygous sickle cell disease have been found to have a lower prevalence of hypertension, apparently because of lower peripheral vascular resistance (Hatch et al,1989). Nonetheless, even high-normal levels of pressure are associated with a much higher prevalence of stroke among patients with sickle cell disease (Rodgers et al, 1988).

## Hispanics

In a survey of a random sample of 1288 Hispanics and 929 Anglos living in three socially distinct neighborhoods in San Antonio, Texas,

overall age-adjusted prevalence rates of hypertension were similar for the men and slightly lower for the Hispanic women (Franco et al, 1985). Since Hispanics tend to be more obese, when adjustments were made for obesity, Hispanics were found to have lower rates of hypertension.

## Asians in the United States

In a survey of Asians and Pacific Islanders living in California, Filipinos were found to have higher rates of hypertension and Japanese and other Asians lower rates of hypertension than found among whites (Stavig et al, 1988).

## American Indians

Surveys taken on large populations of American Indians, including Navajos in New Mexico (DeStefano et al, 1979), Chippewas in Minnesota (Gillum et al, 1984) and Penobscots in Maine (Deprez et al, 1985) show no higher and perhaps a lower prevalence of hypertension than among whites.

### Populations Outside the United States

Many surveys of groups throughout the world have been performed, a large number relating blood pressure to dietary sodium intake. Some of those data are reviewed in Chapter 3. Other studies have followed groups who have migrated from rural to urban locations, including Kenyans (Poulter et al, 1984) and Polynesians (Joseph et al, 1983).

Without going into detail, most surveys of people in industrialized countries show prevalence rates similar to those of the United States white population, whereas most surveys of less acculturated people who consume less sodium find lower rates (see Chapter 3). Additional data can be found in the 6th volume of the Handbook of Hypertension (Amsterdam, Elsevier Press, 1985).

Rather marked differences in the prevalence of hypertension that cannot be easily explained have been noted: A 3-fold variation was noted among 7735 middle-aged men in 24 towns throughout Britain, with higher rates in Northern England and Scotland (Shaper et al, 1988).

### INCIDENCE OF HYPERTENSION

Much less is known about the incidence of newly developed hypertension than about the prevalence of established disease. The Framingham study provides one data base (Kannel, 1989) and the National Health Epidemiologic Follow-up Study another (Cornoni-Huntley et al, 1989). In the latter, 14,407 participants in the 1971–75 NHANES I study were followed up an average of 9.5 years later. Unfortunately, only a single blood pressure was taken in the NHANES I survey and only the first of three taken in the follow-up was used in the analysis to provide comparability. Therefore, the incidence rates are likely considerably higher than would be noted with more careful assessment involving multiple sets of readings to ascertain persistence of hypertension.

Nonetheless, the 9.5-year incidence rates of either SBP of 160 and/or DBP of 95 or higher for white men and women show an approximate 5% increase for each 10-year interval of age at baseline except for the 65- to 74-year-old group (Fig. 1.10). Blacks had incidence rates at least twice as high as the whites. The high incidence rates in the older two groups likely represent a considerable proportion of isolated systolic hypertension since the diagnosis of hypertension

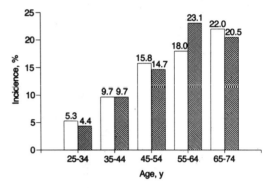

**Figure 1.10.** Incidence rates of hypertension for white men (*open bars*) and women (*cross-hatched bars*) with average follow-up of 9.5 years (follow-up study National Health Epidemiologic Follow-up Study (NHEFS). (From Cornoni-Huntley J, LaCroix AZ, Havlik RJ: *Arch Intern Med* 149:780, 1989).

was based on either systolic or diastolic elevation.

### CLASSIFICATION OF HYPERTENSION

Hypertension should be categorized both as to severity and as to cause in order to facilitate diagnosis and therapy.

#### Classification by Severity

The division of diastolic blood pressure into mild, moderate, and severe has been recommended in the JNC-4 report (Table 1.7). Although, as previously noted, systolic levels have been shown to be even more predictive of risk than diastolic levels (Rutan et al, 1988) and are used in the portrayal of all risk factors from the Framingham study, most continue to use diastolic levels for diagnostic, prognostic, and therapeutic purposes.

The term "accelerated-malignant" is used for the presence of very severe hypertension, usually DBP above 140 mm Hg, with hemorrhages and exudates or papilledema in the fundi (Chapter 8).

An estimate of the number of people with varying degrees of diastolic hypertension can be made from the data of the Hypertension Detection and Follow-up Program (HDFP, 1977), wherein 159,000 people, aged 30 to 69, were initially examined in their homes in 14 communities throughout the United States (Fig. 1.11). More than 80% of all of those with a DBP above 90 are in the mild category, whereas moderate hypertension is present in about 15% and severe in less than 5%. The actual prevalence figures are likely too high since these are the second

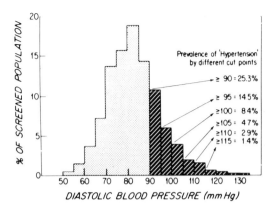

**Figure 1.11.** Frequency distribution of diastolic blood pressure at home screen (158,906 persons, 30 to 69 years of age). (From the Hypertension Detection and Follow-up Program Cooperative Group: The hypertension detection and follow-up program: A progress report. *Circ Res* 40(Suppl 1):106, 1977, and by permission of the American Heart Association, Inc.)

measurements taken on the initial home visit. When these people were reexamined, their pressures were usually lower; among the white men with a DBP of 95 to 104 on the first screen, 44% were below 90 on the second screen. Nonetheless, the relative distribution of various levels should be correct.

As we shall examine further in the next chapter, not only does the blood pressure often come down on repeated measurements but also it is quite variable. Nonetheless, this type of classification is useful to assess risk for the individual patient and to compare groups of patients as to their course and response to therapies. Obviously, within each category, the risk increases with every increment in blood pressure. A patient with a diastolic of 104 is at greater risk than one with 90, though both are in the "mild" category. Black (1988) has proposed a different classification, with "mild" covering DBP of 90 to 99 and moderate 100 to 109, with "low-risk" and "high-risk" subgroups in each category.

In addition to the level of blood pressure, three other factors determine the severity of the individual patient's hypertension: (1) certain demographic features—age, sex, and race; (2) the extent of vascular damage induced by the high blood pressure, as reflected in target organ involvement; and (3) the presence of other risk factors for premature cardiovascular disease. These will be discussed more fully in the next chapter.

## Labile and Borderline Hypertension

In view of the usual variability of the blood pressure, the term "labile" is meaningless whereas "borderline" may be used for those patients whose pressures only occasionally go up into the "mild" range, i.e., DBP above 90. Since multiple ambulatory readings have been recorded over the full 24 hours, the marked variability of virtually all people's blood pressure has become obvious as will be seen in Chapter 2. All people have labile blood pressure, and labile hypertension is not a useful or meaningful term.

People whose blood pressures vary between normal and high, i.e., below and above 140/90, have a greater likelihood of developing persistently elevated blood pressure than do those with uniformly normal readings, but this progression is by no means certain: In a review of long-range follow-up studies, the approximate figure was around 20% (Julius et al, 1980). In one study of a particularly fit, low-risk group of air cadets with borderline pressures, only 12% developed sustained hypertension over the subsequent 20 years (Madsen and Buch, 1971).

## Classification by Cause

This list of causes of hypertension is quite long (Table 1.10). However, more than 90% of hypertension is of unknown cause (primary, essential, or idiopathic). The proportion of cases secondary to some identifiable mechanism has been debated considerably as more of these secondary causes have been recognized. Claims that one or another are responsible for up to 20% of all hypertension repeatedly appear from investigators who are particularly interested in that category of hypertension and therefore see a highly selected population.

Surveys of populations more typical of ordinary clinical practice are available (Table 1.11). Those shown by Gifford (1969) are based on patients referred specifically for evaluation and would therefore be expected to include fewer with typical, mild essential hypertension. The patients of Berglund et al (1976) were unselected but included only men between the ages of 47 and 54. Moreover, their blood pressures had to be above 175/115 on two readings so that many with mild essential hypertension may have been excluded. Despite the likely exclusion of some people with milder hypertension, among whom secondary forms of hypertension are even

**Table 1.10. Types of Hypertension**

| | |
|---|---|
| I. Systolic and diastolic hypertension<br>  A. Primary, essential, or idiopathic<br>  B. Secondary<br>    1. Renal<br>      a. Renal parenchymal disease<br>        1. Acute glomerulonephritis<br>        2. Chronic nephritis<br>        3. Polycystic disease<br>        4. Connective tissue diseases<br>        5. Diabetic nephropathy<br>        6. Hydronephrosis<br>      b. Renovascular<br>      c. Renin-producing tumors<br>      d. Renoprival<br>      e. Primary sodium retention (Liddle's<br>        syndrome, Gordon's syndrome)<br>    2. Endocrine<br>      a. Acromegaly<br>      b. Hypothyroidism<br>      c. Hyperthyroidism<br>      d. Hypercalcemia (Hyperparathyroidism)<br>      e. Adrenal<br>        1. Cortical<br>          (a) Cushing's syndrome<br>          (b) Primary aldosteronism<br>          (c) Congenital adrenal hyper-<br>             plasia<br>        2. Medullary: pheochromocytoma<br>      f. Extraadrenal chromaffin tumors<br>      g. Carcinoid<br>      h. Exogenous hormones<br>        1. Estrogen<br>        2. Glucocorticoids<br>        3. Mineralcorticoids: licorice<br>        4. Sympathomimetics |         5. Tyramine-containing foods and<br>          monamine oxidase inhibitors<br>    3. Coarctation of the aorta<br>    4. Pregnancy-induced hypertension<br>    5. Neurological disorders<br>      a. Increased intracranial pressure<br>        1. Brain tumor<br>        2. Encephalitis<br>        3. Respiratory acidosis<br>      b. Sleep apnea<br>      c. Quadriplegia<br>      d. Acute porphyria<br>      e. Familial dysautonomia<br>      f. Lead poisoning<br>      g. Guillain-Barre syndrome<br>    6. Acute stress, including surgery<br>      a. Psychogenic hyperventilation<br>      b. Hypoglycemia<br>      c. Burns<br>      d. Pancreatitis<br>      e. Alcohol withdrawal<br>      f. Sickle cell crisis<br>      g. Postresuscitation<br>      h. Postoperative<br>    7. Increased intravascular volume<br>    8. Alcohol, drugs, etc.<br>II. Systolic hypertension<br>  A. Increased cardiac output<br>    1. Aortic valvular insufficiency<br>    2. A-V fistula, patent ductus<br>    3. Thyrotoxicosis<br>    4. Paget's disease of bone<br>    5. Beriberi<br>    6. Hyperkinetic circulation<br>  B. Rigidity of aorta |

less common, note that essential hypertension was the diagnosis in 90% or more of the patients.

The 1000 patients reported by Danielson and Dammstrom (1981) were all of those referred from the southeastern suburbs of Stockholm to a hospital hypertension unit from 1974 to 1979. The evaluation included isotopic renography in 16%, pyelography in 22%, renal aortography in 4%, urinary catechols in 15%, and plasma renins in 10%, all done for "particular suspicion of secondary hypertension," so it seems unlikely that many of these were missed. Despite the referral base for this population, the overall frequency of secondary diseases was less than 5%.

Similarly the 3783 patients reported by Sinclair et al (1987) had been referred to the Glasgow Blood Pressure Clinic and included a large proportion of complicated or difficult to treat patients. They, too, seldom were found to have a secondary cause except for the presence of

**Table 1.11. Frequency (%) of Various Diagnoses in Hypertensive Subjects[a]**

| | Gifford | Berglund | Rudnick | Danielson | Sinclair |
|---|---|---|---|---|---|
| Essential hypertension | 89 | 94 | 94 | 95.3 | 92.1 |
| Chronic renal disease | 5 | 4 | 5 | 2.4 | 5.6 |
| Renovascular disease | 4 | 1 | 0.2 | 1.0 | 0.7 |
| Coarctation | 1 | 0.1 | 0.2 | | |
| Primary aldosteronism | 0.5 | 0.1 | | 0.1 | 0.3 |
| Cushing's syndrome | 0.2 | | 0.2 | 0.1 | 0.1 |
| Pheochromocytoma | 0.2 | | | 0.2 | 0.1 |
| Oral contraceptive-induced | | (Men only) | 0.2 | 0.8 | 1.0 |
| No. of patients | 4339 | 689 | 665 | 1000 | 3783 |

[a]Compiled from Gifford RW, Jr: *Milbank Mem Fund Q* 47:170, 1969; Berglund G, Andersson O, Wilhelmsen L: *Br Med J* 2:554, 1976; Rudnick KV, Sackett DL, Hirst S, et al: *Can Med Assoc J* 117:492, 1977; Danielson M, Dammstrom BG: *Acta Med Scand* 209:451, 1981; Sinclair AM, Isles CG, Brown I, et al: *Arch Intern Med* 147:1289, 1987.

renal insufficiency that could have been either the cause or the effect of the hypertension.

Perhaps the best data for what would be expected in a medical practice of middle class whites come from the study by Rudnick et al (1977), which involved 655 patients found to be hypertensive in a family practice in Hamilton, Canada, from 1965 to 1974. The patients had a complete workup, including an intravenous pyelogram. Notice again, in this relatively unselected population, the rarity of secondary types of hypertension. Those series reporting higher frequencies deal with highly selected populations. As we shall see, some secondary causes for hypertension are more frequent in elderly hypertensives.

## HYPERTENSION IN THE YOUNG AND THE OLD

Within the population at large, two groups deserve special consideration because their hypertension often involves different causes, risks, and management.

### Hypertension in the Elderly

#### Prevalence

If 140 mm Hg systolic or 90 diastolic is used as the criterion for hypertension, about 50% of whites and 60% of blacks over age 65 have either systolic or diastolic hypertension (Fig. 1.8). The use of higher levels, as suggested previously, would reduce these numbers but they, too, would identify many elderly people as hypertensive. Recall that ''pseudohypertension'' due to rigid arteries that do not collapse under the cuff may lead to an overdiagnosis of hypertension in the elderly.

#### Diastolic Hypertension in the Elderly

The mechanisms of diastolic hypertension in the elderly will be covered in more detail in Chapter 3, the various complications in Chapter 4, and therapy in Chapter 7. For now, note should be taken of a few general features about hypertension in people over age 65:

—The prevalence of diastolic hypertension tends to fall, because with increasing rigidity of the larger arteries the reduced reservoir capacity causes diastolic pressure to fall from the more rapid emptying of a smaller volume.

—The increased risk for cardiovascular complications persists with a doubling of heart attacks and a quadrupling of strokes noted among 488 noninstitutionalized 75- to 85-year-olds with blood pressure above 140/

90 compared with those with lower blood pressure (Greenberg et al, 1989). However, as noted earlier, overall and cardiovascular mortality in groups of men over age 75 (Langer et al, 1989) and in men and women over age 85 (Mattila et al, 1988) has been found to be *lower* when the blood pressure is *higher*.

—Severe concentric cardiac hypertrophy may accompany the hypertension, leading to a distinct syndrome of hypertrophic cardiomyopathy (Topol et al, 1985).

—Reduction of blood pressure will protect against stroke but has not been found to reduce overall or coronary mortality (Staessen et al, 1988). As will be shown in Chapter 7, therapy of the elderly may pose many problems.

### Isolated Systolic Hypertension (ISH)

The commonly noted rise in systolic pressure in the elderly reflects a loss of compliance within the major arteries, which become progressively thicker and more rigid from atherosclerosis. When the cardiac output is ejected into the less distensible aorta, the systolic pressure rises as a steeper slope. Thus, ISH in the elderly results not from a change in the amount or rate of cardiac output but from loss of arterial compliance (Abrams, 1988).

More about the course of ISH and its treatment will be covered in Chapters 4 and 7, respectively.

### Evaluation of the Elderly Hypertensive

In the next chapter, the evaluation of the newly discovered hypertensive will be covered. If the diastolic blood pressure is found to be very high in a previously normotensive elderly person, the likelihood of renovascular hypertension from atherosclerotic stenosis of a main renal artery should be strongly considered (Chapter 10). Some other forms of secondary hypertension may also be more common in the elderly. Of 128 patients over age 60 seen in Copenhagen with diastolic pressures over 110 mm Hg, 14% had chronic renal disease, and 7% had renovascular hypertension (Hansen et al, 1982).

### Hypertension in Children

Hypertension used to be considered quite rare and usually very severe in people below age 20. In the past few years, large groups of presumably normal children and adolescents have been found to have mildly elevated blood pressures and, as they have been recognized, the usual picture of childhood hypertension has changed. A leading worker in this field, Dr. Ellin Lieberman, addresses this area, which is becoming a major part of clinical hypertension, in Chapter 16.

### Systolic Hypertension in the Young

Isolated systolic hypertension may occur in the young as well as the elderly. The hemodynamics and pathogenesis are different: The young have a hyperkinetic circulation with a fast heart rate, increased cardiac output, and "normal" peripheral resistance; the old have a tight vascular bed with a shrunken plasma volume (Messerli et al, 1983). As will be detailed in Chapter 3, the hyperkinetic state in the young may precede the development of diastolic hypertension.

## POPULATION RISK FROM HYPERTENSION

Now that the definition of hypertension and its classes has been provided along with various estimates of its prevalence, the impact of hypertension on the population at large can be considered. As noted, for the individual patient, the higher the level of blood pressure, the greater the risk of morbidity and mortality. However, for the population at large, the greatest burden from hypertension occurs among those with only minimally elevated pressures—because there are so many of them. This can be seen when the death rate observed with each increment of blood pressure, as found in the Framingham Study, is multiplied by the number of people with each level to obtain the percentage of excess deaths attributable to hypertension by each blood pressure level (Fig. 1.12). Almost 60% of the excess risk associated with hypertension in the population as a whole occurs among those with diastolic blood pressure between 90 and 104 mm Hg, the level often referred to as "mild" hypertension.

### Strategy for the Population

The recognition of this disproportionate risk for the population at large from relatively mild hypertension bears strongly on the question as to how to achieve the greatest reduction in the risks of hypertension. In the past, most effort has been directed at the high risk group with the highest levels of blood pressure. However, this "high risk" strategy, as effective as it may be for those affected, does little to reduce total morbidity and mortality if the "low risk" pa-

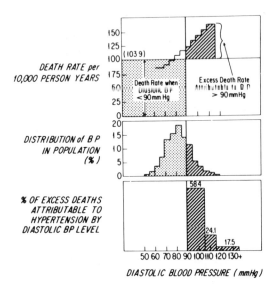

**Figure 1.12.** The percentage of excess deaths attributable to hypertension by diastolic blood pressure level (*bottom*), based upon the death rate observed in Framingham (*top*) and the distribution of the blood pressure found in the HDFP population (*middle*). (From the Hypertension Detection and Follow-up Program Cooperative Group: The hypertension detection and follow-up program: A progress report. *Circ Res* 40(Suppl 1):106, 1977, and by permission of the American Heart Association, Inc.)

tients, who comprise the largest share of the population burden, are ignored (Rose, 1981).

As we shall see in Chapter 5, the active treatment with antihypertensive drugs of many more of the "low risk" individuals is now being aggressively pursued. However, as emphasized by Rose (1981), a more effective strategy would be to lower the blood pressure level of the entire population, as might be accomplished by reduction of sodium intake. Rose calculates that if this were to result in only a 2- to 3-mm Hg-lowering of the entire distribution of blood pressure, it would be as effective in reducing the overall risks of hypertension as would be current antihypertensive drug therapy given to all whose diastolic (Phase 4) blood pressure is 105 mm Hg or higher.

The broad approach advocated by Rose is almost certainly correct on epidemiological grounds. However, until such mass strategies can be implemented, we are left with the need to better control those with established hypertension. Let us now see how we are doing in this more narrowly directed approach.

## DETECTION AND CONTROL OF HYPERTENSION IN THE POPULATION

In the national survey done in 1960 to 1962, fewer than half of the hypertensives in the United

States were diagnosed, and only one in six had their blood pressure under control (Table 1.8). Findings as bad or worse were reported from surveys done in the 1970s in Australia (Prineas et al, 1973), England (Heller et al, 1978), and Israel (Rosenfeld and Silverberg, 1979).

## Current Status

However, the situation in the United States, relative to the number of hypertensives aware of their disease, improved markedly in the 1970s (Table 1.8). This improvement resulted from major efforts by the federal government through the National High Blood Pressure Education Program, voluntary health agencies such as the American Heart Association and Red Cross, medical societies, pharmaceutical companies, neighborhood organizations, and many individual practitioners, all of whom have found the public increasingly aware of the need (National Center for Health Statistics—Schoenborn, 1988).

The number of patients under good control has also increased nationwide from around 12 to 16% in 1960 to 1962 to as high as 34% in 1976 to 1980 (Table 1.8). More recent data support continued overall improvements. A household survey of a representative sample of the United States population in 1985 found these results among adults, aged 18 years and over (National Center for Health Statistics—Schoenborn, 1988):

—More than 90% were aware that high blood pressure increases the risk of heart disease.
—85% had their blood pressure checked within the past year.
—61% of men and 70% of women previously diagnosed as hypertensive were currently taking antihypertensive medication.
—41% of men and 37% of women previously diagnosed as hypertensive reported that their last blood pressure reading was below 140/90.

Even better data have been reported from surveys done in 1983 in two cities in Ontario, Canada (Birkett et al, 1986). Of 6258 adults chosen as a representative sample of the population and who were examined at their homes, 70% of those found to be hypertensive were being treated and were controlled with DBP below 90 mm Hg. Only 6% were undetected, 6% detected but untreated, and 17% treated but uncontrolled. These better figures from Canada than those reported in the United States may reflect the

more organized national health care system providing easier access and follow-up care.

## Continued Problems

Clearly, most United States adults know that hypertension is a threat and have had their blood pressures taken recently. Nonetheless, the number of people found to be hypertensive whose blood pressure is not well controlled remains high. What we find is not unexpected: The massive campaign to inform people that hypertension is a danger and that blood pressure should be measured every year has been successful. However, the adequate management of the large hypertensive population has proved to be more difficult. Part of this reflects the less than adequate health care provided the poor in the United States, a group with a large proportion of blacks who have the highest prevalence of hypertension and the largest percentage of uncontrolled disease (Blendon et al, 1989). Even when programs in community health centers serving low-income patients are successful in increasing the number of identified hypertensives, as many as 30% are soon lost to follow-up (Vallbona et al, 1985). Presumably as a reflection of less adequate management of hypertension and other cardiovascular risk factors, the overall decline in coronary heart disease mortality from 1976 to 1985 has slowed among black men and women compared with the continued significant decline in white men (Sempos et al, 1988).

The continued difficulties in maintaining adequate follow-up and management of the poor are not by any means unique to the United States. Similar problems have been noted in England, where a nationalized health care system should overcome the economic impediments to adequate blood pressure management. There, too, the fall in cerebrovascular and coronary heart disease mortality from 1979 to 1983 has been far greater in nonmanual occupational classes than in manual workers, further widening the gap between them (Marmot and McDowall, 1986).

More than just income levels and educational status are obviously involved in these inequities. However, we in the United States need to consider the probable deleterious effects of our political decision made during the Reagan administration to cut back on federally funded health care for the poor, a group that has a particularly high prevalence of hypertension. The improvement in overall and cardiovascular mortality since 1968 could, at least in part, reflect the greater access to health care provided to the indigent and elderly by Medicare and Medicaid, which were introduced in 1965. Recent cutbacks in such programs have been shown to affect health adversely, specifically the level of blood pressure control (Lurie et al, 1986). Whatever else we do, we should not lose sight of the higher prevalence and severity of hypertension among the indigent and the elderly and of the need to ensure that their access to health care is not curtailed further.

### Proposed Solutions

Beyond improving the availability and utilization of needed medical services to the poor, there are various ways to extend the benefits of adequate management of hypertension. As noted in surveys in California, the major need now is not to educate or screen but to improve adherence to treatment by maintaining contact and encouraging follow-up care (Bohnstedt et al, 1987).

Improvements in long-term management can be made both by large-scale and individual provider actions. Examples of successful large-scale approaches include:

—the North Karelia, Finland control program with intensive community education, hypertension dispensaries run by specially trained nurses, and more widespread use of both non-drug and drug therapies (Nissinen et al, 1988);
—rural control programs such as organized in Kentucky, providing education at various levels and a network for both screening and monitoring of blood pressure through multiple community resources (Kotchen et al, 1986);
—utilization of the work site for follow-up care (Rudd et al, 1987);
—nurse-run outpatient hypertension clinics such as in Skaraborg, Sweden, which have improved the effectiveness of blood pressure management (Råstam et al, 1986b).

Among the techniques found useful by individual providers are these:

—use of a computer to characterize patients' cardiovascular risk status and their progress, and to provide reminders of appointments (Robson et al, 1989);
—provision of a special nurse or physician assistant (Bass et al, 1986) to screen and monitor patients' progress;
—performance of careful blood pressure measurement as part of periodic health examinations (Oboler and LaForce, 1989);

—utilization of home blood pressure monitoring (Stahl et al, 1984);
—use of community health workers to maintain contact with patients seen in the emergency room (Bone et al, 1989).

### Consequences of Improved Control of Hypertension

At least partly as a result of the improved control of hypertension, more people are avoiding disability and premature death. There has been a steady decrease in cardiovascular mortality both for coronary heart disease and, even more so, for stroke, in the United States, starting in 1968, with a steeper decline than seen for noncardiovascular disease (Fig. 1.13). The decrease in hypertension-related mortality has been observed in both men and women, black and white, although as noted previously the decline from 1976 to 1985 has been less steep for blacks than for whites (Sempos et al, 1988). As a result of the decline in cardiovascular mortality, life expectancy for adults in the United States has risen about 3 years since 1970, the most dramatic improvement in adult life expectancy noted since such statistics have been collected (Feinleib, 1984).

Similar falls in mortality from heart disease have been noted in other countries, particularly

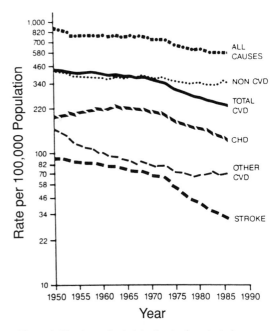

**Figure 1.13.** Age-adjusted death rates for selected causes of death in the United States, 1950 to 86. (From Kannel WB: Risk factors in hypertension. *J Cardiovasc Pharmacol* 13(Suppl 1):S4, 1989.)

some of those (e.g., Finland, Australia) that, like the United States, have had very high rates (Thom et al, 1985). On the other hand, in some countries (e.g., Poland, Yugoslavia, Norway) mortality from heart disease has been rising fast, likely because of increased consumption of cigarettes and saturated fat (Stamler and Liu, 1983). There has been an almost universal fall in death rates for heart disease among women compared with the variable changes in men.

## Contribution of Hypertension Control

The explanation for the reduced mortality from CVD in the United States remains uncertain (Kannel and Thom, 1984). A careful analysis of the comparative effects of various medical interventions and changes in life style concluded that the latter were responsible for the larger part of the decline in coronary mortality (Goldman and Cook, 1984) (Table 1.12). Note that only 8.5% of the fall in coronary mortality from 1968 to 1976 was attributed to improved control of hypertension.

Stroke is more closely related to hypertension than is coronary disease, and the fall in stroke mortality would logically be ascribable to improved control of hypertension. In the population of Rochester, Minnesota, the incidence of stroke has been found to be closely (inversely) connected to the control of hypertension, more so in women than in men (Garraway and Whisnant, 1987). Analysis of vital statistics for the entire United States, on the other hand, shows no correlation between the fall in stroke mortality and improved antihypertensive therapy (Klag et al, 1989). Moreover, in Framingham, the incidence of stroke has *risen* from 1953 through 1983 despite declines in the prevalence

**Table 1.12. Estimated Benefit of Interventions on Coronary Heart Disease Mortality (1968 to 1976)[a]**

| Medical Intervention | No. of Lives Saved | % of Decline in Mortality |
|---|---|---|
| Coronary care | 85,000 | 13.5 |
| Prehospital CPR | 25,000 | 4 |
| Coronary bypass surgery | 23,000 | 3.5 |
| Medical Rx of CHD | 61,000 | 10 |
| Rx of hypertension | 55,000 | 8.5 |
| Total | 249,000 | 39.5 |
| Changes in Life Style | | |
| Decrease in serum cholesterol | 190,000 | 30 |
| Decrease in cigarette | 150,000 | 24 |
| Total | 340,000 | 54 |

[a]Data from Goldman L, Cook EF: *Ann Intern Med* 101:825, 1984.

of hypertension and average levels of blood pressure (Wolf et al, 1989). Similar increases in the prevalence of CHD in the Framingham cohort have been observed despite declines in blood pressure, LVH, cigarette smoking, and cholesterol levels (Kannel et al, 1989). More obesity and diabetes have been noted and these may be responsible for the higher stroke and CHD rates.

Thus, we have to look elsewhere than improved control of hypertension to explain much of the good that has occurred in both coronary and cerebrovascular mortality since 1968. An intriguing, direct relation between stroke mortality and maternal mortality has been noted in England and Wales (Barker and Osmond, 1987). These data have been taken to support a connection between the recent decrease in stroke mortality and the improvement in maternal health whereas the increase in coronary disease mortality until recently is considered to be a reflection of greater affluence and a richer diet.

Nonetheless, the increased treatment of hypertension has almost certainly played some role: Among the Framingham population, the 8-year predicted risk of coronary heart disease declined 2.3 events per 100 more among the treated hypertensives than among the untreated hypertensives (Shea et al, 1985). As we shall explore further in Chapter 5, the evidence for protection against stroke and heart failure by drug therapy of hypertension seems strong. However, there remain serious doubts about the benefits of therapy for prevention of coronary disease. Of particular concern is the continued high frequency of sudden death, responsible for almost 300,000 deaths per year in the United States. Although it is clearly increased among hypertensives with left ventricular hypertrophy, its risk was increased an additional 2-fold among those receiving antihypertensive drug therapy in the same Framingham population (Kannel et al, 1988).

We obviously have a long way to go, both in the United States and elsewhere in the world. As we work to prolong healthy survival to the presumed ideal (Fries et al, 1989), we need to address the issues of hypertension in the individual patient, as will be done in the next chapter, before considering its mechanisms and management in the following chapters.

## Potential for Prevention

A greater awareness of the causes and accelerators of hypertension may provide in-

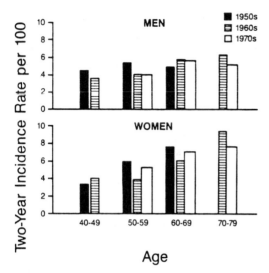

Age

**Figure 1.14.** Trends in 2-year incidence of definite hypertension per 100 by sex and age based on examinations 2–6, 7–11, and 12–16 (Framingham cohort). (From Kannel WB: Risk factors in hypertension. *J Cardiovasc Pharmacol* 13(Suppl 1):S4, 1989.)

have done little that might prevent its onset. The incidence of hypertension in the Framingham population has remained quite stable over the past 30 years (Kannel, 1989) (Fig. 1.14). Among the offspring of the original Framingham cohort, increases in blood pressure have been associated with weight gain, increases in alcohol consumption in men, and beginning oral contraceptive use in women (Hubert et al, 1987). In other populations as well, obesity stands out as a major correlate to a rise in blood pressure (Buck and Donner, 1987; Daniels et al, 1988). As we shall see in Chapter 3, obesity, particularly distributed in the upper body, may be a major causal factor and should be a primary focus in our attempts to prevent hypertension. Unfortunately, the prevalence of obesity in the United States has progressively risen from 1960 to 1980, both in adults (Harlan et al, 1988) and even more disturbingly in children among whom more obesity-related hypertension has also been noted (Gortmaker et al, 1987). More about obesity and hypertension will be covered in Chapter 3, but we should keep the goal of prevention in mind as we consider the overall problems of hypertension for the population in this chapter and for the individual patient in the next.

sights into the real goal—prevention. Despite the more "aggressive" management of millions of people who have developed hypertension, we

## References

Abrams WB: *Am J Med* 85 (Suppl 3B):7, 1988.

Agner E: *Acta Med Scand* 214:285, 1983.

Akinkugbe OO: *J Clin Hypertens* 3:1S, 1987.

Amery A, Birkenhäger WH, Brixko P, et al: *Lancet* 11:589, 1986.

Anderson NB, Myers HG, Pickering T, et al: *J Hypertension* 7:161, 1989.

Barker DJP, Osmond C: *Br Med J* 295:83, 1987.

Barrett-Connor E, Suarez L, Khaw KT, et al: *J Chron Dis* 37:903, 1984.

Bass MJ, McWhinney IR, Donner A: *Can Med Assoc J* 134:1247, 1986.

Berglund G, Andersson O, Wilhelmsen L: *Br Med J* 2:554, 1976.

Birkenhäger WH, de Leeuw PW: *J Hypertension* 6 (Suppl 1):S21, 1988.

Birkett NJ, Donner AP, Maynard MD: *CMAJ* 136:595, 1987.

Birkett NJ, Evans CE, Haynes RB, et al: *J Hypertension* 4:369, 1986.

Black HR: *Diagnosis* 10:20, 1988.

Blendon RJ, Aiken LH, Freeman HE, et al: *JAMA* 261:278, 1989.

Bohnstedt M, Leonard AR, Trudeau MJ, et al: *Am J Prev Med* 3:200, 1987.

Bone LR, Mamon J, Levine DM, et al: *Am J Emerg Med* 7:16, 1989.

Brett AS: *Am J Med* 76:557, 1984.

Buck CW, Donner AP: *CMAJ* 136:357, 1987.

Bulpitt CJ: *Br J Clin Pharmacol* 13:73, 1982.

Coope J, Warrender TS, McPherson K. *J Human Hypertens* 2:79, 1988.

Cornoni-Huntley J, LaCroix AZ, Havlik RJ: *Arch Intern Med* 149:780, 1989.

Curb JD, Schneider K, Taylor JO, et al: *Hypertension* 11 (Suppl II):II-51, 1988.

Daniels SR, Heiss G, Davis CE, et al: *Hypertension* 11:249, 1988.

Danielson M, Dammstrom BG: *Acta Med Scand* 209:451, 1981.

Dannenberg AL, Drizd T, Horan MJ, et al: *Hypertension* 10:226, 1987.

Dawber TR: *The Framingham Study. The Epidemiology of Atherosclerotic Disease*. Cambridge: Harvard University Press, 1980.

Deprez RD, Miller E, Hart SK: *Am J Public Health* 75:653, 1985.

DeStefano F, Coulehan JL, Wiant MK: *Am J Epidemiol* 109:335, 1979.

Doyle AE: *Clin Sci* 63:431s, 1982.

Dyer AR: *J Chron Dis* 28:571, 1975.

Dyer AR, Stamler J, Paul O, et al: *Circulation* 56:1067, 1977.

Ekbom T, Lindholm L, Oden A, et al: *J Hypertension* 6 (Suppl 4):S626, 1988.

Farchi G, Menotti A, Conti S: *Am J Epidemiol* 126:400, 1987.

Feinleib M: *Am J Cardiol* 54:2C, 1984.

Folsom AR, Gomez-Marin O, Sprafka JM, et al: *Am Heart J* 114:1199, 1987.

Franco LJ, Stern MP, Rosenthal M, et al: *Am J Epidemiol* 121:684, 1985.

Fries JF, Green LW, Levine S: *Lancet* 1:481, 1989.

Garcia-Palmieri MR, Costas R Jr: In: Yu PH, Goodwin JF (eds). *Progress in Cardiology*, Volume 14. Philadelphia: Lea and Febiger, 1986:101.

Garraway WM, Whisnant JP: *JAMA* 258:214, 1987.

Gifford RW Jr: *Milbank Mem Fund Q* 47:170, 1969.

Gifford RW, Borhani N, Krishan I, et al: *JAMA* 250:3171, 1983.

Gillum RF: *Stroke* 19:1, 1988.

Gillum RF, Gillum BS, Smith N: *Am Heart J* 107:765, 1984.

Goldman L, Cook EF: *Ann Intern Med* 101:825, 1984.

Gortmaker SL, Dietz WH Jr, Sobol AM, et al: *AJDC* 141:535, 1987.

Greenberg S, Guzik H, Frishman W, et al: *JACC* 13:37A, 1989.

Guttmacher S, Teitelman M, Chapin G, et al: *Hastings Center Report* 11:12, 1981.

Hansen AG, Jensen H, Laugesen LP, et al: Ninth International Society of Hypertension, Feb 21, 1982 (abstr).

Hansson L: *Am J Hypertens* 1:414, 1988.

Harlan WR, Landis JR, Flegal KM, et al: *Am J Epidemiol* 128:1065, 1988.

Hatch FE, Crowe LR, Miles DE, et al: *Am J Hypertens* 2:2, 1989.

Helgeland A: *Am J Med* 69:752, 1980.

Heller RF, Rose G, Pedoe HDT, et al: *J Epidemiol Community Health* 32:235, 1978.

Hubert HB, Eaker ED, Garrison RJ, et al: *Am J Epidemiol* 125:812, 1987.

Hypertension Detection and Follow-up Program Cooperative Group: *Circ Res* 40 (Suppl 1):106, 1977.

Irvine MJ, Garner DM, Olmsted MP et al: *Psychosom Med* 51:537, 1989.

Jachuck SJ, Brierley H, Jachuck S, et al: *J Royal Coll Gen Practitioners* 32:103, 1982.

Johnson JL, Heineman EF, Heiss G, et al: *Am J Epidemiol* 123:209, 1986.

Johnston ME, Gibson ED, Terry CW, et al: *J Chron Dis* 37:417, 1984.

Joint National Committee on Detection, Evaluation, and Treatment of High Blood Pressure: *Arch Intern Med* 148:1023, 1988.

Joseph JG, Prior IAM, Salmond CE, et al: *J Chron Dis* 36:507, 1983.

Julius S, Hansson L, Andren L, et al: *Acta Med Scand* 208:481, 1980.

Kagan A, Harris BR, Winkelstein W: *J Chron Dis* 27:345, 1974.

Kannel WB: *J Cardiovasc Pharmacol* 13 (Suppl 1):S4, 1989.

Kannel WB, Cupples LA, D'Agostino RB: 25th Conference on Cardiovascular Epidemiology, Cardiovascular Disease Epidemiology Newsletter, No. 37. Dallas, TX, American Heart Association, p 34, 1985 (abstr).

Kannel WB, Cupples LA, D'Agostino RB, et al: *Hypertension* 11 (Suppl II):II-45, 1988.

Kannel WB, D'Agostino RG, Belanger A: *JACC* 13:35A, 1989.

Kannel WB, Thom TJ: *Circulation* 70:331, 1984.

Kannel WB, Wolf PA, McGee DL, et al: *JAMA* 245:1225, 1981.

Kaplan NM: *Ann Intern Med* 98:705, 1983.

Kaplan NM: *Am J Med* 77:1, 1984.

Kirkendall WM, Hammond JJ: *Arch Intern Med* 140:1155, 1980.

Klag MJ, Whelton PK, Seidler AJ. *Stroke* 20:14, 1989.

Kotchen JM, McKean HE, Jackson-Thayer S, et al: *JAMA* 255:2177, 1986.

Langer RD, Ganiats TG, Barrett-Connor E: *Br Med J* 298:1356, 1989.

Lefebvre RC, Hursey KG, Carleton RA: *Arch Intern Med* 148:1993, 1988.

Levy D, Kannel WB: *Am Heart J* 116:266, 1988.

Liebman M, Chopin LF, Carter E, et al: *Hypertension* 8:843, 1986.

Lindholm L, Lanke J, Bengtsson B: *Family Practice* 3:3, 1986.

Lurie N, Ward NB, Shapiro MF, et al: *N Engl J Med* 314:1266, 1986.

MacDonald LA, Sackett DL, Haynes RB, et al: *J Chron Dis* 37:933, 1984.

MacMahon S, Peto R, Cutler J, et al: *Lancet*, 335:765, 1990.

Madsen PER, Buch J: *Aerospace Med* 42:752, 1971.

Marmot MG, McDowall ME: *Lancet* 2:274, 1986.

Mattila K, Haavisto M, Rajala S, et al: *Br Med J* 296:887, 1988.

Medical Research Council Working Party: *Br Med J* 296:1565, 1988.

Messerli FH, Ventura HO, Glade B, et al: *Lancet* 2:983, 1983.

Miall WE: *Clin Exp Hyper Theory and Practice* A4:1121, 1982.

Morrison JA, Khoury P, Kelly K, et al: *Am J Epidemiol* 111:156, 1980.

Murphy JK, Alpert BS, Walker SS, et al: *Hypertension* 11:208, 1988.

Myers MG, Carruthers SG, Leenen FHH, et al: *CMAJ* 140:1141, 1989.

National Center for Health Statistics. Koch H and Knapp DA: Advance Data From Vital and Health Statistics, No. 134. Department of Health and Human Services Pub. No. (PHS) 87-1250. Public Health Service Hyattsville, MD, May 19, 1987.

National Center for Health Statistics. McLemore T, DeLozier J: Advance Data From Vital and Health Statistics, No. 128. Department of Health and Human Services Pub. No. (PHS) 87-1250. Public Health Service. Hyattsville, MD, January 23, 1987.

National Center for Health Statistics. Schoenborn CA: Vital and Health Statistics. Series 10, No. 163. Department of Health and Human Services Pub. No. (PHS) 88-1591. Public Health Service. Washington: United States Government Printing Office, February 1988.

Neaton JD, Kuller LH, Wentworth D, et al: *Am Heart J* 108:759, 1984.

Neaton JD, Wentworth D, Sherwin R, et al: *Circulation* 80:II-300, 1989.

Nissinen A, Tuomilehto J, Korhonen HJ, et al: *Am J Epidemiol* 127:488, 1988.

Oboler SK, LaForce FM: *Ann Intern Med* 110:214, 1989.

Oliver MJ: *Am Heart J* 114:1011, 1987.

Perry HM Jr, McFate Smith W, McDonald RH, et al: *Stroke* 20:4, 1989.

Pickering G: *Am J Med* 52:570, 1972.

Pooling Project Research Group: *J Chron Dis* 31:201, 1978.

Poulter N, Khaw KT, Hopwood BEC, et al: *Hypertension* 6:810, 1984.

Prineas RJ, Stephens WB, Lovel RRH: *Clin Sci Mol Med* 45:47s, 1973.

Rabkin SW, Mathewson FAL, Tate RB: *Ann Intern Med* 88:342, 1978.

Råstam L, Berglund G, Isacsson S-O, et al: *Acta Med Scand* 219:243, 1986a.

Råstam L, Berglund G, Isacsson S-O, et al: *Acta Med Scand* 219:261, 1986b.

Reid DD, Hamilton PJS, McCartney P, et al: *Lancet* 2:979, 1976.

Report of the British Hypertension Society Working Party: *Br Med J* 298:694, 1989.

Ribeiro AB, Ribeiro MBD: *Drugs* 31 (Suppl 4):23, 1986.

Roberts J, Maurer K: Blood Pressure Levels of Persons 6-74 Years, Vital and Health Statistics, Department of Health, Education, and Welfare Pub. No. (HRA) 78-1648, Series 11, No. 203, 1977.

Robson J, Boomla K, Fitzpatrick S, et al: *Br Med J* 298:433, 1989.

Rodgers CP, Walker EC, Podgor MJ: *Clin Res* 36:432A, 1988 (abst).

Rose G: In: Marshall AG, Barritt DW (eds). *The Hypertensive Patient*. Kent, England: Pitman Medical Press, 1980.

Rose G: *Br Med J* 282:1847, 1981.

Rosenfeld JB, Silverberg DS: *Israel J Med Sci* 15:1014, 1979.

Rowland M, Roberts J: NCHS Advance Data, Vital and Health Statistics of the National Center for Health Statistics, No. 84, October 8, 1982. Washington, D.C., United States Department of Health and Human Services.

Rudd P, Price MG, Graham LE, et al: *Hypertension* 10:425, 1987.

Rudnick KV, Sackett DL, Hirst S, et al: *Can Med Assoc J* 117:492, 1977.

Rutan GH, Kuller LH, Neaton JD, et al: *Circulation* 77:504, 1988.

Sempos C, Cooper R, Kovar MG, et al: *Am J Public Health* 78:1422, 1988.

Shaper AG, Ashby D, Pocock SJ: *J Hypertension* 6:367, 1988.

Shea S, Cook EF, Kannel WB, et al: *Circulation* 71:22, 1985.

Shulman NB: *J Clin Hypertens* 3:85S, 1987.

Sinclair AM, Isles CG, Brown I, et al: *Arch Intern Med* 147:1289, 1987.

Smith WM: *Circ Res* 40(Suppl 1):I-98, 1977.

Society of Actuaries and Association of Life Insurance Medical Directors of America: Blood Pressure Study, 1979 and 1980.

Sprafka JM, Folsom AR, Burke GL, et al: *Am J Public Health* 78:1546, 1988.

Staessen J, Fagard R, Van Hoof R, et al: *J Cardiovasc Pharmacol* 12(Suppl 8):S33, 1988.

Stahl SM, Kelley CR, Neill PJ, et al: *Am J Public Health* 74:704, 1984.

Stamler J, Liu K: In: Kaplan NM, Stamler J (eds). *Prevention of Coronary Heart Disease*. Philadelphia: WB Saunders, 1983, p 188.

Stamler J, Rhomberg P, Schoenberger JA, et al: *J Chron Dis* 28:527, 1975.

Stavig GR, Igra A, Leonard AR: *Publ Health Reports* 103:28, 1988.

Subcommittee on Definition and Prevalence of the 1984 Joint National Committee: *Hypertension* 7:457, 1985.

Task Force on Blood Pressure Control in Children: *Pediatrics* 79:271, 1987.

The Lipid Research Clinics: *Population Studies Data Book*, Volume 1. *The Prevalence Study*. Bethesda: National Institutes of Health, 1980.

Thom TJ, Epstein FH, Feldman JJ, et al: *Int J Epidemiol* 14:510, 1985.

Topol EJ, Traill TA, Fortuin NJ: *N Engl J Med* 321:277, 1985.

Tverdal A: *Br Med J* 294:671, 1987.

Vallbona C, Yusim S, Scherwitz L, et al: *Am J Prev Med* 1:52, 1985.

Veterans Administration Cooperative Study Group on Antihypertensive Agents: *Circulation* 145:991, 1972.

Vokonas PS, Kannel WB, Cupples LA: *J Hypertension* 6(Suppl 1):S3, 1988.

Waal-Manning JH, Paulin JM, Wallis TA, et al: *J Hypertension* 6 (Suppl 4):S634, 1988.

Weinberger MH: *Arch Intern Med* 145:1102, 1985.

WHO Expert Committee Report 1980: *Arterial Hypertension—Technical Report Series 628*. Geneva: World Health Organization, 1978.

Wilking SVB, Belanger A, Kannel WB, et al: *JAMA* 260:3451, 1988.

Wolf PA, O'Neil A, D'Agostino RB, et al: *Stroke* 20:101, 1989 (abstr).

Working Group on Risk and High Blood Pressure: *Hypertension* 7:641, 1985.

World Health Organization/International Society of Hypertension: *J Hypertension* 7:689, 1989.

Yano K, McGee D, Reed DM: *J Chron Dis* 36:569, 1983.

# 2 Hypertension in the Individual Patient

Now that some of the major issues about hypertension in the population at large have been addressed, let us turn to the primary concern of this text—the evaluation and management of the individual patient with hypertension. First, the measurement of the blood pressure will be covered, with special attention to the factors that affect its variability.

## MEASUREMENT OF THE BLOOD PRESSURE

Great care should be taken in measuring the blood pressure (BP), both to avoid falsely labeling normotensives as hypertensive and to ensure that those who are hypertensive are provided proper therapy. Although most health practitioners likely consider the measurement of BP to be easy and their findings to be accurate, the procedure is "full of pitfalls and is frequently inaccurate" (Special Task Force, 1988). I would venture to guess that, of all of the procedures done in clinical medicine that have important consequences, measurement of BP is likely the one that is done most haphazardly. Beyond all else, multiple readings—perhaps out of the office and surely out of the hospital—should be obtained before the diagnosis is made, unless the initial BP is so high or the evidences of target organ involvement so compelling as to mandate immediate therapy.

### Adverse Effects of False Labeling

There are two main reasons not to falsely label a person as hypertensive on the basis of improper measurement of the BP. First, if the diagnosis is made, therapy will likely follow. As briefly noted in Chapter 1 and as will be discussed more fully in Chapter 7, the decision to institute antihypertensive therapy involves a lifelong commitment to what often is expensive and bothersome, and occasionally hazardous. Despite its drawbacks, such therapy is clearly necessary for most of those with significant hypertension. But such therapy should never be instituted—as it often is today—in people who have only "office" or "white coat" hypertension, transiently elevated BP that is in a safe range almost all of the time.

Second, as noted in Chapter 1, the mere labeling of a person as "hypertensive" may provoke ill effects. Obviously, then, care is needed in taking the BP so that only those who are in need of having something done about their elevated BP are labeled and treated as hypertensive.

### Importance of "Casual" Readings

As we shall see, "casual," noninvasive BP readings vary a great deal and are often not indicative of the average pressure. On the other hand, remember that most of the data showing increased mortality from minimally elevated BP was derived from single casual readings (Stokes et al, 1987). No single reading should be ignored but, to improve reliability, a number of sources of potential error need to be recognized and appropriate steps taken to avoid them.

As noted 60 years ago (Brown, 1930), casual BP taken in the office, even with the greatest of care, is almost always higher than BP recorded at home (White, 1986) (Fig. 2.1). Readings taken by ausculation or oscillometry, being indirect, may vary considerably from those taken by direct intra-arterial measurements. In one

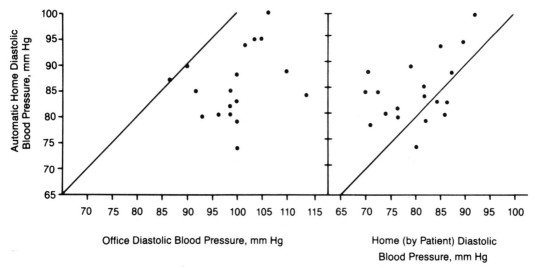

**Figure 2.1.** Relationship between office (physician) or manual home blood pressure and automatic (while awake) blood pressure in patients with office DBP above 90 mm Hg. Lines of identity have been drawn. (From White WB: *Arch Intern Med* 146:2196, 1986, Copyright 1986, American Medical Association.)

comparison, the daytime readings were quite close but the indirect readings tended to be higher than intra-arterial readings during the night (Brigden et al, 1989). Fortunately, indirect readings are more than adequate for both diagnosis and management if some simple precautions are used.

### Guidelines for Measuring the Blood Pressure

Indirect measurement of the BP is based on the finding by Korotkoff in 1905 that the sounds generated over an artery during deflation of an occluding cuff represent the systolic blood pressure (SBP) and diastolic blood pressure (DBP). In practice, the first tapping sound (Korotkoff phase I) is taken as the SBP, and the disappearance of the sounds (Korotkoff phase V) is used for the DBP, although some in England still use the muffling (phase IV) (Bucknall et al, 1986). As noted in Chapter 1, both SBP and DBP need to be considered, both for diagnosis and prognosis.

The use of kilopascals (kPa) instead of mm Hg as the units of the BP, recommended as part of the "metrication" of scientific measurements under the SI system, has little chance of taking over. For conversion to kPa, divide the mm Hg by 7.5.

Use of the guidelines shown in Table 2.1, adopted from those recommended by the American Heart Association (Special Task Force, 1988) and the British Hypertension Society (Petrie et al, 1986), will obviate most errors. By training and testing, observers can take accurate and reproducible BP (Bruce et al, 1988). However, a strong preference for readings ending in the digit 0 is very prevalent even with the use of a random zero sphygmomanometer (Silman, 1985). Such observer bias can be eliminated by use of an electronic recording device with a digital display (Hla et al, 1986).

### Arm and Patient Position (Fig. 2.2)

Although supine readings are often advocated, those obtained with the patient seated comfortably are adequate both for initial and follow-up examinations. The arm should be supported and positioned at the level of the heart: Measurements taken with the arm dependent by the side averaged 8 mm Hg higher than those taken with the arm supported in a horizontal position at heart level (Waal-Manning and Paulin, 1987). When sitting upright on a table without support for the torso or arm, readings may be as much as 10 mm Hg higher presumably because of the isometric exertion needed to support the body and arm (Cooper et al, 1988). For all readings, the arm and position should be noted, e.g., 140/90, right arm, seated.

Initially, the BP should be taken in both arms. Though differences between the two arms are noted only rarely (Gould et al, 1985), if the reading is higher in one arm, that arm should be used for future measurements. Lower pressures, usually in the left arm, are seen in patients with subclavian steal caused by reversal of flow down a vertebral artery distal to an obstructed

**Table 2.1. Guidelines in Measuring Blood Pressure**

I. Conditions for the patient
  A. Posture
    1. Some prefer readings after patient has been supine for 5 minutes. Sitting pressures usually are adequate.
    2. Patient should sit quietly with back supported for 5 minutes and the arm supported at the level of the heart.
    3. For patients who are over age 65, diabetic, or receiving antihypertensive therapy, check for postural changes by taking readings immediately and 2 minutes after patient stands.
  B. Circumstances
    1. No caffeine for preceding hour.
    2. No smoking for preceding 15 minutes.
    3. No exogenous adrenergic stimulants, e.g., phenylephrine in nasal decongestants or eye drops for pupillary dilation.
    4. A quiet, warm setting.
    5. Home readings taken under varying circumstances and 24-hour ambulatory recordings may be preferable and more accurate in predicting subsequent cardiovascular disease.

II. Equipment
  A. Cuff size: The bladder should encircle and cover two-thirds of the length of the arm; if not, place the bladder over the brachial artery; if bladder is too small, spuriously high readings may result.
  B. Manometer: Aneroid gauges should be calibrated every 6 months against a mercury manometer.
  C. For infants, use equipment employing ultrasound, e.g., the Doppler method.

III. Technique
  A. Number of readings
    1. On each occasion, take at least two readings, separated by as much time as is practical. If readings vary by more than 5 mm Hg, take additional readings until two are close.
    2. For diagnosis, obtain 3 sets of readings at least a week apart.
    3. Initially, take pressure in both arms; if pressure differs, use arm with higher pressure.
    4. If arm pressure is elevated, take pressure in one leg, particularly in patients below age 30.
  B. Performance
    1. Inflate the bladder quickly to a pressure of 20 mm Hg above the systolic, as recognized by disappearance of the radial pulse.
    2. Deflate the bladder 3 mg Hg every second.
    3. Record the Korotkoff phase V (disappearance) except in children, in whom use of phase IV (muffling) is advocated.
    4. If Korotkoff sounds are weak, have the patient raise the arm, open and close the hand 5 to 10 times, after which the bladder should be inflated quickly.

subclavian artery. This was noted in 9% of 500 patients with asymptomatic neck bruits (Bornstein and Norris, 1986). On the other hand, pressures may be slightly higher in the paretic arms of stroke patients (Yagi et al, 1986).

After supine or seated measurements, readings should then be taken immediately and 2 minutes after standing to check for spontaneous or drug-induced postural changes. In most people, SBP falls and DBP rises a few millimeters of mercury (mm Hg) on change from supine to standing (Tell et al, 1988). In 128 patients with untreated, mild hypertension, both the immediate and 2-minute standing DBP averaged 8.1% higher than sitting DBP (Hall et al, 1977).

In the elderly, significant postural falls of 20 mm Hg or more in SBP are more common, occurring in about 10% of ambulatory people over age 65 (Mader et al, 1987) and even more frequently in those with systolic hypertension (Lipsitz et al, 1985) (Fig. 2.3). Note the increasingly greater postural fall, the higher the supine level. This suggests that poor baroreceptor function may be responsible both for the postural fall and for the persistence of elevated pressure in the supine position. Standing pressures should routinely be taken in the elderly to recognize such postural falls, particularly before institution of antihypertensive therapy.

If the arm reading is elevated, particularly in a patient below age 30, the BP should be taken in one leg to rule out coarctation. The technique is described in the next section.

**Sphygmomanometer**

*Cuff Size (Fig. 2.4).* The width of the cuff should be equal to about two-thirds of the distance from the axilla to the antecubital space, a 15-cm-wide cuff being adequate for most adults. The bladder within the cuff should be long enough to encircle at least 80% of the arm. Erroneously high readings may arise from the use of a cuff that is either too narrow or too short (van Montfrans et al, 1987) (Fig. 2.5).

Most sphygmomanometers sold in the United States have a cuff with a bladder 12 cm wide and 23 cm long, but the bladder sizes in the cuffs sold by the three major manufacturers differ considerably, and none matches the recommendations of the most recent American Heart Association report (Special Task Force, 1988). The 12- × 23-cm adult cuff is too short for patients with a large arm circumference greater than 33 cm, whether fat or muscular. As noted in Figure 2.4, for most adults the best procedure is to use the obese cuff with a 15- × 33- to 35-cm bladder routinely; for those with arm circumference greater than 41 cm, the thigh cuff with a 18- × 36- to 42-cm bladder should be used (Linfors et al, 1984). Another way to avoid "cuff hypertension" would be to use the longer "balanced" cuffs marketed by Pymah (Somer-

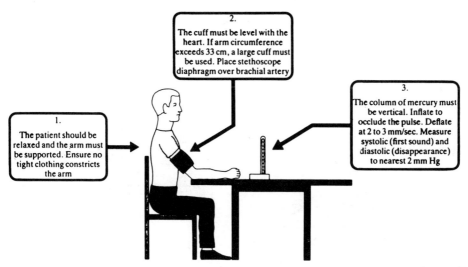

**Figure 2.2.** Technique of blood pressure measurement recommended by the British Hypertension Society. (From *J Hypertens* 3:293, 1985.)

**Figure 2.3.** Relationship between basal supine systolic blood pressure and postural change in systolic blood pressure for old subjects (mean age = 87 ± 7 years). (From Lipsitz LA, Storch HA, Minaker KL, et al: *Clin Sci* 69:337, 1985.)

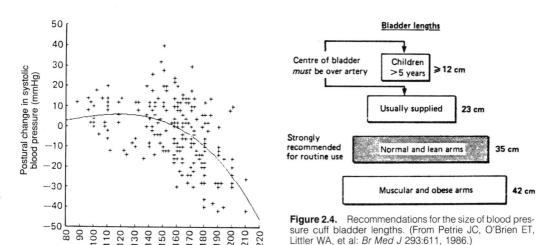

**Figure 2.4.** Recommendations for the size of blood pressure cuff bladder lengths. (From Petrie JC, O'Brien ET, Littler WA, et al: *Br Med J* 293:611, 1986.)

ville, NJ). Simply stated, if the cuff fits on the arm, it is not too large, and the more of the arm encircled by the bladder, the more likely is the reading to be correct.

*Cuff Position.* If the bladder within the cuff does not completely encircle the arm, particular care should be taken that it is placed over the brachial artery. The lower edge of the cuff should be about 2.5 cm above the antecubital space. In extremely fat people, a more accurate reading may be obtained by placing the cuff on the forearm and listening over the radial artery.

*Manometer.* Two types of manometers are in use: aneroid and mercury, and a number of electronic devices are available for semiautomatic recordings out of the office setting (Evans et al, 1989). If aneroid manometers are used, they should be checked every few months by using a Y-tube to connect a bladder to both the aneroid and a mercury manometer. With mercury manometers the reservoir should be full, the meniscus should read zero when no pressure is applied, and the column should move freely when pressure is applied. The filter and vent to the mercury column should be cleaned yearly.

Random-zero manometers have been used to

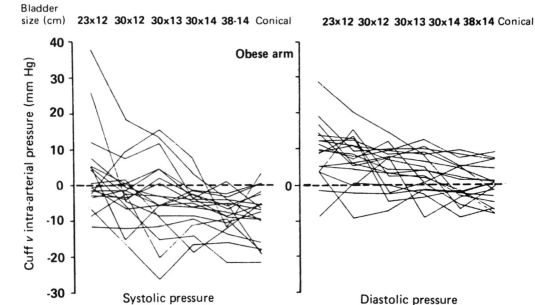

**Figure 2.5.** Individual differences between systolic and diastolic ausculatory (cuff) blood pressures minus intra-arterial blood pressures in 19 subjects with obese arms (circumference ≥ 34 cm) and 18 with normal sized arms. Figure compares six different cuffs with increasing bladder width. Each measurement point represents mean of three comparisons in one subject for one cuff. (From van Montfrans GA, van der Hoeven GMA, Karemaker JM, et al: *Br Med J* 295:354, 1987.)

reduce observer bias, but they underestimate the BP slightly (De Gaudemaris et al, 1985).

*New Devices.* Beyond the various automatic devices to be described that also depend upon compression of the brachial artery, there are other ways to measure the BP. They include two devices that measure the pressure in one finger, providing systolic pressure only (Close et al, 1986) or both systolic and diastolic pressure, the FINAPRES device (Parati et al, 1989). Caution is needed with such digital devices since they have been reported to be quite inaccurate (Watkins-Pitchford and Szocik, 1989) although Parati et al (1989) found the beat-to-beat recordings with the FINAPRES device to be quite close to those simultaneously measured by intraarterial monitoring. In addition, analysis of the external brachial pulse recorded during cuff deflation by use of a transducer may provide more accurate measurements than the auscultatory technique (Blank et al, 1988).

## Technique for Measuring the Blood Pressure (Table 2.1)

As noted in Table 2.1, care should be taken to raise the pressure in the bladder above the systolic level as checked by disappearance of the radial pulse since patients may have an aus-

cultatory gap—a temporary disappearance of the sound after it first appears. The measurement may be repeated after as short an interval as 15 seconds without significantly affecting the accuracy (Shekelle et al, 1981).

For most observers, disappearance of the sound (phase V) is a more reliable and reproducible end point than is the muffling (phase IV) (Hense et al, 1986), and it is closer to the true intraarterial DBP (Nielsen, 1982). In some patients without organic heart disease but with a hyperkinetic circulation (e.g., anemia), the sounds do not disappear, and the muffled sound is heard well below the expected DBP, sometimes near zero. This can also be caused by the stethoscope being held too tightly over the artery (Londe and Klitzner, 1984). If this is not the case, the point wherein muffling began should be taken as the DBP.

In some elderly patients with very rigid, calcified arteries, the bladder may not be able to collapse the brachial artery, giving rise to falsely high readings or "pseudohypertension" (Finnegan et al, 1985). The possibility of pseudohypertension should be suspected in elderly people whose vessels feel rigid, who have little vascular damage in the retina or elsewhere despite seemingly high BP readings, and who suffer inordinate postural symptoms despite cautious therapy. An indication of pseudohypertension can be gained by Osler's maneuver: If during BP measurement with a sphygmomanometer the radial pulse is still palpable after the pressure in the balloon has occluded the brachial artery, i.e., the Korotkoff sounds have disappeared, the true intraarterial pressure was found to be 10 to 54 mm Hg lower than the cuff pressure (Messerli et al, 1985). As simple as it seems, there was such marked intra- and interobserver disagreement in performing Osler's maneuver that it has little utility for identifying the few patients with pseudohypertension (Hla et al, 1989). If one is suspicious, a direct intraarterial reading should settle the issue, but an automatic infrasonic recorder may be as accurate (Hla and Feussner, 1988).

If arrhythmias are present, additional readings may be required to estimate the average systolic and diastolic BP.

### Ways to Improve the Sounds

If the sounds are hard to hear, first be sure you are listening over the brachial artery. Second, try some tricks based upon the fact that the loudness and sharpness of the Korotkoff sounds depend in part upon the pressure differential between the arteries in the forearm and those beneath the bladder. To increase the differential, and thereby increase the loudness of the sounds, one can either decrease the amount of blood or increase the capacity of the vascular bed in the forearm. The amount of blood can be decreased by rapid inflation of the bladder, shortening the time when venous outflow is prevented but arterial inflow continues, or by raising the arm for a few seconds to drain out venous blood before inflating the bladder. The vascular bed capacity can be increased by the vasodilation induced by muscular exercise, specifically by having the patient open and close the hand 10 times before the bladder is inflated. As a corollary, do not stop between the systolic and diastolic readings—reinflate and start all over again. The vessels will have been partially refilled and the sounds thereby altered.

### Taking the Pressure in the Thigh

This should be done as part of the initial workup of every hypertensive, particularly in the young, in whom coarctation is more commonly found. Normally, the SBP is higher, the DBP a little lower at the knee than in the arm because of the contour of the pulse wave (Remington and O'Brien, 1970).

*Use only a thigh cuff.* The use of cuffs with bladders too small and narrow for the size of the leg is another reason that the BP is usually recorded as higher in the legs. With the patient lying on the abdomen and the leg bent and cradled by the observer, listen with the stethoscope for the Korotkoff sounds in the popliteal fossa.

### Taking Blood Pressure in Infants and Children (See Chapter 16)

If the patients can be kept quiet and relaxed, the same technique used for adults should be used with children, except for utilizing smaller and narrower cuffs. However, as in adults, the bladder should encircle the upper arm so as not to over-read the level (Vyse, 1987). Diastolic readings tend to be more variable in children, so that systolic levels have been found to be more useful for screening children under age 13 (Rosner et al, 1987).

If the child is disturbed, the best procedure may be simply to determine the SBP by palpating the radial pulse as the cuff is deflated. In small infants, instruments using ultrasound are much easier to use (Laaser and Labarthe, 1986).

## Blood Pressure During Exercise

The SBP typically rises significantly during isotonic exercise and both SBP and DBP rise during isometric exercise. Care should be taken in measuring indirect BP during isotonic exercise since it may underestimate the true intraarterial change (Gould et al, 1985). The response to isometric exercise may be more accurately ascertained. The DBP tends to rise above 100 mm Hg after either isotonic or isometric effort in patients with borderline hypertension (Cantor et al, 1987), and such a response may be indicative of the development of soon-to-be persistent hypertension.

The prognostic implications of exercise-associated rises in BP for the subsequent development of hypertension in normotensive subjects have not been well delineated, but preliminary studies suggest that a particularly high rise during exercise may be predictive of the development of hypertension. Among a group of 341 people who had normal (less than 140/90) resting BP but a rise during a treadmill exercise test to above 225/90, the relative risk of developing a high resting BP over the next 32 months was 2.28 times higher than among those with a lesser rise during the exercise test (Wilson and Meyer, 1981).

Others have also shown a greater likelihood but by no means a certainty for the development of persistent hypertension some years after an exaggerated pressure response to exercise, i.e., SBP > 200 (Dlin et al, 1983; Chaney and Eyman, 1988). Moreover, normotensive children with a positive family history of hypertension, who are known to be at higher risk for developing the disorder, tend to have a significantly greater rise in SBP after exercise than do normotensive children without a positive family history (Di Tullio et al, 1983; Molineux and Steptoe, 1988). Such children may also have greater left ventricular mass on echocardiography, further supporting the supernormal exercise response as an important predictor of subsequent hypertension (Mahoney et al, 1988).

Though few would consider it purely exercise, coitus will raise everyone's BP. Those who have untreated hypertension may experience peak values as high as 300/175 at the time of orgasm (Mann et al, 1982).

### Final Caution

In whatever manner the BP is taken, notation should be made of the conditions so others can compare the findings or interpret them properly. This is particularly critical in scientific reports; yet, most articles about hypertension in prestigious medical journals have failed to indicate the type of sphygmomanometer, the diastolic end point, the position of the subject, or the number of readings (Lehane et al, 1980).

## VARIABILITY OF THE BLOOD PRESSURE

### Sources of Variation

As delineated by Rose (1980), BP readings are often variable, either because of factors working within the patient ("biological" variation) or because of problems involving the observer ("measurement" variation). Considerable variability has been noted even with the same well-trained observer using a calibrated sphygmomanometer under controlled circumstances (Watson et al, 1987) (Fig. 2.6). In this study of 32 patients, 12 sets of duplicate readings were obtained over a 3-month interval. Two major findings are shown in Fig. 2.6: first, the initial sets of readings tend to be higher; second, considerable variability may be seen between the readings at each visit. Watson et al found that

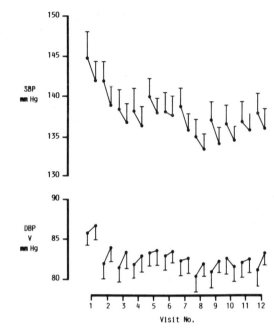

**Figure 2.6.** Mean values (± SEM) of the first and second readings of systolic blood pressure (*SBP*) and diastolic blood pressure (*DBP*; phase V) recorded on 12 visits of 32 patients. (From Watson RDS, Lumb R, Young MA, et al: *J Hypertens* 5:207, 1987.)

the chance of a 5-mm Hg or greater differences being noted between the average stable BP and that recorded at visit 4 was 50% for the systolic and 32% for the diastolic. If the number of visits was increased to eight, the chance of such a clinically relevant difference being noted was 13% for systolic and 2% for diastolic. By Bayesian analysis, the predictive value of the average of two diastolic readings above 90 mm Hg for the presence of "true" DBP above 90 is only 52% (Schechter and Adler, 1988). If the average of eight readings is above 90, the sensitivity or percentage of positive predictive value goes up, but only to 73%.

### Variations Within the Patient: Random and Systemic

Random variations are uncontrollable but can be reduced simply by repeating the measurement as many times as needed. Systematic variations are introduced by something affecting the patient and, if recognized, controllable. If the cause of systematic variation is not recognized, it cannot be reduced by multiple readings. An example of a systematic variation is that related to environmental temperature: A fall in maximal daily temperatures of 12°C was associated with a rise of 5 to 10 mm Hg in mean diastolic daytime BP among 22 mildly hypertensive subjects (Giaconi et al, 1989). This difference would not be reduced by repeating the measurements at any given time but, if recognized, it can be taken into account.

The degree of random variation of the BP is most apparent from continuous intraarterial measurements (Fig. 2.7). Obviously, considerable differences in readings can be seen at different times of the day. Beyond these variations, between-visit variations in BP can be substantial. Among the 32 subjects studied by Watson et al (1987) (Fig. 2.6), after the first three visits the standard deviation of the differ-

ence in BP from one visit to another was 10.4 mm Hg for systolic and 7.0 mm Hg for diastolic BP.

## Types of Variability

As delineated by Conway (1986), BP variability can be usefully looked at in three ways: short-term, daytime, and diurnal. *Short-term* variability at rest is affected by respiration and heart rate under the influence of the autonomic nervous system. *Daytime* variability is mainly determined by the degree of mental and physical activity and is modified by baroreflexes that operate through adjustments in heart rate and peripheral resistance. *Diurnal* variability is substantial, with an average 30% fall in pressure

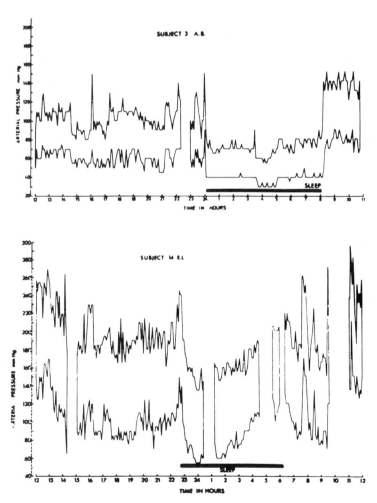

**Figure 2.7.** Systolic and diastolic pressure recorded at 5-minute intervals in a normotensive (*top*) and hypertensive (*bottom*) subject with an intra-arterial device. The high pressures in the normotensive subject at 1600 and 2400 are due to a painful stimulus and coitus, respectively. (Reprinted by permission from Bevan AT, Honour AJ, Stott FH: *Clin Sci* 36:329, copyright 1969, The Biochemical Society, London.)

during sleep, and is partly induced by increased baroreflex sensitivity that decreases sympathetic nervous activity.

The overriding influence of activity on diurnal variations was nicely demonstrated in a study of 461 untreated hypertensive patients whose BP was recorded with a portable noninvasive device over 24 hours, every 15 minutes during the day and every 30 minutes at night (Clark et al, 1987). In addition, five readings were taken in the clinic before and another five after the 24-hour recording. When the mean DBP readings for each hour of the 24 hours was plotted against each patient's mean clinic BP, considerable variations were noted, with lowest pressures in early morning and highest near mid-day (Fig. 2.8, *left*). The patients recorded in a diary the location where their BP was taken, i.e., home, work, or other, and what they were doing at the time, with 16 choices of activity. An analysis of covariance model was then used to correct for the observed effects of the various combinations of location and activity upon the BP. The average effects of the various activities relative to the BP recorded while relaxing are shown in Table 2.2. When the estimated effects of the various combinations of location and activity were then subtracted from the individual readings obtained throughout the 24 hours, very little residual effect of the time of day was found (Fig. 2.8, *right*). The authors conclude "that there is no important circadian rhythm of BP which is independent of activity."

## Sleep and Awakening

It is likely that the usual changes in BP during sleep, a fall during the first portion and then a rise before awakening, largely reflect changes in sympathetic nervous activity. They are not seen either in patients with transplanted denervated hearts (Wenting et al, 1986) or in patients whose hearts are constantly under intense sympathetic stimulation because of congestive heart failure (Caruana et al, 1988). Patients with endogenous or exogenous glucocorticoid excess lose their nocturnal fall in BP, and this too may involve an increase in sympathetic nervous activity (Imai et al, 1989).

The usual fall in BP at night is the result of sleep and inactivity rather than of the time of day: If people stay awake at night, the pressure falls very little; if they sleep during the day, the pressure falls as expected (Sundberg et al, 1988). The fall in nocturnal pressure may cause harm by inducing myocardial ischemia in patients with long-standing hypertension who have hypertrophied ventricles or coronary artery disease and therefore impaired coronary vasodilator reserve (Floras, 1988). This nocturnal fall in perfusion pressure may be particularly ominous when superimposed on inadvertent overtreatment with antihypertensive drugs.

The BP usually begins to rise in the early morning before awakening and before rising out of bed, as seen in the *right portion* of Fig. 2.8. This rise in BP occurs even in patients whose

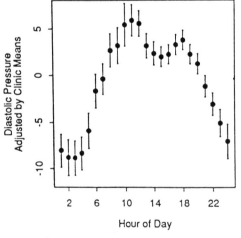
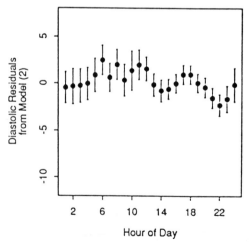

**Figure 2.8.** *Left,* plot of diastolic pressure readings adjusted by individual clinic means. *Right,* plot of the diastolic pressure hourly mean residuals after adjustments for various activities by a time-of-day model. The hourly means (*solid circles*) ± 2 SE (*whiskers*) are plotted versus the corresponding time of day. (Reprinted with permission from Clark LA, Denby L, Pregibon D, et al. A quantitative analysis of the effects of activity and time of day on the diurnal variations of blood pressure, *J Chronic Dis* 40:671, copyright 1987, Pergamon Press PLC.)

**Table 2.2. Average Changes of Blood Pressure Associated with Commonly Occurring Activities Related to Blood Pressure While Relaxing[a]**

|  | Systolic | Diastolic |
|---|---|---|
| Meetings | + 20.2 | + 15.0 |
| Work | + 16.0 | + 13.0 |
| Transportation | + 14.0 | + 9.2 |
| Walking | + 12.0 | + 5.5 |
| Dressing | + 11.5 | + 9.7 |
| Chores | + 10.7 | + 6.7 |
| Telephone | + 9.5 | + 7.2 |
| Eating | + 8.8 | + 9.6 |
| Talking | + 6.7 | + 6.7 |
| Desk work | + 5.9 | + 5.3 |
| Reading | + 1.9 | + 2.2 |
| Business (at home) | + 1.6 | + 3.2 |
| Television | + 0.3 | + 1.1 |
| Relaxing | 0 | 0 |
| Sleeping | − 10.0 | − 7.6 |

[a]Data adapted from Clark et al: *J Chron Dis* 40:671, 1987 by Pickering TG: *Am Heart J* 116:1141, 1988a.
  Changes are shown relative to blood pressure while relaxing.

heart rates are fixed by ventricular demand pacemakers (Davies et al, 1984). This early morning rise in BP may also be harmful. In concert with an increase in platelet aggregation, it may be involved in the higher rate of fatal strokes and heart attacks noted between 6 and 10 a.m. (Muller et al, 1989).

**Stress of the Measurement**

As noted in Figure 2.6, the initial BP measurements tend to be higher than subsequent ones. Clearly, the measurement of the BP may invoke a stress reaction, a reaction that may be only transient in most patients but that may persist in others. The stress reaction may be partially related to the environment but is more related to the measurer.

*The Environment.* Most patients show a progressive and often dramatic fall in BP after admission to a hospital (Nishimura et al, 1987) that may be related both to regression toward the mean and reduction of anxiety (Hossmann et al, 1981). As noted, home readings are usually lower than in the office or clinic and much closer to the average BP recorded by noninvasive ambulatory monitors (White, 1986) (Fig. 2.1).

*The Measurer.* The presence of a doctor usually causes the BP to rise, and the rise may be very impressive (Mancia et al, 1987b) (Fig. 2.9). These data were obtained from patients who underwent a 24-hour intraarterial Oxford recording after 5 to 7 days in the hospital. When the intraarterial readings were stable, BP was taken in the noncatheterized arm by both a male

physician and a female nurse, half of the time by the physician first, the other half by the nurse first. These personnel were previously unknown to the subjects but their visits were forewarned. When the physician took the first of three sets of readings, the pressures uniformly rose, as much as 74 mm Hg systolic, an average of 22/14 mm Hg. Similar rises were seen during three subsequent visits. The rises seen with the nurses' first readings were about half as great as the physicians' and they usually returned to near the baseline reading when taken again after 5 and 10 minutes.

These striking pressure rises invoked by the presence of a doctor reflect an alarm reaction and were dampened but not extinguished after 10 min. They were not related to the patients' ages, sex, overall BP variability, or BP levels and were not closely related to changes in heart rate.

These findings are in keeping with a great deal more data, clearly indicating a marked tendency for most patients' BP to fall in repeated measurements with little effect of the time interval between readings (van Loo et al, 1986). They strongly suggest that nurses and not physicians should take the BP and that at least three sets of readings be taken before labeling the patient as hypertensive and deciding upon the need for treatment.

The acute pressor response to a physician may persist for many years. In a study of 292 patients whose DBP had been repeatedly noted to be between 90 and 104 mm Hg during multiple office visits over an average 6-year duration, 21% had persistently normal readings during a 24-hour ambulatory recording taken under usual life conditions (Pickering et al, 1988). These "white coat" hypertensives had considerably lower office readings taken by the female technicians than by the male physicians, showing that it was not the office setting but the white-coated physician that served as a pressor stimulus. The "white coat" hypertensives were more likely to be younger, nonobese women with shorter duration of hypertension. Thus, the acute pressor response to a physician's measurement of the BP may occur indefinitely, presumably as a conditioned reflex that increases sympathetic nervous arousal each time the pressure is taken.

The same problem occurs in elderly patients with isolated systolic hypertension. Among 81 who had SBP above 160 on three consecutive visits at weekly intervals, the mean awake am-

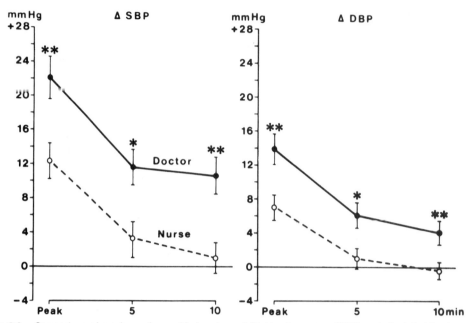

**Figure 2.9.** Comparison of maximum (or peak) rises in systolic blood pressure (SBP) and diastolic blood pressure (DBP) occurring in 30 subjects during a physician's and a nurse's visits. The rises occurring at the 5th and 10th minutes of the visits are shown. Data are expressed as mean (± SEM) changes from a control value taken 4 minutes before each visit. (From Mancia G, Parati G, Pomidossi G, et al: *Hypertension* 9:209, 1987a, by permission of the American Heart Association, Inc.)

bulatory SBPs were normal in 42% (Ruddy et al, 1988).

As I shall indicate, the problems of overdiagnosis and treatment engendered by "office" or "white coat" hypertension can be avoided by more widespread use of home recordings and ambulatory monitoring.

It is important to try and minimize the BP changes that arise because of variations within the patient. Even little things may have an impact: Both SBP and DBP may rise 10 mm Hg with a distended urinary bladder (Fagius and Karhuvaara, 1989) or during relaxed conversation (Silverberg and Rosenfeld, 1980). The pressure rises more when talking to someone perceived to be of higher status (Long et al, 1982), which may be part of the reason that physicians tend to record higher BP than their nurses. Interestingly, the BP rises in deaf people when they use sign language, suggesting that communication, independent of vocalization, effects the cardiovascular system (Malinow et al, 1986).

### Other Factors Affecting Variability

Beyond the level of activity and the stresses related to the measurement, a number of other factors affect BP variability. These include the sensitivity of baroreflexes (Conway, 1986) and

the level of BP, with more variability the higher the pressure (Watson et al, 1980). This latter relationship is probably responsible for the widespread perception that the elderly have more variable BP. When younger and older hypertensives with comparable BP levels were studied, variability was not consistently related to age (Brennan et al, 1986).

On the other hand, elderly patients with less reactive baroreceptors may be more susceptible to falls in BP when assuming the upright posture or after decreases in effective circulating blood volume because of splanchnic pooling after a heavy meal (Lipsitz et al, 1986).

*Smoking.* Acutely, the surge of nicotine causes a rise in both SBP and DBP that may last for 5 to 10 minutes (Benowitz et al, 1984), likely mediated by release of norepinephrine from adrenergic nerves (Cryer et al, 1976).

Chronically, smokers have generally been found to have no more hypertension than nonsmokers. However, smokers have higher death rates from hypertension (Doll and Peto, 1976) and a 5-fold greater incidence of malignant hypertension (Isles et al, 1979). These associations may reflect adverse effects of the carbon monoxide and other toxins in smoke upon the vascular system.

The use of smokeless tobacco is also associated with higher BP (Schroeder and Chen, 1985), perhaps because of its very high sodium content, as much as 3% of snuff or chewing tobacco, in addition to its nicotine content (Hampson, 1985).

When smokers quit, a trivial rise in BP may occur, probably reflecting the gain in weight that frequently accompanies the cessation of smoking (Seltzer, 1974).

*Caffeine.* Acutely, caffeine raises the BP and levels of both renin and catecholamines in people who do not normally ingest caffeine-containing beverages. Within a few days, complete tolerance to all of these effects occurs so that the habitual intake of caffeine-containing beverages is unlikely to affect the BP (Robertson et al, 1981).

*Alcohol.* The acute effects of ethanol upon the BP are variable but chronic alcohol intake beyond 2 ounces per day may lead to considerable and persistent rises in BP. Acutely, when 0.75 g/kg body weight of ethanol was consumed by a group of young normotensives in 15 minutes so that the blood alcohol level rose quickly to almost 100 mg/dl, a definite rise in BP occurred (Potter et al, 1986). As is shown in Chapter 3, chronic heavy alcohol intake may be the most common cause of reversible hypertension.

Beyond the acute effects of nicotine, caffeine, and alcohol, more chronic effects are related to a variety of other factors including stress, obesity, and hyperinsulinemia. These are covered in Chapter 3.

## Variations Involving the Measurer

Some of the errors in measurement related to the measurer are shown in Table 2.3. They are more common than most realize and require regular and frequent retraining of personnel to overcome (Bruce et al, 1988). For example, readings taken by physicians in a clinic differed an av-

**Table 2.3. Sources of Potential Error in Taking Blood Pressure**

1. Improper equipment
   a. Bladder too small for size of arm
   b. Aneroid manometer inaccurate
2. Inaccurate reading
   a. Bladder not centered over brachial artery
   b. Using the wrong values
      1) Missing an auscultatory gap
      2) Confusion over use of muffling (phase IV) for diastolic pressure
   c. Variations due to arrhythmias
   d. Position of arm not at level of heart
   e. Arm or torso held without support
   f. Too slow bladder inflation
   g. Too rapid bladder deflation
3. Observer bias with digit preference

erage of 14/6 mm Hg from those taken by a trained observer, with 14% of the readings having an error in excess of 15 mm Hg diastolic (Scherwitz et al, 1982). Nurses' readings were somewhat more accurate but still incorrectly identified patients' DBP as over or under 90 mm Hg on 25% of occasions.

## Dealing with Variability

In view of the rather marked variability of the BP, changing literally minute to minute, how can we decide what an individual's BP is? From both short-term observations on the degree of variability (Rosner and Polk, 1979) and long-term follow-up of the cardiovascular risks (Kannel et al, 1980), these guidelines seem appropriate:

—Since all blood pressures are variable, there is no justification for the term "labile hypertension." Those whose pressures broach the arbitrary dividing line between "normal" and "high" are best considered "borderline," to be more carefully watched and advised to follow sensible health habits. But they have blood pressures that fall on a continuum between normotensive and persistently hypertensive patients with no more lability than either (Horan et al, 1981).

—At every visit, two BP measurements should be made. The first reading will likely be higher but, before discarding it, remember that most of the available data on eventual risk are based upon such readings. The eventual risk is more closely related to the average than either the highest or lowest readings taken repeatedly over 24-hour periods (Sokolow et al, 1966). In Framingham, the mean, minimum, and maximum of three readings taken during an examination were equally efficient predictors of subsequent cardiovascular disease (Kannel et al, 1980). As expected, the probability of subsequent disease was higher at any given level of BP if that reading was the lowest value obtained at that examination, rather than the highest reading, but the same general relationship held with either the lowest or the highest readings (Kannel, 1977).

—To establish the patient's current BP status, three sets of readings should be taken, preferably weeks apart. If the initial readings are very high, i.e., above 180/120, the best course may be to start evaluation and treatment at that time. But if the patient is under stress, repeated readings should be obtained within a few days before doing anything else.

—If the pressures are coming down, more readings should be obtained. Home BP measurements will avoid the need for frequent office visits. The home readings will likely be at least 5 to 10 mm Hg lower than those taken in the office (Pickering ct al, 1985) and usually show a progressive fall with time as noted with office readings (Fig. 2.6). Ambulatory 24-hour recordings will likely be used more and more, particularly since they are more accurate predictors of future cardiovascular risk (Perloff et al, 1983).

—If multiple home or office readings are used to follow the effects of therapy, it is appropriate to have some taken under the same circumstances and at about the same time of day, in view of the effects of activity, posture, etc. Additional readings may be useful to ascertain the degree and duration of effect from antihypertensive therapy. On the other hand, if multiple readings are being taken to decide whether the patient is hypertensive, they should be taken under various circumstances and at different times.

## HOME AND AMBULATORY MEASUREMENTS

From the preceding, it is clear that pressures recorded in the hospital or office are often affected by both acute and chronic stress reactions and conditioned reflexes that tend to raise the BP, giving rise to significant white coat hypertension. Two techniques that have been long recognized to obviate these problems, home measurements and ambulatory blood pressure monitoring (ABPM), are being more widely advocated and utilized. I believe they will become standard practices in the clinical management of many patients as well as mandated practices in the evaluation of new antihypertensive agents.

## New Drug Evaluation

There are multiple reasons why ABPM should be a major part of the evaluation of new drugs, beyond the greater accuracy it provides as to efficacy (O'Brien et al, 1989). First, drugs may differ in their effect on office versus ambulatory readings. In one study, the response to a beta-blocker and a calcium entry blocker based on office readings was equal but, with ABPM, only the beta-blocker was effective (Waeber et al, 1988). Second, there is a need to ensure the duration of action of whatever regimen is being tested. Clearly, the level of drug in the blood does not necessarily predict the extent or duration of the antihypertensive effect of the drug. The only way to know how long and how much a drug works is to measure its effect in living ambulating patients, going through their usual activities. Third, ABPM is the only way to ascertain the efficacy of the drug during the early morning hours when the pressure spontaneously begins to rise and, likely, is at least partly responsible for the increase in strokes and heart attacks in the 6 to 10 a.m. period (Sirgo et al, 1988).

For all of these reasons, ABPM will certainly be more widely utilized in the evaluation of new drugs (White and Morganroth, 1989). Actually, the data obtained by self-recorded home BP measurements will provide much the same, more accurate data as does ABPM and at far less cost (Gould et al, 1986; Ménard et al, 1988). The self-recorded measurements, of course, cannot assess what goes on during sleep and before awakening, which represents an advantage for the ambulatory technique. Use of either of the out-of-the office measurements is superior to the traditional use of occasional clinic readings.

## Home Measurements in Clinical Practice

Far beyond their value in the evaluation of new drugs, home BP measurements can provide information of great value for the clinical management of many patients (Table 2.4). Except for the additional information provided by measurements taken during sleep and the inability

---

**Table 2.4. Indications for Home Blood Pressure Monitoring**

1. For diagnosis:
   a. Recognize initial, short-term elevations in blood pressure
   b. Identify persistent "white-coat" hypertension
   c. Determine usual blood pressure levels in borderline hypertension

2. For prognosis: Inadequate data except for relation to LVH

3. For therapy:
   a. Monitor response to therapy
      1) Ensure adequate blood pressure control during awake hours
      2) Evaluate effects of increasing or decreasing amounts of therapy
      3) Ascertain whether poor office blood pressure response to increasing treatment represents overtreatment or true resistance
      4) Identify periods of poor control when office readings are normal but target organ damage progresses
      5) Identify relations of blood pressure levels to presumed side effects of therapy
   b. Involve patient to improve adherence

of a few patients to measure their own BP, self-recorded home measurements will give almost all of the information provided by 24-hour ABPM. The average BP levels obtained by multiple home and *awake* ambulatory measurements are quite close, whereas the self-recorded levels will almost always be higher than the full 24-hour ambulatory average since that will include the pressures taken during sleep, which are almost always lower. Both the home and ambulatory readings are usually considerably lower than those obtained in the office (James et al, 1988) (Table 2.5). Note, as well, the closeness of the average levels in the two sets of repeated home and ambulatory readings taken 2 weeks apart, in keeping with the excellent reproducibility of the procedures noted in many studies.

The multiple uses for self-recorded measurements will be reviewed, followed by some information about the currently available equipment and guidelines for its use.

## Diagnosis

As perhaps first clearly recognized by Ayman and Goldshine in 1940, home recordings are generally lower than office readings and much closer to the levels noted by "basal" and ABPM. Home recordings obviously overcome much of the error caused by the acute and persistent pressor-stress response that is responsible for most white coat hypertension. They are particularly useful in providing a more representative long-term assessment of the large population of patients with minimally elevated pressures on initial screening. With proper motivation and instruction, most patients are willing and able

**Table 2.5. Average Pressures in Hypertensive Subjects as Determined by Three Methods of Measurement Compared Over the 2 Weeks[a]**

| Measurement | Ambulatory (Awake and Asleep) | Home | Clinic |
|---|---|---|---|
| Systolic BP (mm Hg) | | | |
| Initial | 134 ± 11 | 140 ± 14 | 158 ± 23* |
| Second | 132 ± 12 | 143 ± 13 | 152 ± 20 |
| Diastolic BP (mm Hg) | | | |
| Initial | 85 ± 10 | 86 ± 12 | 93 ± 11 |
| Second | 86 ± 10 | 87 ± 12 | 91 ± 10 |

[a]From James GD, Pickering TG, Yee LS, et al. The reproducibility of average ambulatory, home, and clinic pressures. Hypertension 11:545, 1988, by permission of the American Heart Association, Inc.
Values are average ± SD. BP = blood pressure. *p < 0.05, significantly different from second reading.

to effectively utilize home recordings (Gould et al, 1982).

## Prognosis

There are few data documenting the validity of self-recorded home measurements for ascertainment of the long-term prognosis of any level of BP (Abe et al, 1987). Presumably they will prove equal to ABPM, which, as will be seen, appears to provide an excellent guide to prognosis.

## Therapy

Home recording will be increasingly used to monitor the short- and long-term response to therapy (Table 2.4). Rather than depending on occasional office visits, with their propensity to make the level of hypertension appear to be worse than it is during usual life circumstances, patients should be encouraged to monitor their course with a home device. Perhaps the greatest benefit will be in the avoidance of inadvertent overtreatment.

A striking example of the potential of overtreatment by use of only office readings was reported by Waeber et al (1987). Although they compared office readings with ABPM, it is likely that the values reported by the ABPM would be close to that of home recordings since they used only the daytime values. In this study, 17 of 34 hypertensives with office diastolic readings above 95 mm Hg despite antihypertensive therapy were noted to have average daytime ambulatory readings below 90 mm Hg. They were given additional treatment on the basis of their office readings and, as a result, some ended up with considerably lower BPs than desired (Fig. 2.10).

Patients whose BPs are lowered too much by overtreatment based on only office readings may suffer nocturnal myocardial ischemia when the usual further fall in BP during sleep is superimposed (Floras, 1988). The results of multiple trials showing an increase in coronary mortality when office DBPs are reduced below 85 to 90 mm Hg (Cruickshank, 1988) point to the need to ensure that patients are not receiving too much therapy based on spuriously elevated office recordings.

The other benefits provided by home recordings in regard to the monitoring of therapy that are listed in Table 2.4 further validate the need for much more widespread use of the technique. In particular, by involving the patient more actively and providing instant reinforcement of the

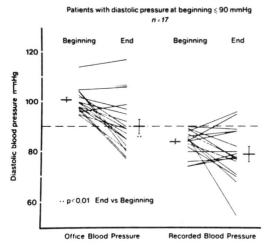

Patients with diastolic pressure at beginning ≤ 90 mmHg
n - 17

**Figure 2.10.** Office and ambulatory (*recorded*) diastolic BP at beginning and end of study in 17 patients with ambulatory diastolic blood pressure of 90 mm Hg or lower at beginning despite office readings above 95 mm Hg. (From Waeber B, Scherrer U, Petrillo A, et al: *Lancet* 2:732, 1987.)

value of therapy, home readings may improve compliance (Stahl et al, 1984).

### Equipment

Three types of devices are available for self-recorded or home measurement in addition to stationary automated machines found at various public places. All three are attached to a cuff having a D-ring or a leaf-spring that allows one-handed self-placement on the arm. Mercury sphygmomanometers with a stethoscope will provide accurate home readings but are usually too cumbersome. Mechanical aneroid instruments, also used with a stethoscope, are easier to handle and use but may become inaccurate and need to be calibrated regularly by comparing the air gauge with a mercury manometer by means of Y tube (Hahn et al, 1987). Battery-operated electronic devices with a built-in microphone or oscillometric sensor to pick up the Korotkoff sounds and a digital display (some providing a printout) to record the readings are becoming increasingly popular. The devices with a microphone appear to provide more accurate systolic readings, those with an oscillometric sensor more accurate diastolic readings (Imai et al, 1988).

The digital devices vary from less expensive models ($50 to $80) that require manual inflation and deflation to more expensive ones ($75 to $200) that inflate and deflate the cuff automatically. A thorough testing of 23 home BP devices found that 11 were not acceptable (Evans et al, 1989). The three models that were least expensive, most accurate, and easy to use were: Radio Shack Model 63-661 ($49.95); Sunbeam Model 7620 ($50); and Lumiscope Model 100-048 ($65). My preference is the Radio Shack model, a battery-operated electronic device that must be manually inflated but automatically deflates and uses an oscillometric sensor so that careful placement of the cuff is not critical. A device such as this, costing around $50, will provide accurate home readings for most patients.

Caution is needed with devices that purport to measure the BP without use of a balloon cuff, i.e., Healthcheck Cuffless Model CX-1-060020. This device, which measures the pressure in one finger, is being widely marketed but was found to be totally inaccurate (Watkins-Pitchford and Szocik, 1989).

### Technique

All of the details concerning posture, circumstances surrounding the measurement, etc. that are needed for office readings (Table 2.1) need to be followed with home readings. The accuracy of the device and the patient (or whoever takes the home readings) should be checked by a simultaneous measurement on the other arm in the office with a mercury manometer. These points should be made to the patient:

1. Do not be concerned by fluctuations of 5, 10, or even 20 mm Hg, but do inform the physician's office if the pressures are going up progressively over a period of a week or longer. If the home readings are being taken to determine whether borderline levels are persistent, the checks should be made at variable times when the patient is either relaxed or stressed, anytime throughout the day or evening (Gould et al, 1983). It may be particularly instructive and helpful to visualize the effects of anger and anxiety.
2. If the readings are being taken to determine the adequacy of antihypertensive therapy, take the readings at the same times of day. Readings should occasionally be taken during the interval of a dose of therapy to ascertain both the peak effect and the duration of effect.
3. Encourage the patient to take the BP of family and friends, advising those with readings above 140/90 to seek medical attention.
4. Recheck the accuracy of the equipment every 6 to 12 months.

Self-measurement of BP is being more widely advocated for use in more patients (Canadian Coalition for High Blood Pressure Prevention and Control, 1988; World Hypertension League, 1988). If home readings are used to manage patients, new guidelines as to what level of pressure is the goal of therapy will need to be established. Home readings will usually be about 10 mm Hg lower systolic and 5 mm Hg lower diastolic than office readings, and the differences usually persist over time (Jyothinagaram et al, 1988). Therefore 130/85 may need to be the goal, rather than 140/90. More about this issue will be addressed in Chapter 6.

### Stationary Automated Recording

Stationary machines for automated measurements of the pressure are widely located in public places, either coin-operated or free of charge. They remove only the errors related to the observer's recording of the BP, while substituting "the technical faults to which all complex equipment is subject and the need for maintenance" (O'Brien et al, 1985). Without going into details, the overall impression is that virtually all devices presently available may be inaccurate (Barker et al, 1984). Most underestimate the systolic and overestimate the diastolic pressure (Hunyor et al, 1978).

### Ambulatory Blood Pressure Monitoring (ABPM)

As noted earlier, 24-hour ABPM is being more widely advocated for various reasons (Table 2.6). The use of this technique, first utilized in England with direct intraarterial recording (Bevan et al, 1969), has become clinically feasible with the general availability of noninvasive monitoring equipment using a cuff. Except for a large-scale study by Sokolow and coworkers with a

**Table 2.6. Indications for Ambulatory Blood Pressure Monitoring**

1. For diagnosis: same as for home blood pressure measurements plus
   a. Patients unable to obtain self (home)-measurements
   b. Need for immediate ascertainment
   c. Measure sleep blood pressure levels
2. For prognosis:
   a. Provide better correlation with target organ damage
   b. Identify role of sleep blood pressure
3. For therapy:
   a. Same as for home measurements plus identification of effects during sleep
   b. Establish duration and degree of effect of new agents

semiautomatic device that had to be inflated by the patient, the Remler M2000, little additional work was done until the early 1980s. Since that time the field has expanded markedly, as detailed in the proceedings of a symposium published as a supplement to the October, 1988 American Heart Journal (Weber, 1988a).

Most of what has subsequently been reported was well described much earlier by Sokolow and his coworkers. They showed the value of ABPM in establishing the diagnosis (Perloff and Sokolow, 1978), the prognosis (Sokolow et al, 1966; Perloff et al, 1983), and the need for therapy (Sokolow et al, 1973). Since they used a device that had to be activated by the patient, they could not study what went on during sleep. That information has assumed an important role.

The overall place of ABPM was succinctly described in an editorial by O'Brien and O'Malley (1988):

> The development of non-invasive techniques for measuring ambulatory blood pressure has made it possible to study blood pressure as it changes, which offers advantages over the conventional practice of measuring it sporadically, often under artificial and stressful circumstances, by a technique replete with potential inaccuracies. It soon became evident that ambulatory measurement gave lower readings than blood pressure measured by family practitioners, hospital staff, and patients themselves. Moreover, the technique may predict cardiovascular morbidity and mortality more accurately than the casual measurement of blood pressure.

Perhaps the most important use of ABPM is to ensure the diagnosis. As noted by Pickering et al (1988):

> Faced with a patient with borderline hypertension, the doctor should be slow to diagnose hypertension until some attempt has been made to categorize the behaviour of blood pressure over time; ambulatory blood pressure measurement is the best way to do this.

### Equipment

The noninvasive 24-hour ABPM systems now available use a standard arm cuff that is inflated at predetermined intervals, usually every 15 to 30 minutes during the day and every hour during the night, by a small pump that is carried on a shoulder strap or attached to the belt. The BP is ascertained either by auscultation through a small microphone placed under the cuff over the brachial artery or by oscillometry that recognizes small changes in air pressure within the inflated cuff, records the systolic and mean BPs, and calculates the diastolic pressure. Some of the units using auscultation remove artifact sounds by accepting only those sounds that are accompanied by an R-wave recorded from a simultaneous electrocardiogram.

The individual BPs measured throughout the 24 hours are stored in the unit worn by the patient and read out by interfacing with a computer that prints out the entire set of readings (Fig. 2.11) along with an analysis of the readings over various periods of time and the mean ± standard deviations.

### Interpretation

The patient is usually asked to keep a diary of activities throughout the 24 hours in view of the often marked associated changes in BP (see Table 2.2). A computer-assisted diary has been described, wherein the patient marks boxes on a computer-readable card to indicate the time, location, body position, activity, and mood associated with each reading (Van Egeren and Madarasmi, 1988).

As noted by Weber (1988b), there are problems inherent in the multiple recordings throughout ambulatory activity. Although it has been shown that the automatic recordings do not induce an alarm reaction that raises the BP (Parati et al, 1985), the simple wearing of the device makes the 24 hours different from the usual day. Moreover, as Weber (1988b) states,

. . . the complexity of interpreting whole-day blood pressure monitoring data reflects our attempt to measure two separate parameters at one time: the intrinsic characteristics of the patient's blood pressure and the responsiveness of the blood pressure to environmental and emotional stimuli. It is probably invalid to interpret responses to stimuli in an individual without first obtaining a meaningful baseline reflective of the innate blood pressure pattern and variability. . . . Unfortunately, issues of practicality and cost make it unlikely that whole-day blood pressure monitoring in controlled environments will easily become a reality. Nevertheless, the establishment of a standardized and partly restricted program of activity probably would add to the reproducibility of the technique and make its findings more interpretable.

In an attempt to overcome some of the methodological problems of dealing with literally hundreds of readings, some advocate the use of shorter periods of ABPM (Drayer et al, 1985). However, others find that the average reading over a few hours may not provide a precise estimate of the day-time or entire 24-hour average (Di Rienzo et al, 1985).

Most would use the average value of all readings obtained throughout the 24 hours, recognizing that night-time readings are normally considerably lower and therefore the full 24-hour average will be lower than the day-time. Since virtually all "normotensive" people have occasional high readings and virtually all "fixed hypertensive" patients have some normal readings (Horan et al, 1981), some advocate using the "load," i.e., the percentage of ambulatory pressures higher than 140 systolic or 90 diastolic, as

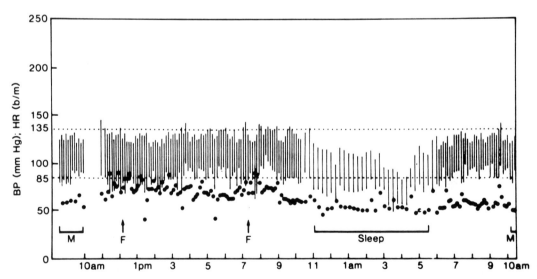

**Figure 2.11.** Ambulatory blood pressure monitoring for 24 hours beginning at 10 a.m. in a normal 40-year-old man with no evidence of hypertension or other cardiovascular disease. •, heart rate; *F*, time of food intake; *M*, simultaneous machine and mercury readings of supine, sitting, and standing blood pressure. (From Zachariah PK, Sheps SG, Smith RL. *Diagnosis* 10:39, 1988a.)

a way to diagnose hypertension (Zachariah et al, 1988b), to decide upon the need for therapy (White et al, 1989), or to ascertain the response to therapy (White and Morganroth, 1989).

## Validity

ABPM is remarkably reproducible (Weber, 1988b) and closely comparable to either intraarterial or sphygmomanometer measurements (Graettinger et al, 1988). The noninvasive ambulatory devices tend to underestimate systolic and overestimate DBP, but the correlations between the intraarterial, routine, and ambulatory readings are highly significant. Since only the noninvasive technique is generally available, "it is the technique likely to prevail in the foreseeable future." Since it provides useful information for the diagnosis, prognosis, and treatment of hypertension, the use of ABPM will almost certainly grow. This is particularly likely in view of the availability of smaller, less expensive models that can literally be worn in a shirt pocket and provide instant data at a relatively small cost. Four such models—Avionics PIV, Novacor Diasys 200, Spacelabs 90202, and Takeda TM2420—were found to provide excellent precision and reliability (De Gaudemaris et al, 1989).

## Diagnostic Use

In view of the marked variability of BP, the question as to what level or pattern should be used to diagnose "hypertension" has been asked but not answered. The data from Framingham and other prospective studies have shown clear relationships between various levels of "casual" BP and cardiovascular events, so that the limits of normality for casual readings have been reasonably well established. However, no such body of data yet exists for ambulatory pressures and its complexity foretells major trouble in trying to establish such relationships.

Nonetheless, a steadily expanding number of readings in normal subjects has provided some approximate criteria (Table 2.7). But, as Weber (1988a) points out:

> The strength of this technique is to establish that BP is truly at a given level within the individual patient. Once this is established, the excellent prognostic data established by previous studies with casual BPs can be used for clinical decision making. . . . Those who advocate the prognostic strength of casual BP should not forget that its strength derives from pooled data accumulated from huge sample sizes (whereas) . . . casual BP in the clinical setting may not be an entirely reliable basis for the important diagnostic and therapeutic decisions that must be made in the individual patient.

The ability of ABPM to identify the 20% of white coat hypertensives is a case in point.

## Prognostic Use

Ambulatory pressures appear to predict the risk for target organ damage and cardiovascular events better than do casual or office readings. As for target organ damage, most of the data are cross-sectional, i.e., they show that the extent of left ventricular hypertrophy by echocardiography is more closely correlated to 24-hour ambulatory pressure than casual pressure in multiple studies (Devereux and Pickering, 1988; White et al, 1989). This closer correlation with ambulatory pressure has also been shown for other indices of target organ damage including changes in the optic fundi and renal function (Floras et al, 1981; Parati et al, 1987).

Even more supportive of the prognostic value of ABPM are the data of Perloff et al (1983). They examined 1076 patients both with multiple office BPs on three visits and with ambulatory readings taken every 30 minutes while the patients were awake over a 1- to 2-day period. The average of the office readings for all patients was 161/101, whereas the ambulatory readings averaged 146/92. In 78% of the patients, the ambulatory readings were lower. The patients were followed for up to 16 years, with the mean duration being 5 years. Life table analyses of their massive set of data showed a significantly greater cumulative 10-year incidence of both fatal and nonfatal cardiovascular events among those patients with higher ambulatory BP than among those with lower ambulatory BP as compared with their office BP readings (Fig. 2.12).

Further prospective data, albeit of a smaller and shorter extent, has been provided by Mann et al (1985) who followed 137 patients for a mean of 2 years and noted that ABPM readings provided better prognostic evidence than did clinic values.

*Nocturnal Blood Pressure.* Nocturnal BPs recorded during sleep are almost always considerably lower than those recorded during the awake period. Higher nocturnal BPs may be a particularly ominous prognostic sign. In a group of 21 elderly hypertensive patients, the presence of both left ventricular hypertrophy (LVH) and atherosclerotic cardiovascular disease was considerably more common in those who did not have the usual decline in nocturnal BP (Korbin et al, 1984) (Table 2.8).

Others have also observed that high nocturnal BP is associated with greater degrees of LVH

**Table 2.7. Ambulatory Blood Pressure Upper Ranges in Normal Subjects**

| Author | Criterion[a] | Group | Blood Pressure (mm Hg) | | |
|---|---|---|---|---|---|
| | | | 24-hr | Day | Night |
| Kennedy et al (1983) | +2 SD | Men (<30 yr) | 133/72 | 129/81 | 131/67 |
| | | Men (>30 yr) | 138/88 | 140/92 | 130/84 |
| Wallace ot al (1984) | +2 SD | Men (<30 yr) | 130/82 | 137/89 | 124/76 |
| | | Men (>30 yr) | 134/88 | 141/95 | 123/78 |
| | | Women (<30 yr) | 123/85 | 129/90 | 117/79 |
| | | Women (>30 yr) | 116/83 | 123/85 | 109/75 |
| Drayer et al (1985) | +2 SD | Men | 144/90 | 152/94 | 131/85 |
| Pickering et al (1985) | 90%ile | 70% Men | 132/90 | 140/94 (work) | 112/80 |
| | | | | 125/90 (home) | |
| DeGaudemaris et al (1989) | 90%ile | Men (20–29) | | 145/91 | |
| | daytime | Men (30–39) | | 138/92 | |
| | only | Men (40–49) | | 141/98 | |
| | | Women (20–29) | | 131/87 | |
| | | Women (30–39) | | 132/87 | |
| | | Women (40–49) | | 140/96 | |

[a]a+2 SD = standard deviations above the mean; 90%ile means that 90% of normal subjects had values below this level of blood pressure.

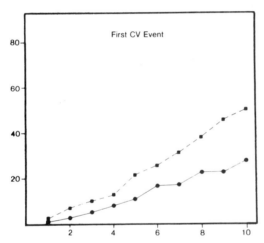

**Figure 2.12.** Estimated cumulative incidence of cardiovascular morbidity and mortality over 10 years among patients classified according to the difference between their observed ambulatory systolic blood pressure and that obtained from their office blood pressures. The *dashed line (above)* represents those whose ambulatory SBP was less than 10 mm Hg lower than the office reading, the *solid line (below)* those with ambulatory SBP more than than 10 mm Hg lower than the office reading, derived from regression of ambulatory BP on office BP. *CV,* cardiovascular. (From Perloff D, Sokolow M, Cowan R: *JAMA* 249:2792–2798, 1983, copyright 1983, American Medical Association.)

**Table 2.8. Nocturnal Blood Pressure and Hypertensive Complications[a]**

| Group | LVH (%) | CVD (%) |
|---|---|---|
| Normal decline in night-time BP | 21 | 43 |
| Lack of nocturnal decline in BP | 56 | 100 |

[a]Diurnal variations of blood pressure in elderly patients with essential hypertension, by Korbin I, Oigman W, Kuman W, et al. *J Am Geriatr Soc* 1984;32:896–9. Reprinted with permission from the American Geriatrics Society.

greater cardiovascular morbidity suffered by black hypertensives.

**Therapeutic Response**

Earlier in this section, the usefulness of ABPM in establishing the extent and duration of antihypertensive drug action was emphasized. With its use, some drugs thought to have a duration of action long enough to allow for once-a-day dosing may turn out not to (Floras et al, 1982), whereas other drugs that are thought to be relatively shorter acting such as captopril (Mancia et al, 1987b) and prazosin (Weber et al, 1987) may be capable of sustained once-a-day effectiveness.

In addition to improving the accuracy of efficacy trials and eliminating the placebo response (Dupont et al, 1987), ABPM can be particularly helpful in assessing individual patients' apparent resistance to increasing therapy (Garrett et al, 1987). As noted (see Fig. 2.10), some patients who appear to be resistant in the office are found to be responsive at home. Pickering (1988b) has proposed a rational approach

in treated (Gosse et al, 1988) and untreated (Lang et al, 1988) hypertensive patients. Moreover, among a group of white and black subjects whose daytime BP readings were similar, the blacks had less BP decline at night (Murphy et al, 1988). The authors suggest that these higher nocturnal BPs could be related to the well-recognized to the evaluation of apparent resistant hypertension. It involves first home BP measurements and, if they are considerably lower, then 24-hour ABPM (Fig. 2.13).

## Summation

All in all, ABPM is likely to be more and more widely used, with applicability to both children (Egger et al, 1987) and the elderly (Torriani et al, 1988). However, it should not be used promiscuously, both because of its cost and because of the unresolved issues about its proper interpretation. When used appropriately it may be very cost effective, as in the evaluation of patients with minimally elevated casual pressures, many of whom will thereby be recognized as nonhypertensive and saved the multiple and considerable costs of having the diagnosis falsely made (Krakoff et al, 1988).

## EVALUATION OF THE NEW HYPERTENSIVE

Now that various factors affecting the BP have been delineated and the guidelines for its ac-

EVALUATION OF "RESISTANT" HYPERTENSION
BY AMBULATORY AND HOME BP MONITORING

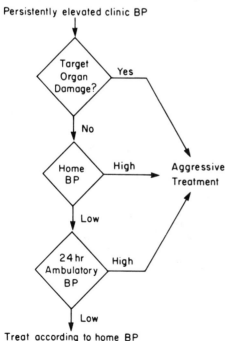

**Figure 2.13.** Proposed schema of blood pressure measurement for patients with apparently resistant hypertension. (From Pickering TG: *Hypertension* 11 (Suppl II):II-96, 1988b, by permission of the American Heart Association, Inc.)

curate measurement described, let us turn to the patient found to have a persistently elevated BP. The first decision to be considered is the extent of the diagnostic workup.

There are three main reasons to evaluate patients with hypertension: (1) to determine the type of hypertension, specifically looking for secondary causes; (2) to assess the impact of the hypertension upon target organs; and (3) to estimate the patient's overall risk profile for the development of premature cardiovascular disease. This can be done with relative ease and should be part of the initial evaluation of every newly discovered hypertensive (Gifford et al, 1989). The younger the patient and the higher the BP, the more aggressive should be the search for secondary causes. Among the middle-aged and older, greater attention will be directed to the overall cardiovascular risk profile, since they are more susceptible to immediate catastrophes unless preventive measures are taken.

### History and the Physical Examination

The history should focus on the duration of the BP and its treatment, the use of various drugs that may raise the blood pressure, and symptoms of target organ dysfunction (Table 2.9). The physical examination should include a careful search for damage to target organs and for features of various secondary causes (Table 2.10). In view of the high prevalence of sleep apnea among even minimally overweight hypertensives, as described further in Chapter 15, both historical and physical features of the syndrome—difficult sleep with loud snoring, morning headaches, and daytime somnolence—should be sought.

Though not usually considered part of the initial workup, attention should be directed toward the patient's psychosocial status, looking for such information as the degree of knowledge about and awareness of hypertension, the willingness to take medication and to make necessary changes in life style, and the family and job situation. An obvious area of great importance, but often neglected until it arises after antihypertensive therapy is given, is sexual function. Impotence, often attributed to antihypertensive drugs, may be present in as many as one-third of untreated hypertensives and likely is related to their underlying vascular disease, not their treatment (Bansal, 1988).

On the basis of only the history and physical examination, most of the secondary diseases can be excluded and the nature of the patient's hy-

**Table 2.9. Important Aspects of the History**

1. Duration of the hypertension
   a. Last known normal blood pressure
   b. Course of the blood pressure
2. Prior treatment of the hypertension
   a. Drugs: types and doses
   b. Side effects
3. Intake of agents that may cause hypertension
   a. Estrogens
   b. Sympathomimetics
   c. Adrenal steroids
   d. Excessive sodium intake
4. Family history
   a. Hypertension
   b. Premature cardiovascular disease or death
   c. Familial diseases: pheochromocytoma, renal disease, diabetes, gout
5. Symptoms of secondary causes
   a. Muscle weakness
   b. Spells of tachycardia, sweating, tremor
   c. Thinning of the skin
   d. Flank pain
6. Symptoms of target organ damage
   a. Headaches
   b. Transient weakness or blindness
   c. Loss of visual acuity
   d. Chest pain
   e. Dyspnea
   f. Claudication
7. Sexual function
8. Features of sleep apnea
   a. Early morning headaches
   b. Daytime somnolence
   c. Loud snoring
   d. Erratic sleep

**Table 2.10. Important Aspects of the Physical Examination**

1. Accurate measurement of blood pressure
2. General appearance: distribution of body fat, skin lesions, muscle strength, alertness
3. Funduscopic
4. Neck: palpation and ausculation of carotids, thyroid
5. Heart: size, rhythm
6. Lungs: rhonchi, rales
7. Abdomen: renal masses, bruits over aorta or renal arteries, femoral pulses
8. Extremities: peripheral pulses, edema

pertension and overall cardiovascular status largely determined. Too often, particularly in the United States, the history and physical examination are given too little attention, with an immediate rush to obtain laboratory data (Epstein et al, 1984).

## Search for Secondary Causes

The frequencies of secondary hypertension shown in Table 1.11 in Chapter 1 are likely much too high for the larger population with mild, asymptomatic hypertension. Among 5485 participants in the Hypertension Detection and Follow-up Program, only about 1% had laboratory or historical evidence for curable hypertension (Lewin et al, 1985). Even though only a few can be cured, every patient should receive

a certain basic workup for these forms when feasible. This assumption is based on these points: First, competent physicians want to apply the most current diagnostic procedures with a reasonably high potential for yielding useful information and low potential for harming the patient, i.e., there is fulfillment in the search, for despite significant advances in drug therapy of hypertension, a lifetime of taking pills is an unattractive prospect; drugs cost money and produce side effects, and many patents will not keep taking them. Second, both physicians and patients are attracted to the drama of a cure. Certainly the immediate correction of a renal arterial lesion is a more attractive prospect than a lifetime of pills. Third, the search for curable or secondary forms of hypertension may also involve uncovering information of value in establishing prognosis and the need for therapy. The minimal workup needed to rule out the secondary causes of hypertension will also help to determine the degree of target organ damage.

I wrote the following in 1969, and it still seems valid:

. . . the workup of patients with only moderately elevated blood pressure which appears after age 35 and does not rapidly progress to cause organ involvement can probably be limited to the following: history, physical exam, urine analysis, blood urea nitrogen or serum creatinine, serum electrolytes, and an intravenous pyelogram (IVP). [I would now omit the IVP and add the ECG.] In patients with more severe hypertension or other significant clinical features, a more thorough evaluation is indicated. However, the workup should be based upon the assumption that it is unrewarding to look for diagnoses for which therapy is not indicated. (Kaplan, 1969)

A great deal more concerning the workup of these various secondary diseases is included in their respective chapters. Table 2.11 is an overall guide to the workup of hypertensive patients. The special diagnostic procedures need be done only if there is evidence from the history, physical examination, or initial urinalysis and blood chemistries that a secondary disease may be present. If so, the studies listed as "initial" will usually serve as adequate screening procedures. They are readily available to every practitioner. If they are abnormal, the "additional" procedures should be obtained along with whatever else is needed to confirm the diagnosis.

### Need for Limitation

In our teaching hospitals, the performance of all of these procedures and more on virtually every hypertensive patient is sometimes taught

**Table 2.11.  Overall Guide to Workup of Hypertension**

| Diagnosis | Diagnostic Procedure | |
|---|---|---|
| | Initial | Additional |
| Chronic renal disease | Urinalysis, serum creatinine, sonography | Isotopic renogram, renal biopsy |
| Renovascular disease | Bruit, plasma renin before and 1 hr after captopril | Aortogram, isotopic renogram 1 hr after captopril |
| Coarctation | Blood pressure in legs | Aortogram |
| Primary aldosteronism | Plasma potassium, plasma renin and aldosterone (ratio) | Urinary potassium, plasma or urinary aldosterone after saline load |
| Cushing's syndrome | AM plasma cortisol after 1 mg dexamethasone at bedtime | Urinary cortisol after variable doses of dexamethasone |
| Pheochromocytoma | Spot urine for metanephrine | Urinary catechols; plasma catechols, basal and after 0.3 mg clonidine |

and practiced. In ambulatory settings, practitioners in the United States perform 4 to 40 times more laboratory tests on uncomplicated chronic hypertensives than practitioners in England (Epstein et al, 1984). Those who practice in larger groups—a trend that is rapidly expanding in the United States—do twice as many laboratory tests as those who are in solo practice (Epstein et al, 1983).

A great deal has been written about the need to limit the use of laboratory procedures, mainly to control costs (Evans, 1983). As we will see when intravenous pyelography is considered, there is another aspect involved in the costs of laboratory procedures that is perhaps even more expensive than the actual performance of various screening tests: When numerous tests are done, particularly in search of rare disease, more and more false-positives will be reported, thereby generating more and more unnecessary tests.

Attempts at rationalizing the indications and interpretation of various test procedures are being made by applying quantitative analyses largely based on Bayes' theorem (Sackett et al, 1985; Sox, 1986). The concept involves not only the sensitivity and specificity of the test but also takes the prevalence of the disease into account in order to provide more valid and meaningful data as to what a positive or negative test means. When applied to the use of intravenous pyelography, the results are revealing (Table 2.12): Assuming a 2% prevalence of renovascular hypertension in the hypertensive population, a positive IVP has a predictive value of only 10.4%, i.e., only 10.4% of hypertensives with an IVP suggestive of renovascular hypertension will have the disease. If the prevalence is 4%, as it might be in young hypertensives, a positive IVP has a 19.1% value. If the prevalence is 10%, as it might be in a very selected population such as

**Table 2.12.  Predictive Value of the IVP for Renovascular Hypertension**

| Prevalence of Renovascular Hypertension | Predictive Value of IVP | |
|---|---|---|
| | Positive Test | Negative Test |
| 2% | 0.104 | 0.996 |
| 4% | 0.191 | 0.992 |
| 10% | 0.386 | 0.980 |
| Sensitivity = 0.85 | | |
| Specificity = 0.85 | | |

young women with an abdominal bruit, the predictive value rises to 38.6%. With any of these prevalence figures, a negative IVP is 98 to 99.6% predictive that renovascular hypertension is not present. A nomogram for Bayes' formula (Fig. 2.14) can be used to determine these predictive values if the sensitivity (i.e., false-negatives), specificity (i.e., false-positives), and prevalence of the disease are known (Møller-Petersen, 1985).

The application of decision analysis adds an interesting dimension to the broad use of screening tests, a dimension rarely considered by clinicians. The main lesson is that with diseases having low prevalence rates, such as all of the secondary forms of hypertension, a positive screening test is neither proof nor even strong evidence for the existence of the disease. There needs to be a greater awareness of this approach toward the sensible interpretation of all clinical data. Publications of an extensive review of the rationale and clinical use of the predictive value of test procedures (Griner et al, 1981) along with continued emphasis on its practical use (Wolf et al, 1985; Sox, 1986; Balla et al, 1989) should help increase this awareness.

For the IVP and renovascular disease, the guidelines seem fairly clear: As will be shown in Chapter 10, the IVP has probably outlived its usefulness. For almost all patients being

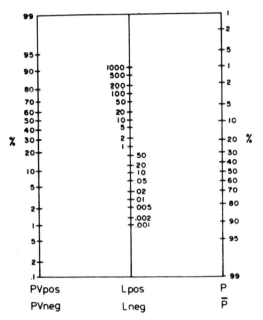

PVpos             Lpos           P

PVneg            Lneg           P̄

**Figure 2.14.** Nomogram to calculate predictive values, both positive (*PVpos*) and negative (*PVneg*), knowing the prevalence of disease (*P*) and values of sensitivity (*Lpos*) and specificity (*Lneg*). For a positive predictive value, a line is drawn from P on the right through Lpos to give PVpos on the left. For a negative predictive value, P̄, Lneg, and PVneg are used. (From Møller-Petersen J: Lancet 1:348, 1985; adapted by permission from Fagan TJ: *N Engl J Med* 293:257, 1975.)

screened for various secondary causes of hypertension, all one needs to do is obtain a brief history and perform a selective physical examination, urine analysis, blood chemistries, and ECG. Additional studies should be limited to those patients who have features considered "inappropriate" for primary or idiopathic hypertension (Table 2.13).

### Ambulatory Monitoring and Echocardiography

Two more complicated and expensive procedures—ABPM and echocardiography—likely will be performed more frequently as part of the workup of some hypertensives. Neither should be "routine" but, as noted earlier in this chapter, ABPM, if performed under appropriate circumstances, may provide very useful information not available by any other technique and may save money by avoiding unnecessary therapy. As will be noted later in this chapter, echocardiography may also be more widely utilized, but a great deal more information about its meaning is needed before it can be recommended as a routine procedure.

**Table 2.13. Features of "Inappropriate" Hypertension**

1. Age of onset: before 20, after 50
2. Level of blood pressure > 180/110 mm Hg
3. Organ damage
   a. Funduscopy grade II or beyond
   b. Serum creatinine > 1.5 mg%
   c. Cardiomegaly or LVH by ECG
4. Presence of features indicative of secondary causes
   a. Unprovoked hypokalemia
   b. Abdominal bruit
   c. Variable pressures with tachycardia, sweating, tremor
   d. Family history of renal disease
5. Poor response to effective therapy

## Determining the Consequences of the Hypertension

Once having established the diagnosis, it is necessary to determine the impact of the hypertension on those organs most vulnerable—the eyes, heart, brain, and kidneys. Thereby, prognosis can be determined and a decision made concerning the need for and type of therapy.

### Funduscopic Examination

Only in the optic fundi can small blood vessels be seen with ease, but this requires dilation of the pupil, a procedure that should be more commonly practiced. With the use of the short-acting mydriatic, tropicamide 1%, excellent dilation can be achieved in almost 90% of patients within 15 minutes (Steinmann et al, 1987). The presence of retinopathy is an independent indicator of mortality (Schouten et al, 1986) and should be determined in every hypertensive patient as part of the initial examination and yearly thereafter.

Damage to the fundal vessels in hypertensive patients was recognized as early as 1859, but not until Keith, Wagener, and Barker classified the changes according to severity in 1939 did the funduscopic examination become a clinically useful guide. Two separate but related vascular diseases are demonstrable: hypertensive neuroretinopathy (hemorrhages, exudates, and papilledema) and arteriosclerotic retinopathy (diffuse narrowing, arteriovenous nicking, silver wiring) (Sapira, 1984). The original Keith-Wagener-Barker grouping mixed the two. The retinopathy of diabetes—punctate hemorrhages and hard exudates—is seen in twice as many diabetics with hypertension as without (Knowler et al, 1980).

*Mild and Moderate Hypertension.* Changes in light reflex, vessel caliber and tortuosity, and arteriovenous crossing defects reflect thickening of the walls of retinal arterioles, which narrows the column of blood. The evidence of sclerosis and narrowing—widened light reflex, copper wiring, silver wiring, and arteriovenous crossing defects—are more related to age than to the presence of hypertension (van Buchem et al, 1964).

When these features were carefully assessed in 25 untreated hypertensives, they were found to have no relation to BP determined by clinic or ABPM, measures of left ventricular mass by echocardiography, or urinary microalbumin excretion (Dimmitt et al, 1989). The authors conclude that "Direct ophthalmoscopy was not clinically useful in the assessment of mild to moderate hypertension."

*Severe Hypertension.*  The group III and IV changes—flame-shaped hemorrhages, soft exudates, and papilledema—are clearly indicative of very severe hypertension. The evolution of retinal vascular lesions has been meticulously followed during life and correlated with the pathological findings in a group of severe hypertensives (Harnish and Pearce, 1973). Various lesions were demonstrated, including reversible narrowing, sheathing, arterial occlusion, and collateral vessels. The same initial vasoconstriction followed by "breakthrough" dilation shown to occur in the cerebral vessels (Strandgaard, 1976) has been incriminated as being responsible for the retinal hemorrhages and exudates (Garner and Ashton, 1979).

## Cardiac Involvement

As will be noted in Chapter 4, the most common mode of death in patients with hypertension is cardiac. Before antihypertensive therapy was available, death was often by congestive failure. Now that failure, strokes, and renal damage have been reduced by therapy, most deaths are by coronary artery disease with myocardial infarction.

Cardiac involvement is usually evident long before failure or infarction occur. Such evidence would include:

—the presence of an S4 gallop;
—left atrial enlargement by electrocardiogram or echocardiogram (Miller et al, 1988);
—left ventricular enlargement by x-ray;
—left ventricular hypertrophy by echocardiogram (Hammond et al, 1988). In 234 patients with mild to moderate hypertension (mean BP = 150/95), 61% had an echocardiographic abnormality (Savage et al, 1979). The ECG is

just as specific but much less sensitive in recognizing left ventricular hypertrophy (LVH) (Reichek and Devereux, 1981).
—changes in left ventricular function measured by cineangiography. These include prolonged diastolic relaxation and filling rate (Fouad, 1987), higher systolic ejection phase indices (de Simone et al, 1988), and subnormal functional response to exercise stress (Heber et al, 1988).

Hypertensive patients have more coronary artery disease but in addition may have symptoms of myocardial ischemia because of limited coronary reserve from ventricular hypertrophy and systolic wall stress (Strauer, 1987). The differential between the two processes may require thallium-201 stress imaging or positron tomography (Prisant et al, 1987). For most hypertensives, none of these high-tech procedures should be needed.

## Cerebral Involvement

Cerebral function should be tested, but it is not possible to relate cerebral dysfunction to the severity of the BP unless hypertension has become accelerated, with resultant encephalopathy. The earlier recognition of cerebrovascular disease may be possible by Doppler ultrasonography of the carotid vessels (Safar et al, 1988) and estimation of regional cerebral blood flow by [133]Xenon inhalation. As with cardiac testing, such procedures should only very rarely be needed in the evaluation of hypertensive patients.

## Renal Involvement

Renal dysfunction may be recognized much earlier than previously noted. In the past, only a loss of concentrating ability, manifested as nocturia, was usually identified until overt renal insufficiency from nephrosclerosis supervened. However, early in the course of hypertension, glomerular filtration rates may be above normal (Odutola et al, 1988) and microalbuminuria may appear because of a rise in filtration fraction from increased efferent arteriolar resistance. The hyperfiltration from increased glomerular capillary hydraulic pressure is thought to be responsible for progressive glomerular sclerosis and nephron loss. An inability to increase the glomerular filtration rate by an infusion of amino acids has been claimed to be an early marker of hyperfiltration (Losito et al, 1988).

As renal dysfunction worsens, heavier proteinuria may develop and rarely may reach the nephrotic range (Narvarte et al, 1987). In addition, creatinine clearance falls and serum creatinine levels rise.

### Renin Levels and Prognosis

In 1972, a retrospective analysis found a relation between plasma renin levels and the frequency of heart attacks and strokes (Brunner et al, 1972). There had been no heart attacks or strokes in the preceding 7 years among the 59 hypertensive patients with low renin, 14 episodes among the 124 with normal renin, and five among the 36 with high renin.

Subsequently, a number of studies have examined this relationship. Though there are multiple methodological differences between Brunner's study and most of the subsequent ones, the majority have found no relationship between renin status and prognosis of hypertension (Kaplan, 1975), and the presumed protection offered by a low renin has not been confirmed (Berglund et al, 1976; Russell et al, 1980). The reason for the discrepancy may be the largely retrospective na-

ture of the original study. In one prospective study, equal numbers of heart attacks and strokes were found among those with initially low renin levels as among those with normal levels, but renin levels rose *after* a vascular complication (Birkenhager et al, 1977). Therefore, in a retrospective study, those who had low renins but suffered a vascular accident would now likely be in the normal or high categories. A preliminary report of another prospective study described fewer heart attacks but not strokes among those with low PRA (Alderman et al, 1989).

More about the various prognostic and other implications of renin levels will be provided in Chapter 3.

### Overall Cardiovascular Risk

Once having documented the cause and consequences of the hypertension, it is necessary to assess the patient's overall cardiovascular risk status. The need for such an assessment—as a guide for preventive measures—is obvious: Most

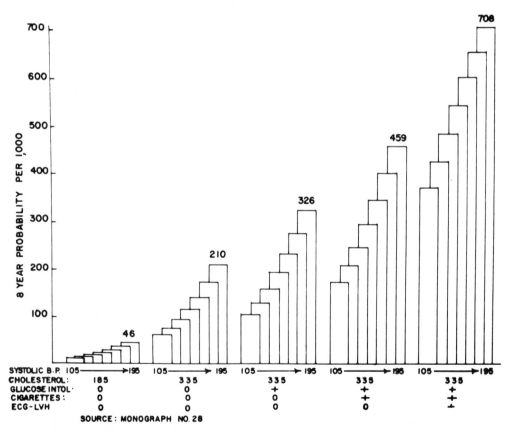

**Figure 2.15.** The 8-year risk of cardiovascular disease for 40-year-old men in Framingham according to progressively higher systolic blood pressure at specified levels of other risk factors. (From Kannel WB: In: Kaplan NM, Stamler J (eds). *Prevention of Coronary Heart Disease.* Philadelphia: WB Saunders, 1983.)

coronary deaths are sudden and unexpected, occurring in patients without evidence of prior clinical heart disease (Gordon and Kannel, 1971), and both heart attacks and sudden death are more common among hypertensives, particularly if they have LVH (Schatzkin et al, 1984). With readily available measurements, the predictability of cardiovascular disease is excellent: The larger share will occur in those at greatest identifiable risk (Kannel, 1983).

The ingredients for the most precise assessment, based upon the 24-year follow-up data from Framingham, are these: age, sex, SBP, serum total cholesterol and high density lipoprotein (HDL)-cholesterol, history of cigarette smoking, glucose tolerance, and the presence of LVH by ECG. Using these measurements, it is possible to obtain a number indicating the likelihood of a major cardiovascular event developing within the next 8 years. Booklets for determining the risk of coronary disease and stroke are available from the American Heart Association (AHA).

An example of the data for 40-year-old men is shown in Figure 2.15. Notice that as each additional risk factor is added, the probability of a major cardiovascular catastrophe for any given level of BP rises progressively. A 40-year-old "low risk" man with a SBP of 195 has a 4.6% chance of having a major cardiovascular event in the next 8 years. The chances in a "high risk" 40-year-old with the same BP increases to 70.8%.

## Purpose of Determining Overall Risk

The proper management of a hypertensive patient should involve attention to all of the risk factors that can be altered. Those at high risk should be counseled and helped to reduce all of their risks. Since for most the BP is the easiest of the risks to control, this may be the first priority.

By using the overall risk profile, we may be able to decide upon the need for therapy and the goal of therapy on a more rational basis than by the use of an arbitrary BP level. Using the Framingham data, it can be shown that lowering the SBP from 165 to 135 over a 15-year period for 35-year-old women at low risk will protect only about 1 in 50 since their overall risk is so small (Alderman and Madhaven, 1981). On the other hand, reducing the SBP from 165 to 135 for high risk 35-year-old men will protect about one in five from premature cardiovascular disease. If their other risk factors can also be reduced, such patients could benefit even more.

More about the potential benefits of antihypertensive therapy will be covered in Chapter 5. As for now, the need for a complete assessment of cardiovascular risk—a simple and inexpensive undertaking—should be obvious for the proper management of all hypertensives.

We will next turn to an in-depth analysis of the process that affects 95% of those with hypertension so that—based upon our understanding of pathophysiology—we can then turn to the most appropriate course of management.

## References

Abe H, Yokouchi M, Saitoh F, et al: *J Clin Hypertens* 3:661, 1987.
Alderman MH, Madhaven S: *Hypertension* 3:192, 1981.
Alderman MH Madhavan S, Ooi WL, et al: *Circulation* 80(Suppl II):II-101, 1989.
Ayman D, Goldshine AD: *Am J Med Sci* 200:465, 1940.
Balla JI, Elstein AS, Christensen C: *Br Med J* 298:579, 1989.
Bansal S: *Hypertension* 12:1, 1988.
Barker WF, Hediger ML, Katz SH, et al: *Hypertension* 6:85, 1984.
Benowitz NL, Kuyt F, Jacob P III: *Clin Pharmacol Ther* 36:74, 1984.
Berglund G, Mattias A, Wikstrand J, et al: *Acta Med Scand* 199:243, 1976.
Bevan AT, Honour AJ, Stott FH: *Clin Sci* 36:329, 1969.
Birkenhager WH, Kho TL, Schalekamp MADH, et al: *Acta Clin Belg* 32:168, 1977.
Blank SG, West JE, Muller FB, et al: *Circulation* 77:1297, 1988.
Bornstein NM, Norris JW: *Lancet* 2:303, 1986.
Brennan M, O'Brien E, O'Malley K: *J Hypertens* 4 (Suppl 6):S269, 1986.
Brigden GS, Cashman PMM, Broadhurst P, et al: *J. Hypertens* 7(Suppl 6): S354, 1989.
Brown GE: *Ann Intern Med* 3:1177, 1930.

Bruce NG, Shaper AG, Walker M, et al: *J Hypertens* 6:375, 1988.
Brunner HR, Laragh JH, Baer L, et al: *N Engl J Med* 286:441, 1972.
Bucknall CA, Morris GK, Mitchell JRA: *Br Med J* 293:739, 1986.
Canadian Coalition for High Blood Pressure Prevention and Control: *Can Med Assoc J* 138:1093, 1988.
Cantor A, Gueron GM, Cristal N, et al: *Cardiology* 74:141, 1987.
Caruana MP, Cashman PMM, Altman DG, et al: *Am J Cardiol* 62:755, 1988.
Casadei R, Parati G, Pomidossi G, et al: *J Hypertens* 6:797, 1988.
Chaney RH, Eyman RK: *Am J Cardiol* 62:1058, 1988.
Clark LA, Denby L, Pregibon D, et al: *J Chronic Dis* 40:671, 1987.
Close A, Hamilton G, Muriss S: *Br Med J* 293:775, 1986.
Conway J: *J Hypertens* 4:261, 1986.
Cooper KM, Horne RA, Cushman WC: Abstract 28th Conference on Cardiovascular Epidemiology, March 17, 1988. *AHA CVD Epid Epidemiology Newsletter* No. 43, 1988.
Cox JP, England R, Cox T, et al: *J Hypertens* 7(Suppl 6):S82, 1989.
Cruickshank JM: *Br Med J* 297:1227, 1988.

Cryer PE, Haymond MW, Santiago JV: *N Engl J Med* 295:573, 1976.
Davies AB, Gould BA, Cashman PMM, et al: *Br Heart J* 52:93, 1984.
De Gaudemaris R, Deloraine A, Courturier P, et al: *Am J Hypertens* 2(5 Part 2):121A, 1989
De Gaudemaris R, Folsom AR, Prineas RJ, et al: *Am J Epidemiology* 121:282, 1985.
de Simone G, Di Lorenzo L, Costantino G, et al: *Hypertension* 11:457, 1988.
Devereux RB, Pickering TG: *Am Heart J* 116:1124, 1988.
Di Rienzo M, Parati G, Pomidossi G, et al: *J Hypertens* 3:343, 1985.
Di Tullio M, Radice M, Alberti D, et al: *J Hypertens* 1 (Suppl 2):302, 1983.
Dimmitt SB, West JNW, Eames SM, et al: *Lancet* 1:1103, 1989.
Dlin RA, Hanne N, Silverberg DS, et al: *Am Heart J* 106:316, 1983.
Doll R, Peto R: *Br Med J* 2:1525, 1976.
Drayer JIM, Weber MA, Hoeger WJ: *Arch Intern Med* 145:271, 1985.
Dupont AG, van der Niepen P, Six RO: *Br J Clin Pharm* 24:106, 1987.
Egger M, Bianchetti MG, Gnadinger M, et al: *Arch Dis Childhood* 62:1130, 1987.
Epstein AM, Begg CB, McNeil BJ: *N Engl J Med* 309:464, 1983.

Epstein AM, Hartley RM, Charlton JR, et al: *JAMA* 252:1723, 1984.

Evans CE, Haynes RB, Goldsmith CH, et al: *J Hypertens* 7:133, 1989.

Evans RW: *JAMA* 249:2047, 1983.

Fagan TJ: *N Engl J Med* 293:257, 1975.

Fagius J, Karhuvaara S: *Hypertension* 14:511, 1989.

Finnegan TP, Spence JD, Wong DG, et al: *J Hypertens* 3:231, 1985.

Floras JS, Jones JV, Hassan MO: *Lancet* 2:107, 1981.

Floras JS: *Lancet* 2:994, 1988.

Floras JS, Jones JV, Hassan MO, et al: *Br Med J* 285:1387, 1982.

Fouad FM: *Circulation* 75(Suppl I):I-48, 1987.

Garner A, Ashton N: *J R Soc Med* 72:362, 1979.

Garrett BN, Dosa S, Thompson AM: *Clin Res* 35:441A, 1987.

Giaconi S, Ghione S, Palombo C, et al: *Hypertension* 14.22, 1989.

Gifford RW Jr, Kirkendall W, O'Connor DT, et al: *Hypertension* 13:283, 1989.

Gordon T, Kannel WB: *JAMA* 215:1617, 1971.

Gosse P, Campello G, Roudaut R, et al: *Am J Hypertens* 1:195S, 1988.

Gould BA, Hornung RS, Altman DG, et al: *Br Heart J* 53:611, 1985.

Gould BA, Hornung RS, Kieso HA, et al: *Hypertension* 8:267, 1986.

Gould BA, Hornung RS, Raftery EB: *J Hypertens* 1 (Suppl 2):293, 1983.

Gould BA, Kieso HA, Hornung R, et al: *Br Med J* 285:1691, 1982.

Graettinger WF, Lipson JL, Cheung DG, et al: *Am Heart J* 116:1155, 1988.

Griner PF, Mayewski RJ, Mushlin AI, et al: *Ann Intern Med* 94:553, 1981.

Hall WD, Douglas MB, Blumenstein BA: *Clin Res* 25:264A, 1977.

Hammond IW, Devereux RB, Alderman MH, et al: *J Am Coll Cardiol* 12:996, 1988.

Hampson NB: *N Engl J Med* 312:919, 1985.

Hahn LP, Folsom AR, Sprafka JM, et al: *Am J Pub Health* 77:1459, 1987.

Harnish A, Pearce ML: *Medicine* (Baltimore) 52:483, 1973.

Heber ME, Brigden GS, Prince H, et al: *Hypertension* 11:464, 1988.

Hense H-W, Stieber J, Chambless L: *Int J Epidemiol* 15:513, 1986.

Hla KM, Feussner JR: *Arch Intern Med* 148:673, 1988.

Hla KM, Stoneking HT, Samsa GP, et al: *Clin Res* 37:776A, 1989.

Hla KM, Vokaty KA, Feussner JR: *Arch Intern Med* 146:2373, 1986.

Horan MJ, Kennedy HL, Padgett NE: *Ann Intern Med* 94:466, 1981.

Hossmann V, FitzGerald GA, Dollery CT: *Hypertension* 3:113, 1981.

Hunyor SN, Flynn JM, Cochineas C: *Br Med J* 2:159, 1978.

Imai Y, Abe K, Sasaki S, et al: *J Hypertens* 7:113, 1989.

Imai Y, Abe K, Sasaki S, et al: Abstract 12th International Society of Hypertension Meeting, June 1988. Kyoto, Japan, Abstract #338.

Isles C, Brown JJ, Cumming AMM, et al: *Br Med J* 1:579, 1979.

James GD, Pickering TG, Yee LS, et al: *Hypertension* 11:545, 1988.

Jyothinagaram SG, Flapan AD, Campbell A, et al: *J Hypertens* 6:942, 1988.

Kannel WB: In: Genest J, Koiw E, Kuchel O (eds): *Hypertension: Physiopathology and Treatment*. New York: McGraw-Hill, 1977.

Kannel WB: In: Kaplan NM, Stamler J (eds). *Prevention of Coronary Heart Disease*. Philadelphia: WB Saunders, 1983, p. 1.

Kannel WB, Sorlie P, Gordon T: *Circulation* 61:1183, 1980.

Kaplan NM: Curable hypertension. In: Stollerman GH (ed). *Advances in Internal Medicine*, New York: Year Book Medical Publishers, 1969, vol. 15, p. 95.

Kaplan NM: *JAMA* 231:167, 1975.

Keith NM, Wagener HP, Barker NW: *Am J Med Sci* 268:336, 1974.

Knowler WC, Bennett PH, Ballintine EJ: *N Engl J Med* 302:645, 1980.

Korbin I, Oigman W, Kumar A, et al: *J Am Geriatr Soc* 32:896, 1984.

Krakoff LR, Eison H, Phillips RH, et al: *Am Heart J* 116:1152, 1988.

Lang RM, Borow KM, Weinert L, et al: *Circ* 78 (Suppl II):II-517, 1988.

Laaser U, Labarthe R: *Clin Exp Hypertens* A8:903, 1986.

Laughlin KD, Fisher L, Sherrard DJ: *Am Heart J* 98:629, 1979.

Lehane A, O'Brien ET, O'Malley K: *Br Med J* 281:1603, 1980.

Lewin A, Blaufox D, Castle H, et al: *Arch Intern Med* 145:424, 1985.

Linfors EW, Feussner JR, Blessing CL, et al: *Arch Intern Med* 144:1482, 1984.

Lipsitz LA, Pluchino FC, Wei JY, et al: *Am J Cardiol* 58:810, 1986.

Lipsitz LA, Storch HA, Minaker KL, et al: *Clin Sci* 69:337, 1985.

Londe S, Klitzner TS: *West J Med* 141:193, 1984.

Long JM, Lynch JJ, Machiran NM, et al: *J Behavior Med* 5:165, 1982.

Losito A, Fortunati F, Zampi I, et al: *Br Med J* 296:1562, 1988.

Mader SL, Josephson KR, Rubenstein LZ: *JAMA* 258:1511, 1987.

Mahoney LT, Schieken RM, Clarke WR, et al: *Hypertension* 12:206, 1988.

Malinow KL, Lynch JJ, Foreman PJ, et al: *Psychosom Med* 48:95, 1986.

Mancia G, Parati G, Pomidossi G, et al: *Hypertension* 9:209, 1987a.

Mancia G, Parati G, Pomidossi G, et al: *J Hypertens* 5(Suppl 5):S591, 1987b.

Mann S, Millar-Craig MW, Gould BA, et al: *Br Heart J* 47:84, 1982.

Mann S, Millar-Craig MW, Raftery EB: *Clin Exp Hypertens* A7:279, 1985.

Mazze RS, Shamoon H, Pasmantier R, et al: *Am J Med* 77:211, 1984.

McNeil BJ, Varady PD, Burrows BA, et al: *N Engl J Med* 293:216, 1975.

Ménard J, Serrurier D, Bautier P, et al: *Hypertension* 11:153, 1988.

Messerli FH, Ventura HO, Amodeo C: *N Engl J Med* 312:1548, 1985.

Miller JT, O'Rourke RA, Crawford MH: *Am Heart J* 116:1048, 1988.

Molineux D, Steptoe A: *J Hypertens* 6:361, 1988.

Møller-Petersen J: *Lancet* 1:348, 1985.

Muller JE, Tofler GH, Stone PH: *Circulation* 79:733, 1989.

Murphy MB, Nelson KS, Oliner CM, et al: *Circ* 78 (Suppl II):II-569, 1988.

Narvarte J, Prive M, Saba SR, et al: *Am J Kidney Dis* 10:408, 1987.

Nielsen PE: *Acta Med Scand* (Suppl 670):75, 1982.

Nishimura H, Nishioka A, Kubo S, et al: *Clin Sci* 73:135, 1987.

O'Brien E, Cox JP, O'Malley K: *J Hypertens* 7:243, 1989.

O'Brien E, Fitzgerald D, O'Malley K: *Br Med J* 290:729, 1985.

O'Brien E, O'Malley K: *Br Med J* 297:1211, 1988.

Odutola TA, Ositelu SB, D'Almeida EA, et al: *J Hum Hypertens* 2:133, 1988.

Parati G, Casadei R, Groppelli A, et al: *Hypertension* 13:647, 1989.

Parati G, Pomidossi G, Albini F, et al: *J Hypertens* 5:93, 1987.

Parati G, Pomidossi G, Casadel R, et al: *Hypertension* 7:597, 1985.

Perloff D, Sokolow M: *Cardiovasc Med* June:655, 1978.

Perloff D, Sokolow M, Cowan R: *JAMA* 249:2792, 1983.

Petrie JC, O'Brien ET, Littler WA, et al: *Br Med J* 293:611, 1986.

Pickering TG: *Am Heart J* 116:1141, 1988a.

Pickering TG: *Hypertension* 11 (Suppl II):II-96, 1988b.

Pickering TG, Harshfield GA, Devereux RB, et al: *Hypertension* 7:171, 1985.

Pickering TG, James GD, Boddie C, et al: *JAMA* 259:225, 1988.

Polk BF, Rosner B, Feudo R, et al: *Hypertension* 2:221, 1980.

Potter JF, Watson RDS, Skan W, et al: *Hypertension* 8:625, 1986.

Prisant LM, Frank MJ, Carr AA, et al: *Hypertension* 10:467, 1987.

Puddey IB, Beilin LJ, Vandongen R: *Lancet* 1:647, 1987.

Reichek N, Devereux RB: *Circulation* 63:1391, 1981.

Remington JW, O'Brien LJ: *Am J Physiol* 218:437, 1970.

Robertson E, Wade D, Workman R, et al: *J Clin Invest* 67:1111, 1981.

Rose G: In: Marshall AJ, Barritt DW (eds). *The Hypertensive Patient*. Kent, England: Pitman Medical Press, 1980.

Rosner B, Cook NR, Evans DA, et al: *Am J Epidemiol* 126:1115, 1987.

Rosner B, Polk BF: *J Chron Dis* 32:451, 1979.

Ruddy MC, Bialy GB, Malka ES, et al: *J Hypertens* 6(Suppl 4):S412, 1988.

Russell GI, Bing RF, Thurston H, et al: *Q J Med* 195:385, 1980.

Sackett DL, Haynes RB, Tugwell P: In: *Clinical Epidemiology. A Basic Science for Clinical Medicine*. Boston: Little, Brown, 1985.

Safar ME, Laurent S, Benetos A, et al: *Stroke* 19:1198, 1988.

Sapira JD: *Disease-A-Month* 30:39, 1984.

Savage JM, Dillon MJ, Taylor JFN: *Arch Dis Child* 54:184, 1979.

Schatzkin A, Cupples LA, Heeren T, et al: *Am Heart J* 107:1300, 1984.

Schechter CB, Adler RS: *Med Decis Making* 8:182, 1988.

Scherwitz LW, Evans LA, Hennrikus DJ, et al: *Med Care* 20:727, 1982.

Schouten EG, Vandenbroucke JP, van der Heide-Wessel C, et al: *Int J Epidemiol* 15:234, 1986.

Schroeder KL, Chen MS Jr: *N Engl J Med* 312:919, 1985.

Seltzer CC: *Am Heart J* 87:558, 1974.

Shekelle SA, Raynor WJ Jr, Gale MB, et al: Presented at National Conference on High Blood Pressure Control, New York, 1981, Abstract A-108.

Silman AJ: *Br Med J* 290:1781, 1985.

Silverberg DS, Rosenfeld JB: *Israel J Med Sci* 16:41, 1980.

Sirgo MA, Mills RJ, DeQuattro V: *Arch Intern Med* 148:2547, 1988.

Sloan PJM, Zezulka A, Davies P, et al: *J Hypertens* 2:547, 1984.

Sokolow M, Perloff D, Cowan R: *Clin Sci Mol Med* 45:195s, 1973.

Sokolow M, Werdegar D, Kain HK, et al: *Circulation* 34:279, 1966.

Sox HC Jr: *Ann Intern Med* 104:60, 1986.

Special Task Force Appointed by the Steering Committee, American Heart Association: *Hypertension* 11:209A, 1988.

Stahl SM, Kelley CR, Neill PJ, et al: *Am J Public Health* 74:704, 1984.

Steinmann WC, Millstein ME, Sinclair SH: *Ann Intern Med* 107:181, 1987.

Stokes J III, Kannel WB, Wolf PA, et al: *Circulation* 75 (Suppl V):V-65, 1987.

Strandgaard S: *Circulation* 53:720, 1976.

Strauer BE: *Am Heart J* 114:948, 1987.

Sundberg S, Kohvakka A, Gordin A: *J Hypertens* 6:393, 1988.

Task Force on Automated Blood Pressure Measuring Devices for Mass Screening: Department of Health, Education and Welfare Publication No. (NIH) 76-929, 1976.

Tell GS, Prineas RJ, Gomez-Marin O: *Am J Epidemiol* 128:360, 1988.

Torriani S, Waeber B, Petrillo A, et al: *J Hypertens* 6(Suppl 1):S25, 1988.

van Buchem FSP, v.d. Heuvel-Aghina JWMTh, v.d. Heuvel JEA: *Acta Med Scand* 176:539, 1964.

Van Egeren LF, Madarasmi S: *Am Heart J* 1:179s, 1988.

van Loo JM, Peer PG, Thien TA: *J Hypertens* 4:631, 1986.

van Montfrans GA, van der Hoeven GMA, Karemaker JM, et al: *Br Med J* 295:354, 1987.

Vyse TJ: *Lancet* 1:561, 1987.

Waal-Manning HJ, Paulin JM: *J Clin Hypertens* 3:624, 1987.

Waeber B, Scherrer U, Petrillo et al: *Lancet* 2:732, 1987.

Waeber G, Beck G, Waeber B, et al: *J Hypertens* 6:239, 1988.

Watkins-Pitchford JM, Szocik J: *JAMA* 261:1153, 1989.

Watson RDS, Lumb R, Young MA, et al: *J Hypertens* 5:207, 1987.

Watson RDS, Stallard TH, Flinn RM, et al: *Hypertension* 2:333, 1980.

Weber MA: *Am Heart J* 116:1118, 1988a.

Weber MA: *Hypertension* 11:288, 1988b.

Weber MA, Cheung DG, Graettinger WF, et al: *JAMA* 259:3281, 1988.

Weber MA, Tonkon MJ, Klein RC: *J Clin Pharmacol* 27:751, 1987.

Wenting GJ, van den Meiracker AH, Ritsema van Eck HJ, et al: *J Hypertens* 4 (Suppl 6):S78, 1986.

White WB: *Arch Intern Med* 146:2196, 1986.

White WB, Morganroth J: *Am J Cardiol* 63:94, 1989.

White WB, Dey HM, Schulman P: *Am Heart J* 118:782, 1989.

White WB, Schulman P, McCabe EJ, et al: *JAMA* 261:873, 1989.

Wilson NV, Meyer BM: *Prev Med* 10:62, 1981.

Wolf FM, Gruppen LD, Billi JE: *JAMA* 253:2858, 1985.

World Hypertension League: *J Hypertens* 6:257, 1988.

Yagi S, Ichikawa S, Sakamaki T, et al: *N Engl J Med* 315:836, 1986.

Young MA, Rowlands DB, Stallard TJ, et al: *Br Med J* 286:1235, 1983.

Zachariah PK, Sheps SG, Ilstrup DM, et al: *Mayo Clin Proc* 63:1085, 1988b.

Zachariah PK, Sheps SG, Smith RL: *Diagnosis* 10:39, 1988a.

# 3 Primary Hypertension: Pathogenesis

As noted in the previous chapters, as much as 95% of all hypertension is of unknown cause. In the absence of a known cause, there is no obvious name for the disease. "Essential" may be mistakenly interpreted to infer an essential need for higher pressure to push blood through vessels narrowed by age. The term "benign" has been buried along with the millions of unfortunate victims of uncontrolled hypertension. "Idiopathic" seems a bit unwieldy, so I have chosen "primary" simply to distinguish it from all of the remainder, which are "secondary" to known causes.

## GENERAL CONSIDERATIONS

Since the actual pathogenesis remains unknown, all one can do is take separate pieces of data from studies on humans and animals and try to construct reasonable hypotheses. Enough is known to provide logical schemes that offer, at least, a better integration of the reams of seemingly disparate experimental data and, at best, models with rather broad explanatory powers.

In considering the evidence about various mechanisms that may be responsible for sustained hypertension, a few disclaimers must be acknowledged:

—The relevance of data from animal models is highly questionable. Despite the many thousands of papers written and the many millions of dollars spent on the spontaneously hypertensive rat (SHR), any relevance of that model or any other small animal to the human condition is highly unlikely. One example: SHR rats given alcohol to drink from 1 to 4 months of age do not develop hypertension (Howe et al, 1989). However, as we shall see, alcohol is among the most common exogenous causes of hypertension in man. On a more basic level, sensitivity to calcium is increased in resistance vessels of SHR but decreased in resistance vessels of hypertensive patients, leading Bing et al (1987) to conclude: "the SHR is not an appropriate model for studying the role of calcium in the pathogenesis of human hypertension." Therefore, whenever possible, this discussion will examine data only from human studies.

—Few analytical techniques are available to measure accurately and repetitively the possibly small changes in various hemodynamic functions that may be involved. Moreover, few investigators or patients have been willing or able to do repetitive studies over the many years it may take for subtle changes to become manifest. Cross-sectional observations may never be able to uncover the sequential changes that might be revealed by longitudinal studies.

—Even when studies are done among adolescent and "borderline" hypertensives, the beginnings may have already been missed. By the time hypertension is detectable, the initiating factors may be obscured by adaptations invoked by the rising pressure. In the absence of a marker to identify the "prehypertensive" individual before the blood pressure has risen, we may be viewing the process after the initiating factor(s) is no longer recognizable.

—Though the search for a single underlying abnormality that begins the hemodynamic cascade toward sustained hypertension continues to attract the imagination and energies of numerous investigators, there may be no such single defect. In view of the multiple factors involved in the control of the blood pressure, the concept of a multifaceted mosaic, introduced by Irvine Page (1963), may be more appropriate, as unattractive as it may be to those who prefer to believe that for every biological defect there should be a single specific cause. An editorial some time ago in the *Lancet* (1977) describes the situation aptly:

Blood pressure is a measurable end product of an exceedingly complex series of factors including those which control blood-vessel calibre and responsiveness, those which control fluid volume within and outside the vascular bed, and those which control cardiac output. None of these factors is independent: they interact with each other and respond to changes in blood pressure. It is not easy, therefore, to dissect out cause and effect. Few factors which play a role in cardiovascular control are completely normal in hypertension: indeed, normality would require explanation since it would suggest a lack of responsiveness to increased pressure.

—The search may be misdirected: In looking for the mechanisms of primary hypertension, we may need to separate the disease into many distinct syndromes, each with its own mechanisms. Fifty years ago, almost all hypertension not obviously secondary to intrinsic renal disease was lumped under the term "essen-tial." Since then, coarctation, pheochromocytoma, Cushing's syndrome, renovascular disease, and primary aldosteronism have been identified and a small but significant percentage of hypertensive patients put into each category. Additional parts of what is now called primary may be separated into other specific categories. However, as of 1990, no basis for such further division is apparent even though, as we shall see, more and more differences are being identified within the population of patients with primary hypertension. For now, unifying hypotheses seem appropriate, with the recognition that there may be considerable variations in the role of various components at different times and stages and in different people.

Before examining the specific hypotheses that may explain the development of hypertension, the contribution of heredity will be considered.

## ROLE OF HEREDITY

The level of blood pressure is strongly familial. Among 16,400 Utah families, normotensive males aged 20 to 39 had a 2.5 greater relative risk for future hypertension "if they had one first-degree relative with hypertension and a 3.8 greater relative risk with two or more hypertensive first-degree relatives" (Williams et al, 1988a). However, there are only a few clues as to what specifically may be transmitted genetically.

### Genetic Contribution

Studies of families and of twins have provided estimates of the genetic contribution to the variability of blood pressure (Table 3.1) (Williams et al, 1988a). Correlation is poor for those who share only environments but strengthens progressively as genetic sharing increases.

These estimates lead Williams et al to con-

**Table 3.1. Familial Blood Pressure Correlations[a]**

| Comparison | Number of Pairs | Correlation Coefficient | |
|---|---|---|---|
| | | Systolic | Diastolic |
| Spouses | 1433 | 0.08 | 0.06 |
| Parent-adoptees | 379 | 0.03 | 0.09 |
| Parent-offspring | 831 | 0.18 | 0.16 |
| Sibling-sibling | 2618 | 0.18 | 0.14 |
| Dizygotic twins | 264 | 0.25 | 0.27 |
| Monozygotic twins | 248 | 0.55 | 0.58 |

[a]Combined data from Framingham, MA, Tecumseh, MI, and Evans Co., GA, plus Canadian adoption, and National Heart, Lung, and Blood Institute twin studies. (From Williams RR, Hunt SC, Hasstedt SJ, et al: *J Cardiovasc Pharmacol* 12(Suppl 3:S7, 1988a).

clude that "blood pressure per se is a largely polygenic trait with an overall heritability estimate of approximately 50% with some mild effects due to shared common environment and assortative mating." With data from individual populations, the genetic contribution to blood pressure variability has been estimated to be as little as 25% (Havlik and Feinleib, 1982), to 40% (Friedlander et al, 1988) to 61% (Mongeau et al, 1986).

## Mode of Inheritance

Back in the late 1950s and early 1960s, Pickering and Platt engaged in a heated argument about whether hypertension was explainable by a single gene, providing a bimodal distribution of blood pressure in the population (the Platt view) or a polygenic inheritance of a quantitative trait, providing a unimodal distribution with a slightly positive skew for those with very high pressures (the Pickering view). McManus (1983) applied more sophisticated statistical models than were available to Pickering and Platt to a population sample of almost 68,000 people originally described in 1957 by Bøe et al, and concluded that the best fit of the data is the logarithm of a bimodal distribution, with a subpopulation of hypertensives in a separate mode.

However, as Camussi and Bianchi (1988) point out, "the debate between bimodalists and unimodalists has now lost much of its importance, since the shape of a distribution is not sufficient to prove the existence of a few or many segregating genes, at least if the environmental conditions cannot be controlled."

Obviously, without knowledge of the specific cause of the disease, without marker genes to identify those who are susceptible, and without a link between a genetic alteration and a physiological dysfunction, the inheritance of primary hypertension cannot be clearly defined.

## Search for Markers

The search for possible biochemical or physiological markers to identify those people with a genetic predisposition continues in hope of proceeding backward to find DNA markers and thereby prove the existence of major gene-hypertension interactions (Dzau et al, 1989). The extent of the search is seen in a partial list of tests reported to show differences, either positive or negative, between normotensive subjects with or without a positive family history for hypertension (Table 3.2).

As Williams et al (1988a) conclude:

**Table 3.2. Tests Reported to Differentiate Normotensive People with or without a Positive Family History for Hypertension**

Blood pressure
  Resting
  Exercise: bicycle, isometric grip
  Forearm vasodilation
Reactivity to stress
  Mental arithmetic
  Cold pressor
  Noise
  Platelet norepinephrine efflux
Sodium handling
  Modulation of adrenal and renal responses to varying $Na^+$ intake
  $Na^+$ excretion after saline infusion
  Whole body $^{22}Na^+$ turnover
  Plasma renin activity
  Urinary kallikrein excretion
  Haptoglobin phenotype (marker for salt sensitivity)
Membrane cation flux
  Intralymphocytic $Na^+$
  RBC concentration of $Na^+$, $Ca^{2+}$
  $Na^+$-$Li^+$ countertransport
  $Na^+$-$K^+$ cotransport
  Circulating $Na^+$-$K^+$ ATPase pump inhibitors
  $Na^+$-$K^+$ ATPase pump activity
  Plasma ionized calcium
Dyslipidemia
Blood group antigens MN

We wish to find traits that allow direct classification of persons into genotypes without overlap. Familial dyslipidemic hypertension, urinary kallikrein, nonmodulation, and gene markers such as MN and haptoglobin types may fit this picture. Others may be useful as quantitative risk factors for hypertension but have too much overlap to allow clear separation into groups. Sodium-lithium countertransport and intracellular sodium probably fit this picture.

We are, then, left with a number of provocative clues but little that is certain about the role of heredity in the pathogenesis of hypertension. It obviously has a role but how large the role is and the manner by which the role is played remain uncertain.

## OVERVIEW OF PATHOGENESIS

The pressure required to move blood through the circulatory bed is provided by the pumping action of the heart (cardiac output) and the tone of the arteries (peripheral resistance). Each of these primary determinants of the blood pressure is, in turn, determined by the interaction of the "exceedingly complex series of factors" referred to in the *Lancet* editorial (1977) and displayed in part in Figure 3.1.

Hypertension has been ascribed to abnormalities in virtually every one of these factors. Each of the major factors shown in Figure 3.1 will be examined, and attempts will be made along the way to integrate them into logical hy-

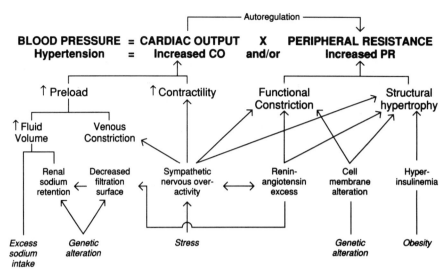

**Figure 3.1.** Some of the factors involved in the control of blood pressure that affect the basic equation: Blood pressure = cardiac output × peripheral resistance.

potheses. Multiple hypotheses may prove to be correct since the hemodynamic hallmark of primary hypertension, a persistently elevated vascular resistance, may be reached through a number of different paths. Before the final destination, these may converge into either structural thickening of the vessel walls or functional vasoconstriction by an increase in intracellular calcium. Whatever else is involved, heredity must play a role, along with varying contributions of at least three environmental factors for which there is strong support: sodium, stress, and obesity. Throughout the remainder of this chapter each of these environmental factors will be repeatedly touched upon, but just how they interact to induce hypertension remains uncertain. Insights are being rapidly uncovered. For example, obese hypertensives often have increased intracellular sodium concentrations that may, in turn, be related to insulin resistance (Modan et al, 1985).

Before considering these individual factors, a brief overview of the manner in which they may enter a final common pathway should be helpful.

Regardless of what starts the process, the perpetuation of hypertension clearly depends upon the development of vascular hypertrophy. Such structural hypertrophy explains the hemodynamics of established hypertension as shown by Folkow (1987) and is responsible for the increased tone and enhanced contractility in response to various pressor agents that are believed to play a functional role in the pathogenesis of

hypertension. Small resistance vessels from subcutaneous tissue from hypertensive subjects have an average 29% increase in the media thickness:lumen diameter ratio (Aalkjaer et al, 1987b). The in vitro responses of these vessels to various pressor agents are either unchanged or depressed, suggesting that the increased contractility induced by pressor agents in vivo is due to the increased muscle mass. As noted by Swales (1988), "In hypertension, there (is) no evidence for an overactive calcium second messenger system or indeed for any form of hyperresponsiveness, despite claims to the contrary over the preceding three decades. Instead, the conspicuous abnormality is hypertrophy giving rise to a generalized increase in contractility."

The search for the pathogenesis of sustained hypertension has increasingly focused on vascular hypertrophy particularly since the recognition that multiple pressor substances serve as growth or trophic factors for vascular hypertrophy. This has come, in part, from the study of the secondary forms of endocrine hypertension, including pheochromocytoma, primary aldosteronism, and renovascular disease. Each of these secondary forms of hypertension is known to arise from the direct effect of a specific pressor hormone. What has now become obvious is that, regardless of the initial hormonal effect, whether it be volume retention as with primary aldosteronism or vasoconstriction as with pheochromocytoma or renovascular disease, maintenance of hypertension derives from vascular hypertrophy that increases peripheral resistance, the process referred to as the "slow mechanism" by Anthony Lever (1986).

Lever starts with the original proposal of Folkow (Fig. 3.2) wherein hypertension is initiated by a minor overactivity of a specific fast-acting pressor mechanism (A), e.g., angiotensin II, that raises blood pressure slightly and initiates a positive feedback (BCB) that induces vascular hypertrophy and maintains the hypertension. The amplification (BCB) is "slowly progressive, ultimately large and probably nonspecific. Thus, different forms of chronic hypertension may resemble each other because part of the hypertension in each has the same mechanism" (Lever, 1986). Lever adds the action of an abnormal or reinforced genetically determined hypertrophic response to pressure (D). Obviously, an inherited abnormality in the cell membrane could serve as this reinforced hypertrophic response to pressure. More importantly, there is an additional contribution of one or more trophic mechanisms (E) for hypertrophy.

This scheme, involving both an immediate pressor action and a slow hypertrophic effect, is thought to be common to the action of various pressor-growth promoters (Heagerty and Ollerenshaw, 1987). In the majority of hypertensive patients, no marked excess of any of the known pressor hormones is identifiable. Nonetheless, a lesser excess of one or more may have been responsible for initiation of the process that is sustained by the positive feedback postulated by Folkow (1987) and the trophic effects empha-

sized by Lever (1986). This sequence encompasses a variety of specific initiating mechanisms that accentuate and maintain the hypertension by a nonspecific feedback-trophic mechanism. If this double process is involved in the pathogenesis of primary hypertension, as seems likely, the difficulty in recognizing the initiating, causal factor is easily explained. In the words of Lever (1986):

> The primary cause of hypertension will be most apparent in the early stages; in the later stages, the cause will be concealed by an increasing contribution from hypertrophy. . . . A particular form of hypertension may wrongly be judged to have "no known cause" because each mechanism considered is insufficiently abnormal by itself to have produced the hypertrophy. The cause of essential hypertension may have been considered already but rejected for this reason.

With this overview in mind, let us now examine the various hemodynamic factors that may be involved in the pathogenesis of hypertension.

## CARDIAC OUTPUT

An increased cardiac output has been found in some early, borderline hypertensives, some of whom display a hyperkinetic circulation. If it is responsible for the hypertension, the increase in cardiac output could logically arise in two ways, either from an increase in fluid volume (preload) or from an increase in neural stimulation of the heart. However, if it is involved in the initiation of hypertension, the increased cardiac output likely does not persist,

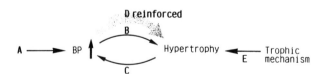

**Figure 3.2.** Hypotheses for the initiation and maintenance of hypertension: (a) Folkow's first proposal that a minor overactivity of a pressor mechanism *A* raises blood pressure slightly, initiating positive feedback (*BCB*) and a progressive rise of blood pressure. (b) As in (a) with two additional signals: *D*, an abnormal or "reinforced" hypertrophic response to pressure and *E*, increase of a humoral agent causing hypertrophy directly. (From Lever AF: *J Hypertension* 4:515, 1986.)

since the typical hemodynamic finding in established hypertension is an elevated peripheral resistance and normal cardiac output (Egan and Schmouder, 1988).

## Hyperkinetic Hypertensives

Numerous investigators have described hypertensives, mostly young, who have definitely high cardiac outputs (Werko and Lagerlof, 1949; Sannerstedt, 1966; Julius and Conway, 1968; Frohlich et al, 1969). Some of these patients displayed a hyperkinetic circulation with variable blood pressure, fast pulse, awareness of the heartbeat, and an increased responsiveness to beta-adrenergic stimulation.

Most of these features could reflect anxiety over both the knowledge that they were hypertensive (Rostrup et al, 1989) and the invasive procedures used in the studies. When such studies have been repeated within a year, cardiac outputs are usually normal (Birkenhäger and de Leeuw, 1984). However, it is likely that a high cardiac output is seen at least in some: Using noninvasive echocardiography to study 83 mild hypertensives whose average age was 53, a subgroup of 19 had increased resting cardiac performance independent of afterload or left ventricular hypertrophy (Lutas et al, 1985). Thus, the hypertension in some middle-aged hypertensives may continue to reflect increased cardiac output. Such patients may be recognized by a high pulse pressure, above 60 mm Hg (Safar et al, 1987).

## Cardiac Hypertrophy

Even if such overtly hyperkinetic patients are rare, the availability of noninvasive echocardiography has made it possible to identify the presence of cardiac hypertrophy in a large portion of early, mild hypertensives (Devereux, 1989) and even in the normotensive children of hypertensive parents (Radice et al, 1986; Celentano et al, 1988). Such hypertrophy, which will be described in greater detail in the next chapter dealing with the cardiac complications of hypertension, has been generally considered to be a compensatory mechanism to an increased vascular resistance (afterload). However, it could also reflect a primary response to repeated neural stimulation and, thereby, could be an initiating mechanism for hypertension (Julius et al, 1989).

## Increased Neural Stimulation

Both heart rate and stroke volume were increased in one group of hyperkinetic borderline hypertensives (Julius and Esler, 1975). These and the other hemodynamic findings in such patients have been explained by neurogenic mechanisms that could be both an increased sympathetic and a decreased parasympathetic drive (Julius, 1988). Tarazi and coworkers found that the high output is attributable to increased cardiac contractility, which in turn is attributed to a heightened adrenergic drive. This mechanism, rather than an increased preload, has been favored since, as we shall see, these workers repeatedly found intravascular blood volume to be normal or reduced (Tarazi et al, 1983).

### Distribution of Blood Volume

Even without an expanded total volume, blood may be redistributed so that more is in the central or cardiopulmonary component because of greater peripheral vasoconstriction. Such a distribution has been reported both in borderline (Messerli et al, 1978) and sustained (London et al, 1978) hypertension and has been attributed to an increased sympathetic stimulation causing peripheral venous constriction. Venous return to the heart would thereby be increased and could mediate an increased cardiac output. However, serious reservations have been expressed, both about the methodology used to measure cardiopulmonary blood volume and the theoretical concept that, if it were increased, it would persist rather than be quickly normalized so that cardiac output is increased only transiently (Birkenhäger and de Leeuw, 1984).

### Increased Fluid Volume

A second mechanism that could induce hypertension by increasing cardiac output would be an increased circulating fluid volume (preload). However, in most studies, patients with established hypertension have a lower blood volume and total exchangeable sodium than do normal subjects (Tarazi, 1976; Beretta-Piccoli and Weidmann, 1984).

### Relation of Blood Volume to Blood Pressure

However, when the blood pressure was compared with the total blood volume (TBV) in 48 normal subjects and 106 patients with fairly early and mild primary hypertension, an interesting relationship was observed (London et al, 1977b) (Fig. 3.3). A negative correlation was found in the normals but not in the hypertensives, with 80% of the hypertensives being outside the 95% confidence limits of the normal curve. The au-

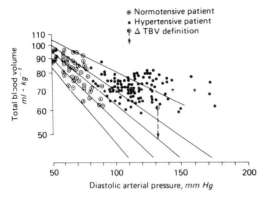

**Figure 3.3.** Relation between diastolic blood pressure and total blood volume (*TBV*) in 48 normotensive (*open circles*) and 106 hypertensive (*solid circles*) subjects. Only 20% of the hypertensive patients fell within the 95% confidence limits of the normal curve. The "ΔTBV definition" represents the degree of the pressure-volume disturbance. (From London GM, Safer ME, Weiss YA, et al: *Kidney Int* 11:204, 1977b.)

thors interpret their data to indicate a quantitative disturbance in the pressure-volume relationship in primary hypertension, i.e., a plasma volume that is inappropriately high for the level of blood pressure. Thus, even if absolute values are reduced, a relatively expanded blood volume may be involved in the maintenance of hypertension.

*Translocation into Interstitial Space.* One logical explanation for the lower intravascular volume would be the translocation of fluid across the capillary bed into the interstitial space, in keeping with the higher capillary filtration pressure (Ulrych, 1973). In general, the higher the blood pressure, the higher the interstitial fluid volume (Simon et al, 1979).

*Intracellular Fluid Volume.* Beyond the relative increase in interstitial fluid, there may also be an increase in intracellular fluid volume in established primary hypertension. In one of the few studies that simultaneously measured red blood cell mass, plasma volume, extracellular fluid volume, and total body water in a sizable number of patients with fairly mild hypertension, there was a significant absolute increase of 1.5 liters/m$^2$ in intracellular fluid (total body water minus extracellular fluid) among the hypertensives, compared with that of age-matched normotensive controls (Bauer and Brooks, 1979). In a larger population, a significant positive relationship between systolic blood pressure and exchangeable sodium was found in men, but not women, with primary hypertension (Beretta-Piccoli et al, 1984).

Beyond the ambiguous findings with these static measurements, Hollenberg (1983) and Simpson (1983) have presented a cogent argument that people with a relatively high sodium intake have a total body sodium content that is above the "set-point," the physiologically normal level. This set-point is reached when sodium intake is markedly lowered and averages about 150 mmol below the body sodium content on a higher sodium intake (Fig. 3.4). That the normal set-point is lower is supported by the finding that, when a small sodium load is taken in while sodium intake is very low, it is excreted within a few days, rather than being retained as it would be if the body sodium content on the low sodium intake were below normal. On the other hand, when a true sodium deficit is induced by a diuretic, a similar sodium load is retained to reestablish the normal body sodium content. Thus, most people ingesting today's usual diet may have a surfeit of body sodium that, in those who are otherwise susceptible, may be enough to mediate hypertension.

This brings us to the final feature about cardiac output: Even if it is involved in the initiation of hypertension, once hypertension is established, cardiac output is usually not increased, but peripheral resistance is elevated.

### Autoregulation

A changing pattern of initially high cardiac output giving way to a persistently elevated peripheral resistance has been observed in a few people and many animals with experimental hypertension. When animals with markedly reduced renal tissue are given volume loads, the blood pressure rises initially as a consequence of the high cardiac output, but within a few days, peripheral resistance rises, and cardiac output returns to near the basal level (Guyton,

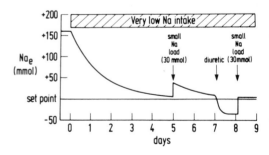

**Figure 3.4.** Body sodium (theoretical) when a very low Na diet is started. The effects of a small Na load before and after a single dose of diuretic is also shown. (From Simpson FO: *NZ Med J* 96:907, 1983.)

1986) (Fig. 3.5). The changeover has been interpreted to reflect an intrinsic property of the vascular bed to regulate the flow of blood depending upon the metabolic need of tissues, a process called *autoregulation* that was described by Borst and Borst-de Geus (1963) and demonstrated experimentally by Guyton and Coleman (1969). With an increased cardiac output, more blood flows through the tissues than is required; the increased flow delivers extra nutrients or removes additional metabolic products; in response, the vessels constrict, decreasing blood flow and returning the balance of supply and demand to normal. Thereby, peripheral resistance increases and thereafter remains high by the rapid induction of structural thickening of the resistance vessels.

Similar conversion from initially high cardiac output to later increased peripheral resistance has been shown in some hypertensive people (Eich et al, 1966; Lund-Johansen, 1977, 1989; Julius et al, 1983). In Lund-Johansen's study, younger (17- to 29-year-old) and older (30- to 39-year-old) mild hypertensives were restudied

both at rest and during exercise after 10 and then 20 years without intervening therapy. As the overall blood pressures rose, the cardiac output fell and peripheral resistance increased (Fig. 3.6).

### Problems with the Autoregulation Model

Autoregulation of tissue blood flow has been documented in the forearm of humans (Blake et al, 1985) and in conscious dogs where it has been shown to amplify the pressor responses to vasoconstrictor agents (Metting et al, 1989). However, the role of autoregulation in the conversion of a high cardiac output to a high peripheral resistance has been questioned. First, most young hypertensives do not have increased cardiac outputs (Hofman et al, 1982). Second, those found to have an increased cardiac output also have an increased oxygen consumption, rather than the lower level that should be seen if there were overperfusion of tissues as entailed in the autoregulation concept (Julius, 1988). Third, hypertension can be induced purely by an increase in resistance without a rise in cardiac

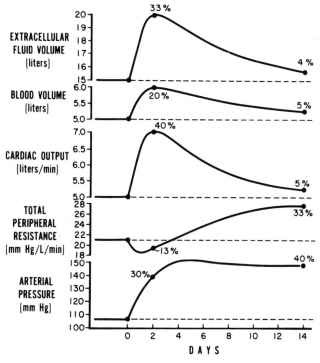

**Figure 3.5.** Progressive changes in important circulatory system variables during the first few weeks of volume-loading hypertension. The initial rise in cardiac output is the basic cause of the hypertension. Subsequently, the autoregulation mechanism returns the cardiac output almost to normal while at the same time causing a secondary increase in total peripheral resistance. (From Guyton AC: *Textbook of Medical Physiology*, Seventh Edition. Philadelphia: WB Saunders Company, 1986:265.)

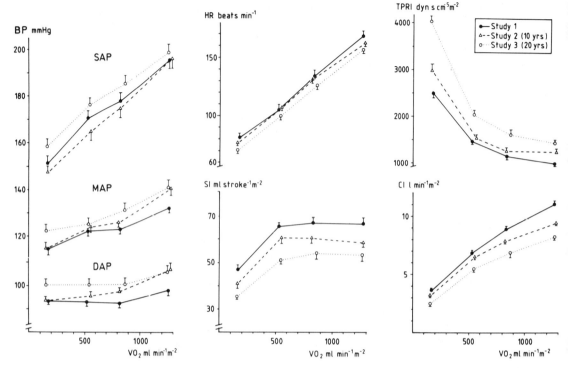

**Figure 3.6.** Central hemodynamic at rest and during exercise in age group 1 (17 to 29 years) at first study and at restudies after 10 and 20 years. Mean values: *SAP*, systolic arterial blood pressure; *MAP*, mean arterial blood pressure; *DAP*, diastolic arterial blood pressure; *HR*, heart rate; *SI*, stroke index; *TPRI*, total peripheral resistance index; *CI*, cardiac index; *VO₂*, oxygen consumption. Note the marked increase in TPRI from study I to study III and also the reduction in SI and CI from study I to study III. (From Lund-Johansen P: *J Hypertension*, 7(Suppl 6):S52, 1989.)

output (Fletcher et al, 1976). Fourth, the cardiac output can be raised without bringing about a subsequent increase in peripheral resistance (Korner et al, 1980). Ledingham (1989) discounts these objections and defends autoregulation as the "dominant factor" leading to the rise in peripheral resistance in hypertension.

Julius (1988) considers autoregulation to be an unlikely explanation for the switch from high cardiac output to increased peripheral resistance and offers another: structural changes that decrease the cardiac responses to nervous and hormonal stimuli but enhance the vascular responses. He proposes "This hemodynamic transition can be explained by a secondary response to elevated blood pressure. The heart becomes less responsive as a result of altered receptor responsiveness and decreased cardiac compliance, whereas the responsiveness of arterioles increases because of vascular hypertrophy, which leads to changes in the wall-to-lumen ratio."

Before discarding the autoregulatory model, we should recognize that it explains the course of hypertension in animals and in people given

a volume load, particularly in the presence of reduced renal mass (Fig. 3.5). As another example of volume overload hypertension that follows this sequence, patients with primary aldosteronism were followed after discontinuation of the aldosterone antagonist, spironolactone, which had normalized their blood pressure (Schalekamp et al, 1985). As their hypertension reappeared, they had an initial overexpansion of plasma volume and increase in cardiac output that then, in some of the patients, returned toward normal while peripheral resistance rose progressively.

Admittedly, these experimental and clinical models do not portray the usual picture of primary hypertension. However, there is more evidence in favor of volume expansion in the pathogenesis of the disease, based upon presumed alterations in renal function.

## RENAL SODIUM RETENTION

The first suggestion that hypertension might be a homeostatic response to impaired renal excretory function was likely made by Traube in

1871. The link remained vague until the early 1960s when Guyton (1961) laid out the concept and, soon thereafter, Ledingham et al (1962) in animals and Borst and Borst-de Geus (1963) in a patient independently documented the long-term role of renal excretory function on blood pressure regulation and the presence of expanded fluid volume and cardiac output in the development of hypertension. Guyton and his collaborators have, over the last 30 years, provided an impressive body of experimental and analytical data supporting the central role of renal pressure-natriuresis in the regulation of the normal circulation and its functional resetting in the pathogenesis of hypertension. More recently, Sealey et al (1988a) and Brenner et al (1988) have proposed primary structural changes in the kidney that lead to sodium retention and, thereby, to hypertension. Evidence for each of these three hypotheses will be considered.

## Resetting of Pressure-Natriuresis

In normal people, when blood pressure rises, renal excretion of sodium and water increases, shrinking fluid volume and returning the pressure to normal, the phenomenon of *pressure-natriuresis*. Therefore, in hypertensives, even a normal blood volume is inappropriately high. This was noted in the data of London et al shown in Figure 3.3. Only 20% of their hypertensives fit within the negative slope of the blood pressure to blood volume relationship observed in normotensives.

According to the pressure-natriuresis relationship, if volume and cardiac output are high in the presence of an elevated blood pressure, the kidneys must be at fault. Since the regulation of body fluid volume by the kidneys is considered to be the dominant mechanism for the long-term control of blood pressure, if hypertension develops, something must be amiss with this renal-body fluid pressure control mechanism (Guyton, 1987).

### Experimental Support

The concept is based upon a solid foundation: When arterial pressure is raised, the normal kidney excretes more salt and water, i.e., pressure-natriuresis (Selkurt, 1951; Shipley and Study, 1951). The curve relating arterial pressure to sodium excretion is very steep (Fig. 3.7). A small change in perfusion pressure causes a very large change in the rate of sodium and water excretion, acting as a powerful negative feedback stabilizer of systemic arterial pressure. Un-

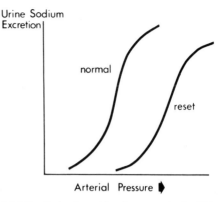

**Figure 3.7.** Derived renal function curve for the kidneys in people with normal blood pressure and primary hypertension. The resetting of the pressure-natriuresis curve in primary hypertension is shown. (From Guyton AC, Coleman TG, Cowley AW Jr, et al: *Am J Med* 52:584, 1972.)

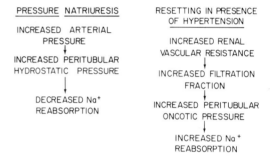

**Figure 3.8.** Origin of pressure-natriuresis (*left*) and its resetting in the presence of essential hypertension (*right*). (From Brown JJ, Lever AF, Robertson JIS, et al: *Lancet* 2:320, 1974.)

der normal conditions, the perfusion pressure is around 100 mm Hg, sodium excretion is about 150 mEq per day, and the two are in a remarkably balanced state. The mechanism is considered to reflect transmission of increased arterial pressure into peritubular capillaries (Azar et al, 1974), wherein the increased hydrostatic pressure would reduce sodium reabsorption and increase sodium excretion (Kaloyanides et al, 1971). Extracellular fluid (ECF) and plasma volume would presumably shrink enough to lower the blood pressure back to its previous level.

### Resetting of Pressure-Volume Control

In patients with primary hypertension, a rightward or resetting of this pressure-sodium excretion curve prevents the return of pressure to normal (Fig. 3.8). The process starts with increased renal vascular resistance, reflecting a preferential constriction of efferent arterioles, perhaps by a humoral stimulus with renin-angiotensin being an obvious candidate. The decrease in renal blood flow increases filtration fraction. The peritubular capillary blood, with less sodium and water, will have a higher oncotic pressure, favoring sodium reabsorption. The retained sodium and water overfills the vascular bed, raising blood pressure further. Once a certain level is reached, the higher set pressure-sodium excretion relation comes back into play, returning sodium excretion to balance intake—but at the cost of a persistently elevated blood pressure. This resetting of the renal perfusion pressure-sodium excretion control mechanism has been shown experimentally (Tobian et al, 1975; Roman and Cowley, 1985) and in patients with two forms of secondary hypertension, primary aldosteronism and renovascular hypertension (Kimura et al, 1987). When the hypertension was relieved in these patients, the curves shifted leftward, back toward normal.

Guyton (1987) lists many factors, some intrinsic to the kidney, others extrinsic, that may alter the renal pressure-natriuresis curve. As shown in Figure 3.8, the resetting of the pressure-natriuresis curve involves an increase in filtration fraction, the proportion of renal blood flow that is filtered, determined by dividing glomerular filtration rate (GFR) by renal plasma flow (RPF). In normal people, this would be about 120 ÷ 600 or 0.20. Numerous studies have shown that in early hypertension, GFR is usually well maintained but RPF is reduced, thereby increasing the filtration fraction (Brod, 1960; de Leeuw and Birkenhäger, 1983; London et al, 1984). A lower RPF has even been found in the normotensive offspring of hypertensive parents (van Hooft et al, 1989). This selective decrease in renal blood flow reflects an increased resistance within the renal circulation affecting the efferent arterioles more than the afferent arterioles.

Radioxenon measurements of renal blood flow (RBF) have provided strong evidence for a reversible intrarenal vasoconstriction in early hypertension that may be mediated by increased sympathetic nervous activity since it usually could be reversed by the adrenergic blocker phentolamine (Hollenberg et al, 1978).

A greater level of activity of the renin-angiotensin system may also be involved. A group of hypertensives put through a mild emotional stress had a much greater fall in RBF than did a group of normotensives (Hollenberg et al, 1981). The changes in RBF were inversely related to changes in plasma renin activity (PRA) levels, with the greatest falls in RBF occurring in those hypertensives with the greatest rises in PRA.

## Experimental Support

Although norepinephrine and angiotensin II will constrict both afferent and efferent arterioles (Carmines et al, 1986), greater constriction of the renal efferent vessels has been found, particularly with AII (Heller and Horácek, 1986), thereby reducing RBF and increasing GFR and the filtration fraction. This may reflect a protective vasodilation of afferent arterioles by AII-stimulated prostaglandin production (Hura and Kunau, 1988).

The data supporting a preferential constriction of the renal efferent arterioles in response to both catecholamines and AII provide a basis for an increased renal vascular resistance and filtration fraction that would be responsible for the resetting of pressure-natriuresis in hypertensives. As we shall see, it is likely that hypertensives are exposed to increased levels of both catechols and angiotensin.

The reset pressure-natriuresis curve restores the balance between sodium intake and excretion—but at the cost of persistently elevated blood pressure (Fig. 3.9). If the pressure were to fall, sodium retention would resume, a phenomenon repeatedly observed with the use of a number of antihypertensive agents. When they lower the blood pressure, fluid retention frequently follows and, unless volume expansion is countered by a diuretic, their antihypertensive action may be blunted or lost.

## Inherited Defect in Renal Sodium Excretion

The alteration in renal function responsible for the resetting of the pressure-natriuresis curve may be inherited. Beyond the data previously noted from study of normotensive children of hypertensive parents, most of the evidence comes from rats, bred to spontaneously develop hypertension when given a high sodium diet.

Using rats bred to be either sensitive (S) or resistant (R) to the hypertensive action of dietary sodium, Dahl and Heine (1975) showed the primacy of the kidney in the development of hypertension by a series of transplant experiments. These studies show that the blood pressure follows the kidney: When a kidney from a normotensive (R) donor was transplanted to hypertensive (S) host, the blood pressure of the recipient fell to normal (Fig. 3.10). Conversely, when a hypertensive (S) kidney was trans-

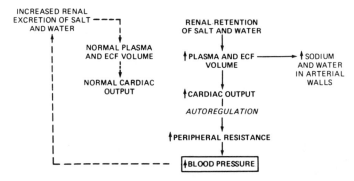

**Figure 3.9.** Hemodynamics of established essential hypertension. The elevated pressure is shown by the *dash lines* to increase renal excretion of salt and water, thereby returning plasma volume and cardiac output to normal.

planted into a normotensive (R) host, the blood pressure rose.

### Evidence in Humans

The same may be true in people. Curtis et al (1983) observed long-term remission of hypertension after renal transplantation in six black male patients who likely developed renal failure solely as a consequence of primary hypertension. Since five of these patients had remained hypertensive after removal of their native kidneys, their hypertension was presumably not of renal pressor origin. The most likely explanation for the reversal of hypertension in these patients was the implantation of normal renal tissue that provided control of body fluid volume, something their original kidneys had been unable to manage.

Of further interest, the exaggerated natriuresis seen in patients with primary hypertension was not found among hypertensive patients who had received "normotensive" kidney transplants but who remained hypertensive (Mimran et al, 1983), further evidence that there is an inherited defect in the native kidneys of those who develop primary hypertension.

Both the animal and the human data indicating that "blood pressure follows the kidney" can also be explained by mechanisms other than resetting of the pressure-natriuresis curve.

### Reduction in Filtration Surface

Brenner et al (1988) have proposed that hypertension may eventuate from a congenital reduction in the number of nephrons or in the filtration surface area (FSA) per glomerulus, either of which limits the ability to excrete sodium, raising the blood pressure and setting off a vicious cycle whereby systemic hypertension

begets glomerular hypertension, which begets more systemic hypertension (Fig. 3.11). These investigators point out that as many as 40% of the entire population under age 30 have fewer than the presumably normal number of nephrons, i.e., fewer than 800,000 per kidney, and "speculate those individuals whose congenital nephron numbers fall in the lower range constitute the population subsets that exhibit enhanced susceptibility to the development of essential hypertension." Similarly, a decrease in filtration surface area, reflected in a decreased glomerular diameter or capillary basement membrane surface area, may be responsible for an increased susceptibility to hypertension even in the presence of a normal nephron number. Either or both would reduce total surface area available for filtration and thereby enhance sodium retention.

Brenner et al (1988) invoke this congenital decrease in filtration surface as a possible explanation for "observed differences in susceptibility to hypertension, irrespective of dietary factors, which characterize different genetic populations" as well as blacks, women, and older people, all of whom may have smaller kidneys or fewer functioning nephrons. As will be described in Chapter 9, these investigators have developed a similar hypothesis for the progression of renal damage that is commonly observed among diabetics and patients with most forms of acquired kidney disease.

### Nephron Heterogeneity

Sealey et al (1988a) have provided another hypothesis for the renal contribution to the pathogenesis of primary hypertension based upon the presence of "a subpopulation of nephrons that is ischemic from either afferent arteriolar

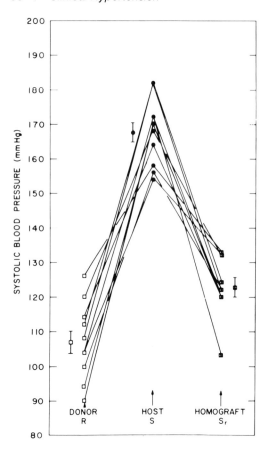

**Figure 3.10.** Effect of transplanting a "normotensive" kidney from the *Donor R* (resistant) rats to hypertensive *Host S* (sensitive) rats. The resultant blood pressure levels at a median time of 17 weeks after surgery are on the *right*. The mean blood pressure ± SE is indicated for each group. (From Dahl LK, Heine M: *Circ Res* 36:692, 1975, and by permission of the American Heart Association, Inc.)

vasoconstriction or from an intrinsic narrowing of the lumen. Renin secretion from this subgroup of nephrons is tonically elevated. This increased renin secretion then interferes with the compensatory capacity of intermingled normal nephrons to adaptively excrete sodium and, consequently, perturbs overall blood pressure homeostasis."

This hypothesis is similar to that proposed by Goldblatt who believed that "the primary cause of essential hypertension in man is intrarenal obliterative vascular disease, from any cause, usually arterial and arteriolar sclerosis, or any other condition which brings about the same disturbance of intrarenal hemodynamics" (Goldblatt, 1958). When Goldblatt placed the clamp on the main renal arteries of his dogs, he was trying to explain the pathogenesis of primary (essential) hypertension rather than what he ended up explaining—the pathogenesis of renovascular hypertension (Goldblatt et al, 1934). Although unable to place minuscule clamps on small arterioles, his experimental concept, nonetheless, is the basis for the more modern model of Sealey et al (Table 3.3). The elevated renin from the ischemic population of nephrons, although diluted in the systemic circulation, provides the "normal" renin levels that are usual in patients with primary hypertension who otherwise would be expected to shut down renin secretion and have low levels. These diluted levels are still high enough to impair sodium excretion in the nonischemic hyperfiltering nephrons but are too low to support efferent tone in the ischemic nephrons, thereby reducing sodium excretion in them as well.

Sealey and associates' concept of nephron heterogeneity differs from Brenner and associates' concept of nephron scarcity but Sealey et al agree that "a reduction in nephron number related to either age or ischemia could amplify the impaired sodium excretion and promote hypertension" (Sealey et al, 1988a).

Sealey et al expand their model to explain the varying plasma renin levels seen in both normals at different ages and patients with primary hypertension as well as the high renin levels with renovascular hypertension (RVH) and the low renin levels with primary aldosteronism (1° Aldo) (Fig. 3.12).

Note that even the low renin form of essential hypertension is shown to involve a few ischemic nephrons since "*any* renin secretion in the presence of arterial hypertension is abnormal and it works in the same way to impair salt excretion and raise arterial pressure" (Sealey et al, 1988a).

This imaginative amplification of Goldblatt's original concept brings us to a consideration of the renin-angiotensin mechanism.

## RENIN-ANGIOTENSIN SYSTEM

As seen in Figure 3.12, plasma renin levels vary within both the normal and hypertensive populations. Renin may play a critical role in the pathogenesis of most hypertension, a view long espoused by John Laragh and coworkers (Laragh and Resnick, 1988). Others give it less credit, but all agree that it is a major player in the control of blood pressure.

Figure 3.13 is a schematic overview of the renin-

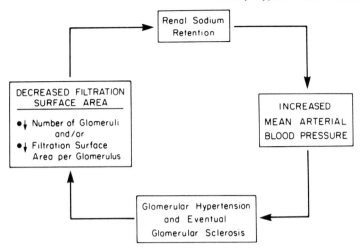

**Figure 3.11.** Relationship between decreased filtration surface area (FSA) and mean arterial pressure. Decreased FSA, due to decreased nephron number and/or FSA per glomerulus, leads to renal sodium retention, and thereby to increased mean arterial pressure. Systemic hypertension in turn promotes glomerular hypertension and eventual sclerosis further decreasing the functioning filtration surface area. (From Brenner BM, Garcia DL, Anderson S: *Am J Hypertens* 1:335, 1988.)

**Table 3.3. Hypothesis: There Is Nephron Heterogeneity in Essential Hypertension**[a]

1. There are ischemic nephrons with impaired sodium excretion intermingled with adapting hyperfiltering hypernatriuretic nephrons.
2. Renin secretion is high from ischemic nephrons and very low from hyperfiltering nephrons.
3. The inappropriate circulating renin-angiotensin level impairs sodium excretion because:
   a. In the adapting hypernatriuretic nephrons:
      i. It increases tubular sodium reabsorption.
      ii. It enhances tubuloglomerular feedback-mediated afferent constriction.
   b. As the circulating renin level is diluted by nonparticipation of adapting nephrons it becomes inadequate to support efferent tone in hypoperfused nephrons.
4. A loss of nephron number with age and from ischemia further impairs sodium excretion.

[a]From Sealey JE, Blumenfeld JD, Bell GM, et al: *J Hypertens* 6:763, 1988a.

angiotensin system showing its major components, the regulators of renin release and the primary effects of angiotensin II (AII) (Dzau and Pratt, 1986). It is of interest that, unlike other endocrine glands, the kidney releases into blood the processor enzyme renin rather than the active peptide AII. As Lever (1989) points out:

A possible reason for this is that AII released from the kidney could not act on the peripheral vasculature without causing marked effects within the kidney at the same time. The concentration of AII needed in renal blood to produce a peripheral effect would be too high. Thus, endocrine and paracrine renal mechanisms for renin could only operate independently because the pro-

cessor enzyme, which is without direct vasoconstrictor effect, is released from the kidney.

## Nature of Renin

Renin was the name given in 1898 by Tigerstedt and Bergman to the pressor material in extracts of rabbit kidneys. Page and Helmer (1940) and Braun-Menéndez et al (1940) showed that this material was renin, which acts upon a protein, angiotensinogen, to release angiotensin. Renin is stored and secreted from the renal juxtaglomerular (JG) cells located in the wall of the afferent arteriole, which is contiguous with the macula densa portion of the same nephron (Churchill and Churchill, 1988) (Fig. 3.14).

The human renin gene has been elucidated (Hardman et al, 1983), pure human renal renin purified and characterized (Do et al, 1987) and the structure of recombinant human renin determined (Sielecki et al, 1989). As reviewed by Dzau et al (1988) and Inagami et al (1988), the molecular biology of the renin-angiotensin system has been found to be increasingly more complicated as its intricacies have been revealed.

### Forms of Renal Renin

The first product of the translation of renin mRNA is preprorenin, which is processed in the endoplasmic reticulum to a 47-kDa prorenin. Prorenin may be secreted directly from the JG cell or packaged into immature granules where it is further processed to the active 41-kDa ma-

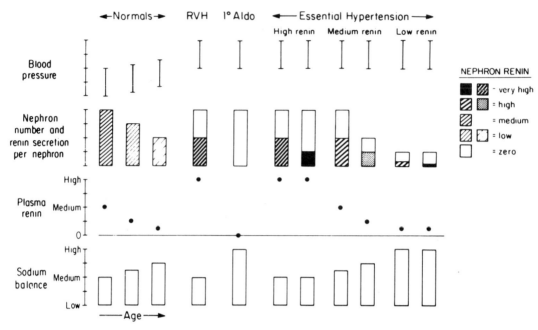

**Figure 3.12.** Renin secretion, plasma renin, sodium balance, and proportions of ischemic and hyperfiltering nephrons and nephron number in normal subjects with age, in unilateral renovascular hypertension, in primary aldosteronism, and in the three renin subgroups of essential hypertension. Relative values shown are derived from data and the hypothetical model reviewed in the text. (From Sealey JE, Blumenfeld JD, Bell GM, et al: *J Hypertension* 6:763, 1988a.)

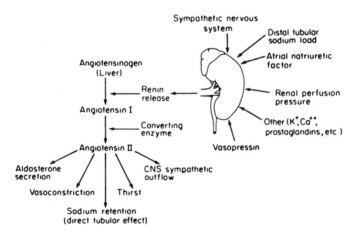

**Figure 3.13.** Schematic representation of the renin-angiotensin system showing major regulators of renin release, the biochemical cascade leading to AII, and the major effects of AII. (From Dzau VJ, Pratt RE: In: Fozzard HA et al, eds. *The Heart and Cardiovascular System.* New York: Raven Press, 1986.)

ture (active) renin, which is a glycolsylated single-chain polypeptide (Dzau et al, 1988).

### Secretion of Renal Renin

Both inactive prorenin and active renin are secreted from the JG cells, apparently by two pathways. Prorenin is secreted mainly via a constitutive (nonstimulable) pathway directly from the Golgi complex (Kawamura et al, 1988) whereas active renin is released from the mature secretory granules in a regulated manner. The rate of release of these two forms can be shown to differ with various acute stimuli (Toffelmire et al, 1989).

The manner by which active renin is secreted from its storage granules differs from most secretory processes. For one, the granules contain lysosomal enzymes, unlike other secretory gran-

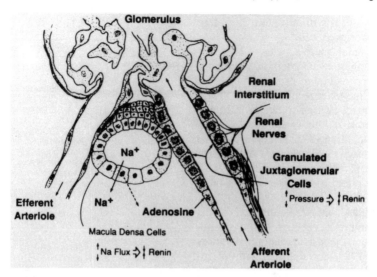

**Figure 3.14.** Juxtaglomerular apparatus (JGA), consisting of three cell types: JG cells, macula densa cells, and interstitial or mesangial cells. The renin-secreting JG cells are found primarily in the media of the afferent arteriole and act as intrarenal "baroreceptors" in that renin secretion is inversely related to transmural pressure across the arteriole or to some function of it such as stretch. In addition, these cells are innervated by the sympathetic nervous system and have many types of receptors. The macula densa cells are tubular epithelial cells found at the end of the loop of Henle and the beginning of the distal tubule of the nephron. These cells act as intrarenal "chemoreceptors" in that renin secretion is inversely related to the reabsorptive flux of sodium across them. Macula densa cells synthesize adenosine in direct proportion to sodium transport and the adenosine acts to inhibit the renin secretory activity of neighboring JG cells. Interstitial or mesangial cells surround both JG and macula densa cells, and they probably play no role in renin secretion. (From Churchill PC, Churchill MC: *ISI Atlas of Science: Pharmacology,* 1988.)

ules (Hackenthal et al, 1987). But what is really distinctive is the "calcium paradox" of renin secretion: Unlike almost all other secretory processes wherein calcium is essential for stimulus-secretory coupling, increases of intracellular calcium *inhibit* the secretion of renin (Fray et al, 1987). The trigger for the secretion of active renin is a lowering of cytosolic calcium, which in some manner leads to a fusion of granules that release renin into the cytoplasmic space from which it escapes the cell.

### Control of Renal Renin Secretion

By its location, the JG apparatus is capable of responding to changes in both vascular and tubular influences within the kidney. In addition, it is richly innervated with adrenergic nerves (Barajas and Powers, 1984). It should be noted that JG cells are, in fact, modified smooth muscle cells, with a continuous transition between the two cell types along the afferent arteriole and some cells containing both contractile elements and renin granules (Taugner et al, 1984).

The multiple factors that can alter renin secretion include those shown in Figure 3.14, changes in pressure within the afferent arte-

rioles, and sodium concentration in the macula densa. In addition, circulating and intrarenal angiotensin II exerts a direct "short loop" feedback suppression. Prostacyclin ($PGI_2$) stimulates renin secretion, whereas other products of the lipoxygenase pathway are potent inhibitors (Antonipillai et al, 1987). Keaton and Campbell (1980) reviewed the influence of multiple other factors on renin release.

### Prorenin and Inactive Renin

Prorenin is the molecular precursor for active renin and is also released from the JG cells. Detectable levels of prorenin remain in the blood after bilateral nephrectomy, suggesting—along with other evidence—that prorenin is secreted from extrarenal tissues as well (Sealey and Rubattu, 1989). Although it constitutes 80 to 90% of the renin in human plasma, no physiological or pathogenetic role for prorenin has as yet been established (Nielsen and Poulsen, 1988). When recombinant human prorenin was infused in large amounts to rhesus monkeys, no effects on cardiovascular or renal functions were noted (Sealey et al, 1989). It does not appear to be converted within the circulation into active renin but such conversion may occur within tissues, including the heart (Skinner et al, 1986).

On the other hand, there appears to be a separate prorenin-angiotensin system that functions locally within reproductive organs whose role has not been defined. Large amounts of prorenin have been found in ovarian follicular fluid and its synthesis localized to ovarian theca cells (Sealey and Rubattu, 1989). Prorenin has also been found in testes (Sealey et al, 1988b) along with AII receptors (Millan and Aguilera, 1988), supporting a possible role of this system there too.

The only disease states wherein high levels of inactive prorenin have been found are nephroblastomas and other malignant renal tumors (Carachi et al, 1987) and diabetes with microvascular complications (Luetscher et al, 1989). In a prospective study of diabetic patients, Luetscher et al have observed elevations of plasma prorenin to appear 1 to 2 years before the signs of vascular complications, usually starting with microalbuminuria. Higher plasma levels of active renin have also been noted in those teenage type I diabetics who develop albuminuria than in those who do not (Paulsen et al, 1989).

### Extrarenal Renin

Beyond these possible special sites of prorenin synthesis, a large number of other tissues have been found to have the various components of the renin-angiotensin system. Some investigators believe that multiple local renin-angiotensin systems exist and exert multiple effects, both autocrine (acting within the cell of origin) and paracrine (acting on neighboring cells) (Table 3.4). Others, including Sealey and Rubattu (1989) and Campbell (1989), believe that, although angiotensin is certainly produced in various peripheral tissues, the renin (except for that within reproductive organs) comes from the kidney, having been taken into the other tissues from the blood.

The issue is not just academic, since the physiological effects of the system and the actions of various pharmacological inhibitors upon the system may relate directly to where the system is located.

### Tonin and Other Proteases

Another protease enzyme, tonin, has been purified from rat submaxillary glands (Ikeda et al, 1981) and found in human plasma. It is said to be unique in directly forming angiotensin II from renin substrates without first forming an-

**Table 3.4. Diversity of Tissue Renin-Angiotensin Systems and Their Possible Functions**[a]

| Tissue | Documented and Putative Functions |
| --- | --- |
| Kidney | Renal blood flow, glomerular filtration rate, glomerular haemodynamics, sodium reabsorption |
| Blood vessel | Vascular tone, vascular hypertrophy |
| Heart | Myocardial metabolism, hypertrophy, and contractility |
| Adrenal | Aldosterone secretion, catecholamine release (?) |
| Brain | Thirst, behavior, blood pressure, vasopressin and catecholamine release |
| Pituitary | ACTH, gonadotropin hormone, prolactin release |
| Ovary | Ovulation (?), estrogen production (?) |
| Testes | Androgen production (?) |
| Uterus | Uteroplacental flow, contractility |
| Chorion-amnion | Unknown |
| Placenta | Uteroplacental flow, placental hormone production (?) |
| Gut (jejunum) | Absorption of ions and water |
| Salivary gland | Unknown |

[a]Adapted by Dzau VJ: *J Hypertens* 6(Suppl 3):S7, 1988, from Linz W, Scholkens BA, Han YF: *J Cardiovasc Pharmacol* 8(Suppl 10):S91, 1986.

giotensin I. Though there are experimental data in support of tonin (Boucher et al, 1978), its possible physiological role remains in question.

### Actions of Renin

Renin acts as an aspartyl proteinase that catalyzes the hydrolytic release of the decapeptide angiotensin I from its alpha-globulin substrate, angiotensinogen (Fig. 3.13). As it courses through the circulation, the two end amino acids histidyl and leucine are removed by a converting enzyme present on the plasma membrane of endothelial cells, forming the eight amino acid polypeptide angiotensin II. Conversion occurs throughout the body (Erdos, 1977), particularly in the lung. AII exerts the primary physiological effects of the system. Renin itself probably is without effect other than by its activation of angiotensin.

AII is inactivated by a series of peptidase enzymes, angiotensinases, present in most tissues and in very high concentrations in red blood cells.

### Angiotensinogen

The amount of the renin substrate, angiotensinogen, in the plasma may vary considerably and its level may play some role in the overall function of the renin-angiotensin system (Gordon, 1983). Estrogens and other stimulators of hepatic microsomal enzyme activity will increase renin substrate levels.

With the cloning and sequencing of the human angiotensinogen gene, it has been possible to identify angiotensinogen mRNA in many tissues in addition to the liver, its major site of synthesis (Clauser et al, 1989). These multiple sites, in addition to providing support for the existence of local renin systems, suggest possible other roles for angiotensinogen beyond being the renin substrate.

## Angiotensin Activity

The activity of the final product of this system, AII, is the physiologically important one. This activity reflects complicated interactions.

### Angiotensin Receptors

In a manner comparable to that of other peptide hormones, the action of AII is triggered by its interaction with receptors on the plasma membrane of the tissues responsive to the hormone (Ullian and Linas, 1989).

The binding of circulating AII to its receptors on vascular smooth muscle is impaired during sodium depletion (Brunner et al, 1972) as a result of prior occupancy of the receptor sites by increased levels of endogenous hormone generated both in the plasma and locally within the blood vessel walls (Thurston, 1976). Thereby, any given level of AII exerts a lesser response with less vasoconstriction and less of a rise in blood pressure (Kaplan and Silah, 1964). In adrenal tissue, both sodium deprivation and potassium loading independently increase aldosterone synthesis along with the number of

specific AII receptor sites in a manner independent of circulating AII levels (Rogacz et al, 1987). These opposite effects of sodium deprivation upon the response to AII—a lesser rise in blood pressure, a greater increase in aldosterone synthesis—are physiologically sensible, enabling sodium to be retained without a rise in blood pressure. As we shall see, this modulation of adrenal and vascular responsiveness to angiotensin II with changes in sodium intake has been shown to be altered in 30 to 50% of patients with primary hypertension who are "nonmodulators" (Hollenberg and Williams, 1988).

### Sites of Action of AII

Beyond the vascular smooth muscle and the adrenal cortex, AII acts with the central nervous system, at the adrenergic nerve endings, and at the adrenal medulla. These actions mainly amplify its vasoconstrictive effects on the peripheral vascular system (Fig. 3.15). The presence of AII at these various sites likely results from its local synthesis and not from its deposition from the circulation (Campbell, 1989).

### Effects of Inhibition of Renin-Angiotensin

There are four sites wherein intervention in the renin-angiotensin system is now feasible (Fig. 3.16). Studies in humans and animals using agents that work at these various sites have provided a great deal of the preceding information about the functions and controls of the renin-angiotensin system. The mechanisms by which agents can act to inhibit the system will be covered in

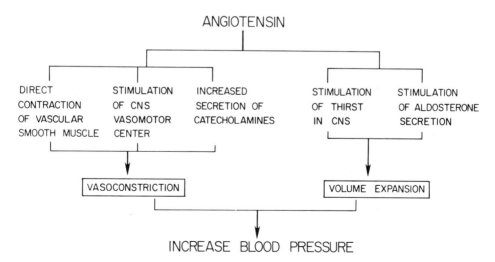

**Figure 3.15.** Most of the various actions of angiotensin are shown to be directed toward an increase in the blood pressure.

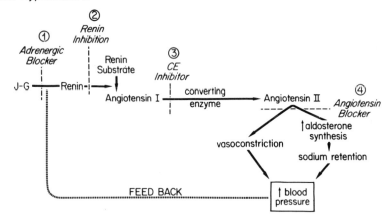

**Figure 3.16.** The four sites of action of the currently available inhibitors of the renin-angiotensin system.

detail in Chapter 7, along with practical considerations about their use to treat hypertension.

Since these various inhibitors provide temporary inhibition of the renin-angiotensin system without the need to remove vital organs, they have been extensively used in attempts to unravel the functions of the system in health and disease. From what has been learned, most find little evidence that the renin-angiotensin system is of much importance under normal conditions (Brunner and Gavras, 1980). However, when certain perturbations are imposed—volume depletion, sodium restriction, hypotension—the system comes into play and may be essential for survival (Dzau and Pratt, 1986).

Another global question has been addressed through evidence derived from use of these inhibitors: What role does the renin-angiotensin system play in primary hypertension? This question will be addressed after a brief review of the measurements of these hormones.

### Plasma Measurements

Direct assays of renin, AI, and AII are available but are technically difficult (Nussberger et al, 1988). Therefore, as of now, it is easier to measure renin "activity" for most clinical purposes.

### Clinical Use of Renin Assays

Considering all of the factors affecting the level of renin and the methodological problems in its measurement, it is a wonder that any clinical sense can be made from plasma renin assays. In fact, more agreement than not has been seen in the clinical use of PRA measurements: Almost all patients with primary aldosteronism

have suppressed values; most with renovascular or accelerated-malignant hypertension have elevated levels; and the incidence of suppressed values among patients with essential hypertension is surprisingly similar in different series (Fig. 3.17). The PRA values obtained with an assay run at pH 6.0, shown in Table 3.5, are representative of many sets of published data.

The lesson, though, is clear: Plasma renin assays should be obtained under proper and controlled conditions, assayed in a laboratory that is capable of performing radioimmunoassays and has established its own normal values, and interpreted in light of the variables already mentioned as well as those to follow. Despite these cautions, it is comforting to know that Helmer's original data with a very crude bioassay correctly identified most of the important relationships between renin and hypertension (Helmer, 1964).

The listing in Table 3.6 is not intended to cover every known condition and disease in which

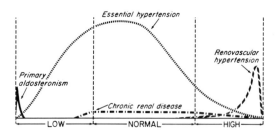

**Figure 3.17.** Schematic representation of plasma renin activity in various hypertensive diseases. The approximate number of patients with each type of hypertension is indicated along with their proportion of low-, normal-, or high-renin levels. (From Kaplan NM: *JAMA* 238:611,1977, Copyright 1977, American Medical Association.)

**Table 3.5. Values for PRA[a]**

| Condition | No. of Patients | Supine | Upright |
|---|---|---|---|
| | | *ng/ml/hr* | |
| Control patients | 200 | 1.34 ± 0.27 | 3.09 ± 0.41 |
| Essential hypertension | 113 | 1.21 ± 0.08 | 1.92 ± 0.17 |
| Primary hypertension | 12 | 0.26 ± 0.04 | 0.35 ± 0.05 |
| Renovascular hypertension | 42 | 9.17 ± 1.48 | 19.50 ± 3.23 |
| Anephric (male) | 6 | 0.00 ± 0.08 | |
| | | (Range) | |

[a]From Fyhrquist F, Soveri P, Puutala L, et al: *Clin Chem* 22:250, 1976.

a renin assay has been performed, but the more clinically important ones are listed in an attempt to categorize them by mechanism. Some could well fit in two or more categories—e.g., upright posture may involve a decreased effective plasma volume, a decreased renal arterial pressure, or catecholamine excess.

The mechanism by which renin levels fall with increasing age is listed as a decrease of renal tissue. The mechanism responsible for lower renin levels in blacks, whether normotensive or hypertensive (Kaplan et al, 1976), is unknown.

The prudent clinician will take as many of the known variables into account as possible, recognizing the vagaries of PRA, taking care neither to ascribe more certainty to a given level than is justified nor to make important diagnostic, prognostic, or therapeutic decisions based upon small differences.

Specific information about the use of PRA assays in the evaluation of various secondary forms of hypertension is provided in their respective chapters.

## Role of Renin-Angiotensin

Patients with primary hypertension tend to have lower PRA levels than do age- and sex-matched normotensives (Meade et al, 1983), although levels of circulating AII and of plasma aldosterone (reflecting one of the major actions of AII) are usually normal. The average PRA levels tend to fall with age in patients with hy-

**Table 3.6. Clinical Conditions Affecting Renin Levels**

| Decreased PRA | Increased PRA |
|---|---|
| *Expanded fluid volume* | *Shrunken fluid volume* |
| Salt loads, oral or IV | Salt deprivation |
| Primary salt retention (Liddle's syndrome, Gordon's syndrome) | Fluid losses |
| Mineralocorticoid excess | Diuretic-induced |
| Primary aldosteronism | Gastrointestinal losses |
| Congenital adrenal hyperplasia | Hemorrhage |
| Cushing's syndrome | Salt-wasting renal disease |
| Licorice excess | *Decreased effective plasma volume* |
| Deoxycorticosterone (DOC), 18-hydroxy-DOC excess | Upright posture |
| *Catecholamine deficiency* | Adrenal insufficiency |
| Autonomic dysfunction | Cirrhosis with ascites |
| Therapy with adrenergic neuronal blockers | Nephrotic syndrome |
| Therapy with β-adrenergic blockers | *Decreased renal perfusion pressure* |
| *Hyperkalemia* | Therapy with peripheral vasodilators |
| *Decreased renin substrate (?)* | Renovascular hypertension |
| Androgen therapy | Accelerated-malignant hypertension |
| *Decrease of renal tissue* | Chronic renal disease (renin-dependent) |
| Hyporeninemic hypoaldosteronism | Juxtaglomerular hyperplasia (Bartter's syndrome) |
| Chronic renal disease (volume-dependent) | *Catecholamine excess* |
| Anephric | Pheochromocytoma |
| Increasing age | Stress: hypoglycemia, trauma |
| *Unknown* | Exercise |
| Low renin essential hypertension | Hyperthyroidism |
| | Caffeine |
| | *Hypokalemia* |
| | *Increased renin substrate* |
| | Pregnancy |
| | Estrogen therapy |
| | *Autonomous renin hypersecretion* |
| | Renin-secreting tumors |
| | *Acute damage to JG cells* |
| | Acute renal failure |
| | Acute glomerulonephritis |
| | *Unknown* |
| | High-renin essential hypertension |

pertension, though plasma aldosterone levels remain normal.

Some attach a great deal of significance to the various PRA levels found in patients with primary hypertension (Laragh, 1973). According to this view, the levels of renin can identify the relative contributions of vasoconstriction (peripheral resistance) and body fluid volume expansion to the pathogenesis of hypertension. According to the "bipolar vasoconstriction-volume analysis," arteriolar vasoconstriction by AII is predominantly responsible for the hypertension in patients with high renin, whereas volume expansion is predominantly responsible in those with low renin.

This conceptual breakthrough, as original and clever as it was and still is, has not been confirmed by actual measurements. When PRA levels have been obtained along with hemodynamic measurements, no such relation has been found (Tarazi, 1976; Fagard et al, 1977; London et al, 1977a; Schalekamp et al, 1977; Julius, 1988). In fact, in each of these studies, the higher the renin levels, the lower the peripheral resistance, the reverse of the relationship predicted by the "bipolar analysis."

### Nonmodulators

Nonetheless, for many hypertensives, the renin-angiotensin system is "inappropriately" normal, higher than expected for the circumstance of a high blood pressure that should suppress release of renin from the JG cells. An explanation for the "inappropriately" normal renin levels in the majority of patients with primary hypertension has been sought beyond the higher levels expected in a normal Gaussian distribution curve. Two logical explanations have been presented: Sealey and associates' (1988a) proposal for nephron heterogeneity with a population of ischemic nephrons contributing excess renin, and Julius' (1988) concept of a state of increased sympathetic drive, a concept that will be explored later in this chapter.

A third explanation for "normal" renin levels when low levels are to be expected has been proposed by Gordon Williams and Norman Hollenberg on the basis of a series of studies that began in 1970, studies indicating that as many as half of normal-renin and high-renin hypertensive patients have a defective feedback regulation of renin-angiotensin within the kidney and the adrenal.

*Defective Feedback Mechanism.* Normal subjects modulate the responsiveness of their AII target tissues with the level of dietary sodium intake: With sodium restriction, the adrenal secretion of aldosterone is enhanced whereas vascular responses are reduced; with sodium loading, the adrenal response is suppressed, and vascular responses are enhanced, particularly within the renal circulation. With sodium restriction, renal blood flow is reduced, facilitating sodium conservation; with sodium loading, RBF increases, promoting sodium excretion. These changes are mediated mainly by changes in AII, increasing with sodium restriction and decreasing with sodium loading.

Williams, Hollenberg, and their coworkers have found that about one-half of normal to high renin hypertensives are *nonmodulators*, as shown by these differences from normals:

—After volume depletion, the adrenal secretion of aldosterone in response to AII is blunted despite higher renin-angiotensin levels (Williams et al, 1970).

—On a high sodium intake, renal blood flow does not increase, less of the sodium is excreted, and the blood pressure rises (Hollenberg et al, 1986) (Fig. 3.18). Renin suppression is blunted with volume expansion (Rabinowe et al, 1987) and during exogenous AII infusion (Seely et al, 1989).

These findings have been attributed to an abnormally regulated and rather fixed level of tissue AII that, in the adrenal, does not increase aldosterone secretion in response to sodium restriction and, in the renal circulation, does not allow renal blood flow to increase with sodium loading. The hypothesis that there is an abnormally regulated fixed local AII concentration in these nonmodulators received support from the correction of both the adrenal and renal defect after suppression of AII by use of converting enzyme inhibitors (Dluhy et al, 1989).

In the overall view of this intriguing set of observations, nonmodulation in the face of relatively high dietary sodium intake could both explain the pathogenesis of "sodium-sensitive" hypertension and provide a more targeted, rational therapy for its correction. Apparently, a blunted adrenal responsiveness to exogenous AII, part of the nonmodulation profile, is very common in black hypertensives, which may contribute to their sodium sensitivity (Cordero et al, 1989).

The investigators have begun a search for proof

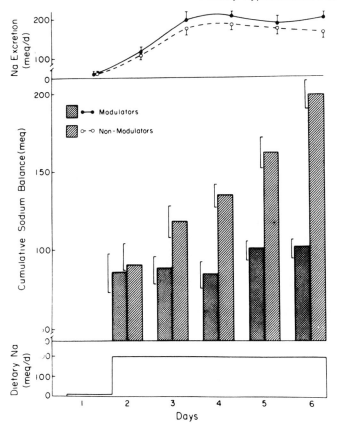

**Figure 3.18.** Documented shifts in sodium balance in patients with essential hypertension, classified as to modulating status, with a shift in sodium intake from 10 to 200 mEq per day. Note that the nonmodulators take a longer time to achieve external sodium balance and show more positive sodium balance when they do so. The weight gain in each group was congruent with the degree of positive sodium balance, and the nonmodulators increased their blood pressure significantly, whereas the modulators did not. (From Hollenberg NK, Moore T, Shoback D, et al: *Am J Med* 81:412, 1986.)

that nonmodulation is inherited with the following findings:

—a higher prevalence of nonmodulation in hypertensives with a positive family history of hypertension than in those with a negative family history (Lifton et al, 1989);
—nonmodulating features in the normotensive offspring of hypertensives (Blackshear et al, 1987; Beretta-Piccoli et al, 1988);
—nonmodulation and basal renal blood flow aggregate in families, independent of sodium intake (Dluhy et al, 1988);
—higher red blood cell lithium-sodium countertransport in nonmodulators than in modulators, although there is considerable overlap (Redgrave et al, 1989).

Clearly, these observations point strongly to a hereditary defect in the pathogenesis of hypertension in a sizeable part of the population, those with normal-renin, sodium-sensitive hypertension.

## Low-Renin Primary Hypertension

We have, then, numerous possible explanations for normal-renin hypertension, the usual finding. Even though low-renin levels are to be expected in the absence of one or another of the previously described circumstances, a great deal of work has also been done to elucidate special mechanisms, prognosis, and therapy for this subgroup. This concern may be largely unfounded since the presence of low or suppressed renin levels in a certain portion of the hypertensive population, as previously argued, most likely represents a Gaussian distribution curve that is shifted toward the low side by the larger proportion of blacks and older people who are hypertensive and is not indicative of a peculiar form of primary hypertension (Fig. 3.17). Nonetheless, the known presence of low renin levels in other hypertensive diseases associated with mineralocorticoid excess or volume expansion (Chapter 13) prompted extensive search for such a mechanism in low-renin primary hypertension. In addition, some believe that patients with low renin levels may have a better prognosis and special therapeutic needs.

*Diagnosis.* The possible mechanisms for low-renin hypertension go beyond volume expansion with or without mineralocorticoid excess as shown in the left side of Table 3.6. But an expanded body fluid volume is a logical explanation for low-renin hypertension. Though such expansion has been reported in some patients, the majority of careful analyses fail to indicate any abnormality (Lebel et al, 1974).

If volume expansion were responsible, a logical mechanism would be an excess of mineralocorticoid hormone. The possibility that lower renin levels in hypertension might reflect a subtle deficiency of the adrenal 11-hydroxylase enzyme has been raised (De Simone et al, 1985). Higher levels of deoxycorticosterone (DOC) and deoxycortisol were found in both basal and post-ACTH stimulation blood samples obtained from 15 hypertensive patients than were found in those from 15 normotensive subjects. An even more intriguing possibility has been raised by the recognition of a deficiency of the enzyme 11-β-hydroxysteroid dehydrogenase (11-β-OHSD) in the kidney as the mechanism for the syndrome of "apparent mineralocorticoid excess" (see Chapter 13). A partial deficiency of 11-β-OHSD has been found in a few low-renin hypertensives (Lewicka et al, 1989).

Despite this and prior claims that there is an excess of one or another mineralocorticoids, most studies have failed to document either an excess amount or the mineralocorticoid potency of the putative hormone (Gomez-Sanchez et al, 1985). A relatively simple explanation for low renin levels is an increased adrenal sensitivity to angiotensin II, as has been demonstrated in some patients (Wisgerhof and Brown, 1978; Wambach et al, 1984). Thus, they would need less renin-angiotensin to maintain normal aldosterone levels and volume control.

The lower PRA levels in a group of black hypertensives were abolished after 2 months of potassium supplementation suggesting a low potassium intake as a reason for their lower levels (Langford et al, 1989).

*Prognosis.* A retrospective analysis of the number of strokes and heart attacks over a 7-year interval showed that patients with low renin hypertension had none, whereas 11% of normal-renin and 14% of high-renin patients had experienced one of these cardiovascular complications (Brunner et al, 1972). High renin levels most likely indicate more severe intrarenal vascular damage, so that the higher rate of complications among the high-renin group is not surprising. However, the data of Brunner et al posed the possibility of vasculotoxic effects of presumably normal levels of renin.

A number of subsequent studies failed to document an improved prognosis in low-renin hypertension (Kaplan, 1975). One prospective study found equal numbers of heart attacks and strokes among those with initially low renin levels as among those with initially normal levels (Birkenhäger et al, 1977). A rise in renin levels was noted after a vascular complication, providing a plausible explanation for those few retrospective studies that have reported a lower incidence of complications in low-renin hypertensives. Alderman et al (1989) have found fewer heart attacks but not strokes in patients with low renin.

*Therapy.* In keeping with their presumed volume excess, patients with low-renin essential hypertension have been found to have a greater fall in blood pressure when given diuretics than do normal-renin patients (Vaughan et al, 1973). However, others find no difference between the response to diuretics in the two groups (Hunyor et al, 1975; Woods et al, 1976; Ferguson et al, 1977).

If low-renin hypertensive patients do respond better to diuretics, the response does not necessarily indicate a greater volume load. Patients with low renin, by definition, are less responsive to stimuli that increased renin levels, including diuretics, and they therefore experience a lesser rise in PRA with diuretic therapy. Less renin and AII would result in less compensatory vasoconstriction and aldosterone secretion, so that volume depletion would proceed and the blood pressure would fall further in low-renin hypertensive patients given a diuretic.

In summary, the evidence that patients with low renin are unique in the spectrum of primary hypertension seems slim.

## SODIUM TRANSPORT

Now that the roles of cardiac output and fluid volume, renal sodium retention and the renin-angiotensin system have been examined, we will turn to more detailed analysis of the specific element upon which these mechanisms focus—sodium. The presence of excess sodium—within the circulation or within cells or both—is widely held to be a necessary though not sufficient basis for the development of primary hypertension. The resetting of the pressure-natriuresis curve that prevents a shrinkage of fluid volume from self-correcting a rise in blood pressure may be looked upon as essential for the maintenance of hypertension, whatever initiates the rise in pressure. However, the renal retention of sodium may be the fundamental defect and may not play just an essential supporting role. The idea has evolved from multiple sources, but the lifelong work of Lewis Dahl and his colleagues is the basis for much of what follows. Based upon their work on salt-sensitive rats, Dahl and co-workers (1969) first proposed that permanent hypertension might evolve through this path: high sodium intake + genetic defect in renal sodium excretion → increase in body fluid volume → increase in a "sodium-excreting hormone" → hypertension.

From this rather skimpy evidence, a new hypothesis for the genesis of hypertension has evolved based upon a combination of concepts proposed by Haddy and Overbeck in 1976, Blaustein in 1977, and deWardener and MacGregor in 1980. Added to the findings of Jones and Hart (1975) and Friedman et al (1975) on altered movement of sodium and potassium in the vascular smooth muscle of rats as they developed hypertension, a complete hypothesis has been constructed linking an inhibitor of the sodium pump to an increased intracellular sodium concentration to an increase in free intracellular calcium that, in turn, is responsible for heightened contraction of vascular tissue (Fig. 3.19).

Simultaneously, a series of observations by European and American investigators (Postnov, 1975; Garay and Meyer, 1979; Canessa et al, 1980) demonstrated various abnormalities in the transport of various ions across cell membranes that did not depend upon the presence of an acquired inhibitor of sodium transport. As of early 1990, it remains uncertain as to whether the increase in cellular sodium—which is likely present in hypertensives (Hilton, 1986)—develops as a primary defect in permeability across the cell membrane (Furspan and Bohr, 1988) or as a secondary effect of endogenous sodium pump inhibitors (Poston, 1987).

The scheme drawn in Figure 3.19 comes from multiple sources, starting with Dahl and including the more recent reviews by deWardener and MacGregor (1983), Haddy (1987), and Blaustein (1988), among many others. Without regard to chronological order of discovery, let us examine each piece of the scheme in sequence.

The scheme indicates that stress may be one of the primary initiators of the sequence by increasing sympathetic nervous system activity that directly or through stimulation of renin-angiotensin would constrict renal efferent arterioles and lead to volume retention. In addition to the prior coverage of the renal events, more about stress and sympathetic activity will follow the description of the remaining steps in the sequence.

## Excess Dietary Sodium

After reviewing the available evidence about sodium intake and hypertension to be summarized in the following sections, I conclude that dietary sodium excess is intimately involved in the pathogenesis of primary hypertension. Others reviewing the same evidence do not, stating that "it is misguided to claim epidemiological or physiological evidence that the present intake of salt in Western countries causes high blood pressure" (Brown et al, 1984). Still others accept a role for sodium but question its primacy (Dustan and Kirk, 1989).

The view that excess sodium intake is intimately involved reflects the belief of a large number of investigators perhaps most completely summarized by Denton in the last 87 pages of his book *The Hunger for Salt* (1982). To quote Denton's nearly final words: "There are good grounds, but by no means a proven case, for suspecting excess salt intake, probably associated with reduced potassium intake, in the aetiology of hypertension in Western-type communities."

My interpretation of these "good grounds" can be summarized thusly: Western diets contain many times the daily adult sodium requirement. Only part of the population may be susceptible to the deleterious effects of this high sodium intake, presumably because they have the inherited renal defect in sodium excretion. As portrayed in Figure 3.20, almost everyone ingests an excess of sodium beyond the threshold needed to induce hypertension. Therefore, among such populations, it may not be possible to show a relationship between sodium intake and blood pressure; the absence of such a relationship in no way detracts from the possible

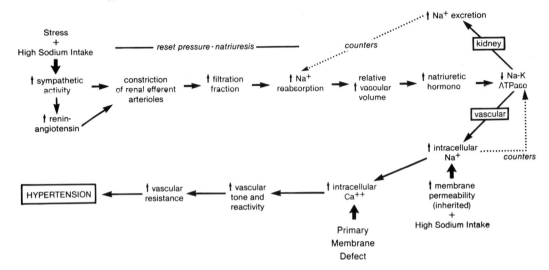

**Figure 3.19.** Hypothesis for the pathogenesis of primary (essential) hypertension, starting from one of three points, shown as *heavy arrows*. The first, starting on the *top left*, is the combination of stress and high sodium intake, which induces an increase in natriuretic hormone and thereby inhibits sodium transport. The second, at the *bottom right*, invokes an inherited defect in sodium transport to induce an increase in intracellular sodium. The third, at the *bottom middle*, suggests a primary membrane defect that directly leads to increased free intracellular calcium. (From Kaplan NM: Systemic hypertension: mechanisms and diagnosis. In: Braunwald E, ed. *Heart Disease*, Philadelphia: WB Saunders, 1988:833.)

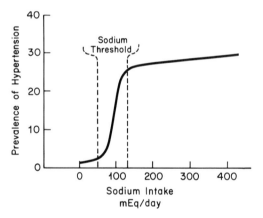

**Figure 3.20.** Probable association between usual dietary sodium intake and the prevalence of hypertension in large populations. (From Kaplan NM: *JAMA* 251:142, 1984, Copyright 1984, American Medical Association.)

role of excess dietary sodium in causing hypertension.

### Evidence for a Role for Excess Sodium

The evidence for this role will now be provided along with some of the data to the contrary. Before going into the evidence, note should be taken of studies suggesting that chloride, and not just sodium, may be involved. In two classic rat models of "sodium-dependent" hyperten-

sion, hypertension could be induced with sodium chloride but not with sodium bicarbonate or ascorbate, supporting a role of the chloride anion in sodium sensitivity (Kurtz and Morris, 1983; Whitescarver et al, 1984). In people, too, the blood pressure (BP) rises more with NaCl than with NaHCO$_3$ (Morgan, 1982) or Na citrate (Kurtz et al, 1987). On the other hand, excess chloride without sodium failed to induce hypertension in rats (Whitescarver et al, 1984) so that it may require both sodium and chloride in concert.

These preliminary studies suggest that both the experimental and epidemiological evidence about sodium excess and the therapeutic implications of sodium restriction need to take the anion into account. The issue is largely academic since chloride is the major anion accompanying sodium in the diet and in the body fluids. Most of what is known considers only sodium, though in almost all instances the sodium is in the form of the chloride salt. These data include:

—Primitive, unacculturated people from widely different parts of the world who do not eat sodium have no hypertension, nor does the blood pressure rise with age as it does in all "civilized" populations (Page, 1979). As an example, the Yanomamo Indians of northern Brazil, who excrete only about 1 mEq of sodium per day, have an average BP of 107/67 among men and 98/62 among women aged 40 to 49 (Oliver et al, 1975).

—The lack of hypertension may be attributable to other differences in life style, but comparisons made in groups living under similar conditions relate the BP most directly to the level of dietary sodium intake (Lowenstein, 1961; Prior et al, 1968; Page et al, 1981). Moreover, when unacculturated people, free of hypertension, adopt modern life styles, including increased intake of sodium, their BP rises (Rikimaru et al, 1988), and hypertension appears (Maddocks, 1967; Prior et al, 1968; Poulter et al, 1984).

—In large populations, significant correlations between the level of salt intake and the frequency of hypertension have been found by most (Kesteloot et al, 1988; Khaw and Barrett-Connor, in press; Poulter et al, 1988) but not by some (Smith et al, 1988). In the largest study, 10,079 men and women aged 20 to 59 in 52 places around the world had a 24-hour urine analyzed for electrolytes and BP measured (Intersalt Cooperative Research Group, 1988). For all 52 centers, there was a positive correlation between sodium excretion and both systolic (SBP) and diastolic (DBP) blood pressure but an even more significant association between sodium excretion and the slope of BP with age (Fig. 3.21). Unfortunately, the levels of 24-hour sodium excretion included four that were very low and the remaining 48 that were all above 100 mmol.

Therefore, the data shed no light on what may be the critical range, between 50 and 100 mmol/day as shown in Figure 3.20.

—When hypertensives are sodium restricted, their BP falls. As perhaps most graphically shown by Kempner with his rice diet containing less than 8 mEq of sodium per day, dramatic falls in BP may follow rigid sodium restriction (Kempner, 1974). Less rigid restriction to a level of 75 to 100 mEq per day has been found to lower BP modestly in most, but not all, studies (Staessen et al, 1989).

—Though it may never be possible to show conclusively that salt intake causes hypertension in people, it is fairly easy to do so in animals. As in people, there must be a genetic predisposition. In those with the genetic lesion, exposure to sodium leads to hypertension—the more sodium and the earlier it is added to the diet, the higher the BP (Dahl et al, 1972; Louis et al, 1971). It may not be possible to perform long-term intervention studies starting with infants and children to confirm that sodium restriction can prevent hypertension or that sodium excess can cause it in humans. A short-term 6-month study on almost 500 newborn infants showed that the half whose sodium intake was reduced by about one-half had a 2.1 mm Hg lower SBP at the end of the 6 months than did the half who were on the higher sodium intake (Hofman et al, 1983).

—A high sodium intake may activate a number

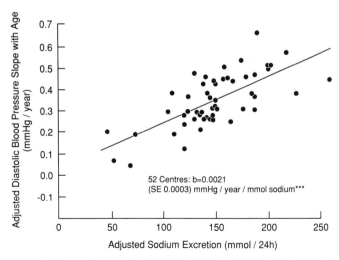

**Figure 3.21.** Cross center plots of diastolic blood pressure slope with age and median sodium excretion and fitted regression line for 52 centres, also adjusted for body mass index and alcohol intake. ***p < 0.001. (From Intersalt Cooperative Research Group: *Br Med J* 297:319, 1988.)

of pressor mechanisms. Data from animal models show increased pressor responses to exogenous AII, which may reflect increased numbers of vascular receptors to AII (Catt et al, 1984). A number of features in salt-loaded animals suggest a hyperadrenergic state that could reflect a release from central alpha₂-adrenergic inhibitory mechanisms (Gavras, 1986). The signal by which sodium loading induces hypertension may be swelling of neural tissue near the volume control centers (Lee et al, 1989).

## Sodium Sensitivity

Since almost everyone in Western countries ingests a high sodium diet, the fact that only 20% or so will develop hypertension suggests a variable degree of sodium sensitivity, though obviously heredity and other environmental exposures may be the major determinants. Short periods of high sodium intake, in most studies involving 200 to 400 mmol per day for 10 to 30 days, will cause the BP to rise in some but not all normotensive or borderline hypertensive people. Those whose blood pressure rises by 10% or by 10 mm Hg are usually called "sodium sensitive," the others "sodium resistant" (Kawasaki et al, 1978). Weinberger et al (1986) define sodium sensitivity as a 10-mm Hg or greater decrease in mean blood pressure the morning after 1 day of a 10-mEq sodium diet during which three oral doses of furosemide were given at 1000, 1400, and 1800. They found that half of hypertensives were sodium sensitive, twice more than seen among normotensives (Fig. 3.22). Whether the world can be divided neatly into two such populations remains to be seen, the more likely situation being a continuously progressing responsiveness that may be heightened with increasing age (Weinberger et al, 1986). However, a large number of altered responses have been reported among the sodium-sensitive group while on a high sodium intake, including these:

—greater increase in cardiac output from a higher sympathetic drive (Fujita et al, 1980);
—a reduced ability to excrete a sodium load, related to a lesser fall in renal blood flow and lesser renal vascular response to infused AII (Hollenberg and Williams, 1988);
—less suppression (Gill et al, 1988) and higher levels of plasma norepinephrine, both on a regular and a high sodium intake (Koolen and van Brummelen, 1984a);

—increased pressor response to exogenous norepinephrine (Skrabal et al, 1984);
—higher levels of atrial natriuretic factor (Kohno et al, 1987);
—a fall in forearm blood flow and rise in forearm vascular resistance (Koolen and van Brummelen, 1984a);
—lower venous capacitance (Sullivan and Ratts, 1988);
—less rise in dopamine excretion (Sowers et al, 1988);
—greater suppression of serum calcium and a greater rise in intracellular free calcium (Oshima et al, 1988);
—greater increase in intracellular [red blood cell (RBC)] sodium concentration (Oshima et al, 1989).

Beyond these altered responses on a high sodium diet, the sodium-sensitive patients have been found to have lower baseline renin levels (Weinberger et al, 1986) and a lesser activation of their renin-aldosterone system when put on a sodium-restricted diet (Koolen and van Brummelen, 1984b; Sullivan and Ratts, 1988). Thus, in most ways, sodium-sensitive hypertensives appear to be relatively, if not absolutely, volume expanded, with a suppressed, less responsive renin-aldosterone mechanism.

Whatever the mechanism, it appears that sodium sensitivity is heritable, with close mother-offspring resemblance in blood pressure change with sodium restriction (Miller et al, 1987). A genetic contribution is further supported by an association with haptoglobin 1-1 phenotype (Weinberger et al, 1987).

Beyond all of these experimental and clinical findings, a high sodium intake may cause hypertension by activating a natriuretic hormone that works to raise the BP in a manner that will soon be described as the next major step in this pathogenetic scheme.

### Potential Benefit of Sodium Restriction

These observations and many more provide adequate evidence, admittedly in large part circumstantial, to indict excess sodium as a probable factor in the genesis of hypertension. Though some are not convinced (Brown et al, 1984), most believe that no harm and a great deal of potential good could come from a reduction in dietary sodium intake to a level of 60 to 80 mEq per day.

Brown et al (1984) have attempted to justify their concern about sodium restriction by calling

SODIUM SENSITIVITY AND RESISTANCE IN NORMAL AND HYPERTENSIVE SUBJECTS

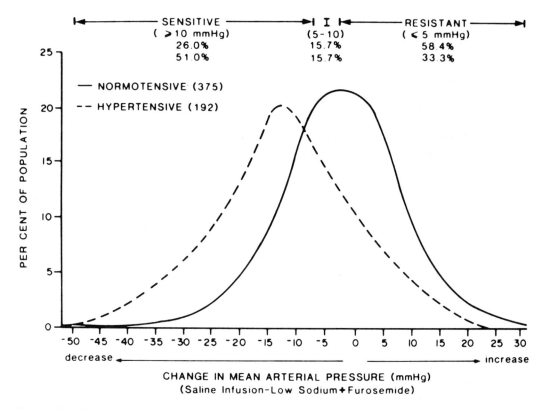

**Figure 3.22.** Blood pressure responses to the maneuvers in (——) normotensive (n = 375) and (---) hypertensive (n = 192) subjects. The definitions are identified. The hypertensives are significantly (p < 0.001) more sodium sensitive than the normotensives. The distributions are Gaussian. (From Weinberger MH, Miller JZ, Luft FC, et al: Definitions and characteristics of sodium sensitivity and blood pressure. *Hypertension* 8(Suppl II):II-127, 1986, and by permission of the American Heart Association, Inc.)

attention to studies of "normal rats [that] show a rise of blood pressure with salt restriction" (Seymour et al, 1980) and experiments with rats wherein sodium restriction stunts growth (Toal and Leenen, 1983) and increases susceptibility to the effects of hemorrhage (Göthberg et al, 1983) or raises the BP (Ott et al, 1989). However, when the designs of these studies are examined, they are seen not to be applicable to people, since they all used markedly low sodium diets—less than 1% (Ott et al, 1989), 3% (Seymour et al, 1980), 6% (Toal and Leenen, 1983), or 10% of normal (Göthberg et al, 1983)—far below what anyone has suggested for the treatment or prevention of hypertension in the human. Moreover, the rats made hypertensive with the 3% of normal sodium intake by Seymour et al (1980) were uninephrectomized. So let no one be concerned about the potential harm of moderate restriction of dietary sodium intake. None

has been shown in animals, much less in man. For instance, no ill effects or loss of exercise capability were noted among a group of normotensives who consumed a 50-mmol/d sodium-restricted diet for 2 weeks while exercising strenuously in a hot environment (35°C) (Hargreaves et al, 1989).

Those who question the wisdom of such a reduction should remember that our current high sodium-low potassium intake is a recent phenomenon, beginning perhaps 2000 years ago and accelerated by modern food processing that adds sodium and removes potassium. In the usual diet, as little as 15% of total sodium consumption is discretionary, the rest already added to the food we purchase (Sanchez-Castillo et al, 1987). Our herbivorous ancestors probably consumed less than 10 mEq of sodium per day, whereas our carnivorous ancestors might have eaten 30 mEq per day (Eaton et al, 1988) (Table 3.7).

Much of our current preference for a high sodium intake likely is an acquired taste, one that may be acquired early in childhood (Beauchamp, 1987). As pointed out by Meneely and Battarbee (1976), this increase in sodium intake has been so recent that genetic adaptation has not been possible. Since evolutionary changes to preserve Darwinian fitness are not needed if new environmental factors only produce disability or death after the reproductive years, modern people may simply not be able to adapt successfully to their high sodium exposure (Trowell, 1980).

## Sodium Retention—Increase in ECF Volume

With more than enough sodium in the diet and many mechanisms to explain sodium sensitivity, let us consider the hypothesis that patients with primary hypertension are in "a state of continuous correction of a slightly expanded extracellular fluid volume" (deWardener and MacGregor, 1980).

### Increased Inhibitor of Sodium Transport

The next step in this scheme is based on an observation by Dahl and coworkers in the late 1960s that was incorporated into an expanded hypothesis by deWardener and MacGregor (1980, 1983). As part of their multiple studies on salt-sensitive and salt-resistant rats, Dahl and coworkers joined one of each type together by parabiosis, in which two animals are chronically united by an area of skin and subcutaneous tissue (Knudsen et al, 1969). When a salt-sensitive rat was joined to a nephrectomized salt-resistant

rat, the BP of the salt-resistant animal rose slowly and progressively. Dahl and coworkers explained the development of this hypertension by postulating that a "hypertensinogenic" substance made in the salt-sensitive rat had crossed over into the salt-resistant animal. Without specific evidence for the nature of this substance, Dahl et al (1969) postulated that it was a "sodium-excreting hormone" produced by the salt-sensitive rat to compensate for its genetically driven increase in renal sodium retention, a hormone that also had the capacity to induce hypertension.

The search for a "sodium-excreting hormone," i.e., a natriuretic hormone, had already begun in patients with renal failure (Welt et al, 1964), but not until the last few years have investigators provided evidence linking a natriuretic hormone with the genesis of hypertension, as proposed by Dahl et al.

## Ion Transport Across Membranes

Before proceeding, a brief description will be provided of the cell membrane and the transport systems that control the movement of sodium, potassium, calcium, and other ions across these membranes (Fig. 3.23). These transport systems are needed to maintain the marked differences in concentration of these ions on the outside and inside of cells as well as to provide the electrochemical gradients needed for various cell functions. Abnormalities of the physical properties of the membrane or of one or more of the transport systems have been implicated in the pathogenesis of hypertension. Most of what follows relates to vascular smooth muscle cells but, since such cells are not available for study in humans, surrogates such as red and white blood cells have mainly been used. Fortunately, at least for leucocytes, intrinsic characteristics of cell membrane transport are similar to those seen in human vascular smooth muscle (Aalkjaer et al, 1986). Since white cells have transport systems much closer to other body cells than do red cells, data from them seem more likely to be physiologically pertinent (Hilton, 1986).

At the onset, it should be noted that the literature on cell transport in hypertension is clouded by inadequate attention in many studies to the multitude of environmental and technical factors that can give erroneous data, as described by Williams et al (1988) and Bianchi et al (1988). For example, inadequate matching of hypertensive subjects and normotensive controls for age and weight can lead to false-positive results on

**Table 3.7. Estimated Diet of Late Paleolithic Man Versus That of Contemporary Americans[a]**

|  | Late Paleolithic Diet (Assuming 35% Meat) | Current American Diet |
|---|---|---|
| Total dietary energy (%) |  |  |
|   Protein | 33 | 12 |
|   Carbohydrate | 46 | 46 |
|   Fat | 21 | 42 |
| Polyunsaturate:saturate fat ratio | 1.41 | 0.44 |
| Sodium (mg) | 690 | 3400 |
| Potassium (mg) | 11000 | 2400 |
| K:Na ratio | 16:1 | 0.7:1 |
| Calcium (mg) | 1500-2000 | 740 |

[a]From Eaton SB, Konner M, Shostak M: *Am J Med* 84:739, 1988.

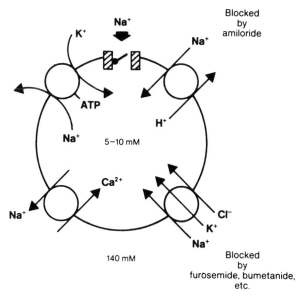

**Figure 3.23.** Sodium transport systems. *Clockwise from the top,* these include the sodium channel, $Na^+/H^+$ antiport exchange, $Na-K$ cotransport, $Na^+-Ca^{2+}$ exchange, and the $Na^+-K^+$ ATPase pump. (From Lazdunski M: *Am J Med* 84(Suppl 1B):3, 1988.)

intracellular cations and transport (Bramley et al, 1986). Even one of the widely accepted "facts," i.e., intracellular sodium is increased, has been questioned, with data showing that under appropriate experimental conditions erythrocyte intracellular sodium concentration is *reduced* in human hypertension (Simon, 1989). On the other hand, most have found that white cell sodium concentration is elevated (Hilton, 1986). Obviously, caution is needed in interpreting data about any of these highly dynamic and interrelated functions that are obtained by static and often highly artificial techniques.

### Defects of Sodium Transport

After an increase in intracellular sodium was recognized as a common feature of three forms of experimental hypertension, Vanatta (1951) suggested that "this might be a fundamental chemical disturbance of this disease state." Soon thereafter, working at the same medical school (where, I am proud to say, the author was a student at the time and remains a faculty member), Tobian and Binion (1952) provided the first demonstration of an increased concentration of sodium within tissue from hypertensive humans, namely the renal arteries obtained from hypertensive patients at necropsy. Losse et al (1960) next reported an increase in sodium within the red cells of patients with hypertension. These same investigators then reported an increased

net passive influx of radiolabeled sodium into red cells of hypertensive patients (Wessels et al, 1967). The observations seemed to elicit little interest until 1975 when Edmundson et al reported both an elevated sodium content and a lower active sodium efflux rate in the white cells of 17 patients with uncomplicated primary hypertension.

Since then, additional defects in sodium transport have been reported, mostly in the red and white blood cells of patients with primary hypertension and, in some studies, in their normotensive relatives (Table 3.8). The defects are not found with secondary forms of hypertension.

As will be seen, many of these abnormalities in ion transport across membranes are thought to induce hypertension by increasing the concentration of free calcium within vascular smooth muscle cells either directly or indirectly through an increase in intracellular sodium concentration.

### Cell Membrane

The cell membrane, composed of proteins and lipids, is semipermeable and allows for the passive movement of some ions. However, its structure protects against much passive movement and provides the framework for a number of receptor pumps and other devices that control ionic fluxes (Freidman, 1983). The basic mo-

**Table 3.8.   Transport Defects in Red and White Blood Cells Reported in Patients with Hypertension**

| Measurement | Defect | Reference |
|---|---|---|
| Red blood cells | | |
|   Intracellular Na content | Increased | Losse et al, 1960 |
|   Passive Na influx | Increased | Wessels et al, 1967 |
|   Na efflux (ouabain-resistant) | Increased | Postnov et al, 1977 |
|   Na efflux rate constant | Increased | Fitzgibbon et al, 1980 |
|   Na efflux (ouabain-sensitive) | Decreased | Walter and Distler, 1982 |
|   Na-K cotransport | Decreased efflux of Na[a] | Garay and Meyer, 1979 |
|   Na-Li countertransport | Increased rate[a] | Canessa et al, 1980 |
|   K-Na countertransport | Increased K efflux | Adragna et al, 1981 |
|   Na-K pump (ouabain-sensitive) Rb uptake | Increased Rb influx[a] | Woods et al, 1981 |
|   Calcium binding | Decreased[a] | Postnov et al, 1977 |
|   Calcium pump activity | Decreased | Devynck et al, 1981 |
|   Cell-membrane fluidity | Decreased | Orlov et al, 1982 |
| White blood cells | | |
|   Intracellular Na content | Increased | Edmundson et al, 1975 |
|   Na influx | Increased[a] | Nielsen et al, 1989a |
|   Na-K pump (ouabain-sensitive) | Decreased Na[+] efflux | Edmundson et al, 1975 |
|   Membrane permeability | Increased | Forrester and Alleyne, 1981 |
|   Intracellular calcium | Increased | Oshima et al, 1988 |

[a]Defect also found in normotensive relatives of patients with primary hypertension.

lecular structures of multiple ion channels are now partly known, and considerable work is being done to define them completely (Catterall, 1988).

*Defects in Hypertension.*   An increase in the permeability to sodium has been found to be a generalized characteristic of membranes in sodium-dependent forms of hypertension in animals and in man (Furspan and Bohr, 1988). In addition, the structure of the erythrocyte membrane both in spontaneously hypertensive rats and in patients with primary hypertension has been found to be altered (Postnov and Orlov, 1985), and increased turnover of inositol phospholipids has been found in the erythrocyte membranes of the normotensive children of hypertensive parents (Riozzi et al, 1987a). These findings suggest that defects in membrane physiochemical function are genetically determined and could be involved in the pathogenesis of primary hypertension.

Beyond these and other structural changes, the red blood cells of both genetically hypertensive rats (Devynck et al, 1981) and patients with essential hypertension (Postnov et al, 1984) have been shown to handle calcium abnormally. The membranes do not bind calcium as avidly and do not pump calcium out of cells as efficiently. More about calcium handling will be considered later in this chapter since a primary defect in the membrane handling of calcium has been proposed as a mechanism that secondarily increases sodium permeability (Swales, 1983).

**Sodium Pump**

Since the ionic concentrations on the two sides of the cell membrane are so unequal, energy must be continuously expended to maintain these inequalities. Specific pumps for $Na^+$, $K^+$, $Ca^{2+}$, and $Mg^{2+}$ are known and, of these, those that control the active transport of sodium may consume as much as half of the body's energy expenditure.

The extrusion of sodium from within cells is the primary task of the membrane-bound, magnesium-dependent enzyme $Na^+$, $K^+$-ATPase, the $Na^+$ pump. This enzyme catalyzes the breakdown of adenosine triphosphate (ATP) to provide the energy for ionic movements. The activity of the pump is stimulated by an increase of sodium on the inside or of potassium on the outside of the cell membrane and is inhibited by cardiac glycosides. Ouabain is usually used to inhibit the pump in experimental work, the difference between sodium movement before and after ouabain being taken as the level of pump activity.

*Defects in Hypertension.*   A *decrease* in the activity of the sodium pump, measured as the rate of ouabain-sensitive sodium efflux, has been found in the leucocytes of patients with essential hypertension (Edmundson et al, 1975) and in some of their first-degree relatives (Heagerty et al, 1982). Subsequently, erythrocyte sodium pump activity has been reported to be either *normal* (Ringel et al, 1987; Tuck et al, 1987) or *increased* (Simon and Engel, 1987; Smith et al, 1989a) in hypertensive subjects. Beyond these disparate data, kinetic studies have shown a minority of hypertensives to have a decreased apparent affinity of the RBC pump for internal Na$^+$ (Diez et al, 1987). With leucocytes, increased pump activity (Nielsen et al, 1988a) and an increased number of pumps (Nielsen et al, 1989b) have been found in young male offspring of hypertensive parents. A similar increase in sodium pump activity in the renal tubules would increase sodium reabsorption and thereby initiate volume expansion.

*An Acquired Pump Inhibitor.* With volume expansion, partial inhibition of the sodium pump had been seen in experimental animals (Haddy and Overbeck, 1976) and attributed to the production of a circulating pump inhibitor (Haddy, 1984). Blaustein (1977) postulated that such a circulating pump inhibitor could induce hypertension by inhibiting the sodium-calcium exchange in vascular tissue. Subsequently, deWardener and MacGregor (1980, 1983) put together the hypothesis that the pump inhibitor was the same as the hypertensinogenic substance postulated by Dahl et al (1969) to be responsible for the hypertension in their sodium-sensitive rats. They proposed that the pump inhibitor, then, was the natriuretic hormone and proposed the hypothesis shown in Figure 3.24.

Despite the initial results with volume-expanded hypertensive animals showing inhibition of the pump, subsequent studies with both spontaneous and induced forms of hypertension in the rat have shown an *increased* Na-K pump activity (Freidman, 1979; Pamnani et al, 1980; Overbeck et al, 1988) in a similar manner as

shown in humans. To reconcile the increased pump activity (which should reduce the intracellular sodium content) with the measured increase in intracellular sodium, Pamnani et al (1980) suggested that the increased pump activity was a secondary compensatory response to increased passive penetration of sodium into the cell. An increase in the number of pump molecules may also be an attempt to compensate for the inhibition by a circulating inhibitor of sodium pump activity in vivo, i.e., a natriuretic hormone. Thus, hypotheses may need to accommodate either an increase or a decrease in pump activity.

## Evidence for a Natriuretic Hormone

There is strong evidence for endogenous sodium pump inhibitors, although both their basic mode of action (Kelly and Smith, 1989) and their role in the pathogenesis of hypertension (Poston, 1987) remain uncertain. Part of the evidence for their existence is indirect, namely, the exaggerated natriuresis when hypertensives are given an acute sodium load (Baldwin et al, 1958). The rate of natriuresis is the highest in those with the lowest PRA levels who presumably are the most volume expanded (Krakoff et al, 1970). A higher rate of sodium excretion has also been found in eight of the 20 normotensive sons of hypertensive parents (Wiggins et al, 1978), suggesting that increased amounts of natriuretic hormone may be involved in the pathogenesis of the disease and may not just be secondary to the elevated BP.

In the face of continued evidence that plasma from volume-expanded animals and people does inhibit the sodium pump (Overbeck et al, 1988; Deray et al, 1987; Haupert, 1988), an intensive search by numerous investigators over the past 30 years has failed to prove the presence of the putative natriuretic factor. However, the search may soon be over, as a variety of digitalis-like factors that inhibit the sodium pump have been isolated (Hamlyn et al, 1989; Eliades et al, 1989; Goto et al, 1989). There may turn out to be several. Among the candidates are long chain fatty acids (Tamura et al, 1987), unstable peroxides (Masugi et al, 1988), peptides (Mir et al, 1988), and steroids (Hamlyn et al, 1989).

## Source of Natriuretic Hormone

The source of the natriuretic factor(s) is unknown, but considerable evidence from animal studies points to an origin in the brain, specifically the hypothalamus (Haupert et al, 1984;

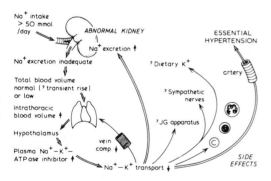

**Figure 3.24.** Sequence of events to explain a postulated inherited defect in the ability of the kidneys to excrete sodium, the observed rise in the concentration of a circulating sodium-transport inhibitor, the salt intake, and the rise in peripheral resistance in essential hypertension. *JG,* juxtaglomerular; *vein comp.,* venous compliance. (From de Wardener HE, MacGregor GA: *Lancet* 1:450, 1982.)

Mir et al, 1988). In the rat, the area of periventricular tissue surrounding the anteroventral third ventricle (AV3V) has been identified as the probable source (Brody et al, 1978).

To recapitulate, according to the hypothesis proposed by deWardener and MacGregor (1980):

Essential hypertension in man is due to an inherited variability in the ability of the kidney to eliminate sodium. This variability becomes increasingly obvious the greater the sodium intake. The difficulty in eliminating sodium increases the concentration of a circulating sodium transport inhibitor. This substance affects sodium transport across cell membranes. In the kidney, it adjusts urinary sodium excretion so that sodium balance is near that of normal subjects on the same intake of sodium, thus making it difficult to demonstrate an increase in extracellular fluid volume. In the arteriole, it causes a rise in intracellular sodium concentration, which in turn raises the intracellular calcium concentration and thus increases vascular reactivity (Fig. 3.24).

## Atrial Natriuretic Peptide

Although the search for a natriuretic hormone has been unproductive thus far, peptides have been isolated from atrial tissue that exert a potent natriuretic effect (de Bold et al, 1981). Unlike the putative factor involved in hypertension, the atrial natriuretic factor (ANF), a 24 to 28 amino acid peptide, does not inhibit $Na^+,K^+$-ATPase and is vasodilatory (Espiner and Richards, 1989). Its role in hypertension remains uncertain, but it could be involved in the exaggerated natriuresis of primary hypertension (Sørensen et al, 1989). In hypertensives, basal levels of ANF are likely normal (Hedner et al, 1989) but ANF secretion may be exaggerated during exercise (Saito et al, 1988).

Regardless of the eventual role of ANF in pathogenesis, it may have a therapeutic role since it will effectively lower BP (Janssen et al, 1989). Although, in most ways, the infusion of ANF mimics what is seen by injection of furosemide, the lure of a more "physiological" therapy—if it can be given orally—may lead to the use of ANF itself or of ANF enhancers in the treatment of hypertension.

### Brain Natriuretic Peptide

ANF-like immunoreactivity is present in the brain, suggesting that it may function as a neurotransmitter (Saper et al, 1985). In addition, another similar but definitely distinct 26 amino acid peptide has been isolated from porcine brain and called brain natriuretic peptide (Sudoh et al, 1988). This peptide is also present in cardiac tissue and appears to share many of the functions of ANF (Nakao et al, 1989).

## Other Transport Defects

Beyond the possible role of ANF et al, the hypothesis that an acquired natriuretic factor arises in response to, rather than being the cause of, volume retention remains an attractive one. However, there is also an extensive body of evidence for other, presumably primary, defects in sodium transport that could start the cascade that eventuates in hypertension as shown at the bottom right of Figure 3.19. These involve changes in membrane permeability and in various of the other known transport systems (Fig. 3.25). Since changes in some of these should not alter intracellular sodium concentration, they may serve only as markers for primary abnormalities in membrane structure and function. Beyond those shown in Figure 3.25, there may also be defects in the $Na^+/Ca^{2+}$ or $Na^+/H^+$ bidirectional antiport systems.

### Cotransport

The cotransport system involves the simultaneous inward and outward coupled movements of sodium and potassium. A decrease in furosemide-sensitive Na-K cotransport was initially reported to provide complete separation between patients with primary and secondary hypertension (Garay and Meyer, 1979). Unfortunately, subsequent experience with the procedure has shown variable results, some finding as few as 5% of hypertensives to be below the normal range, whereas others find 100% to be below the normal range (Garay et al, 1983). More recently it has been noted in up to 40% of hypertensive patients (de la Sierra et al, 1989) and found to be related to high vascular resistance (Weder and Egan, 1988).

### Countertransport

This process involves the movement of one ion in one direction coupled to the movement of another ion in the opposite direction. The technique used to measure countertransport has involved loading red cells with lithium and measuring its efflux in the presence and absence of external sodium. Though the RBC $Na^+$-$Li^+$ countertransport is purely a laboratory phenomenon, it has been accepted as a measure of $Na^+$-$Na^+$ countertransport across the plasma membrane in vivo (Swales, 1983). Since the exchange of $Na^+$ for $Na^+$ is on a 1:1 basis, it

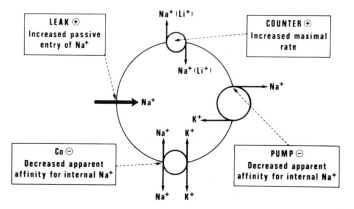

**Figure 3.25.** Stable Na$^+$ transport abnormalities found in erythrocytes from essential hypertensive patients: (1) *Leak* (+), increased passive entry of Na$^+$, (2) *Co* (−), decreased apparent affinity of the Na$^+$−K$^+$ cotransport system for internal Na$^+$, (3) *Counter* (+), increased maximal rate of Na$^+$−Li$^+$ countertransport, (4) *Pump* (−), a decreased apparent affinity of the Na$^+$−K$^+$ pump for internal Na$^+$. (From Diez J, Hannaert P, Garay PP: *Am J Physiol* 252(*Heart Circ Physiol* 21):H1, 1987.)

cannot affect intracellular sodium concentration.

Aronson (1982) proposed and Weder (1986) showed that Na$^+$-Li$^+$ countertransport is mediated by the same transporter as sodium-hydrogen exchange in the renal proximal tubule. However, Na$^+$/H$^+$ exchange is sensitive to amiloride but Na$^+$-Li$^+$ countertransport is not (Kahn, 1987). Moreover, hypertensives with higher Na$^+$-Li$^+$ countertransport do not appear to have increased proximal but rather increased distal tubular sodium reabsorption (Weinberger et al, 1989).

*Defects in Hypertension.* An increased rate of Na$^+$-Li$^+$ countertransport was originally reported in 100% of hypertensives (Canessa et al, 1980), but subsequent experience has shown it to be present in perhaps half (de la Sierra et al, 1988). Nonetheless, it may turn out to be a marker: Two distinct distributions have been found in large populations (Turner et al, 1989); it is more likely elevated in patients with a positive family history for hypertension (Carr et al, 1989); and, it aggregates among the nonmodulating subset who also are more likely to have a familial concordance (Redgrave et al, 1989).

## Sodium-Hydrogen Exchange and Intracellular pH

Another countertransport mechanism involves the exchange of external Na$^+$ ions for intracellular H$^+$ ions, the Na$^+$/H$^+$ antiport (*top right* of Fig. 3.23). This exchange is mediated by the same transporter as Na$^+$-Li$^+$ countertransport (Canessa et al, 1988) and is present in all cell membranes. Among its possible multiple major functions are regulation of intracellular pH, the entry of sodium into cells and the transfer of solutes across epithelial cells (Seifter and Aronson, 1986). In rat vascular smooth muscle, Na$^+$/H$^+$ exchange accounts for about 80% of basal sodium influx (Little et al, 1986). With the recent cloning and sequencing of the cDNA of the human Na$^+$/H$^+$ antiporter (Sardet et al, 1989), a great amount of information about this mechanism should be forthcoming.

Increased Na$^+$/H$^+$ exchange has been found in platelets of patients with primary hypertension using an indirect assay (Livne et al, 1987). With the same technique, Na$^+$/H$^+$ exchange was found to be elevated in platelets from both white and black hypertensives with no significant correlation to RBC Na$^+$-Li$^+$ countertransport (Schmouder and Weder, 1989). With more specific assays involving isotopic sodium influx into leucocytes, hypertensives have been noted to have raised total sodium influx (Ng et al, 1988). Moreover, Na$^+$/H$^+$ antiport activity, measured indirectly, was higher in leucocytes from hypertensives than in age-, sex-, weight-matched normotensives (Ng et al, 1989).

One of the major functions of Na$^+$/H$^+$ exchange may be the control of intracellular pH: If Na$^+$/H$^+$ exchange and sodium influx are increased, intracellular pH would be expected to be higher, i.e., more alkaline. The regulation of cell pH in turn is intimately involved with the control of cell growth and proliferation (Pouyssegur, 1985). Growth factors such as angiotensin II activate the antiporter so that the cytoplasm becomes more alkaline and cell growth is stimulated (Vallega et al, 1988). Arterioles from young hypertensive SHR rats were more alkaline than those taken from normotensive WKY rats at a time when vascular hypertrophy was occurring (Izzard and Heagerty, 1989). Both platelets (Astarie et al, 1989) and leucocytes (Ng et al, 1989) of hypertensives have been found to have a more alkaline pH than the cells of normotensives. Not only would such higher pH stimulate cell growth, but it would also raise cytosolic free calcium by releasing it from intracellular stores (Siskind et al, 1989) and enhance the affinity of myosin for calcium, increasing the sensitivity of vascular smooth muscle to vasoconstrictors (Danthuluri and Deth, 1989). Lever (1986) has provided a simplified scheme for these effects of AII or other growth factors on vascular cells (Fig. 3.26). More about this will be covered under Vascular Hypertrophy.

## Membrane Permeability

The increase in sodium influx via the $Na^+/H^+$ exchange should be differentiated from the passive "leak" of sodium into cells first noted by Wessels et al in 1967 and more recently confirmed by more specific techniques (Diez et al, 1987). Such an increased influx of sodium has been thought to be of little consequence since the $Na^+/K^+$ pump would presumably correct any change. However, this self-correction would not necessarily follow influx that is the consequence of specifically regulated bio-chemical processes such as the $Na^+/H^+$ antiport (Bobik et al, 1987). As noted, this influx could stimulate both contraction and hypertrophy.

In whatever manner it arises, variations in intracellular sodium have been found to predict the subsequent course of the blood pressure (Ambrosioni et al, 1988). In a 5-year follow-up of 80 young borderline hypertensives, these investigators observed striking correlation between initial lymphocyte sodium concentration and the diastolic blood pressure 5 years later.

Among others, Freidman (1983) believes that "salt-dependent forms of hypertension evolve from an increased membrane fluidity that allows ions to move more freely down their concentration gradients and enhances the activity of mechanisms for extruding $Na^+$ from cells. . . . The overall effect can be described as an increase in $Na^+$ transport activity, but it is not known whether this produces the blood pressure rise directly or indirectly through a decline in transmembrane $Na^+$ and $Ca^{2+}$ gradients.''

## Altered Lipid Composition

We shall examine further the possible connection between increased sodium and calcium, but there is a growing belief that the various changes in sodium transport previously noted are part of more global disturbances in the cell membrane that are more directly related to hypertension by their effect on calcium binding (Bing et al, 1986; Bohr and Webb, 1988).

Numerous abnormalities of membrane func-

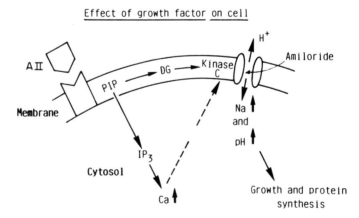

**Figure 3.26.** Schematic representation of the main events in a signaling system activated by growth factors. For example, angiotensin II occupies a membrane receptor; phosphatidylinositol biphosphate (*PIP*) is hydrolyzed by phosphodiesterase in the membrane; inositol triphosphate (*IP₃*) is released into the cytosol and diacylglycerol (*DG*) in the plane of the membrane. The latter activates protein kinase C linked to an amiloride-sensitive $Na^+/H^+$ exchanger whose activity increases. Sodium enters the cell down an electrochemical gradient and protons are extruded. The increased intracellular pH that results promotes growth and protein synthesis. (From Lever AF: *J Hypertension* 4:515, 1986.)

tion and structure have been reported in cells from hypertensive animals and people. These include reduced membrane fluidity (Masuyama et al, 1988), reduced amounts of linoleic acid (Ollerenshaw et al, 1987), increased cholesterol:phospholipid ratio (Benjamin et al, 1988), and increased protein kinase C activity (Kravtsov et al, 1988). With increased awareness of the roles played by membrane lipids in cell function (Yeagle, 1989), the recognition that blood lipid levels are more frequently deranged in hypertensives and that these are associated with changes in cation transport systems (Hunt et al, 1986) takes on even greater significance. An attempt at altering membrane lipids by dietary supplements of linoleic acid was found to decrease ouabain-resistant sodium efflux, but no changes in blood pressure were noted in this short-term study (Robertson et al, 1989). Obviously, a great deal of additional study of membrane structure in hypertension will be forthcoming, along with additional attempts to alter the structure in order to normalize function.

The preceding coverage has suggested that intracellular sodium is increased in hypertension, either through acquired inhibition of the sodium pump or through presumably inherited defects in one or another sodium transport systems. Let us now turn to the next step in the pathogenetic scheme shown in Figure 3.19—an increase in intracellular calcium.

## INCREASED INTRACELLULAR CALCIUM

Increased concentrations of free calcium found within the cytosol of vascular smooth muscle cells are thought to be responsible for the increased contractility of vessels in hypertension. These could be secondary to alterations in calcium entry, binding, or extrusion from the cells (Fig. 3.27). Studies on human cells, mostly platelets and erythrocytes, have shown changes in all three of these mechanisms.

### Increased Entry

No direct evidence is now available to demonstrate an increase in the entry of calcium into cells of hypertensive patients. Although total extracellular calcium levels, as measured in serum, tend to be higher in people with hypertension (Kaplan and Meese, 1986), it is unlikely that such slightly elevated levels could break through the normal protective mechanisms that maintain the usual 1000-fold or greater differential between extracellular and intracellular

calcium concentrations. Moreover, serum ionized calcium, the physiologically potent fraction, is either normal (Shore et al, 1987) or slightly reduced (Folsom et al, 1986) in most patients with primary hypertension.

A component in plasma ultrafiltrates from patients with hypertension has been found to increase free calcium within platelets from normotensive people (Lindner et al, 1987). The nature of this circulating factor in hypertensive patient's blood is unknown, but other investigators have reported a similar effect of a plasma fraction with a molecular weight around 100 to 1500 daltons on calcium uptake into treated human neutrophils (Zidek et al, 1987). It is possible that this plasma factor could be the putative circulating inhibitor of Na,K-ATPase, released presumably from the hypothalamus in response to volume expansion. Rather than increasing calcium entry, inhibition of the sodium pump would raise intracellular sodium and thereby inhibit the sodium-calcium exchange, increasing intracellular calcium levels by reducing calcium efflux (Hannaert et al, 1987).

### Decreased Binding

The evidence is much stronger for a decreased binding of calcium to the inner plasma membrane in both experimental models and human hypertension as first shown by Postnov et al in 1979 and confirmed by many others subsequently (Bing et al, 1987). Multiple mechanisms might work to reduce calcium binding and most involve alterations in the structure of the membrane, as suggested by the finding among hypertensives that platelet cytosolic free calcium concentration was positively correlated with plasma total cholesterol and low-density lipoprotein concentrations (Le Quan-Sang et al, 1987).

### Decreased Extrusion

Two mechanisms are involved in removing calcium in addition to the dynamic processes of release and sequestration of free calcium between cytosol and endoplasmic reticulum and mitochondria (Fig. 3.27). Both the $Ca^{2+}$ pump and $Na^+$-$Ca^{2+}$ exchange may be altered. Activity of the $Ca^{2+}$ pump ATPase was found to be significantly reduced in erythrocyte lysates of hypertensives compared with normotensives (Vincenzi et al, 1986). Blaustein (1988) has shown the importance of $Na^+$-$Ca^{2+}$ exchange for extrusion of calcium after contractile activation and his observation has been amply con-

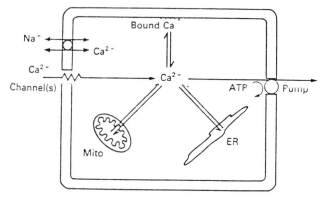

**Figure 3.27.** Mechanisms controlling cytosolic $Ca^{2+}$. Entry is mainly via calcium channels and the Na/Ca exchange; binding is to the cell membrane, mitochondria (*mito*) and endoplasmic reticulum (*ER*); exit is via the Na/Ca exchange and the $Ca^{2+}$ ATPase pump. (From Exton JH: *Kidney Int* 32(Suppl 23):S-68, 1987.)

firmed (Hannaert et al, 1987; Nabel et al, 1988; Smith et al, 1989c). Blaustein proposed in 1977 and has provided confirmatory evidence (Blaustein et al, 1986) that as little as a 5% increase in intracellular sodium via the acquired volume-induced inhibition of the sodium pump would inhibit $Na^+$-$Ca^{2+}$ exchange enough to raise intracellular calcium so that the resting tone of vascular smooth muscle would increase by as much as 50%.

### Unifying Hypothesis

Although abnormalities in calcium entry and extrusion may be involved, the strongest evidence now available supports a primary role for altered calcium binding. Swales (1983) has taken the evidence for decreased calcium binding to cell membranes as evidence for a "global disturbance of membrane function (that) causes elevation of intracellular calcium and reduces sodium pump activity" (Fig. 3.28). Moreover,

an increased intracellular calcium concentration has been shown to enhance sodium and potassium permeability across erythrocytes (Romero and Whittam, 1971). The increase in intracellular sodium would lead to an increase in sodium pump activity so that, overall, sodium pumping could be either increased as a secondary response to increased intracellular sodium or decreased as a primary membrane dysfunction.

To explain this "global disturbance" Swales (1988) invokes a disturbance of the phospholipids of the inner layer of the cell membrane, along the lines shown by Marche et al (1985), which could also be responsible for the increased membrane viscosity demonstrated by Orlov and Postnov (1982). The Swales hypothesis could explain the association of hypertension with hyperlipemia and the antihypertensive effect of polyunsaturated fats if these, in turn, were reflected in changes within the phospholipid structure of the cell membrane.

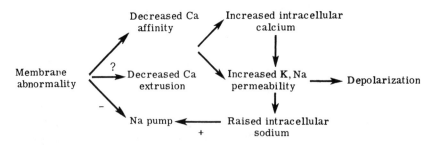

**Figure 3.28.** Sequence of events according to the membrane abnormality hypothesis. A global disturbance of membrane function causes elevation of intracellular calcium and reduces sodium pump activity. That gives rise to a secondary increase in sodium and potassium permeability, with increased intracellular sodium tending to oppose primary reduction in sodium pumping. According to this hypothesis, therefore, sodium pumping might be either elevated or reduced. (From Swales JD: In: Robertson JIS, ed. *Handbook of Hypertension, Volume 1: Clinical Aspects of Essential Hypertension.* Amsterdam: Elsevier Science Publishers, 1983:258.)

## Other Aspects of Calcium

Beyond the probability that an increased intracellular calcium is involved in the pathogenesis of hypertension, there are other fascinating aspects of the relationship between calcium and hypertension. The first relates to serum calcium levels, the second to dietary calcium intake, the third to renal excretion of calcium. Along with the third, the possible involvement of parathyroid hormone also arises.

### Serum Calcium and Hypertension

Hypertension is more common in the presence of hypercalcemia and, in most studies with sizeable numbers of patients, there is a direct relationship between total serum calcium and blood pressure (Kaplan and Meese, 1986). On the other hand, measurements of serum ionized calcium have shown a less uniform relationship to blood pressure: Some find a direct correlation (Hunt et al, 1984), others either no correlation (Strazzullo et al, 1983) or an inverse one (McCarron, 1982a). One group found the relationship to vary with the level of plasma renin activity: inverse in those with low PRA, none with normal PRA, and direct with high PRA (Resnick et al, 1983).

Nonetheless, most of the carefully collected data show a vasoconstrictive effect of increasing extracellular calcium levels, presumably by an increase in calcium influx by mass action and by a stimulation of catecholamine release (Bianchetti et al, 1983). Calcium infusion raises the blood pressure in dogs and humans but not in the hindlimbs of rats, whose arteriolar smooth muscle is relaxed by calcium (Overbeck, 1984).

### Dietary Calcium Intake

Despite the evidence that serum calcium and blood pressure are related in a direct, positive manner, some have reported an inverse relationship between dietary calcium intake and blood pressure (McCarron, 1982b; McCarron et al, 1984; Harlan et al, 1984; Garcia-Palmieri et al, 1984). Beyond numerous methodological problems with the data, others do not find significant differences in calcium intake between normotensive and hypertensive people (Sempos et al, 1986).

### Increased Renal Excretion of Calcium

As first noted by McCarron et al (1980) and confirmed by Strazzullo et al (1986a), hypertensives excrete more calcium both under basal circumstances and during a calcium infusion.

The renal leak could represent a decreased binding of calcium to kidney cells. However, another explanation for an increased calcium excretion in hypertensives is the well-described excess in calcium excretion whenever intravascular volume is expanded and sodium excretion is increased (Suki et al, 1968).

Patients with volume-expansion forms of hypertension, e.g., primary aldosteronism, excrete calcium in excess (Resnick and Laragh, 1985). The simple intake of increased amounts of sodium leads directly to an increase in calcium excretion (Breslau et al, 1982). Whether the development of hypertension is related to excess sodium intake and retention or not, an increase in urine calcium excretion can be identified even in 11-year-old boys whose blood pressures are normal but in the highest quartile of their population (Strazzullo et al, 1987).

### Increased Levels of Parathyroid Hormone (PTH)

Probably as a homeostatic response to their urinary calcium leak, hypertensives tend to have increased levels of plasma PTH (McCarron et al, 1980; Hvarfner et al, 1987). Although not nearly so high as seen with primary hyperparathyroidism (wherein hypertension is frequent), these elevated PTH levels could exert a pressor effect (Hulter et al, 1986) and be involved in the hypertension of volume-expanded states.

This possibility is supported by data from studies in both dogs (Kageyama and Bravo, 1987) and humans (Zemel et al, 1986), wherein volume expansion has been shown to raise blood pressure in association with increases in calcium excretion and falls in serum ionized calcium, which secondarily increased PTH levels. As expected, when extra calcium is given, PTH levels and the blood pressure fall in parallel (Zemel et al, 1986).

### Selective Benefit of Calcium Supplementation

This scenario implies that PTH levels elevated in response to ionized calcium levels that are lowered by hypercalciuria could be responsible for at least some of the hypertension seen in volume-expanded states (Fig. 3.29). This scheme is carried one step further: The provision of additional calcium that would raise plasma calcium (at the price of even more hypercalciuria) would shut off PTH and thereby lower the blood pressure.

The scheme fits clinical practice. Most prop-

Sodium-sensitive, Low-renin Hypertension

$$\text{Volume expansion} \dashrightarrow \uparrow U_{Ca} \dashrightarrow \downarrow \text{plasma}_{Ca} \dashrightarrow \uparrow PTH \dashrightarrow \uparrow BP$$

$$\begin{array}{c}\uparrow Ca \\ \text{intake} \end{array} \dashrightarrow \left[\begin{array}{c}\text{further} \\ \uparrow U_{Ca}\end{array}\right] \dashrightarrow \uparrow \text{plasma}_{Ca} \dashrightarrow \downarrow PTH \dashrightarrow \downarrow BP$$

**Figure 3.29.** A potential explanation for the involvement of parathyroid hormone (*PTH*) in volume-expanded forms of hypertension and for a hypotensive action of increased dietary calcium intake.

erly performed clinical studies have shown little or no overall effect of calcium supplementation among unselected hypertensives (Kaplan and Meese, 1986; McCarron, 1989). However, when patients are identified with one or more of these characteristics—increased urine calcium excretion (Strazzulo et al, 1986b), low ionized calcium (Grobbee and Hofman, 1986), or increased PTH levels (Grobbee and Hofman, 1986)—calcium supplements often cause a significant fall in blood pressure. As discussed further in Chapter 6, until the scheme shown in Figure 3.29 is documented further, caution is advised: Calcium supplements may lower the blood pressure in those who have lower serum calcium and higher PTH levels but with the potential risk of causing kidney stones.

All of the preceding discussion about calcium and hypertension focused on vascular smooth muscle. That focus may overlook the importance of the heart in the pathogenesis and maintenance of hypertension since calcium is obviously of critical importance for cardiac function.

## VASCULAR HYPERTROPHY

The nearly final step in the pathogenetic scheme for hypertension (Fig. 3.19) is an increase in vascular tone and contractility, resulting in increased peripheral resistance. This develops from an increase in intracellular calcium, induced in one of the multiple ways previously described. However, the sequence shown in Figure 3.19 wherein increased vascular resistance is the end result of one or more primary pressor events may not be correct. Rather, vascular hypertrophy may be a primary event, developing early in response to relatively mild neurohumoral stimulation and acting as the major driving force to raise resistance and blood pressure.

This modified view has surfaced in part because data from both animals (Folkow, 1987) and people (Aalkjaer et al, 1987b) have shown that resistance vessels are not more sensitive to

stimulation but rather have an increase in the ratio between wall thickness and lumen diameter that leads to the development of higher wall stress and intraluminal pressure when they are stimulated (Fig. 3.30).

As proposed by Lever (1986) (Fig. 3.2) and Heagerty et al (1988), the main rationale for the modified view is the recognition of trophic mechanisms that may induce vascular hypertrophy either in concert with an initial pressor stimulus or in a manner independent of a rise in pressure. Folkow (1987) has long favored stress-activated sympathetic nervous stimulation as a likely initiating mechanism but, as Lever (1986) points out, a number of other pressor-trophic mechanisms are likely candidates and some of these are shown in Figure 3.31. Angiotensin II is clearly a strong candidate, increasing protein synthesis in an in vitro of aortic cells by 80% in 24 hours (Berk et al, 1989). But the list is expanding explosively with one report showing seven growth factors, including platelet-derived

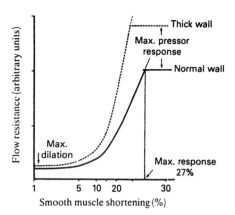

**Figure 3.30.** Increased vascular reactivity in hypertension explained by structural changes. The differences in flow resistance are calculated in a mathematical model assuming a 30% increased wall thickness being the only difference between hypertensive and normal vessels. (Modified from Folkow B: *Am Heart J* 114:938, 1987 by Westerhof N, Huisman RM: *Clin Sci* 72:391, 1987.)

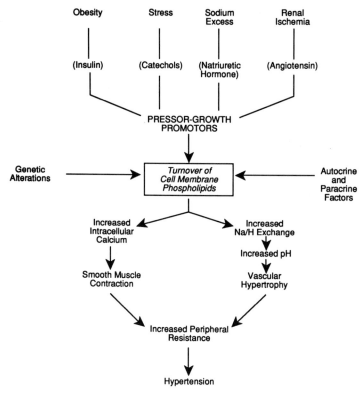

**Figure 3.31.** Scheme for the induction of hypertension by numerous pressor hormones that act as vascular growth promotors.

(PDGF), insulin-like (ILGF), and transforming growth factor-beta (TGF-β), being expressed in aortic cells (Sarzani et al, 1989). Moreover, various factors may be interrelated, e.g., AII induces PDGF in cultured vascular smooth muscle cells (Naftilan et al, 1989).

## Mechanisms of Cellular Proliferation

As seen in Figure 3.26, when a growth factor occupies its membrane receptor it activates phosphodiesterase in the membrane that hydrolyzes the phosphatidylinositol biphosphate (PIP) that comprises 5 to 15% of the total membrane phospholipid content (Berridge, 1988; Heagerty and Ollerenshaw, 1987). This hydrolysis produces two compounds: The water-soluble inositol trisphosphate ($IP_3$) is released into the cytosol, and the hydrophobic 1,2-diacylglycerol (DG) is retained in the membrane. These two compounds have two major, separate functions: $IP_3$ releases calcium from nonmitochondrial organelles, which, in smooth muscle cells, triggers contraction; DG has a second messenger role in the cell membrane, activating protein kinase C, which controls the activity of the ami-

loride-sensitive $Na^+/H^+$ exchanger. As more sodium enters and hydrogen exits, the cell becomes more alkaline; the increased alkalinity is the cell signal to provoke the nucleus to initiate protein synthesis and division. As Heagerty et al (1988) point out, the intricacies of this mechanism may be much beyond those schematically shown in Figure 3.26 and more about these inner workings is rapidly being recognized.

For now, it is clear that various pressor-trophic factors, including AII (Griendling et al, 1987; Lyall et al, 1988) induce this dual effect. These effects are separable: "The constrictor stimulus is short-term and sufficient to initiate contraction but not proliferation. Cellular growth only occurs when the tissue is stimulated excessively for a long time" (Heagerty et al, 1988).

Whether this process is the answer to Folkow's contention, it has great explanatory power, as noted by Heagerty et al (1988): "In a disease such as hypertension where abnormal medial thickening is observed, the process of activation of (the phosphoinositide) system such as by autonomic excess, and the possibility of a genetically inherited abnormal smooth muscle cell reinforcing the stimulus by proliferating more avidly, might hold the key. . . . It is conceivable that an overactive phosphoinositide system could underlie the structural changes in hypertension.''

Beyond the effects of pressor-trophic factors, the elevated pressure *per se* may lead to further structural change. Presumably, even transient rises, such as with stress-induced sympathetic surges, could set off the phosphoinositide system. This was shown in a more chronic setting by inducing coarctation of the aorta in normotensive rats (Ollerenshaw et al, 1988). With the elevated pressures above the coarctation, inositol phosphate accumulated in the aorta and its medial cross-sectional area and thickness increased. Despite the common hormonal milieu, the vessels below the coarctation did not hypertrophy, presumably because their hypertrophic machinery was not turned on by exposure to a higher pressure. Of great significance, the increase in phosphoinositide hydrolysis proximal to the coarctation preceded any significant rise in blood pressure. Thus, hypertrophy appears to have been triggered very early by the stretch induced by the initial load placed upon the aorta and not as a later consequence of high pressure.

### Endothelial Factors

Beyond the effects of pressure per se and of the various known pressor-growth factors, another area of explosive development has been the recognition of various endothelium-derived autocrine and paracrine substances that modulate either relaxation (Furchgott and Zawadzki, 1980; Vanhoutte, 1989) or contraction (Inoue et al, 1989). It is increasingly obvious that endothelial cells, rather than serving as a passive covering for the conduit of blood, are constantly interacting with shear forces, intravascular pressure, circulating hormones, platelet factors, and who knows what else to play a significant role in modulating vascular tone. Clearly, the products arising from within the endothelial cells may act locally to influence both contraction-relaxation and cell growth.

### Endothelin

Although it took some years to (apparently) identify endothelium-derived relaxing factor (EDRF) as nitric oxide (Ignarro, 1989), the amazingly fast recognition and elucidation of endothelin as an endothelial-derived vasoconstrictor (Yanagisawa et al, 1988) is a tribute to the new molecular biology. Its role in pathophysiology remains uncertain, but it is a highly potent vasoconstrictor that appears to be composed of at least three distinct isopeptides (Inoue et al, 1989). Endothelin has been found to stimulate proliferation of vascular smooth muscle cells (Grooms et al, 1989), inhibit renin, stimulate aldosterone secretion (Cozza et al, 1989), release atrial natriuretic factor, and stimulate the myocardium (Inoue et al, 1989).

It is now too soon to know where the place of these "ying and yang" influences will eventually be. Evidence is being presented of impaired endothelium-derived relaxation (Panza et al, 1988) and of imbalances between the vasodilator and vasoconstrictor factors (Lüscher, 1989) in the pathophysiology of hypertension.

### Microvascular Rarefaction

Along with the changes in larger vessel caliber and thickness, the increased resistance and subsequent elevation of pressure in hypertension may also reflect a permanent closure of capillaries and arterioles, i.e., structural rarefaction of microvessels. Such has been seen in animal models (Greene et al, 1989) and muscle biopsies from hypertensive patients (Henrich et al, 1988).

### Insulin As A Growth Factor

Of all the known pressor-growth factors, insulin seems likely to be of signal importance. Hyperinsulinemia is present both in hypertensive patients with upper body obesity and in nonobese hypertensives (Reaven, 1988). Beyond its apparent effects on cation transport across cell membranes (Halkin et al, 1988) insulin, in the presence of euglycemia, may induce hypertension in at least three other ways: renal sodium retention (DeFronzo et al, 1975); catecholamine release (Rowe et al, 1981); and what is particularly pertinent to this discussion, vascular smooth muscle hypertrophy (Stout et al, 1975).

High affinity receptors for insulin and insulin-like growth factors are present in human endothelial (Bar et al, 1988) and arterial smooth muscle cells (Banskota et al, 1989). In vitro, insulin activates the $Na^+/H^+$ exchanger (Rosic et al, 1985) and induces a remarkable growth of endothelial and smooth muscle cells (King et al, 1985). As detailed elsewhere (Kaplan, 1989), the story holds together very well for a major role of hyperinsulinemia in the hypertension, hyperlipidemia, and diabetes so commonly seen with upper body obesity (Fig. 3.32). The presence of hyperinsulinemia with obesity has been

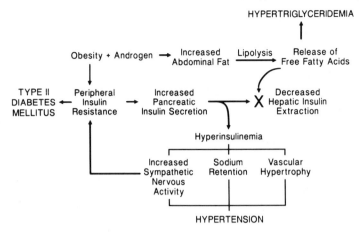

**Figure 3.32.** Overall scheme for the mechanism by which upper body obesity could promote glucose intolerance, hypertriglyceridemia, and hypertension via hyperinsulinemia.

long recognized and easily understood. However, the presence of hyperinsulinemia in non-obese hypertensives came as a surprise. Although known to reflect insulin resistance (Ferrannini et al, 1987; Shen et al, 1988), neither the mechanism responsible for the high insulin levels nor the contribution of these high levels to the hypertensive state is now known.

Among the possible explanations for the peripheral insulin resistance that leads to the hyperinsulinemia seen in non-obese hypertensives are these:

—increased sympathetic nervous system activity which impairs tissue sensitivity to insulin (Deibert and DeFronzo, 1980);
—increased dietary intake of fat, sucrose, or fructose (Reaven et al, 1989);
—differences in muscle fiber composition, with more type IIB fibers which have reduced glucose uptake during insulin infusion (Lillioja et al, 1987) perhaps secondary to their decreased capillary density.

In whatever manner it arises, hyperinsulinemia is associated with an increased prevalence of hypertension as seen even in nondiabetic people with glucose intolerance, independent of age and body mass index (Cederholm and Wibell, 1985). This likely reflects hyperinsulinemia, an association observed with hypertension in multiple groups from childhood (Burke et al, 1986) through old age (Varricchio et al, 1988). Hyperinsulinemia even in the presence of normal glucose tolerance is associated with higher blood pressure (Zavaroni et al, 1989). High insulin levels may contribute to the hypertension both

in non-insulin-dependent patients who are hyperinsulinemic because of insulin resistance and in insulin-dependent patients who are hyperinsulinemic because of exogenous administration. When doses of exogenous insulin are reduced, blood pressure may fall (Tedde et al, 1989).

**Obesity**

The particularly elevated insulin levels seen with obesity may certainly be playing a significant role in the hypertension that is so common—perhaps 3-fold more—in obese people than in nonobese. Since obesity is increasing among both children (Gortmaker et al, 1987) and adults (Harlan et al, 1988) in the United States, attention obviously needs to be directed toward its prevention and control as will be described in Chapter 6.

The risks both for hypertension and for other cardiovascular complications are more severe with predominant upper body obesity (Peiris et al, 1989). As more is learned about the metabolic differences in fat deposited in different locations (Rebuffé-Scrive et al, 1989) and as easier ways to study human adipose tissue become available (Frayn et al, 1989), hopefully it will be possible to counter the serious consequences of what is unfortunately typical in American men, a progressive increase in abdominal fat as they go through middle age.

## STRESS AND SYMPATHETIC NERVOUS OVERACTIVITY

Now that the end of the overall scheme for the pathogenesis of hypertension (Fig. 3.19) has been reached via a number of possible pathways, further consideration will be given to the possible role of sympathetic nervous system overactivity. In Figure 3.19, stress and increased sympathetic activity are shown to interact with high sodium intake to initiate the process that eventuates in persistent hypertension.

The concept has considerable support. Folkow (1989) has concluded that "excitatory psychosocial influences and increased salt intake, which at least partly operate via different genetic elements, are in fact closely intertwined, and are mutually reinforcing as to their actions . . . to gradually elevate the pressure equilibrium until a state of 'established' hypertension is reached." The evidence, even in a partial listing (Table 3.9), strongly indicates increased sympathetic nervous activity in early hypertension and, even more impressively, in the still normotensive offspring of hypertensive parents among whom a large number are likely to develop hypertension.

The place in the overall scheme wherein sympathetic nervous hyperactivity plays its role is uncertain. Clearly, it may be one of the primary

**Table 3.9. Evidence for Increased Sympathetic Nervous System Activity in Hypertension**

*Normotensive Offspring of Hypertensive Parents*
Increased heart rate and blood pressure during stress
  —Perini et al: *J Cardiovasc Pharmacol* 1988;12:S130.
Increased plasma norepinephrine response to mental stress
  —Lenders et al: *J Hypertens* 1989;7:317.
Increased plasma norepinephrine response to exercise
  —Nielsen et al: *J Hypertens* 1989c;7:377.
Decreased vasodilation after exercise
  —Ambrosioni et al: *J Human Hypertens* 1987;1:229.
Increased pressor sensitivity to norepinephrine
  —Bianchetti et al: *Kidney Int* 1986;29:882.
Increased sensitivity of isolated resistance vessels to norepinephrine
  —Aalkjaer et al: *Hypertension* 1987a;9(Suppl 3):III-155.
Increased platelet $\alpha_2$-adrenoreceptor density
  —Michel et al: *J Cardiovasc Pharmacol* 1989;13:432.
Increased WBC sodium transport (ouabain-resistant efflux rate constant) during stress
  —Riozzi et al: *Hypertension* 1987b;9:13.
Decreased sodium excretion during stress
  —Light et al: *Science* (Wash DC) 1983;220:429.
*Early Hypertension*
Elevated plasma norepinephrine levels
  —Goldstein and Lake: *Fed Proc* 1984;43:57.
Increased norepinephrine spillover rate
  —Esler et al: *Am J Hypertens* 1989;2:1405.
Increased muscle sympathetic nerve activity
  —Yamada et al: *Hypertension* 1989;13:870.
Increased heart rate variability
  —Guzzetti et al: *J Hypertens* 1988;6:711.
Increased alpha-adrenergic vasoconstriction
  —Egan et al: *J Clin Invest* 1987;80:812.
Increased vascular reactivity to norepinephrine
  —Laurent et al: *Am J Physiol* 1988;255:H36.

trophic factors shown in Figure 3.31 to lead to vascular hypertrophy as well as serving as a primary pressor mechanism that sets off the entire process. Moreover, the altered transport of sodium described earlier in this chapter is also under the influence of the sympathetic nervous system (Hermsmeyer, 1984). Therefore, it may be inserted early or late in the overall scheme but, one way or another, sympathetic nervous overactivity seems likely to be involved.

Before considering further some of the evidence listed in Table 3.9, a brief review of the pertinent physiology of the sympathetic nervous system will be provided.

## Normal Physiology

A number of peripheral and central nervous structures are interconnected to provide control over the circulation (Izzo, 1984). The vasomotor center activates efferent pathways that innervate sympathetic ganglia. From these, an arborizing network of neurons exerts its effects by release into the synaptic cleft of norepinephrine, which stimulates receptors on target tissues. The central pathways have been mapped only in animals (Brody, 1988), but there is no doubt that similar centers exist in humans. The presence of both inhibitory and stimulatory peripheral pathways is more certain, and increasingly sophisticated techniques are now available to study the physiological consequences of sympathetic activity in man. With such techniques, it has become increasingly obvious that measurement of catecholamine concentrations in peripheral blood may not be an accurate reflection of what happens in the synapse, particularly since what is measured is only an overflow and only portions of the norepinephrine release mechanism may be activated by any given stimulus (Esler et al, 1989).

### Activity Within the Synapse

Sympathetic nerves and their catecholamine secretions induce their effects upon the heart and blood vessels by multiple interactions with both presynaptic and postsynaptic receptors (Langer and Hicks, 1984) (Fig. 3.33).

## Role of Epinephrine

Beyond its well-known role as the mediator of the "fight-or-flight" response to stress, adrenomedullary epinephrine may be involved both in normal physiology and in the pathophysiology of hypertension. The secretion of epinephrine may induce far greater and longer effects

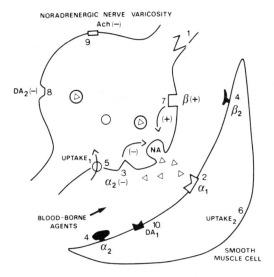

**Figure 3.33.** Schematic representation of the major receptor types of catecholamines as might be found on the innervation of smooth muscle or cardiac muscle. (*1.*) Electrical stimulation leads to depolarization in the terminal varicosities. The sympathetic varicosity releases noradrenaline (*NA*) into the neuromuscular junction. (*2.*) The major sympathetic innervation of smooth muscle cells is the $\alpha_1$-receptor subtype (on cardiac cells it is the $\beta_1$-receptor subtype). (*3.*) Noradrenaline released from the varicosity may act on presynaptic $\alpha_2$-receptors to inhibit the further release of noradrenaline. (*4.*) $\alpha_2$-Receptors located postjunctionally may be activated by noradrenaline released from the varicosities. $\alpha_2$-Receptor stimulation mediates contraction; $\beta_2$-receptor stimulation leads to dilatation of blood vessels. (*5.*) The major route of inactivation of noradrenaline is by active neuronal reuptake (*uptake₁*), which may also take up adrenaline. (*6.*) An extraneuronal uptake mechanism also exists in smooth muscle and cardiac muscle. Both adrenaline and noradrenaline are substrates for this uptake process. (*7.*) $\beta$-receptors are also found on the sympathetic nerve terminals, where their stimulation leads to facilitation of noradrenaline release. These $\beta$-receptors (probably $\beta_2$-receptor subtype) may be activated by adrenaline. (*8.*) Dopamine (*DA₂*) receptors whose stimulation leads to inhibition of noradrenaline release. (*9.*) Muscarinic cholinergic receptors whose stimulation leads to inhibition of noradrenaline release. (*10.*) In certain vascular beds, the smooth muscle possesses dopamine (*DA₁*) receptors that mediate relaxation. (From Langer SZ, Hicks PE: *Br J Anaesth* 56:689, 1984.)

upon the blood pressure than the relatively short "fight-or-flight" response. As shown first in animals (Majewski et al, 1981) but more recently in humans (Blankestijn et al, 1988), after an infusion of epinephrine at levels comparable to those seen during stress, the blood pressure may rise and remain elevated for some time thereafter. Presumably, part of the epinephrine enters the sympathetic nerve endings, (5 in Fig. 3.33) and is rereleased into the synaptic cleft as a cotransmitter during subsequent stimulation of the sympathetic nerves. However, in addition,

this epinephrine acts upon the presynaptic beta₂-receptor to facilitate the release of more norepinephrine (7 in Fig. 3.33). Thus intermittently secreted adrenomedullary epinephrine may invoke a sustained increase in neuronal release of both epinephrine and norepinephrine, in turn causing neurogenic vasoconstriction and a persistent rise in blood pressure (Floras et al, 1988a).

Thus, a mechanism exists for the translation of intermittent stress into more sustained hypertension. As suggested by Folkow (1989), these periods of intermittently elevated blood pressure could rapidly lead to structural changes in the vasculature, thereby inducing permanent hypertension.

### Baroreceptor Dysfunction

Another component of the sympathetic nervous system, the inhibitory baroreceptors, may also be involved in the pathogenesis of hypertension and in the higher levels of circulating catecholamines seen among hypertensive patients. These reflexes, when activated by a rise in blood pressure, normally reduce heart rate and lower blood pressure by vagal stimulation and sympathetic inhibition. As shown by McCubbin et al in 1956, this reflex is reset downward within hours when hypertension is induced so that, despite higher pressures, the afferent neural activity is similar to that seen in normotension.

The lesser sensitivity of the baroreceptors in hypertensive patients is likely the principal determinant of their increased BP variability (Floras et al, 1988b). With longer-standing hypertension, as evidenced by the presence of left ventricular hypertrophy, the contribution of the arterial baroreflex to the regulation of BP is no longer detectable (Floras et al, 1988c).

Beyond rare instances of paroxysmal hypertension in humans with baroreceptor denervation (Aksamit et al, 1987), the effects of the progressive loss of baroreceptor sensitivity as elevated blood pressure persists are uncertain. Even if loss of baroreceptor function were responsible only for a greater increase in minute to minute variability in blood pressure and greater swings during periods of stress, such peaks may be responsible for the structural thickening that may lead to persistent hypertension.

### Hypertension and Stress

Now that we have seen how repeated stress may lead to sustained and perhaps permanent hypertension, let us examine the evidence that people with hypertension and, even more importantly, those likely to develop hypertension either have more stress or respond differently to stress.

## Exposure to Stress

People exposed to repeated psychogenic stresses may develop hypertension more frequently than otherwise similar people not so stressed:

—As an extreme example, the blood pressure remained normal among nuns in a secluded order over a 20-year period whereas it rose with age in women nearby in the outside world (Timio et al, 1988).

—Air traffic controllers, who work under high level psychological stress, annually develop hypertension at a rate 5.6 times greater than do nonprofessional pilots who were initially comparable in physical characteristics (Cobb and Rose, 1973).

—Among blue collar factory workers, stressful work conditions and overall job dissatisfaction were significant predictors of diastolic blood pressure (Matthews et al, 1987).

—Multiple populations living in small, cohesive, protected societies have been found to have low blood pressures that do not rise with aging; those who abandon such an environment and migrate to more urbanized, modern, disorganized societies have higher blood pressures that rise with aging (Cassel, 1974; James, 1987; Sever et al, 1989). Environmental factors such as weight gain and increased sodium intake may be responsible, but in some of these groups, the association between hypertension and social disorganization seems strong (Kaplan et al, 1988).

—The higher prevalence of hypertension among blacks has been attributed to their increased level of discontent (Naditch, 1974) and other social stresses (Harburg et al, 1973). However, the black may not be peculiar in this regard: Whites in the lower social class (Tyroler, 1989) or with lower occupational status (Jenner et al, 1988) or with less formal education (Hypertension Detection and Follow-up Program Cooperative Group, 1987) also have more hypertension and higher mortality associated with it.

## Psychological Makeup

People may become hypertensive not just because they are more stressed but because they respond differently to stress. Greater cardiovas-cular and sympathetic nervous activity has been repeatedly documented in hypertensives to various mental stresses (Brod et al, 1959; Steptoe et al, 1984; Jern, 1986). Although the evidence for a different psychological substrate in hypertensive people is impressive, it should be remembered that most of the data are short-term, cross-sectional observations that may not relate to the underlying pathogenesis of hypertension. In particular there is a need to study psychological status before patients are aware of their diagnosis since they may develop various psychological problems after being labeled as hypertensive (Steptoe and Melville, 1984; Irvine et al, 1989). These may be responsible for the adverse consequences of labeling people as hypertensive (Macdonald et al, 1984).

Nonetheless, there are numerous studies showing a greater intensity of anger and hostility, but at the same time a greater suppression of the expression of the anger among both hypertensives (Schneider et al, 1986; Goldstein et al, 1988) and normotensive offspring of hypertensive parents (Perini et al, 1988). Moreover, hypertensives tend to remain emotionally stressed longer (Melamed, 1987) and to be more disposed to cope actively with stressors (Duijkers et al, 1988).

Higher levels of emotional reactivity and repression of anger and hostility certainly could be responsible for greater activation of the sympathetic nervous system and, thereby, for the development of hypertension. On the other hand, hypertension may lead to a physiological alteration of perception. As one example, hypertensives had a higher threshold to dental pain than did normotensives (Ghione et al, 1988). For another, a higher prevalence of hypertension was found among bus drivers than among men in other less stressful occupations (Ragland et al, 1987), but those bus drivers who were hypertensive perceived their jobs to be less stressful than did those who were normotensive (Winkleby et al, 1988).

Hypertensives have also been reported to display impaired cognitive ability (Elias et al, 1987; Lindgärde et al, 1987), but no such impairment was found in over 2000 participants in the Framingham Study (Farmer et al, 1987).

The association of hypertension with a particular, inappropriate, "hot" reaction to stress (Eliot, 1988) has not been validated in a hemodynamic study of almost 300 subjects (Rüddel et al, 1988).

A high prevalence of hypertension is seen

among patients with overt affective disorders (Yates and Wallace, 1987), and marked rises in pressure are usual during panic attacks (White and Baker, 1987). As noted in Chapter 2, many of the common symptoms noted by hypertensives are caused by recurrent anxiety-induced hyperventilation, during which the blood pressure may rise even further.

### Prehypertension

As noted in Table 3.9, young people who are normotensive but because of a positive family history are genetically predisposed to develop hypertension often can be shown to hyperrespond to various stimuli. An excellent example, shown in Figure 3.34, utilized mental tasks to demonstrate a higher heart rate response and a reduction in urinary sodium excretion among young men with hypertensive parents (Light et al, 1983). Both of these reactions were assumed to reflect sympathetic nervous system hyperresponsiveness.

### Changes With Age

Various indices of sympathetic nervous hyperreactivity are seen exclusively or mainly in younger patients. These include plasma levels of norepinephrine and norepinephrine spillover (Esler et al, 1989). Julius (1988) explains the tendency for previously elevated plasma norepinephrine levels to fall as hypertension becomes established by a negative feedback of the

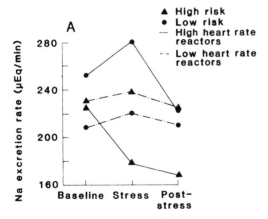

**Figure 3.34.** Rates of sodium excretion during baseline, the stress of competitive mental tasks, and the poststress periods, each of 1 hour duration, in 40 young men. The high-risk subjects had occasional systolic blood pressure above 140 mm Hg or a parental history of hypertension, whereas the low-risk subjects had neither. The high heart rate reactors had mean increases of 13 beats per minutes during the stress, the low reactors less than that. (From Light KC, Koepke JP, Obrist PA, et al: *Science* (Wash DC) 220:430, 1983, and Copyrighted 1983 by the AAS.)

elevated blood pressure per se on the central nervous system. This same explanation is offered for the transition from a high cardiac output to an elevated vascular resistance. In Julius' words: "If the central nervous system seeks to obtain a certain pressure and maintains the high blood pressure in early phases by an elevation in cardiac output, later as structural arteriolar changes evolve and the arterioles become hyperresponsive, the same blood pressure elevation could be achieved with less sympathetic drive, and the plasma norepinephrine values return to the normal range."

### Overview of Sympathetic Activity

These various pieces of evidence add up to make a fairly strong case for a role of increased sympathetic nervous system activity in the pathogenesis of hypertension. Catecholamine-induced constriction of renal efferent arterioles has been previously emphasized as a logical way to explain the pressure-natriuresis phenomenon, which is critical to the renal retention of sodium. Moreover, catechols are leading candidates to be both the pressor mechanism that initiates the rise in blood pressure and the trophic mechanism that maintains hypertension via vascular hypertrophy (Fig. 3.31).

### Neurogenic Mechanisms

In concert with and often related to increases in sympathetic nervous system activity, other neural mechanisms may be involved in hypertension. Most of the evidence for central neural involvement must come from experiments with animals; their relevance to hypertension in people is unknown.

#### Central Neural Mechanisms

The baroreceptor and other cardiopulmonary afferent nerves terminate in the intermediate one-third of the nucleus of the solitary tract (nucleus tractus solitarius, or NTS) in the brain stem. Lesions in this area will lead to varying degrees of hypertension in various animals (Nathan and Reis, 1977). On the other hand, lesions in tissue surrounding the anteroventral third ventricle (AV3V) in the rat prevent the development of hypertension induced by various mechanisms, including damage to the NTS (Brody, 1981). The possible origin of natriuretic hormone in the AV3V region was previously noted.

#### Central Neurotransmitters

Beyond studies involving ablation of various parts of the brain, research is ongoing into the possible role of various neurotransmitters in the control of the blood pressure and the pathogenesis of hypertension. Some of these appear to act via the sympathetic nervous system, including opioid peptides (May et al, 1989), neuropeptide Y (Waeber et al, 1988), and dopamine (Os et al, 1987). Other endogenous substances that may in some manner be involved include serotonin (Hollenberg, 1988), substance P (Petty and Reid, 1981), and human calcitonin gene-related peptide (Gennari et al, 1989).

## OTHER PRESSOR AND DEPRESSOR HORMONES

### Vasopressin

Another pressor hormone that could be involved in primary hypertension is the antidiuretic hormone, vasopressin. High levels of vasopressin have been found in various experimental models of hypertension (Möhring et al, 1979; Crofton et al, 1979), and elevated plasma levels have been reported in patients with low renin primary hypertension (Os et al, 1986).

### Diminished Vasodepressor Hormones

In addition to the considerable evidence for an excess of one or more pressor mechanisms, the other side of blood pressure control—the absence of vasodepressors—should be considered. Beyond the evidence for their role in renoprival hypertension (see Chapter 9), there are some data implicating vasodepressors in primary hypertension.

### Prostaglandins

Most of the members of this family of hormones act locally within tissues and the microcirculation. Recognition of the balance between the vasodilator prostacyclin and the vasoconstrictor thromboxane (Chapter 9) has added greatly to the belief that these hormones may have a role in the control of normal blood pressure and may be involved in the pathogenesis of hypertension. Whereas the majority of prostaglandins (PG) are inactivated within the pulmonary circulation, prostacyclin is not, and it can therefore be considered a circulating hormone.

The major site of prostaglandin action relative to hypertension may be in the kidney. When $PGE_2$ or the precursor arachidonic acid is infused into the renal artery, renal vasodilation, increased renal blood flow, and natriuresis follow. Thus, $PGE_2$ protects against ischemia. When renal blood flow is compromised, both renin and prostaglandins are released. By this mechanism the kidney via renin-angiotensin can raise systemic blood pressure without diminishing renal blood flow, since intrarenal prostaglandins would counteract the effects of intrarenal angiotensin (Hura and Kunau, 1988).

A deficiency of $PGE_2$ might then lead to hypertension by impairing renal function and permitting fluid retention as well as by accentuating the vasoconstrictive effects of renin-angiotensin. Decreased levels of urinary $PGE_2$ have been measured in hypertensive patients and have been related to decreased renal blood flow and urinary sodium excretion (Córdova and Martínez-Maldonado, 1988).

### Renomedullary Lipid

Muirhead and coworkers have considerable experimental support for the secretion of medullipin, a neutral lipid from the renomedullary interstitial cells that is antihypertensive (Muirhead et al, 1989). The possible role of a deficiency of such vasodepressor lipids in the pathogenesis of hypertension in the human remains unknown.

### Kallikrein-Kinin System

The evidence for a possible role of this vasodepressor system in primary hypertension is not impressive. Though lower urinary excretion of kallikrein has been claimed in both hypertensives and their children, more recent data do not show a significant difference when various demographic and methodological factors are taken into account (Córdova and Martínez-Maldonado, 1988).

## ENVIRONMENTAL FACTORS

Hypertension may develop because of too much of some external factors, e.g., calories, sodium, alcohol, or too little of others, e.g., physical activity and potassium.

### Obesity

Most of the environmental factors may aggravate hypertension, but it is unlikely that they are responsible for causing the disease. Obesity may be an exception in view of the strong association between obesity and the prevalence of hypertension and the increasing incidence of hypertension when weight is gained. In the Framingham offspring study, adiposity as measured by subscapular skinfold thickness was the major controllable contributor to hypertension, with estimates of 78% of hypertension in men and

64% in women attributable to obesity (Garrison et al, 1985).

As noted earlier, the distribution of body fat is important since blood pressure as well as blood triglyceride and glucose levels are highest in those with central or abdominal obesity who also have hyperinsulinemia (Kaplan, 1989) (Fig. 3.32).

Without taking into account the distribution of the obesity, the degree of cardiovascular risk for any level of systolic blood pressure has been found to be equal or even greater for obese hypertensives than for lean ones in multiple studies (Kannel et al, 1989) with one exception (Barrett-Connor and Khaw, 1985).

The mechanism by which obesity leads to hypertension likely involves an increase in blood volume, stroke volume, and cardiac output (Raison et al, 1986). Children seem particularly vulnerable to the hypertensive effects of weight gain (Aristimuno et al, 1984), and the best predictor of high blood pressure in young adults was childhood obesity (Higgins et al, 1980). Therefore, avoidance of childhood obesity seems important, with the hope of avoiding subsequent hypertension. The evidence that weight reduction will lower established hypertension will be covered in Chapter 6.

### Sleep Apnea

Obese people have an increased prevalence of obstructive sleep apnea, often identified by snoring. Among habitual snorers, hypertension is more common, as much as 2-fold (Waller and Bhopal, 1989), likely because of its association with obesity and sleep apnea (Hoffstein et al, 1988). Hypertension is commonly seen with sleep apnea (Guilleminault et al, 1981), probably because of the associated excessive sympathetic activation (Fletcher et al, 1987). The prevalence of previously unrecognized sleep apnea in hypertensive patients has been reported to be as high as 30% by some (Kales et al, 1984; Fletcher et al, 1985), but Warley et al (1988) found no excessive arterial hypoxemia among 30 untreated hypertensives.

### Physical Inactivity

People who are physically active and fit may develop less hypertension, and those who are hypertensive may lower their blood pressure by regular isotonic exercise (Jennings et al, 1986). The prevention of hypertension may be one of the ways exercise protects against the development of cardiovascular disease. Among 14,998

Harvard male alumni followed for 16 to 50 years, those who did not engage in vigorous sports play were at 35% greater risk for developing hypertension, whether or not they had higher blood pressures while in college, a family history of hypertension, or obesity, all of which also increased the risk of hypertension (Paffenbarger et al, 1983). In a similar vein, normotensive people who were at a low level of physical fitness, assessed by maximal treadmill testing, had a 52% greater relative risk for developing hypertension over the next 1 to 12 years when compared with people initially at a high level of physical fitness (Blair et al, 1984).

### Potassium, Magnesium, Lead, and Trace Metals

#### Potassium Deficiency

As noted earlier in this chapter when the possible role of a high sodium:low potassium ratio was described, there are considerable data suggesting a lack of potassium as being involved in hypertension (Tobian, 1988). These include population surveys of dietary intake (Khaw and Barrett-Connor, 1988a), particularly among black hypertensives (Veterans Administration Cooperative Study Group, 1987), and lesser total body (Berretta-Piccoli et al, 1984) and skeletal muscle (Ericsson, 1984) potassium in untreated hypertensives. As noted in Chapter 6, potassium depletion will raise blood pressure (Krishna et al, 1989) and potassium supplementation may lower the blood pressure, perhaps by diminishing the pressor hyperresponsiveness to norepinephrine (Bianchetti et al, 1987). The overall potassium intake of modern people has certainly been reduced below that of our ancestors (Table 3.7), so there are logical reasons to advocate a return to a more "natural" higher potassium-lower sodium diet.

#### Magnesium

Magnesium, beyond its role in activation of many critical enzymes involved in intermediary metabolism and phosphorylation, works as a natural antagonist to many of the actions of calcium. Magnesium deficiency in rats induced significant hypertension associated with marked reductions in the size of the lumen of small vessels (Altura et al, 1984). Hypomagnesemia enhances the contractility of several vascular beds and may potentiate the contractile response to numerous pressor hormones.

Nonetheless, in 50 untreated male hypertensive patients, magnesium levels in serum and urine were normal and intracellular levels were higher than in a group of matched normotensives (Kjeldsen et al, 1989).

## Lead

There is a likely relationship between levels of blood lead and blood pressure as reviewed in Environmental Health Perspectives, volume 78, pages 3 to 155, 1988. This relationship was most clearly noted in the second National Health and Nutrition Examination Survey (NHANES II) performed from 1976 to 1980, with a direct relationship found between blood lead and systolic and diastolic pressures for men and women, white and black, aged 12 to 74 (Harlan et al, 1985). In multiple regression analyses, the relationship was independent of other variables for men, though not for women.

Although no such relation has been noted in Welshmen (Elwood et al, 1988), it has been seen in other groups, including Boston policemen (Weiss et al, 1986) and Danes (Grandjean et al, 1989). In this latter group, the association was largely attributable to alcohol intake, which could either alter lead metabolism or, more likely, provide the source for lead exposure.

Although there are conflicting data about the role of lead in human hypertension, the strong association found among the NHANES II sample supports continued efforts to reduce environmental lead exposure.

### Other Trace Metals: Zinc, Cadmium

The same NHANES II data found an inverse relation between serum zinc levels and blood pressure (Harlan et al, 1984). There are considerable data in animals but little in man incriminating a direct relation of blood pressure with cadmium (Saltman, 1983) with the possible exception of patients with renal insufficiency (Geiger et al, 1989). Beyond these, there are no other known significant associations between trace elements and blood pressure.

### Caffeine

People not tolerant to caffeine will have a pressor effect from it, but tolerance develops rapidly so that caffeine does not produce a persistent increase in blood pressure (Myers, 1988).

### Alcohol

The last of the specific possible causes of hypertension, like many of those in the latter sections of this chapter, can only be a factor in

a portion of the hypertensive population. However, the possible role of alcohol, in amounts consumed by a large part of the overall population, needs special emphasis: Even in small quantities, alcohol may raise the blood pressure; in larger quantities, alcohol may be responsible for a significant amount of hypertension.

### Nature of the Relationship

The association was reported in 1915 (Lian, 1915) but not until Klatsky et al (1977) documented it in a large population was alcohol recognized as a pressor substance. As reviewed by MacMahon (1987), about 40% of the many subsequent reports show the pressor effect only when consumption goes beyond two drinks a day, with even lower pressures in those who drink one or two drinks a day than in those who abstain. This relation is seen in a study of 7735 middle-aged men drawn at random from general practices in 24 British towns (Shaper et al, 1988) (Fig. 3.35). This J-shaped pattern parallels the association with total and coronary mortality (Anderson, 1988).

Based upon these associations, as much as 10% of hypertension in men can be directly attributed to alcohol (MacMahon, 1987). Those who quit drinking have blood pressures similar to those who never drank (Klatsky et al, 1977), and those who are hypertensive while consuming 3 or more ounces of ethanol per day will usually become normotensive and stay normotensive if they abstain even for a short time

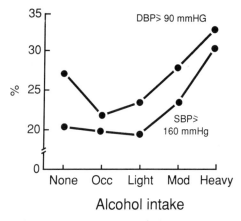

**Figure 3.35.** Age-adjusted prevalence rates (%) of measured systolic and diastolic hypertension by levels of alcohol intake in drinks: occasional, light (one to two daily), moderate (three to six daily), and heavy (more than six daily). (From Shaper AG, Wannamethee G, Whincup P: *J Human Hypertens* 2:71, 1988.)

(Saunders et al, 1981). The pressor effect of alcohol in such patients has been demonstrated under controlled conditions (Puddey et al, 1987).

### Possible Mechanisms (Fig. 3.36)

Higher blood pressures have been noted with intake of all types of alcohol-containing beverages (Criqui et al, 1981). The manner by which alcohol acutely raises blood pressure may reflect sympathetic activation as seen with direct measurement of muscle sympathetic nerve activity (Grassi et al, in press). Plasma calcium levels are lowered (Howes et al, 1986) perhaps reflecting changes in cell membranes that increase calcium entry or decrease calcium extrusion (Arkwright et al, 1984). A few heavy drinkers develop a ''pseudo-Cushing's'' appearance, suggesting a more intense, prolonged stimulation of cortisol secretion (Kirkman and Nelson, 1988).

Those who suddenly withdraw from ethanol may have an even greater rise in blood pressure, likely resulting from marked sympathetic nervous discharge (Linnoila et al, 1987).

### Low Birth Weight

A higher prevalence of hypertension has been noted among people who were growth retarded at birth (Gennser et al, 1988; Barker et al, 1989). The adverse effects of the intrauterine environment obviously could reflect the external environment into which the child was born and raised. Regardless of the cause, growth retardation should be considered to be a risk for the development of hypertension in adult life.

### ASSOCIATIONS WITH HYPERTENSION

In addition to all of these possible mechanisms, there are a number of associations with hypertension that are likely not directly causal but rather reflective of shared mechanisms (e.g., diabetes) or of consequences of the hypertension (e.g., hyperuricemia).

### Diabetes and Hyperinsulinemia

Hypertension is more common in patients with diabetes mellitus. The reason likely differs with the type of diabetes. In insulin-dependent dia-

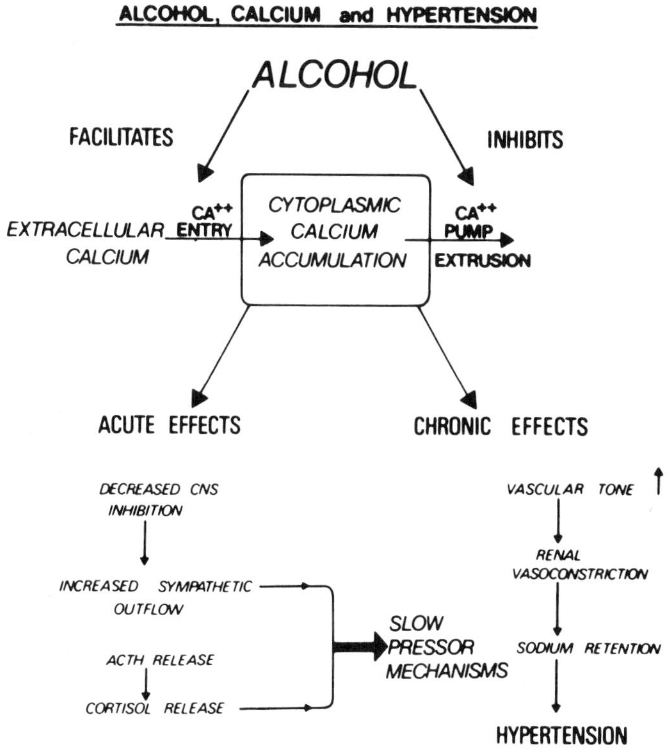

**Figure 3.36.** Schema by which chronic alcohol consumption may lead to hypertension in susceptible individuals. (From Arkwright P, Beilin LJ, Vandongen R, et al: *J Hypertension* 2:387, 1984.)

betes mellitus (IDDM), hypertension is seen primarily among those who develop nephropathy, probably as a familial liability to hypertension that may be responsible for the progression of their renal damage (Viberti et al, 1987). In non-insulin-dependent diabetes mellitus (NIDDM), hypertension is more common from the onset, likely a consequence of the insulin resistance and hyperinsulinemia induced by obesity (Simonson, 1988). The major consequences of diabetic nephropathy will be covered in Chapter 9, and some aspects of the obesity-hyperinsulinemia relationship were covered earlier in this chapter (Fig. 3.32).

When hypertension coexists with diabetes, vascular complications are more severe, including retinopathy (Knowler et al, 1980) and nephropathy (Mogensen and Christensen, 1985). As will be described in Chapter 7, there is renewed interest in tight control of hypertension in diabetics, particularly with angiotensin-converting enzyme inhibitors.

### Gout and Hyperuricemia

Hypertension is more common in patients with gout (Rapado, 1974), and hyperuricemia is found in 25 to 50% of untreated hypertensives, some 5 times the expected incidence (Breckenridge, 1966). This has been attributed to renal disease: In 71 male hypertensives, asymptomatic hyperuricemia was associated with decreased renal blood flow, presumably reflecting nephrosclerosis (Messerli et al, 1980). Diuretics commonly used in the treatment of hypertension frequently raise the serum uric acid level further and may precipitate gout in those who are susceptible. More on this in Chapter 7.

### Polycythemia and Viscosity

Primary polycythemia may be associated with hypertension, since vascular volume is expanded and blood viscosity is increased. Increased whole blood viscosity, not related to higher hematocrits, has been implicated in the hemodynamics of essential hypertension (Devereux et al, 1984) and as a risk factor for both hypertension and other cardiovascular diseases (Koenig et al, 1989). Some hypertensives have a red face, a high hematocrit, contracted plasma volume, and normal red cell mass; the syndrome is associated with a high mortality (Burge et al, 1975) but can be reversed by antihypertensive therapy (Chrysant et al, 1976).

### Sex Hormones

#### Menopause

There is no evidence that hypertension is part of the menopausal syndrome, and it does not appear to explain the increased risk of cardiovascular disease that follows menopause, an increased risk that is likely caused by the cessation of estrogen production per se (Witteman et al, 1989). Women do show a rising incidence of hypertension after menopause but this may primarily reflect an increase of body weight (Grobbee et al, 1988). Another simple but intriguing explanation for the increased incidence of hypertension after menopause is that the monthly menses keeps fluid volume slightly lower in women before menopause so that the hemodynamic cascade toward hypertension is slowed (Seely, 1976).

#### Estrogen

Premenopausal women with hypertension usually have a higher heart rate and cardiac output and a lower peripheral resistance than do men with similar degrees of hypertension (Messerli et al, 1987). These differences logically reflect higher estrogen levels, which have been found to be even higher in premenopausal hypertensive women than normotensive subjects (Hughes et al, 1989). In that same study, estrogen levels were also higher in hypertensive than normotensive men, though still well below those in women.

#### Testosterone

Hypertensive men have also been reported to have lower testosterone levels than normotensives (Khaw and Barrett-Connor, 1988b).

### Other Associations

The following have been said to have an increased association with hypertension:

—senile cataracts (Clayton et al, 1980);
—retinal vein obstruction (Williams et al, 1981);
—color blindness (Morton, 1975);
—uterine fibromyomas (Summers et al, 1971);
—generalized osteoarthritis (Lawrence, 1975);
—blood group MN (Gleiberman et al, 1984);
—HL-A antigens (Gelsthorpe et al, 1975);
—increased levels of the platelet release product beta-thromboglobulin (Kjeldsen et al, 1983);
—aortic stenosis (Beevers et al, 1983);
—pseudoxanthoma elasticum (Goodman et al, 1963);

—cancer mortality (Khaw and Barrett-Connor, 1984) and incidence (Buck and Donner, 1987);
—gastric ulcer and cancer (Sonnenberg, 1988);
—reduced forced vital capacity (Sparrow et al, 1988).

## MECHANISM OF HYPERTENSION IN BLACKS

Now that various possible mechanisms for primary hypertension have been described, let us examine which of these may be involved in the more common occurrence of hypertension in blacks. As noted in Chapter 1, they appear to differ from other racial groups in many ways relative to hypertension.

A number of differences between black and white hypertensives have been offered as explanations for the higher incidence and severity of hypertension among blacks (Table 3.10). Some

of these differences have been noted between normotensive blacks and hypertensive blacks but are similar to what has been observed between normotensive and hypertensive whites (e.g., low socioeconomic status.). Even among normotensive children of hypertensive parents, differences have been noted between blacks and whites: Black children had higher postexercise heart rates and blood pressure, higher urinary sodium and lower urinary potassium excretion, and lower levels of plasma renin activity and kallikrein excretion (Hohn et al, 1983).

As noted in Table 3.10, numerous measures of sodium and calcium transport suggest that there may be a basic difference in the manner of handling the high sodium intake that most blacks and whites ingest. These observations involve various defects in sodium transport described earlier in this chapter as possibly in-

**Table 3.10. Racial Differences Related to Hypertension**

| Characteristic in Hypertensive Blacks | Independent Associations | | References |
|---|---|---|---|
| | Difference from Normotensive Blacks | Difference from Hypertensive Whites | |
| Heredity | | | |
| Darker skin color | Yes | | Harburg et al, 1978 |
| | No | | Keil et al, 1981 |
| Higher proportions of African genes | Yes | | MacLean et al, 1974 |
| Diet | | | |
| Obesity | Yes | Weaker association | Tyroler et al, 1975 |
| Increased sodium intake | | No | Grim et al, 1989 |
| Decreased potassium intake | | Yes | Grim et al, 1980 |
| Decreased calcium intake | Yes | Yes | Sempos et al, 1986 |
| Socioeconomic status | | | |
| Low economic status | Yes | No | Harburg et al, 1973 |
| Low educational status | Yes | No | Hypertension Detection and Follow-up Program Cooperative Group, 1977 |
| Hemodynamics and hormones | | | |
| Blood volume | No | Lower | Mitas et al, 1979 |
| | No | Same | Messerli et al, 1979 |
| | | Higher | Chrysant et al, 1979 |
| Reduced excretion of sodium load | Yes | Yes | Luft et al, 1979 |
| Low plasma renin | Yes | Yes | Kaplan et al, 1976 Berenson et al, 1979 |
| Decreased kallikrein excretion | No | Yes | Holland et al, 1980 |
| Low dopamine $\beta$-hydroxylase | Yes | Yes | Berenson et al, 1979 |
| Greater pressure reactivity to stress | | Yes[a] | Murphy et al, 1988a |
| Greater pressure reactivity to norepinephrine | | Yes | Dimsdale et al, 1987 |
| Responsiveness to drug therapies | | | |
| Greater response to diuretics | | Yes | Holland et al, 1979 |
| Lesser response to $\beta$-blockers | | Yes | Seedat et al, 1980 |
| Sodium and calcium transport | | | |
| Lower RBC $Na^+$ pump activity | | Yes[a] | Aderounmu and Salako, 1979 Woods et al, 1981 |
| Higher RBC $Na^+$ concentration | | Yes[a] | Lasker et al, 1985 |
| Higher $Na^+$ turnover in fibroblasts | | Yes | Kuriyama et al, 1988 |
| Lower $Na^+$-Li countertransport | | Yes[a] | Bunker et al, 1987 |
| Higher $Ca^{++}$ transients in fibroblasts | | Yes[a] | Nakamura et al, 1989 |

[a]These differences have been noted between normotensive whites and blacks.

volved in the pathogenesis of primary hypertension. Whether these cellular sodium transport defects have anything to do with the higher prevalence of hypertension in blacks remains to be seen. However, together with a number of other findings among black hypertensives—the higher frequency of expanded blood volume (Chrysant et al, 1979), the lesser excretion of sodium loads (Luft et al, 1979), the lower plasma renin levels (Kaplan et al, 1976), and the excellent antihypertensive response to diuretics (Holland et al, 1979)—a very attractive case can be constructed, all based upon a genetic defect in sodium excretion that is more prevalent among blacks. Perhaps blacks, who originally lived in hot, arid climates wherein sodium conservation was important for survival, have evolved the physiological machinery that protects them in their original habitat but makes it difficult for them to handle the excessive sodium they ingest when they migrate (Grim et al, 1989).

## POTENTIAL FOR PREVENTION

The preceding coverage in no way exhausts the possible mechanisms for primary hypertension. It should be reemphasized that multiple defects are likely involved and some of the initiating factors may no longer be discernible, having been dampened as the process develops.

Without a certain genetic marker, it is impossible to know whether a normotensive, even with a strongly positive family history, will definitely develop hypertension so that long-term prospective studies could be performed. Subtle defects are demonstrable in such people, e.g., a shift in sensitivity to norepinephrine (Aalkjaer et al, 1987b), but it will be exceedingly difficult to follow the progress from truly normal to definitely hypertensive.

In the absence of certainty about the pathogenesis, it will be difficult to convince many that preventive measures should be undertaken. However, there seems no possible harm and a great deal of potential good to be gained from encouraging moderation in intake of sodium, calories, and alcohol; maintenance of good physical condition; and avoidance of unnecessary stress. The value of these preventive measures has now been demonstrated. The incidence of hypertension over 5 years was reduced from 19.2% among 99 initially normotensive subjects who were simply monitored to 8.8% among 102 who followed such a program (Stamler et al, 1989).

Now that the possible causes of primary hypertension have been examined, we will turn to the natural history and clinical consequences of the disease. Regardless of cause, it must be dealt with.

## References

Aalkjaer C, Heagerty AM, Bailey I, et al: *Hypertension* 9(Suppl III):III-155, 1987a.

Aalkjaer C, Heagerty AM, Parvin SD, et al: *Lancet* 1:649, 1986.

Aalkjaer C, Heagerty AM, Petersen KK, et al: *Circ Res* 61:181, 1987b.

Aderounmu AF, Salako LA: *Curr J Clin Invest* 9:369, 1979.

Adragna N, Canessa M, Bize I, et al: *Clin Sci* 61(Suppl 7):115, 1981.

Aksamit TR, Floras JS, Victor RG, et al: *Hypertension* 9:309, 1987.

Alderman M, Madhavan S, Ooi WL, et al: *Circulation* 80:II-101, 1989.

Altura BM, Altura BT, Gebrewold A, et al: *Science* (Wash DC) 223:1315, 1984.

Ambrosioni E, Borghi C, Boschi S et al: *J Cardiovasc Pharmacol* 12(Suppl 3):S85, 1988.

Ambrosioni E, Borghi C, Costa FV, et al: *J Human Hypertens* 1:229, 1987.

Anderson P: *Br Med J* 297:824, 1988.

Antonipillai I, Nadler JL, Robin EC, et al: *Hypertension* 10:61, 1987.

Aristimuno GG, Foster TA, Voors AW, et al: *Circulation* 69:895, 1984.

Aronson PS: *N Engl J Med* 307:317, 1982.

Arkwright PD, Beilin LJ, Vandongen R, et al: *J Hypertension* 2:387, 1984.

Astarie C, Levenson J, Simon A, et al: *J Hypertension* 7:485, 1989.

Azar S, Tobain L, Johnson MA: *Am J Physiol* 227:1045, 1974.

Baldwin DS, Biggs AW, Goldring W, et al: *Am J Med* 24:893, 1958.

Banskota NK, Taub R, Zellner K, et al: *Diabetes* 38:123, 1989.

Bar RS, Boes M, Dake BL, et al: *Am J Med* 85(Suppl 5A):59, 1988.

Barajas L, Powers K: *J Hypertension* 2(Suppl 1):3, 1984.

Barker DJP, Osmond C, Golding J, et al: *Br Med J* 298:564, 1989.

Barrett-Connor E, Khaw KT: *Circulation* 72:53, 1985.

Bauer JH, Brooks CS: *Am J Cardiol* 44:1163, 1979.

Baxter JS, Schambelan M, Matulich DT, et al: *J Clin Invest* 58:579, 1976.

Beauchamp GK: *Am Sci* 75:27, 1987.

Beevers DG, Sloan PJM, Mackinnon J: *Br Med J* 286:1960, 1983.

Benjamin N, Graham JM, Robinson BF, et al: *J Hypertension* 6(Suppl 4):S706, 1988.

Berenson GS, Voors AW, Webber LS, et al: *Metabolism* 28:1218, 1979.

Beretta-Piccoli C, Pusterla C, Städler P, et al: *J Hypertension* 6:57, 1988.

Beretta-Piccoli C, Weidmann P: *Mineral Electrolyte Metab* 10:292, 1984.

Beretta-Piccoli C, Weidmann P, Brown JJ, et al: *J Cardiovasc Pharmacol* 6:S134, 1984.

Berridge MJ: *Proc R Soc Lond* 234:359, 1988.

Bianchetti MG, Beretta-Piccoli C, Weidman P, et al: *Hyertension* 5(Suppl II):II-57, 1983.

Bianchetti MG, Beretta-Piccoli C, Weidmann P, et al: *Kidney Int* 29:882, 1986.

Bianchetti MG, Weidmann P, Beretta-Piccoli C, et al: *Kidney Int* 31:956, 1987.

Bianchi G, Cusi D, Vezzoli G: *Semin Nephrol* 8:110, 1988.

Bing RF, Heagerty AM, Thurston H, et al: *Clin Sci* 71:225, 1986.

Bing RF, Heagerty AM, Swales JD: *J Hypertension* 5(Suppl 4):S29, 1987.

Birkenhäger WH, de Leeuw PW: *J Hypertension* 2:121, 1984.

Birkenhäger WH, Kho TL, Schalekamp MA, et al: *Acta Clin Belg* 32:168, 1977.

Blackshear JL, Garnie D, Williams GH, et al: *Hypertension* 9:384, 1987.

Blair SN, Goodyear NN, Gibbons LW, et al: *JAMA* 252:487, 1984.

Blake S, Carey M, McShane A, et al: *Hypertension* 7:1003, 1985.

Blankestijn PJ, Man in't Veld AJ, Tulen J, et al: *Lancet* 2:1386, 1988.

Blaustein MP: *Am J Physiol* 232:C165, 1977.

Blaustein MP: *J Cardiovasc Pharmacol* 12(Suppl 5):S56, 1988.

Blaustein MP, Ashida T, Goldman WF, et al: *Ann NY Academy of Sci* 488:199, 1986.

Bobik A, Weissberg PK, Little PJ: *Clin Exp Pharmacol Physiol* 14:191, 1987.

Bohr DF, Webb RC: *Ann Rev Pharmacol Toxicol* 28:389, 1988.

Borst JGG, Borst-De Geus A: *Lancet* 1:7283, 1963.

Boucher R, Garcia R, Gutkowska J, et al: *Clin Sci Mol Med* 55:183s, 1978.

Bramley PM, Paulin JM, Millar JA: *J Hypertension* 4:589, 1986.

Braun-Menendez E, Fasciolo JC, Leloir CF, et al: *J Physiol* (Lond) 98:283, 1940.

Breckenridge A: *Lancet* 1:15, 1966.

Brenner BM, Garcia DL, Anderson S: *Am J Hypertens* 1:335, 1988.

Breslau NA, McGuire JO, Zerwekh JE, et al: *J Clin Endocrniol Metab* 55:369, 1982.

Brod J: *Lancet* 2:773, 1960

Brod J, Fencl V, Hejl Z, et al: *Clin Sci* 23:339, 1959.

Brody MG: *Fed Proc* 40:2257, 1981.

Brody MJ: *Clin Physiol Biochem* 6:230, 1988.

Brody MJ, Fink GD, Buggy J, et al: *Circ Res* (Suppl I):I-2 and 43, 1978.

Brown JJ, Lever AF, Robertson JIS, et al: *Lancet* 2:320, 1974.

Brown JJ, Lever AF, Robertson JIS, et al: *Q J Med* 53:427, 1984.

Brunner HR, Chang P, Wallach R, et al: *J Clin Invest* 51:58, 1972.

Brunner HR, Gavras H: *Am J Med* 69:739, 1980.

Buck C, Donner A: *Cancer* (Phila) 59:1386, 1987.

Bunker CH, Mallinger AG, Adams LL, et al: *J Hypertension* 5:7, 1987.

Burge PS, Johnson WS, Prankerd TAJ: *Lancet* 1:1266, 1975.

Burke GL, Webber LS, Srinivasan SR, et al: *Metabolism* 35:441, 1986.

Campbell DJ: *Am J Hypertens* 1:266, 1989.

Camussi A, Bianchi G: *Hypertension* 12:620, 1988.

Canessa M, Adragna N, Solomon HS, et al: *N Engl J Med* 302:772, 1980.

Canessa ML, Morgan K, Semplicini A: *J Cardiovasc Pharmacol* 12(Suppl 3)S92, 1988.

Carachi R, Lindop GBM, Leckie BJ: *J Pediatr Surg* 22:278, 1987.

Carmines PK, Morrison TK, Navar LG: *Am J Physiol* 251:F610, 1986.

Carr SJ, Thomas TH, Wilkinson R: *Eur J Clin Invest* 19:101, 1989.

Cassel M: *Int J Epidemiol* 3:204, 1974.

Catterall WA: *Science* (Wash DC) 242:50, 1988.

Cederholm J, Wibell L: *Acta Med Scand* 217:363, 1985.

Celentano A, Galderisi M, Garofalo M, et al: *J Hypertension* 6(Suppl 4):S107, 1988.

Chrysant SG, Danisa K, Kem DC, et al: *Hypertension* 1:136, 1979.

Chrysant SG, Frohlich Ed, Adamopoulos PN, et al: *Am J Cardiol* 37:1069, 1976.

Churchill PC, Churchill MC: *ISI Atlas of Science: Pharmacology*, 1988.

Clauser E, Gaillard I, Wei L, et al: *Am J Hypertens* 2:403, 1989.

Clayton RM, Cuthbert J, Phillips CI, et al: *Exp Eye Res* 31:553, 1980.

Cobb S, Rose RM: *JAMA* 224:489, 1973.

Cordero PL, Moore T, Williams GH, et al: *Clin Res* 37:552A, 1989.

Córdova HR, Martínez-Maldonado M: *Semin Nephrol* 8:131, 1988.

Cozza EN, Gomez-Sanchez CE, Foecking MF, et al: *J Clin Invest* 84:1032, 1989.

Criqui MH, Wallace RB, Mishkel M, et al: *Hypertension* 3:557, 1981.

Crofton JT, Share L, Shade RE, et al: *Hypertension* 1:31, 1979.

Curtis JJ, Luke RG, Dustan HP, et al: *N Engl J Med* 309:1009, 1983.

Dahl LK, Heine M: *Circ Res* 36:692, 1975.

Dahl KL, Knudsen KD, Iwai J: *Circ Res* 24 and 25(Suppl I):I-21, 1969.

Dahl KL, Leitl G, Greine M: *J Exp Med* 136:318, 1972.

Danthuluri NR, Deth RC: *Am J Physiol* 256:H867, 1989.

de Bold AJ, Borenstein HB, Veress AT, et al: *Life Sci* 28:89, 1981.

De Fronzo RA, Cooke CR, Andres R, et al: *J Clin Invest* 55:845, 1975.

Deibert DC, DeFronzo RA: *J Clin Invest* 65:717, 1980.

de la Sierra A, Coca A, Aguilera MT, et al: *J Hypertension* 6:931, 1988.

de la Sierra A, Coca A, Aguilera MT, et al: *J Hum Hypertens* 3:1, 1989.

de Leeuw PW, Birkenhäger WH: *J Hypertension* 1:321, 1983.

Denton D: *The Hunger for Salt*. New York: Springer-Verlag, 1982.

Deray G, Rieu M, Devynck MA, et al: *N Engl J Med* 316:575, 1987.

De Simone G, Tommaselli AP, Rossi R, et al: *Hypertension* 7:204, 1985.

Devereux RB: *Am J Hypertens* 2:186S, 1989.

Devereux RB, Drayer JIM, Chien S, et al: *Am J Cardiol* 54:592, 1984.

Devynck MA, Pernollet MG, Nunez AM, et al: *Hypertension* 3:397, 1981.

deWardener HE, MacGregor GA: *Kidney Int* 18:1, 1980.

deWardener HE, MacGregor GA: *Lancet* 1:450, 1982.

deWardener HE, MacGregor GA: *Medicine* (Baltimore) 62:310, 1983.

Diez J, Hannaert P, Garay PP: *Am J Physiol* 252:H1, 1987.

Dimsdale JE, Graham RM, Ziegler MG, et al: *Hypertension* 10:564, 1987.

Dluhy RG, Hopkins P, Hollenberg NK, et al: *J Cardiovasc Pharmacol* 12(Suppl 3):S149, 1988.

Dluhy RG, Smith K, Taylor T, et al: *Hypertension* 13:371, 1989.

Do Y-S, Shinagawa T, Tam H, et al: *J Biological Chem* 262:1037, 1987.

Duijkers TJ, Drijver M, Kromhout D, et al: *Psychosomatic Med* 50:353, 1988.

Dustan HP, Kirk KA: *Hypertension* 13:696, 1989.

Dzau VJ: *J Hypertension* 6(Suppl 3):S7, 1988.

Dzau VJ, Burt DW, Pratt RE: *Am J Physiol* 255:F563, 1988.

Dzau VJ, Paul M, Nakamura N, et al: *Hypertension* 13:731, 1989.

Dzau VJ, Pratt RE: In: Fozzard HA et al (eds). *The Heart and Cardiovascular System*. New York: Raven Press, 1986.

Eaton SB, Konner M, Shostak M: *Am J Med* 84:739, 1988.

Editorial: *Lancet* 1:1088, 1977.

Edmundson RPS, Thomas RD, Hilton PJ, et al: *Lancet* 1:1003, 1975.

Egan B, Fitzpatrick MA, Julius S: *Circulation* 75(Suppl I):I-30, 1987.

Egan B, Schmouder R: *Am Heart J* 116:594, 1988.

Eich RH, Cuddy RP, Smulyan H, et al: *Circulation* 34:299, 1966.

Eichler H-G, Ford GA, Blaschke TR, et al: *J Clin Invest* 83:108, 1989.

Eliades D, Swindall B, Johnston J, et al: *Hypertension* 13:690, 1989.

Elias MF, Robbins MA, Schultz NR Jr., et al: *Hypertension* 9:192, 1987.

Eliot RS: *Am Heart J* 116:583, 1988.

Elwood PC, Yarnell JWG, Oldham PD, et al: *Am J Epidemiol* 127:942, 1988.

Erdos EG: *Fed Proc* 36:1760, 1977.

Ericsson F: *Acta Med Scand* 215:225, 1984.

Esler M, Jennings G, Lambert G: *Am J Hypertens* 2:104S, 1989.

Esler M, Jennings G, Vibiano B, et al: *J Cardiovasc Pharmacol* 8(Suppl 5):39, 1986.

Espiner EA, Richards AM: *Lancet* 1:707, 1989.

Exton JH: *Kidney Int* 32(Suppl 23):S-68, 1987.

Fagard R, Amery A, Reybrouck T, et al: *Clin Sci Mol Med* 52:594, 1977.

Farmer ME, White LR, Abbott RD, et al: *Am J Epidemiol* 126:1103, 1987.

Ferguson RK, Turek DM, Rovner DR: *Clin Pharmacol Ther* 21:62, 1977.

Ferrannini E, Buzzigoli G, Bonadonna R, et al: *N Engl J Med* 317:350, 1987.

Fitzgibbon WR, Morgan TP, Myers JB: *Clin Sci* 59:195s, 1980

Fletcher EC, DeBehnke RD, Lovoi MS, et al: *Ann Intern Med* 103:190, 1985.

Fletcher EC, Miller J, Schaaf JW, et al: *Sleep* 10:35, 1987.

Fletcher PJ, Korner PI, Angus JA, et al: *Circ Res* 39:633, 1976.

Floras JS, Aylward PE, Victor RG, et al: *J Clin Invest* 81:1265, 1988a.

Floras JS, Hassan MO, Jones JV, et al: *Hypertension* 11:273, 1988b.

Floras JS, Hassan MO, Jones JV, et al: *Hypertension* 6:525, 1988c.

Folkow B: *Am Heart J* 114:938, 1987.

Folkow B: *Am J Hypertens* 2:103S, 1989.

Forrester TE, Alleyne GA: *Br Med J* 283:5, 1981.

Fray JCS, Park CS, Valentine AND: *Endocrine Rev* 8:53, 1987.

Frayn KN, Coppack SW, Humphreys SM, et al: *Clin Sci* 76:509, 1989.

Freidlander Y, Kark JD, Stein Y: *Int J Epidemiol* 17:70, 1988.

Freidman SM: *Hypertension* 1:572, 1979.

Freidman SM: *J Hypertension* 1:109, 1983.

Freidman SM, Nakashima M, Friedman CL: *Proc Soc Exp Biol Med* 150:171, 1975.

Frohlich ED, Tarazi RC, Dustan HP: *Arch Intern Med* 123:1, 1969.

Fujita T, Henry W, Bartter F, et al: *Am J Med* 69:334, 1980.

Furchgott RF, Zawadzki JV: *Nature* (Lond) 288:373, 1980.

Furspan PB, Bohr DF: *Clin Physiol Biochem* 6:122, 1988.

Fyhrquist F, Soveri P, Puutala L, et al: *Clin Chem* 22:250, 1976.

Garay RP, Meyer P: *Lancet* 1:349, 1979.

Garay RP, Nazaret C, Hannaert P, et al: *Eur J Clin Invest* 13:311, 1983.

Garcia-Palmieri MR, Costas R, Cruz-Vidal M, et al: *Hypertension* 6:322, 1984.

Garrison RJ, Kannel WB, Stokes J, et al: *Abstract*, 25th Conference Cardiovascular Epidemiology, CVD Epid Newsletter 37, American Heart Association (abstr 50), 1985, vol 3, pp 7–9.

Gavras H: *Hypertension* 8:83, 1986.

Geiger H, Bahner U, Anderes S, et al: *J Human Hypertens* 3:23, 1989.

Gelsthorpe K, Doughty RW, Bing RF, et al: *Lancet* 1:1039, 1975.

Gennari C, Nami R, Agnusdei D, et al: *Am J Hypertens* 2:45S, 1989.

Gennser G, Rymark P, Isberg PE: *Br Med J* 296:1498, 1988.

Ghione S, Rosa C, Mezzasalma L, et al: *Hypertension* 12:491, 1988.

Gill JR, Güllner HG, Lake CR, et al: *Hypertension* 11:312, 1988.

Gleiberman L, Gershowitz H, Harburg E, et al: *J Hypertension* 2:337, 1984.

Goldblatt H, Lynch J, Hanzal RF, et al: *J Exp Med* 59:347, 1934.

Goldblatt H: *Circulation* 17:642, 1958.

Goldstein DS, Lake CR: *Fed Proc* 43:57, 1984.

Goldstein HS, Edelberg R, Meier CF, et al: *Psychosomatic Med* 50:321, 1988.

Gomez-Sanchez CE, Holland OB, Upcavage R: *J Clin Endocrinol Metab* 60:234, 1985.

Goodman RM, Smith EW, Paton D, et al: *Medicine* (Baltimore) 42:297, 1963.

Gordon DB: *Hypertension* 5:353, 1983.

Gortmaker SL, Dietz WH Jr, Sobol AM, et al: *AJDC* 141:535, 1987.

Göthberg G, Lundin S, Aurell M, et al: *J Hypertension* 1(Suppl 2):24, 1983.

Goto A, Yamada K, Ishii M, et al: *Hypertension* 13:916, 1989.

Grandjean P, Hollnagel H, Hedegaard L, et al: *Am J Epidemiol* 129:732, 1989.

Grassi GM, Somers VK, Renk WS, et al: *J Hypertension* 7(Suppl 6):S20, 1989.

Greene AS, Tonellato PJ, Lui J, et al: *Am J Physiol* 256:H126, 1989.

Griendling KK, Berk BC, Ganz P, et al: *Hypertension* 9(Suppl III):III–181, 1987.

Grim CE, Luft FC, Miller JZ, et al: *J Chron Dis* 33:87, 1980.

Grim CE, Wilson TW, Drew CR: *Hypertension* 13:513, 1989 (abst).

Grobbee DE, Hofman A: *Lancet* 2:703, 1986.

Grobbee DE, van Hemert AM, Vandenbroucke JP, et al: *J Hypertension* 6(Suppl 4):S614, 1988.

Grooms A, Mitchel A, Millar JA, et al: *J Hypertens* 7(Suppl 6):S368, 1989

Guilleminault C, Simmons FB, Motta J, et al: *Arch Intern Med* 141:988, 1981.

Guyton AC: *Am J Cardiol* September:401, 1961.

Guyton AC: *Textbook of Medical Physiology*, Seventh Edition. Philadelphia: WB Saunders Company, 1986:265.

Guyton AC: *Hypertension* 10:1, 1987.

Guyton AC, Coleman TG: *Circ Res* 24:1, 1969.

Guyton AC, Coleman TG, Cowley AW Jr, et al: *Am J Med* 52:584, 1972.

Guzzetti S, Piccaluga E, Casati R, et al: *J Hypertension* 6:711, 1988.

Hackenthal E, Metz R, Bührle CP, et al: *Kidney Int* 31(Suppl 2):S4, 1987.

Haddy FJ: *J Cardiovasc Pharmacol* 6:S439, 1984.

Haddy FJ: *N Engl J Med* 316:621, 1987.

Haddy FJ, Overbeck HW: *Life Sci* 19:935, 1976.

Halkin H, Modan M, Shefi M, et al: *Hypertension* 11:71, 1988.

Hamlyn JM, Harris DW, Clark MA, et al: *Hypertension* 13:681, 1989.

Hannaert PA, Galli CE, Diaz AS, et al: *J Hypertension* 5(Suppl 5):S261, 1987.

Harburg E, Erfurt JC, Chape C, et al: *J Chronic Dis* 26:595, 1973.

Harburg E, Gleibermann L, Roeper P, et al: *AJPH* 68:1177, 1978.

Hardman JA, Hort YJ, Catanzaro DF, et al: *DNA* 3:457, 1983.

Hargreaves M, Morgan TP, Snow R, et al: *Clin Sci* 76:553, 1989.

Harlan WR, Hull AL, Schmouder RL, et al: *Am J Epidemiol* 120:17, 1984.

Harlan WR, Landis JR, Flegal KM, et al: *Am J Epidemiol* 128:1065, 1988.

Harlan WR, Landis JR, Schmouder RL, et al: *JAMA* 253:530, 1985.

Haupert GT Jr: *J Cardiovasc Pharmacol* 12(Suppl 3):S70, 1988.

Haupert GT, Carilli CY, Cantley LC: *Am J Physiol* 247:F919, 1984.

Havlik RJ, Feinleib M: *Hypertension* 4(Suppl III):III–121, 1982.

Heagerty AM, Bing RF, Milner M, et al: *Lancet* 2:894, 1982.

Heagerty AM, Izzard AS, Ollerenshaw JD, et al: *Int J Cardiol* 20:15, 1988.

Heagerty AM, Ollerenshaw JD: *J Hypertension* 5:515, 1987.

Hedner T, Hartford M, Caidahl K, et al: *J Intern Med* 225:229, 1989.

Heller J, Horácek V: *Renal Physiol* 9:357, 1986.

Helmer OM: *Can Med Ass J* 90:221, 1964.

Henrich HA, Romen W, Heimgärtner W, et al: *Klin Wochenschr* 66:54, 1988.

Hermsmeyer K: *J Cardiovasc Pharmacol* 6:S10, 1984.

Higgins MW, Keller JB, Metzner HL, et al: *Hypertension* 2(Suppl I):I–117, 1980.

Hilton PJ: *N Engl J Med* 314:222, 1986.

Hoffstein V, Rubinstein I, Mateika S, et al: *Lancet* 2:992, 1988.

Hofman A, Ellison RC, Newburger J, et al: *Br Heart J* 48:377, 1982.

Hofman A, Hazebroek A, Valkenburg HA: *JAMA* 250:370, 1983.

Hohn AR, Riopel DA, Keil JE, et al: *Hypertension* 5:56, 1983.

Holland OB, Chud JM, Braunstein H: *J Clin Invest* 65:347, 1980.

Holland OB, Gomez-Sanchez C, Fairchild C, et al: *Arch Intern Med* 139:1365, 1979.

Hollenberg NK: *Semin Nephrol* 3:171, 1983.

Hollenberg NK: *Ann Rev Pharmacol Toxicol* 28:41, 1988.

Hollenberg NK, Moore T, Shoback D, et al: *Am J Med* 81:412, 1986.

Hollenberg NK, Williams GH: *The Kidney* 21:13, 1988.

Hollenberg NK, Williams GH, Adams DF: *Hypertension* 3:11, 1981.

Howe PRC, Rogers PF, Smith RM: *J Hypertension* 7:387, 1989.

Howes LG, Macgilchrist A, Hawksby C, et al: *Br J Clin Pharmac* 22:521, 1986.

Hughes GS, Mathur RS, Margolius HS: *J Hypertension* 7:181, 1989.

Hulter HN, Melby JC, Peterson JC, et al: *J Clin Hypertens* 4:360, 1986.

Hunt SC, McCarron DA, Smith JB, et al: *Clin Exp Hypertens* A6:1397, 1984.

Hunt SC, Williams RR, Smith JB, et al: *Hypertension* 8:30, 1986.

Hunyor SN, Zweifler AJ, Hansson L, et al: *Aust NZ J Med* 5:17, 1975.

Hura CE, Kunau RT Jr: *Am J Physiol* 254:F734, 1988.

Hvarfner A, Bergström R, Mörlin C, et al: *J Hypertension* 5:451, 1987.

Hypertension Detection and Follow-up Program Cooperative Group: *Am J Epidemiol* 106:351, 1977.

Hypertension Detection and Follow-up Program Cooperative Group: *Hypertension* 9:641, 1987.

Ignarro LJ: *FASEB J* 3:31, 1989.

Ikeda M, Gutkowska J, Thibault G, et al: *Hypertension* 3:81, 1981.

Inagami T, Mizuno K, Nakamaru M, et al: *Cardiovasc Drugs Ther* 2:453, 1988.

Inoue A, Yanagisawa M, Kimura S, et al: *Proc Natl Acad Sci* 86:2863, 1989.

Intersalt Cooperative Research Group: *Br Med J* 297:319, 1988.

Irvine MJ, Garner DM, Olmsted MP, et al: *Psychosom Med* 51:537, 1989.

Izzard AS, Heagerty AM: *J Hypertension* 7:173, 1989.

Izzo JL: *J Cardiovasc Pharmacol* 6:S515, 1984.

James SA: *Circulation* 76(Suppl I):I-60, 1987.

Janssen WMT, de Zeeuw D, van der Hem GK, et al: *Hypertension* 13:640, 1989.

Jenner DA, Puddey IB, Beilin LJ, et al: *J Hypertension* 6(Suppl 4):S605, 1988.

Jennings G, Nelson L, Nestel P, et al: *Circulation* 73:30, 1986.

Jern S: *J Cardiovasc Pharmacol* 8(Suppl 5):S48, 1986.

Jones AW, Hart RG: *Circ Res* 37:333, 1975.

Julius S: *Am Heart J* 116:600, 1988.

Julius S, Conway J: *Circulation* 38:282, 1968.

Julius S, Esler M: *Am J Cardiol* 36:685, 1975.

Julius S, Li Y, Brant D, et al: *Hypertension* 13:422, 1989.

Julius S, Weder AB, Egan BM: In: Gross F, Strasser T (eds). *Mild Hypertension : Recent Advances*. New York: Raven Press, 1983:219.

Kageyama Y, Bravo EL: *Hypertension* 9(Suppl III):III-166-70, 1987.

Kahn AM: *Hypertension* 9:7, 1987.

Kales A, Bixler EO, Cadieux RJ, et al: *Lancet* 2:1005, 1984.

Kaloyanides GJ, Dibona GF, Raskin P: *Am J Physiol* 220:1660, 1971.

Kannel WB, Garrison RJ, Zhang T: *JACC* 13:104A, 1989 (abst).

Kaplan GA, Salonen JT, Cohen RD, et al: *Am J Epidemiol* 128:370, 1988.

Kaplan NM: *JAMA* 231:167, 1975.

Kaplan NM: *JAMA* 238:611, 1977.

Kaplan NM: *JAMA* 251:142, 1984.

Kaplan NM: Systemic Hypertension: Mechanisms and Diagnosis. In: Braunwald E (ed). *Heart Disease*. Philadelphia: WB Saunders, 1988:833.

Kaplan NM: *Arch Intern Med* 149:1514, 1989.

Kaplan NM, Kem DC, Holland OB, et al: *Ann Intern Med* 84:639, 1976.

Kaplan NM, Meese RB: *Ann Intern Med* 105:947, 1986.

Kaplan NM, Silah JG: *J Clin Invest* 43:659, 1964.

Kawamura M, Parmentier M, Inagami T: *Am J Physiol* 255:F100, 1988.

Kawasaki T, Delea CS, Bartter FC, et al: *Am J Med* 64:193, 1978.

Keeton TK, Campbell WB: *Pharmacol Rev* 32:81, 1980.

Keil JE, Sandifer SH, Loadholt CB, et al: *Am J Publ Health* 71:532, 1981.

Kelly RA, Smith TW: *Am J Physiol* 256:C937, 1989.

Kempner W: *Arch Intern Med* 133:758, 1974.

Kesteloot H, Joossens JV: *Hypertension* 12:594, 1988.

Khaw K-T, Barrett-Connor E: *Am J Clin Nutr* 39:963, 1984.

Khaw K-T, Barrett-Connor E: *Circulation* 77:53, 1988a.

Khaw K-T, Barrett-Connor E: *J Hypertension* 6:329, 1988b.

Khaw K-T, Barrett-Connor E, in press.

Kimura G, Saito F, Kojima S, et al: *Hypertension* 10:11, 1987.

King GL, Goodman AD, Buzney S, et al: *J Clin Invest* 75;1028, 1985.

Kirkman S, Nelson DH: *Metabolism* 37:390, 1988.

Kjeldsen SE, Flaaten B, Eide I, et al: *Scand J Clin Lab Invest* 43:15, 1983.

Kjeldsen SE, Sejersted OM, Frederichsen P, et al: *J Hypertension*, 7(Suppl 6):S156, 1989.

Klatsky AL, Friedman GD, Siegelaub AB, et al: *N Engl J Med* 296:1194, 1977.

Knowler WC, Bennett PH, Ballintine EJ: *N Engl J Med* 302:645, 1980.

Knudsen KD, Iwai J, Heine M, et al: *J Exp Med* 130:1353, 1969.

Koenig W, Sund M, Ernst E, et al: *Angiology* 40:153, 1989.

Kohno M, Yasunari K, Murakawa K, et al: *Am J Cardiol* 59:1212, 1987.

Koolen MI, van Brummelen P: *Hypertension* 6:820, 1984a.

Koolen MI, van Brummelen P: *Hypertension* 2:55, 1984b.

Korner PI, Oliver JR, Casley DJ: *Hypertension* 2:794, 1980.

Krakoff LR, Goodwin FJ, Baer L, et al: *Circulation* 42:335, 1970.

Kravtsov GM, Dulin NO, Postnov YV: *J Hypertension* 6:853, 1988.

Krishna GG, Miller E, Kapoor S: *N Engl J Med* 320:1177, 1989.

Kuriyama S, Hopp L, Tamura H, et al: *Hypertension* 11:301, 1988.

Kurtz TW, Al-Bander HA, Morris RC Jr: *N Engl J Med* 317:1043, 1987.

Kurtz TW, Morris RC Jr: *Science* (Wash DC) 222:1139, 1983.

Langer SZ, Hicks PE: *Br J Anaesth* 56:689, 1984.

Langford HG, Cushman WC, Hsu H: *Clin Res* 37:33A, 1989 (abst).

Laragh JH: *Am J Med* 55:263, 1973.

Laragh JH, Resnick LM: *Kidney Int* 34(Suppl 25):S-162, 1988.

Lasker N, Hopp L, Grossman S, et al: *J Clin Invest* 75:1813, 1985.

Laurent S, Juillerat L, London GM, et al: *Am J Physiol* 255:H36, 1988.

Lawrence JS: *Ann Rheum Dis* 34:451, 1975.

Lazdunski M: *Am J Med* 84(Suppl 1B):3, 1988.

Lebel M, Schalekamp MA, Beevers DG, et al: *Lancet* 2:308, 1974.

Ledingham JM: *J Hypertension* 7(Suppl 4):S97, 1989.

Ledingham JM, Cohen RD, Burns RF: *Clin Sci* 22:69, 1962.

Lee JY, Tobian L, Hanlon S, et al: *Hypertension* 13:668, 1989.

Lenders JWM, Willemsen JJ, de Boo T, et al: *J Hypertension* 7:317, 1989.

Le Quan-Sang KH, Levenson J, Simon A, et al: *J Hypertension* 5(Suppl 5):S251, 1987.

Lever AF: *J Hypertension* 4:515, 1986.

Lever AF: *Am J Hypertens* 2:276, 1989.

Lewicka S, Vecsei P, Abdelhamid S, et al: Program 1989, Endocrine Society, June 21, 1989, Seattle, Abstract 413, pg. 126.

Lian C: *Bull Acad Natl Med* 74:525, 1915.

Lifton RP, Hopkins RN, Williams RR, et al: *Hypertension* 13:884, 1989.

Light KC, Koepke JP, Obrist PA, et al: *Science* (Wash DC) 220:429, 1983.

Lillioja S, Young AA, Culter CL, et al: *J Clin Invest* 80:415, 1987.

Lindner A, Kenny M, Meacham AJ: *N Engl J Med* 316:509, 1987.

Lindgärde F, Furu M, Ljung B-O: *J Epidemiol Comm Health* 41:220, 1987.

Linnoila M, Mefford I, Nutt D, et al: *Ann Intern Med* 107:875, 1987.

Linz W, Scholkens BA, Han YF: *J Cardiovasc Pharmacol* 8(Suppl 10):S91, 1986.

Little PJ, Cragoe EJ, Bobik A: *Am J Physiol* 251:C707, 1986.

Livne A, Balfe JW, Veitch R, et al: *Lancet* 1:533, 1987.

London GM, Levenson JA, London AM, et al: *Kidney Int* 26:342, 1984.

London GM, Safar ME, Simon AC, et al: *Circulation* 57:995, 1978.

London GM, Safar ME, Weiss YA, et al: *Arch Intern Med* 137:1042, 1977a.

London GM, Safer ME, Weiss YA, et al: *Kidney Int* 11:204, 1977b.

Losse H, Wehmeyer H, Wessels F: *Klin Wochenschr* 38:393, 1960.

Louis WJ, Tabei R, Spector S: *Lancet* 2:1283, 1971.

Lowenstein FW: *Lancet* 1:389, 1961.

Luetscher JA, Kraemer FB, Wilson DM: *Am J Hypertens* 2:382, 1989.

Luft FC, Rankin LI, Bloch R, et al: *Circulation* 60:697, 1979.

Lund-Johansen P: *Acta Med Scand* (Suppl 603):1, 1977.

Lund-Johansen P: *J Hypertension*, 7(Suppl 6):S52, 1989.

Lüscher TF: *Am J Hypertens* 2:108A, 1989 (abst).

Lutas EM, Devereux RB, Reis G, et al: *Hypertension* 7:979, 1985.

Lyall F, Morton JJ, Lever AF, et al: *J Hypertension* 6(Suppl 4):S438, 1988.

Macdonald LA, Sackett DL, Haynes RB, et al: *J Chron Dis* 37:933, 1984.

MacLean CJ, Adams MS, Leyshon WC, et al: *Am J Hum Genet* 26:614, 1974.

MacMahon S: *Hypertension* 9:111, 1987.

Maddocks I: *Med J Aust* 1:1123, 1967.

Majewski H, Tung LH, Rand MJ: *J Cardiovasc Pharmacol* 3:179, 1981.

Marche P, Koutouzov S, Girard A, et al: *J Hypertension* 3:25, 1985.

Masugi F, Ogihara T, Sakaguchi K, et al: *J Hypertension* 6(Suppl 4):S351, 1988.

Masuyama Y, Tasuda K, Shima H, et al: *J Hypertension* 6(Suppl 4):S266, 1988.

Matthews KA, Cottington EM, Talbott E, et al: *Am J Epidemiol* 126:280, 1987.

May CN, Whitehead CJ, Heslop KE, et al: *Clin Sci* 76:431, 1989.

McCarron DA: *N Engl J Med* 307:226, 1982a.

McCarron DA: *Hypertension* 4(Suppl III):III-27, 1982b.

McCarron DA: *Kidney Int* 35:717, 1989.

McCarron DA, Morris CD, Henry HJ, et al: *Science* (Wash DC) 224:1392, 1984.

McCarron DA, Pingree PA, Rubin RJ, et al: *Hypertension* 2:162, 1980.

McManus IC: *Stat Med* 2:253, 1983.

Meade TW, Imeson JD, Gordon D, et al: *Clin Sci* 64:273, 1983.

Melamed S: *Psychosomatic Med* 49:217:1987.

Messerli FH, DeCarvalho JGR, Christi B, et al: *Circulation* 48:441, 1978.

Messerli FH, DeCarvalho JGR, Christie B, et al: *Am J Med* 67:27, 1979.

Messerli FH, Frohlich ED, Dreslinski GR, et al: *Ann Intern Med* 93:817, 1980.

Messerli FH, Garavaglia GE, Schmieder RE, et al: *Ann Intern Med* 107:158, 1987.

Metting PJ, Stein PM, Stoos BA, et al: *Am J Physiol* 256:R98, 1989.

Michel MC, Galal O, Stoermer J, et al: *J Cardiovasc Pharmacol* 13:432, 1989.

Millan MA, Aguilera G: *Endocrinology* 122:1984, 1988.

Miller JZ, Weinberger MH, Christian JC, et al: *Am J Epidemiology* 126:822, 1987.

Mimran A, Mourad G, Mion CM: *J Hypertension* 1(Suppl 2):55, 1983.

Mir MA, Morgan K, Chappel S, et al: *Clin Sci* 75:197, 1988.

Mitas JA II, Holle R, Levy SB, et al: *Arch Intern Med* 139:157, 1979.

Modan M, Halkin H, Almog S, et al: *J Clin Invest* 75:809, 1985.

Mogensen CE, Christensen CK: *Hypertension* 7(Suppl II):II-64, 1985.

Möhring J, Kintz J, Schoun J: *J Cardiovasc Pharmacol* 1:593, 1979.

Mongeau J-G, Biron P, Sing CF: *Clin Exper Theory and Pract* A8:653, 1986.

Morgan TO: *Clin Sci* 63(Suppl):407s, 1982.

Morton WE: *Arch Intern Med* 135:653, 1975.

Muirhead EE, Byers LW, Capdevila J, et al: *J Hypertension* 7:361, 1989.

Mulvany MJ: *J Hypertension* 5:129, 1987.

Myers MG: *Arch Intern Med* 148:1189, 1988.

Nabel EG, Berk BC, Brock TA, et al: *Circ Res* 62:486, 1988.

Naditch MP: *Soc Psychiatry* 9:111, 1974.

Naftilan AJ, Pratt RE, Dzau VJ: *J Clin Invest* 83:1419, 1989.

Nakamura A, Hatori N, Nakamura M, et al: *Am J Hypertens* 2:105, 1989.

Nakao K, Saito Y, Hosoda K, et al: Endocrine Society Meeting, 1989 (abst).

Nathan MA, Reis DJ: *Circ Res* 40:72, 1977.

Ng LL, Dudley C, Bomford J, et al: *J Hypertension* 7:471, 1989.

Ng LL, Harker M, Abel ED: *Clin Sci* 75:521, 1988.

Nielsen JR, Gram LF, Pedersen PK: *J Hypertension* 7:377, 1989c.

Nielsen AH, Poulsen K: *J Hypertension* 6:949, 1988.

Nielsen JR, Johansen T, Pedersen KE, et al: *J Hypertension* 6:815, 1988.

Nielsen JR, Pedersen KE, Klitgaard NA, et al: *Scand J Clin Lab Invest* 49:293, 1989a.

Nielsen JR, Pedersen KE, Klitgaard NA, et al: *Eur J Clin Invest* 19:72, 1989b.

Nussberger J, Brunner DB, Waeber B, et al: *Life Sci* 42:1683, 1988.

Oliver WJ, Cohen EL, Neel JV: *Circulation* 52:146, 1975.

Ollerenshaw JD, Heagerty AM, Bing RF, et al: *J Human Hypertens* 1:9, 1987.

Ollerenshaw JD, Heagerty AM, West KP, et al: *J Hypertension* 6:733, 1988.

Orlov SN, Gulak PV, Litvinov IS: *Clin Sci* 63:43, 1982.

Orlov SN, Postnov Y: *Clin Sci* 63:281, 1982.

Os I, Kjeldsen SE, Skjøtø, et al: *Hypertension* 8:506, 1986.

Os I, Kjeldsen SE, Westheim A, et al: *J Hypertension* 5:191, 1987.

Oshima T, Matsuura H, Kido K, et al: *J Hypertension* 7:223, 1989.

Oshima T, Matsuura H, Matsumoto K, et al: *Hypertension* 11:703, 1988.

Ott CE, Welch WJ, Lorenz JN, et al: *Am J Physiol* 256:H1426, 1989.

Overbeck HW: *Hypertension* 6:647, 1984.

Overbeck HW, Wallick ET, Shikuma R, et al: *Hypertension* 12:32, 1988.

Paffenbarger RS Jr, Wing AL, Hyde RT, et al: *Am J Epidemiol* 117:245, 1983.

Page IH: *Arch Intern Med* 111:149, 1963.

Page IH, Helmer O: *J Exp Med* 71:29, 1940.

Page LB: In: Hunt JC (ed). *Hypertension Update.* Bloomfield, NJ: Health Learning Systems, 1979.

Page LB, Vandevert DE, Nader K, et al: *Am J Clin Nutr* 34:527, 1981.

Pamnani MB, Clough DL, Hout SJ, et al: *Proc Soc Exp Biol Med* 165:440, 1980.

Panza JA, Quyyumi AA, Epstein SE: *Circulation* 78(Suppl II):II–473, 1988.

Paulsen EP, Seip RL, Ayers CR, et al: *Hypertension* 13:781, 1989.

Peiris AN, Sothmann MS, Hoffmann RG, et al: *Ann Intern Med* 110:867, 1989.

Perini C, Müller FB, Bühler FR: *J Cardiovasc Pharmacol* 12(Suppl 3):S130, 1988.

Petty MA, Reid JL: *Hypertension* 3(Suppl I):I–142, 1981.

Postnov YV: *Cardiology* (Moscow) 15:18, 1975.

Postnov YV, Orlov SN: *Physiological Rev* 65:904, 1985.

Postnov YV, Orlov SN, Pokudin NI: *Pfluegers Arch Eur J Physiol* 379:191, 1979.

Postnov YV, Orlov SN, Reznikova MB, et al: *Clin Sci* 66:479, 1984.

Postnov YV, Orlov SN, Shevchenko A, et al: *Eur J Physiol* 371:263, 1977.

Poston L: *Clin Sci* 72:647, 1987.

Poulter N, Khaw KT, Hopwood BEC, et al: *J Cardiovasc Pharmacol* 6S:197, 1984.

Poulter NR, Shipley MJ, Bulpitt CJ, et al: *J Hypertension* 6(Suppl 4):S611, 1988.

Pouyssegur J: *Trends Biochem Sci* 10:453, 1985.

Prior IAM, Evans JG, Harvey HPB, et al: *N Engl J Med* 279:515, 1968.

Puddey IB, Beilin LJ, Vandongen R: *Lancet* 1:647, 1987.

Rabinowe SL, Redgrave JE, Shoback DM, et al: *Hypertension* 10:404, 1987.

Radice M, Alli C, Avanzini F, et al: *Am Heart J* 111:115, 1986.

Ragland DR, Winkleby MA, Schwalbe J, et al: *Int J Epidemiol* 16:208, 1987.

Raison J, Achimastos A, Asmar R, et al: *Am J Cardiol* 57:223, 1986.

Rapado A: *Advances Exp Med Biol* 41:451, 1974.

Reaven GM: *Diabetes* 37:1595, 1988.

Reaven GM, Ho H, Hoffmann BB: *Hypertension* 14:117, 1989.

Rebuffe-Scrivé M, Andersson B, Olbe L, et al: *Metabolism* 38:453, 1989.

Redgrave J, Canessa M, Gleason R, et al: *Hypertension* 13:721, 1989.

Resnick LM, Laragh JH: *Am J Med* 78:385, 1985.

Resnick LM, Laragh JH, Sealey JE, et al: *N Engl J Med* 309:888, 1983.

Rikimaru T, Fujita Y, Okuda T, et al: *Am J Clin Nutr* 47:502, 1988.

Ringel RE, Hamlyn JM, Hamilton BP, et al: *Hypertension* 9:437, 1987.

Riozzi A, Heagerty AM, Ollerenshaw JD, et al: *Clin Sci* 73:29, 1987a.

Robertson DA, Heagerty AM, Ollerenshaw JD, et al: *J Human Hypertens* 3:117, 1989.

Rogacz S, Hollenberg NK, Williams GH: *Hypertension* 9:289, 1987.

Roman RJ, Cowley AW: *Am J Physiol* 248:F199, 1985.

Romero PJ, Whittam R: *J Physiol* 214:481, 1971.

Rosic NK, Standaert ML, Pollet RJ: *J Biol Chem* 260:6206, 1985.

Rostrup M, Westheim A, Kjeldsen SE, et al: *Am J Hypertens* 2:110A, 1989 (abst).

Rowe JW, Young JB, Minaker KL, et al: *Diabetes* 30:219, 1981.

Rüddel H, Langewitz W, Schächinger H, et al: *Am Heart J* 116:617, 1988.

Safar ME, St. Laurent S, Safavian AL, et al: *J Hypertension* 5:213, 1987.

Saito Y, Nakao K, Sugawara A, et al: *Am Heart J* 116:1052, 1988.

Saltman P: *Ann Intern Med* 98:823, 1983.

Sanchez RA, Marco EJ, Oliveri C, et al: *Am J Cardiol* 59:881, 1987.

Sanchez-Castillo CP, Warrender S, Whitehead TP, et al: *Clin Sci* 72:95, 1987.

Sannerstedt R: *Acta Med Scand* 180(Suppl 458):1, 1966.

Saper CB, Standaert DG, Currie M, et al: *Science* (Wash DC) 227:1047, 1985.

Sardet C, Franchi A, Pouyssegur J: *Cell* 58:271, 1989.

Sarzani R, Brecher P, Chobanian AV: *J Clin Invest* 83:1404, 1989.

Saunders JB, Beevers DG, Paton A: *Lancet* 2:653, 1981.

Schalekamp MADH, Birkenhäger WH, Zaal GA, et al: *Clin Sci Mol Med* 52:405, 1977.

Schalekamp MADH, Man in't Veld AJ, Wenting GJ: *J Hypertension* 3:97, 1985.

Schmouder RL, Weder AB: *J Hypertension* 7:325, 1989.

Schneider RH, Egan BM, Johnson EH, et al: *Psychosomatic Med* 48:242, 1986.

Sealey JE, Blumenfeld JD, Bell GM, et al: *J Hypertension* 6:763, 1988a.

Sealey JE, Goldstein M, Pitarrest, et al: *J Clin Endocrinol Metab* 66:974, 1988b.

Sealey JE, Lenz T, Lappe RW, et al: *Am J Hypertens* 2:59A, 1989 (abst).

Sealey JE, Rubattu S: *Am J Hypertens* 2:358, 1989.

Seedat YK: *Br Med J* 281:1241, 1980.

Seely EW, Moore TJ, Rogacz S, et al: *Hypertension* 13:31, 1989.

Seely S: *Am Heart J* 91:275, 1976.

Seifter JL, Aronson PS: *J Clin Invest* 78:859, 1986.

Selkurt EE: *Circulation* 4:541, 1951.

Sempos C, Cooper R, Kovar MG, et al: *Hypertension* 8:1067, 1986.

Sever PS, Poulter NR, Khaw KT: In: Mathias CJ, Sever PS (eds). *Concepts in Hypertension.* New York: Springer-Verlag, 1989.

Seymour AA, Davis JO, Freeman RH, et al: *Hypertension* 2:125, 1980.

Shaper AG, Wannametheee G, Whincup P: *J Hum Hypertens* 2:71, 1988.

Shen D-C, Shieh S-M, Fuh M-T, et al: *J Clin Endocrinol Metab* 66:580, 1988.

Shipley RE, Study RS: *Am J Physiol* 167:676, 1951.

Shore ACE, Booker J, Sagnella GA, et al: *J Hypertension* 5:499, 1987.

Sielecki AR, Hayakawa K, Fujinaga M, et al: *Science* (Wash DC) 243:1346, 1989.

Simon ACh, Safar ME, Levenson JA, et al: *Clin Exp Hypertension* 1:557, 1979.

Simon G: *Clin Sci* 76:455, 1989.

Simon G, Engel CR: *Hypertension* 9(Suppl III):III–13, 1987.

Simonson DC: *Diabetes Care* 11:821, 1988.

Simpson FO: *NZ Med J* 96:907, 1983.

Siskind MS, McCoy CE, Chobanian A, et al: *Am J Physiol* 256:C234, 1989.

Skinner SL, Thatcher RL, Whitworth JA, et al: *Lancet* 1:995, 1986.

Skrabal F, Herholz H, Neumayr M, et al: *Hypertension* 6:152, 1984.

Smith JB, Wade MB, Fineberg NS, et al: *Hypertension* 13:716, 1989a.

Smith JB, Fineberg NS, Wade MB, et al: *Hypertension* 13:15, 1989b.

Smith JB, Zheng T, Smith L: *Am J Physiol* 256:C147, 1989c.

Smith WCS, Crombie IK, Tavendale RTT, et al: *Br Med J* 297:329, 1988.

Sonnenberg A: *Gastroenterology* 95:42, 1988.

Sørensen SS, Danielsen H, Amdisen A, et al: *J Hypertension* 7:21, 1989.

Sowers JR, Zemel MB, Zemel P, et al: *Hypertension* 12:485, 1988.

Sparrow D, Weiss ST, Vokonas PS, et al: *Am J Epidemiol* 127:731, 1988.

Staessen J, Fagard R, Pijnen P, et al: *J Hypertension* 7(Suppl 1):S19, 1989.

Stamler R, Stamler J, Gosch FC, et al: *JAMA* 262:1801, 1989.

Steptoe A, Melville D: *Lancet* 2:457, 1984.

Steptoe A, Melville D, Ross A: *Psychosomatic Med* 46:33, 1984.

Stout RW, Beirman EL, Ross R: *Circ Res* 36:319, 1975.

Strazzullo P, Cappuccio FP, De Leo A, et al: *J Human Hypertens* 1:155, 1987.

Strazzullo P, Galletti F, Cirillo M, et al: *Clin Sci* 71:239, 1986a.

Strazzullo P, Nunziata V, Cirillo M, et al: *Clin Sci* 65:137, 1983.

Strazzullo P, Siani A, Guglielmi S, et al: *Hypertension* 8:1084, 1986b.

Sudoh T, Kangawa K, Minamino N, et al: *Nature* (Lond) 332:78, 1988.

Suki WN, Schwettmann RS, Rector FC, et al: *Am J Physiol* 215:71, 1968.

Sullivan JM, Ratts TE: *Hypertension* 11:717, 1988.

Summers WE, Watson RL, Wooldridge WH, et al: *Arch Intern Med* 128:750, 1971.

Swales JD: In: Robertson JIS (ed). *Handbook of Hypertension, Vol 1: Clinical Aspects of Essential Hypertension*. Amsterdam: Elsevier Science Publishers, 1983:258.

Swales JD: *J Roy Coll Phys London* 22:11, 1988.

Tamura M, Inagami T, Kinoshita T, et al: *J Hypertension* 5:219, 1987.

Tarazi RC: *Circ Res* 38(Suppl II):II-73, 1976.

Tarazi RC, Fouad FM, Ferrario CM: *Fed Proc* 41:2691, 1983.

Taugner R, Bührle C, Hackenthal E, et al: *Contrib Nephrol* 43:76, 1984.

Tedde R, Sechi LA, Marigliano A, et al: *Am J Hypertens* 2:163, 1989.

Thurston H: *Am J Med* 61:768, 1976.

Timio M, Verdecchia P, Venanzi S, et al: *Hypertension* 12:457, 1988.

Toal CB, Leenen FHH: *Am J Physiol* 245:H1081, 1983.

Tobian L: *J Hypertension* 6(Suppl 4):S12, 1988.

Tobian L, Binion JT: *Circulation* 5:754, 1952.

Tobian L, Johnson MA, Lange J, et al: *Circ Res* 36 and 37(Suppl 1):1, 1975.

Toffelmire EB, Slater K, Corvol P, et al: *J Clin Invest* 83:679, 1989.

Trowell HC: *Lancet* 2:88, 1980.

Tuck ML, Corry DB, Maxwell M, et al: *Hypertension* 10:204, 1987.

Turner ST, Weidman WH, Michels VV, et al: *Hypertension* 13:378, 1989.

Tyroler HA: *Hypertension* 13(Suppl I):I-94, 1989.

Tyroler HA, Heyden S, Hames CG: In: Paul O (ed). *Epidemiology and Control of Hypertension*. Miami: Symposium Specialists, 1975:177.

Ullian ME, Linas SL: *J Clin Invest* 84:840, 1989.

Ulrych M: *Clin Sci Mol Med* 45:173, 1973.

Vallega GA, Canessa ML, Berk BC, et al: *Am J Physiol* 254:C751, 1988.

Vanatta JC: *JAMA* 147:893, 1951.

Van Hooft IMS, Grobbee DE, Derkx FHM: *J Hypertens* 7(Suppl 6):S371, 1989.

Vanhoutte PM: *Hypertension* 13:658, 1989.

Varricchio M, Paolisso G, Torella R, et al: *J Hypertension* 6(Suppl 1):S41, 1988.

Vaughan ED Jr, Laragh JH, Gavras I, et al: *Am J Cardiol* 32:523, 1973.

Veterans Administration Cooperative Study Group on Antihypertensive Agents: *J Chron Dis* 40:839, 1987.

Viberti GC, Keen H, Wiseman MJ: *Br Med J* 295:515, 1987.

Vincenzi FF, Morris CD, Kinsel LB, et al: *Hypertension* 8:1058, 1986.

Waeber B, Aubert J-F, Corder R, et al: *Am J Hypertens* 1:193, 1988.

Waller PC, Bhopal RS: *Lancet* 1:143, 1989.

Walter V, Distler A: *Hypertension* 4:205, 1982.

Wambach G, Meiners U, Bonner G, et al: *Klin Wochenschr* 62:1097, 1984.

Warley ARH, Mitchell JH, Stradling JR: *Q J Med* 68:637, 1988.

Weder AB: *N Engl J Med* 314:198, 1986.

Weder AB, Egan BM: *Hypertension* 12:199, 1988.

Weinberger MH, Miller JZ, Fineberg NS, et al: *Hypertension* 10:443, 1987.

Weinberger MH, Miller JZ, Luft FC, et al: *Hypertension* 8(Suppl II):II-127, 1986.

Weinberger MH, Smith JB, Fineberg NS, et al: *Hypertension* 13:206, 1989.

Weiss ST, Munoz A, Stein A, et al: *Am J Epidemiol* 123:800, 1986.

Weissberg PL: *J Hypertension* 1(Suppl 2):395, 1983.

Welt LG, Sachs JR, McManus TJ: *Trans Assoc Am Physiol* 77:169, 1964.

Werko L, Lagerlof H: *Acta Med Scand* 133:427, 1949.

Wessels VF, Junge-Hulsing G, Losse H: *Z Kreislaufforschung* 56:374, 1967.

White WB, Baker LH: *Arch Intern Med* 147:1973, 1987.

Whitescarver SA, Ott CE, Jackson BA, et al: *Science* (Wash DC) 223:1430, 1984.

Wiggins RC, Basar I, Slater JDH: *Clin Sci Mol Med* 54:639, 1978.

Williams BI, Gordon D, Peart WS: *Lancet* 2:1255, 1981.

Williams GH, Rose LI, Dluhy RG, et al: *Ann Intern Med* 72:317, 1970.

Williams RR, Hunt SC, Hasstedt SJ, et al: *J Cardiovasc Pharmacol* 12(Suppl 3):S7, 1988a.

Williams RR, Hunt SC, Wu LL, et al: *Clin Physiol Biochem* 6:136, 1988.

Winkleby MA, Ragland DR, Syme SL: *Am J Epidemiol* 127:124, 1988.

Wisgerhof M, Brown RD: *J Clin Invest* 61:1456, 1978.

Witteman JCM, Grobbee DE, Kok FJ, et al: *Br Med J* 298:642, 1989.

Woods JW, Pittman AW, Pulliam CC, et al: *N Engl J Med* 294:1137, 1976.

Woods KL, Beevers DG, West M: *Br Med J* 282:1186, 1981.

Yamada Y, Miyajima E, Tochikubo O, et al: *Hypertension* 13:870, 1989.

Yates WR, Wallace R: *J Affective Disorders* 12:129, 1987.

Yanagisawa M, Inoue A, Ishikawa T, et al: *Proc Natl Acad Sci* 85:6964, 1988.

Yeagle PL: *FASEB J* 3:1833, 1989.

Zavaroni I, Bonora E, Pagliara M, et al: *N Engl J Med* 320:702, 1989.

Zemel MB, Gualdoni SM, Walsh MF, et al: *J Hypertension* 4(Suppl 5):S364, 1986.

Zidek W, Sachinidis A, Spieker C, et al: *J Hypertension* 5(Suppl 5):S287, 1987.

Now that the possible causes of primary hypertension have been considered, we turn to its clinical course and complications. We will first view the overall natural history of the disease if left untreated. Then we will examine the specific manner by which hypertension leads to premature cardiovascular damage and the ways such damage is clinically expressed.

## OVERVIEW

The natural history of primary hypertension can be sketched from a few long-term uncontrolled observations, a larger number of short-term controlled studies, and extensive epidemiological data.

In a few words, the higher the blood pressure (BP) and the longer it remains elevated, the greater the morbidity and mortality. Though some with very high untreated BP never have trouble, we have no way to identify those who will have an uncomplicated course, the few who will enter a rapidly accelerating phase (malignant hypertension), and the majority who will more slowly but progressively develop vascular complications (Fig. 4.1).

As detailed in Chapter 1, the level of the BP alone is a rather insensitive guide for determining an individual's cardiovascular risk. However, for the population at large, the risks of untreated hypertension have been well defined. Without question, hypertension is among the leading preventable causes of disability and death in the United States and most of the world today. It is probable that its role is underestimated from morbidity and mortality statistics since in the past it was seldom reported on death certificates even when the physician was aware of its presence (Schweitzer et al, 1965). When a patient

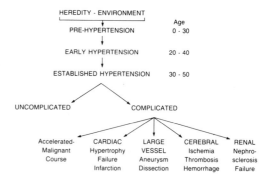

**Figure 4.1.** A representation of the natural history of untreated essential hypertension.

dies from a stroke, a heart attack, or renal failure—all directly attributable to untreated hypertension—the stroke, the heart attack, or the renal failure but not its cause is often listed on the death certificate.

## PREHYPERTENSION

Even before BP becomes persistently elevated, those destined to become hypertensive tend to have higher BP than those who will remain normotensive. This tendency can be identified even in young children (Labarthe, 1989), as will be described further in Chapter 16. It is more likely in children of hypertensive parents, mothers more so than fathers (Munger et al, 1988). Even with normal resting pressures, the children of hypertensives may display greater BP responses to exercise and larger left ventricular dimensions than children of normotensives (Celentano et al, 1988). Children with these features have an increased likelihood of developing hypertension as they grow older (Mahoney et al, 1988).

## Tracking the Blood Pressure

Perhaps the best tracking data come from the Framingham study (Kotchen et al, 1982), which has now been extended into the offspring of the original cohort (Garrison et al, 1987). There is an obvious regression toward the mean between the first examination and the second, 2 years later (Fig. 4.2). Thereafter, those in each segment of BP tend to remain in that segment, with a slow, gradual rise through the 14 years of follow-up. Interestingly, the risk for development of cardiovascular disease in the Framingham study was related to the actual level of the BP at the beginning of the prospective follow-up period, and not to its long-term trend in the more distant past (Hofman et al, 1983). Whether an elevated BP had been persistently elevated for the prior 12 years or had slowly risen up to its current level, the subsequent occurrence of cardiovascular disease over the next 15 years was similar.

Among the Framingham offspring ages 20 to 49, the prevalence of hypertension, defined as BP of 160/95 or higher or the current use of antihypertensive drugs, rose progressively over

the 3 decades, more in men than women. When age was factored out, the major contributors to the occurrence of hypertension were adiposity, heart rate, alcohol intake, hematocrit, blood sugar, serum protein, triglyceride, and phosphorus, the last having a negative correlation (Garrison et al, 1987). As described in Chapter 3, the distribution of body fat played a significant role, with a markedly higher incidence of hypertension among those with greater upper body fat as ascertained by subscapular skinfold thickness (Fig. 4.3). As in all other populations, the strongest predictor was the previous level of BP.

Thus, those whose BP is high now tend to have more of a rise with time but, as noted in Chapter 1, most with ''borderline'' BP will not progress into definite hypertension. The issue is clouded by the marked variability of the BP, but most hypertension develops in a slow, gradual manner. Until something more definitive can be offered, children of hypertensive parents and young adults who are on the higher tracks should be advised to avoid obesity, moderate their intake of sodium and alcohol, and exercise regularly. Among a group of 201 normotensive men and women aged 30 to 44 years who were considered hypertension prone because of high-normal blood pressure, overweight, and/or a rapid resting pulse, the 5-year incidence of hypertension was reduced from 19.2% in the half randomly assigned to only occasional monitoring to 8.8% in the half who moderated their intake of calories, sodium, and alcohol and exercised regularly (Stamler et al, 1989).

## EARLY HYPERTENSION

### Course of the Blood Pressure

In most who become hypertensive the hypertension persists. In fewer than 1%, it progresses to the malignant phase whereas in some the BP may return to normal, presumably not to rise again. Stewart (1971) reported his long-term observations on 53 asymptomatic men, aged 18 to 50, seen soon after the discovery of their elevated BP and who were at that time free of all vascular complications. Of these 53, 13 had normal or equivocally elevated BP on repeated readings, leaving 40 with established essential hypertension. In 12 of these, the diastolic blood pressure (DBP) fell without therapy from an average of 105 to 88 mm Hg over the next 2 to 16 years (average 6.7 years), and only one of the 12 developed a vascular complication. These

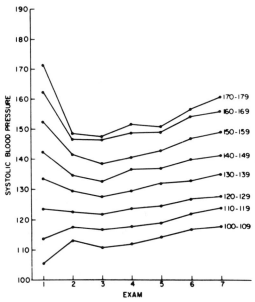

**Figure 4.2.** Mean systolic blood pressure levels measured every 2 years on repeated examinations of Framingham Study men, aged 30 to 59 years, divided into groups by their initial levels of blood pressure. Those taking antihypertensive drugs are excluded. (From Kotchen JM, McKean HE, Kotchen TA: Blood pressure trends with aging. *Hypertension* 4(suppl III):III-128, 1982, and by permission of the American Heart Association.)

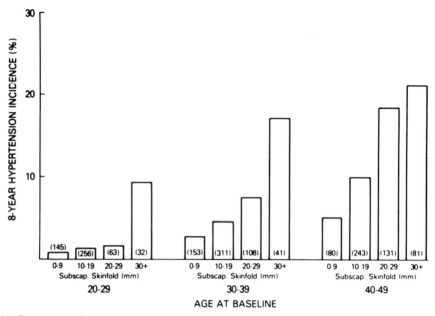

**Figure 4.3.** The age-specific 8-year incidence rates of hypertension by level of subscapular skinfold thickness in women ages 20 to 49 years in the Framingham offspring study. (From Garrison RJ, Kannel WB, Stokes J III, et al: *Prevent Med* 16:235, 1987.)

12 tended to be younger and more physically active, with lower initial levels of hypertension and fewer family members with the disease.

The findings in this small but carefully followed series reaffirm the point made in Chapter 2: Hypertension should be confirmed by multiple readings before the diagnosis is made and therapy is begun. If the second set of readings is considerably lower and the patient is free of obvious vascular complications, the patient should be advised to follow good health habits and to return every few months for repeat measurement or to self-monitor the BP at home. If the tendency toward a falling pressure continues, the patient should be simply followed, hopefully to become and remain normotensive.

The wisdom of this course is further shown by the Australian Therapeutic Trial (Management Committee, 1980): 12.8% of their patients whose DBPs averaged above 95 on two sets of initial readings had a subsequent fall in DBP to below 95 that persisted over the next year so that they could not be entered into the trial. An even larger portion—47.5%—of those who entered the trial with DBP above 95 and who received only placebo tablets for the next 3 years maintained average DBP below 95 mm Hg. A significant portion remained below 90 while on placebo, including 11% of those whose initial DBP was as high as 105 to 109 mm Hg.

## Symptoms

Most hypertension is asymptomatic even after it becomes persistent. This is in a way unfortunate: Too often hypertension is detected only after appearance of overt organ damage, years after the onset of the disease. As shown in Chapter 1, as many as 50% of patients found to have hypertension in surveys of various populations did not know their pressures were elevated.

Even if symptomatic, hypertensives may be less likely to complain, reflecting an unwillingness to disclose information, probably for psychosocial reasons. When two groups of eight male students, one group normotensive, the other identified as hypertensive but untreated, were asked whether they ever had concern over a series of problems occurring during their lives, most hypertensives denied concerns when the questions were asked casually, but more expressed concerns when they were asked in a high pressure, testing situation (Cumes-Rayner and Price, 1989).

### Headaches and Hyperventilation

Of the symptoms that are reported, headache is the most common, but those who complain of headache are more likely to have their BP taken and hypertension discovered (Bauer, 1976a). Stewart (1953) found that only 17% of patients unaware of their hypertension complained of headache but, among patients with similar levels of BP who were aware of their diagnosis, 71% had headaches. This is in keeping with my firm belief that many of the symptoms described by hypertensives are secondary to anxiety over having "the silent killer," as hypertension is frequently described, anxiety often expressed as recurrent acute hyperventilation episodes . Many of the symptoms described by hypertensives, such as band-like headaches, dizziness and lightheadedness, fatigue, palpitations, and chest discomfort reflect recurrent hyperventilation, a common problem among all patients but likely even more common among hypertensives who are anxious over their diagnosis and its implications. The alkalosis that develops during hyperventilation causes vasoconstriction (Rinaldi et al, 1987), thus setting up a vicious cycle: Anxiety over hypertension leads to recurrent hyperventilation, which raises the blood pressure further.

This belief that most symptoms and headache in particular are related not to the level of blood pressure but rather to the anxiety over the diagnosis of hypertension is strengthened by the fact that the prevalence of headache among *newly diagnosed* hypertensives varies little in relation to the level of BP, with 15 to 20% complaining whether their DBPs were as low as 95 mm Hg all the way up to 125 mm Hg (Cooper et al, 1989).

Further evidence that most hypertension is asymptomatic before it is recognized comes from a survey of symptoms present at the time of discovery of hypertension (Table 4.1). Neither headaches nor epistaxis, tinnitus, dizziness, or fainting were more common among those *previously unrecognized* hypertensives than among those with normal blood pressure.

In keeping with my belief that many symptoms attributed to the elevated BP are in fact related to the anxiety induced by the diagnosis, untreated hypertensive patients who *were aware* of their diagnosis complained more frequently of morning headache, depression, blurred vision, and, to a lesser extent, faintness and nocturia than did normotensive people (Bulpitt and Breckenridge, 1976). Some of these symptoms, in particular headaches and unsteadiness, were relieved with lowering of the blood pressure by therapy, which could reflect relief either from the elevated pressure or from the anxiety of having uncontrolled hypertension. On the other hand, once drug therapy is given, a host of additional symptoms may be imposed as reflections either of the nonspecific lowering of the BP or of the side effects of specific antihypertensive agents, as described in Chapter 7.

Clearly with very high BP, headaches become more common. The headache is usually present upon awakening, is felt in the back of the head, may or may not be throbbing in character, and often lasts only a few hours even without analgesic therapy. It should also be noted that sleep apnea is common among even minimally obese hypertensives, as described in Chapter 15, so that early morning headaches may reflect not hypertension but nocturnal hypoxia.

Beyond the symptoms of either the BP per se or the anxiety associated with the diagnosis, hypertensives may display various signs of target organ damage as described in Chapter 2 and later in this chapter. They may be easily flushed and plethoric, reflecting a pseudopolycythemia from a shrunken plasma volume.

## Laboratory Findings

None of the usual blood or urine tests is usually abnormal in the early, uncomplicated phases of essential hypertension. As noted first by Fishberg in 1924, hyperuricemia is found in about a third of untreated hypertensives (Breckenridge, 1966), and this has been shown to reflect underlying nephrosclerosis (Messerli et al, 1980). Two additional tests may indicate significant but unrecognized underlying renal disease, microalbuminuria and increased urinary levels of the enzyme $N$-acetyl-$\beta$-D-glucosaminidase, derived from renal tubules (Opsahl et al, 1988). Microalbuminuria, described by Parving et al (1974) in moderately severe hypertension, is now recognized among many with mild hypertension, likely a marker of glomerular hyperfiltration with a reduced ability to increase filtration further after a protein load (Losito et al, 1988).

**Table 4.1. Percentages of Subjects with Symptoms According to Diastolic Blood Pressure Level**[a]

| | Diastolic Blood Pressure (mm Hg) | | |
|---|---|---|---|
| | <90 | 90–99 | >100 |
| No. of subjects | 5447 | 754 | 383 |
| Symptoms (% affected) | | | |
| Headache | 22 | 21 | 25 |
| Epistaxis | 11 | 9 | 12 |
| Tinnitus | 9 | 9 | 8 |
| Dizziness | 9 | 11 | 11 |
| Fainting | 24 | 21 | 16 |

[a]Reprinted by permission of the *New England Journal of Medicine* 287:631, 1973, and NS Weiss.

Hypertriglyceridemia (Thomas et al, 1977) and, even more threatening, hypercholesterolemia (Hjermann et al, 1978) is found up to twice as frequently in untreated hypertensives as in normotensives (Fig. 4.4). The association may, in turn, reflect the quartet of upper body obesity, hyperlipidemia, and hypertension related to hyperinsulinemia that was described in Chapter 3.

Once therapy is given, a number of biochemical abnormalities may develop, as will be described in Chapter 7. As an example, with diuretics, the frequency of hyperuricemia more than doubles.

## ESTABLISHED HYPERTENSION

### Long-Term Observations

Few have the opportunity to follow a large group of untreated hypertensives over a long period. Three such long-range series have been reported—by Ranges (1949), Perera (1955), and Bechgaard (1967, 1976, 1983). Ranges observed 241 patients with hypertension of undefined severity for an average of 14 years and emphasized their generally benign course, with 79% remaining asymptomatic. Perera followed 500 patients with casual DBP of 90 mm Hg or

higher—150 from before onset and 350 from an uncomplicated phase—until their death. The incidence of complications is given in Table 4.2. The mean age of onset was 32, and the mean survival time was 20 years. Perera summarized his survey of the natural history of hypertension:

> . . .as a chronic illness, more common in women, beginning as a rule in early adult life, related little if at all to pregnancy, and persisting for an average period of two decades before its secondary complicating pathologic features cause death at an average age fifteen to twenty years less than the normal life expectancy. Hypertensive vascular disease may progress at a highly variable rate, but on the whole the patient with this disorder spends most of his hypertensive life with insignificant symptoms and without complications.

One additional point about Perera's data is worth emphasis: Few of his patients experienced the onset of hypertension after age 45. A similar finding was observed in the Cooperative Study of Renovascular Hypertension, wherein the diagnosis of primary hypertension was made with even greater certainty on 1128 patients. Of these, the onset of an elevated BP was documented to be below age 20 in 12% and above age 50 in only 7% (Maxwell, 1975). Thus, hypertension appearing after age 50 should be suspected of being secondary.

On the other hand, in a more recent prospective study of a large, more representative population than the more severely hypertensive patients followed by Perera or seen in the Cooperative Study, 20% of people aged 40 to 69 who became hypertensive over a 5-year period

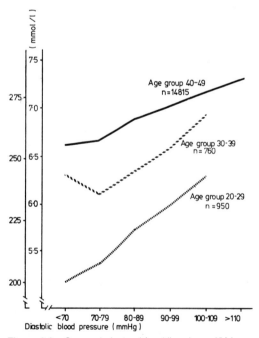

**Figure 4.4.** Serum cholesterol (mg/dl and mmol/L) in relation to diastolic blood pressure in three age groups of healthy men. (From Hjermann I, Helgeland A, Holme I, et al: *J Epidemiol Comm Health* 32:117, 1978.)

**Table 4.2. Complications in 500 Untreated Hypertensives**[a]

| Complication | % Affected | Mean Survival after Onset (Years) |
|---|---|---|
| Cardiac | | |
| Hypertrophy (seen by x-ray) | 74 | 8 |
| Hypertrophy (seen by ECG) | 59 | 6 |
| Congestive failure | 50 | 4 |
| Angina pectoris | 16 | 5 |
| Cerebral | | |
| Encephalopathy | 2 | 1 |
| Stroke | 12 | 4 |
| Renal | | |
| Proteinuria | 42 | 5 |
| Elevated blood urea nitrogen | 18 | 1 |
| Accelerated phase | 7 | 1 |

[a]Reprinted with permission from Perera GA: Hypertensive vascular disease: Description and natural history. *J Chronic Dis* 1:33, copyright 1955, Pergamon Press.

were 60 years of age or older (Buck et al, 1987). Moreover, the rate of developing a significant cardiovascular event among the newly discovered hypertensives was almost as high among those in their 40s as those aged 60 to 65 (Table 4.3). Note that the middle-aged hypertensives were much more likely to develop an event than normotensives of the same age but, as the authors state, "age overtakes hypertension as a cause of cardiovascular disease," so that among those aged 60 to 65, the rate was little different.

Bechgaard monitored the survival of 271 men and 629 women with an initial BP of 160/100 or higher who remained untreated for 45 years. Most of the excess mortality occurred during the first 10 years. Thereafter, survival was similar to that expected in the general population. Despite their average age of 54 at the beginning of the study, 29% of the men and 45% of the women reached the age of 75 and 6% and 11%, respectively, reached the age of 85.

As noted by Bechgaard, most series have shown a better prognosis for women, with fewer entering the accelerated-malignant phase or suffering from coronary artery disease. This lesser incidence of coronary heart disease among women is almost certainly the main reason for their longer survival (Lerner and Kannel, 1986).

## Control Groups in Clinical Trials

We have seen what happened to the patients of Ranges, Perera, and Bechgaard left untreated during the 1940s and 1950s when no effective therapy was readily available. To them, we can add those patients who served as the control populations in the trials of the therapy of hypertension performed in the 1960s, 1970s, and early 1980s. Though these trials were not designed to observe the natural history of hypertension, we can use their data to help define the course of untreated disease (Table 4.4).

The types of patients included in these trials

and the manner in which they were followed differed considerably, so comparisons between them are largely inappropriate. In particular, the European Working Party on High Blood Pressure in the Elderly (EWPHE) trial (Amery et al, 1985) and the trial of Coope and Warrender (1986) included only patients aged 60 years or older and included patients with DBP up to 120 mm Hg. The remainder generally excluded those over 65 and most limited DBP to 110 or 115 mm Hg. The patients also differed as to preexisting cardiovascular disease. All such patients were purposely excluded from the United States Public Health Service, Australian, and Oslo trials but not from the Veterans Administration Cooperative and the two trials in the elderly so the higher rate of complications in those entered in these three trials almost certainly reflects their preexisting target organ damage.

## Veterans Administration Cooperative Study Group on Antihypertensive Agents

The publications on these data [Veterans Administration (VA) Cooperative Study Group on Antihypertensive Agents, 1967, 1970, and 1972] have become landmarks in the field of clinical hypertension. The VA Study involved a selected population—men who were reliable and cooperative—but the data are probably in large part applicable to most moderately severe hypertensives, perhaps with some softening for women, who have a milder course.

*DBP Between 115 and 129.* The first VA study described the course of 70 men with initial DBP between 115 and 129 mm Hg who received only placebo. During their follow-up, which averaged 16 months and ranged up to 3 years, these complications were noted:

—6% (four patients) died, three from ruptured aortic aneurysms.
—24% (17 patients) developed accelerated hypertension, cerebral hemorrhage, severe congestive heart failure, or azotemia.
—9% (six patients) developed myocardial infarction, milder congestive failure, cerebral thrombosis, or transient ischemic attacks.

Thus, in less than 3 years, almost 40% of the patients with DBP between 115 and 129 mm Hg, *but initially without severe complications of their hypertension,* developed severe complications.

*DBP Between 90 and 114.* As surprising as the results described above were at the time, even more dramatic were those in the 194 pa-

**Table 4.3. Five-Year Occurrence of Cardiovascular Events in Newly Diagnosed Hypertensive Subjects and Normotensive Subjects by Age at Baseline**[a]

| Age Group (years) | Rate (per 100) | | Odds Ratio |
| --- | --- | --- | --- |
| | New Hypertensive | Normotensive | |
| 40–49 | 4.6 (239) | 0.9 (4677) | 5.2 |
| 50–59 | 5.6 (288) | 3.2 (3655) | 1.8 |
| 60–65 | 6.5 (153) | 5.7 (1301) | 1.2 |

[a]Number of subjects shown in parentheses. From Buck C, Baker P, Bass M, et al: The prognosis of hypertension according to age at onset. *Hypertension* 9:204, 1987, and by permission of the American Heart Association.

**Table 4.4. Complications Among Control Groups in Trials of Antihypertensive Therapy**

| | VA Cooperative 1967 | VA Cooperative 1970 | USPHS 1970 | Australian Trial, 1980 | Oslo Study, 1980 | MRC Study, 1985 | EWPHE (Amery) 1985[a] | Coope & Warrender 1986[a] |
|---|---|---|---|---|---|---|---|---|
| Range of diastolic blood pressure | 115–129 | 90–114 | 90–115 | 95–109 | 90–110 | 95–109 | 90–119 | 105–120 |
| No. on placebo | 70 | 194 | 196 | 1617 | 379 | 8654 | 424 | 465 |
| Average follow-up (yrs) | 1.3 | 3.3 | 7 | 3 | 5.5 | 5.5 | 4.6 | 4.4 |
| Rate/100 patients for entire trial | | | | | | | | |
| Coronary disease | | | | | | | | |
|   Fatal | 1 | 6 | 2 | 0.4 | 0.5 | 1.1 | 11.8 | 6.0 |
|   Nonfatal | 3 | 1 | 26 | 4.9 | 2.9 | 1.6 | 2.8 | 2.2 |
| Congestive heart failure | 3 | 6 | 1 | 0.1 | 0.2 | | 5.4 | 7.7 |
| Cerebrovascular disease | 16 | 11 | 3 | 1.5 | 1.8 | 1.3 | 13.7 | 9.4 |
| Renal insufficiency | 4 | 2 | 1 | 0.1 | | | 0.5 | 0.2 |
| Progression of hypertension | 4 | 10 | 12 | 12.2 | 17.2 | 11.7 | 6.8 | |
| Total mortality | 6 | 10 | 2 | 1.2 | 2.4 | 2.9 | 35.1 | 14.8 |

[a]Patients were all over age 60.

tients with initial DBP of 90 to 114 mm Hg, a group considered to have mild to moderate hypertension (Veterans Administration Cooperative Study, 1970, 1972). Their initial blood pressures averaged 157/101, and just over half had some evidence of preexisting hypertensive complications. Maximal follow-up was 5.5 years and averaged 3.3 years. The overall risk to these patients of developing a morbid event in a 5-year period was 55%.

All of the various complications except progression into accelerated hypertension occurred more frequently in the older patients (Table 4.5). More than six of 10 patients over age 60 developed some serious complication during this short interval. Perhaps even more striking is the occurrence of such complications in 15% of the younger patients. Another 14% of these younger patients had a significant rise in their DBP to above 124 mm Hg, so that without therapy they would be expected to develop serious complications quickly.

These results showed a more serious and rapidly progressive course of untreated mild to moderate essential hypertension than suggested by most previously reported studies. Morbidity was greater in those with the higher initial BP and preexisting cardiovascular disease. However, even among those who had no preexisting abnormalities attributable to hypertension, 16% developed a major complication in only 5 years.

## United States Public Health Service Hospital Study

In this study (Smith, 1977), 389 patients with milder hypertension than was present among the patients in the VA study were randomly divided into placebo and drug treatment groups and were followed for as long as 7 years. At the onset, none of the patients had evidence of target organ damage, and their mean BP was only 148/99. During the 7-year follow-up, the complications listed in Table 4.4 were noted among the placebo-treated group of truly mild hypertensives.

## Australian Therapeutic Trial

Over 1600 adults with DBP between 95 and 109 mm Hg who were initially free of known cardiovascular disease were kept on placebo for an average of 3 years (Management Committee, 1980). Over this relatively short period, significantly increased morbidity and mortality occurred only in those whose DBP averaged 100 mm Hg or higher during this interval. However, when the course of the BP among these 1617 patients is examined, an interesting point becomes apparent (Fig. 4.5). In this figure, taken from Table 10 of the 1980 *Lancet* paper, the patients given placebo are divided into three

**Table 4.5. Five-Year Morbidity in Untreated Male Hypertensives with Diastolic Blood Pressures of 90 to 114 mm Hg[a]**

| Age | <50 | 50–59 | 60+ |
|---|---|---|---|
| Total no. | 99 | 52 | 43 |
| Percentage with | | | |
|   Cerebral vascular accidents | 5 | 10 | 23 |
|   Congestive heart failure | 1 | 2 | 20 |
|   Accelerated hypertension | 5 | 4 | 0 |
|   Coronary artery disease | 4 | 8 | 12 |
|   Dissecting aneurysm | 0 | 2 | 2 |
| Overall % with morbidity | 15 | 27 | 63 |

[a]From Veterans Administration Cooperative Study Group on Antihypertensive Agents: Effects of treatment on morbidity in hypertension. *Circulation* 45:991, 1972, and by permission of the American Heart Association, Inc.

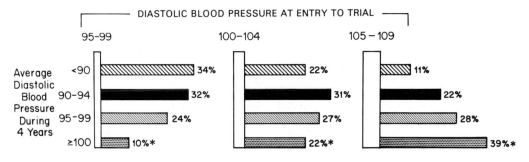

* Excess morbidity and mortality seen only among those with DBP ≥ 100 (22% of the total group), compared to drug treated patients

**Figure 4.5.** The average diastolic blood pressure (DBP) over 4 years in the 1617 hypertensive patients treated with placebo in the Australian Therapeutic Trial. Note that the majority of those with initial DBP from 95 all the way up to 109 ended with DBP below 100 and that excess complications were noted only in those whose end DBP was above 100. (Composed from data in Management Committee: *Lancet* 1:1261, 1980.)

groups by their DBP at entry (95 to 99, 100 to 104, and 105 to 109). The *bars* represent the percentage of each group whose average DBP during the 3 years of observation was below 90, 90 to 94, 95 to 99, and 100 or above. Note that even among those whose entry DBP was 105 to 109, 61% averaged less than 100 while on placebo. For all three groups, 80% had average DBP below 100. During this 3-year interval, no excess morbidity or mortality occurred in that 80% whose DBP averaged less than 100. The average fall over 3 years of placebo therapy was 14/11 mm Hg, and the DBP was below 95 in 47.5% of the patients at the end of the trial (Management Committee, 1982). Though the fall was greatest in those who lost weight, there was a significant decrease in the average BP even among those who gained weight while on placebo.

There are a number of implications that can be drawn from these observations:

—Though placebo may be more effective than no therapy, many patients not given antihypertensive drugs will have a significant fall in their BP, often to levels considered "safe" and not requiring therapy. Remember that another 12.8% of the patients originally screened for this trial whose DBP had averaged above 95 on two occasions had a spontaneous fall in their BP to below 95 during the year before the trial began so that they were excluded.
—On the other hand, recall from Table 4.4 that 12.2% of these patients had a progressive rise in the DBP to above 110 mm Hg, so that continued surveillance is obviously essential.
—Patients who are free of recognizable cardio-

vascular disease and whose DBP are below 100 mm Hg and certainly below 95 mm Hg can safely be left off active drug therapy for at least a few years while being kept under observation.

These conclusions form part of the basis of the approach toward initial management of patients with relatively mild hypertension presented in the next chapter.

### Oslo Trial

This trial (Helgeland, 1980) was similar to the Australian one in that it included only uncomplicated patients free of target organ damage with DBP below 110 and randomly divided them into nontherapy and drug therapy groups. It differed in being smaller in size, involving only men below 50 years of age, and providing no placebo pills to the control group.

The results were quite similar to those of the Australian trial. About half of the nontreated group had a fall in DBP during the first 3 years. Relatively little trouble developed among those whose DBP was initially below 100 mm Hg, whereas 16.4% of those within initial DBP between 100 and 110 mm Hg had a cardiovascular complication. The need for close surveillance is further documented: 17.2% of the nontreated group had a rise in their DBP to above 110 mm Hg.

### European Working Party on High Blood Pressure in the Elderly (EWPHE) Trial

This trial enrolled 840 patients over the age of 60 (average 72) with systolic pressure from 160 up to 240 and DBP from 90 up to 120 mm Hg (Amery et al, 1985). Only 122 of the 424 patients initially assigned to placebo were still on placebo at the end of the trial, the others being dropped either because they developed a "terminating" event or because they left prematurely. Nonetheless, the high rate of death, primarily from heart attack and stroke, in this elderly population is obvious. As will be noted in Chapter 5, this is the only placebo-controlled trial wherein protection against coronary mortality has been demonstrated by drug therapy.

### Elderly Patients in Primary Care

Similar to the EWPHE trial, this trial (Coope and Warrender, 1986) enrolled 884 patients aged 60 to 79 (mean of 69) with BP up to 280 systolic or 120 diastolic, but also included 23% with only systolic elevations. The lower rate of mortality and morbidity in this trial compared with the EWPHE trial could be related to a lesser degree of preexisting cardiovascular disease and the slightly lower average age among the enrolled patients. Here again, untreated elderly patients with fairly severe hypertension are shown to be at considerable risk, particularly from stroke.

### Some Special Groups: Elderly, Diabetic, and Obese

Mention will be made of a few special groups of people whose hypertension may have a different course. The higher prevalence of hypertension and the more rapid progression of cerebral and renal damage among black hypertensives were described in Chapter 3. Two other features that may affect the course were also described: first, the gender, since women have a lower incidence of coronary disease; second, the renin status, which seems to have little influence on the course of the BP.

### Hypertension in the Elderly

The data shown in Tables 4.4 and 4.5 from the three trials that included elderly patients with combined systolic and diastolic hypertension show that they are even more susceptible to cardiovascular risks than are younger patients.

The elderly often have more difficulty in the dynamic regulation of the BP for multiple reasons. A decline in parasympathetic function and baroreceptor sensitivity may decrease the ability to buffer swings in arterial pressure. The reduced responsiveness may lead to a number of problems: significant postural hypotension (de Biase et al, 1988), a marked postprandial fall in BP (Lipsitz et al, 1983), and an exaggerated rise in SBP in response to pressor stimuli (Rowlands et al, 1983). Not only are baroreceptors sluggish, but cerebral autoregulation may be impaired so that, with minor postural falls in BP, cerebral blood flow may decrease inordinately (Wollner et al, 1979).

These age-related circulatory changes may make the elderly more sensitive to natural or drug-induced falls in BP. However, they do not mean that high BP in the elderly should be neglected. They mean that it should be lowered gently and gradually, thus allowing sluggish compensatory responses to come into play while hopefully providing protection from the strokes and heart disease provoked by high SBP.

*Isolated Systolic Hypertension.* As described in Chapter 1, predominantly or isolated systolic hypertension (ISH) is increasingly being seen as the number of elderly people increases. The risks from ISH are at least as great as from diastolic, particularly for stroke, as seen in diverse populations of elderly patients in the United States (Siegel et al, 1987), Sweden (Landahl et al, 1987), throughout Europe (Birkenhäger and de Leeuw, 1988), and Japan (Ueda et al, 1988). The 24-year follow-up data from Framingham portray the problem very well (Kannel, 1989) (see Fig. 1.5, Chapter 1).

The association of cardiovascular risk with ISH is clear. What is not clear is whether ISH is itself a risk or whether it is simply a marker for the risks seen from the atherosclerosis that is responsible for the decrease in arterial compliance that causes the progressive rise in systolic pressures with age.

ISH is likely an independent risk factor (Saltzberg et al, 1988). The markedly increased peripheral resistance that is the hemodynamic profile of ISH puts a major burden on the left ventricle and thereby leads to both coronary ischemia and pump failure (Simon and Levenson, 1987). The high intravascular pressure is responsible for aortic dissection and aneurysms as well as hemorrhagic strokes. The elderly with ISH remain susceptible to the other risk factors for cardiovascular disease as well (Siegel et al, 1987).

Even if the independent risk of ISH seems certain, uncertainty remains as to the ability to reduce the risk by reduction of systolic hypertension. As of now, there is no evidence that long-term reduction of isolated systolic hypertension is beneficial. A proper study, the Systolic Hypertension in the Elderly Program (SHEP), was implemented in early 1985, but the final results will not be available for 3 to 5 years (Perry et al, 1989).

*The Very Old.* The story is different in people over age 80. Most people over age 80 have elevated systolic levels (Danner et al, 1978), but these high levels do not appear to reduce their life expectancy (Anderson and Cowan, 1976). In one large group of people 85 years or older in Finland, all-cause mortality over 2 years was *inversely* related to the height of systolic and diastolic pressure (Mattila et al, 1988). Similar findings—lower all-cause and cardiovascular mortality the higher the pressure—were noted in men over age 75 (Langer et al, 1989).

### Hypertension and Diabetes

Another large group of people have both diabetes and hypertension, with a higher prevalence of each with the other (Simonson, 1988). Their coexistence may be largely predicated on upper body obesity, as described in Chapter 3. Whatever the mechanism responsible, when they coexist the risks for various complications increase markedly. These include retinopathy (Knowler et al, 1980), coronary disease (Jensen et al, 1987), stroke (Abbott et al, 1987), and, in particular, nephropathy (Mogensen and Christensen, 1985). The latter problem is fast becoming the leading cause of death in insulin-dependent diabetics as they escape the infections and ketoacidosis that used to cause early mortality. More about diabetic nephropathy is covered in Chapter 9.

The hyperinsulinemia that is endogenously present in non-insulin-dependent diabetics and that is exogenously supplied in insulin-dependent ones may be the major factor leading to atherosclerosis and coronary disease, a view long held by Stout (1977) and documented more recently (Zavaroni et al, 1989). Diabetics have multiple features that may accentuate atherosclerosis (Colwell and Lopes-Virella, 1988), but hyperinsulinemia may be the major culprit responsible for their high risk for coronary disease (Fontbonne et al, 1988).

### Hypertension and Obesity

Often in association with diabetes, obese people also have a higher prevalence of hypertension. A claim was made that they suffer less from cardiovascular complications than do lean hypertensives (Barrett-Connor and Khaw, 1985), but a large number of better controlled studies document an equal risk for the obese as the nonobese with hypertension (Phillips and Shaper, 1989).

## COMPLICATIONS OF HYPERTENSION

The end of the natural history of untreated hypertension is frequently disability or death from premature cardiovascular disease. Let us now consider the types of organ damage and the causes of death related to hypertension. First, the underlying basis for the arterial pathology caused by hypertension is considered, then the manner in which this pathology is expressed clinically.

### Arterial Pathology

Various structural changes have been described, but the specific manner and sequence in which they arise remain poorly understood. The more easily induced and defined changes of accelerated-malignant hypertension, characterized by extensive hyperplastic arteriosclerosis with endarteritis, particularly noted in the kidney, are described in Chapter 8. The more chronic changes of primary hypertension are similar to, but quantitatively more severe than, the degenerative changes of advancing age. In general, hypertension can be said simply to accelerate the course of the sclerosis of arteries and arterioles that is a feature of aging in people. The progress of the aging process in larger arteries—atherosclerosis—is also accelerated by hypertension. Atherosclerotic plaques appear most commonly where the pressure is highest, such as in the abdominal aorta, rather than in the low pressure pulmonary arteries.

### Mechanism of Arterial Damage

As described in Chapter 3, the pathogenesis of hypertension involves structural changes subsumed under the term hypertrophy, occurring mainly within the smaller resistance arterioles. These same changes almost certainly are also intimately involved in the development of the small vessel arteriosclerosis that is responsible for most of the target organ damage seen in long-standing hypertension. At the same time, the high pressure accelerates large vessel atherosclerosis (Fig. 4.6). Such arterial and arteriolar sclerosis may be considered the secondary consequence of typical combined systolic plus diastolic hypertension, whereas it is the primary mechanism responsible for the development of the predominantly systolic hypertension so common among the elderly.

The development of vascular damage induced by hypertension has been studied after both acute, marked rises in pressure and chronic, slowly progressive increases that more closely mimic the usual human condition. As an example of

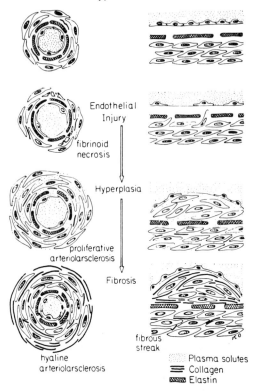

Endothelial
Injury

fibrinoid
necrosis

Hyperplasia

proliferative
arteriolarsclerosis

Fibrosis

fibrous
streak

hyaline
arteriolarsclerosis

Plasma solutes
Collagen
Elastin

**Figure 4.6.** Small vessel arteriosclerosis, or arteriolar-sclerosis (*left*), has many features in common with large vessel atherosclerosis (*right*). This diagram outlines mechanisms whereby both lesions might originate from a common source, endothelial injury, which leads to entry of serum factors that stimulate replication of smooth muscle cells. In the large vessel, the result is accumulation of smooth muscle cells in the intima and formation of an atherosclerotic plaque. In small vessels, the result is hypertrophy, hyperplasia, and fibrosis of the vascular media. (From Schwartz SM, Ross R: *Prog Cardiovasc Dis* 26:355, 1984.)

the acute situation, changes in blood flow pattern and morphology have been seen within the carotid vessels of monkeys as soon as 4 hours after induction of hypertension by surgical coarctation of the thoracic aorta (Hennerici et al, 1989). Such changes presage the multiple effects of hypertension on the macrovasculature (Leitschuh and Chobanian, 1987). Chobanian (1988) summarizes the more chronic process as seen in the aorta of rats made hypertensive by the administration of desoxycorticosterone and sodium:

Morphologic changes in the endothelial cells and irregularities in the intimal surface of the endothelial cell lining are apparent within 1 month. Subsequently, permeability of the arterial wall increases, allowing increased passage of circulating blood cells into the intima, where substantial numbers adhere. Other cells accumulating in the intima appear to be

arterial smooth muscle cells that have migrated from the arterial media and probably proliferated in the intima. With accumulation of the smooth muscle cells, the media becomes thickened, connective tissue deposition increases, and the vessel wall thickens.

Many of these changes are also seen in atherosclerotic lesions. However, Schwartz and Reidy (1987) point out the following:

This increase in medial smooth muscle mass differs from changes in atherosclerosis because it contributes to the function of the vessel wall, that is, its ability to contract. Unlike atherosclerosis, hypertension produces an increase in the mass, or the number, of smooth muscle cells without causing those cells to migrate into the tunica intima. It may be correct to refer to hypertensive atherosclerosis as an adaptive change that increases the ability of the vessel wall to maintain an elevated pressure. Conversely, we might also imagine the "adaptive" change itself becoming a cause of the maintenance of elevated peripheral resistance.

Obviously hypertension accelerates atherosclerosis but is not essential for its development. Ross (1986) proposes that intimal smooth-muscle proliferative lesions arising in response to injury may develop by at least two pathways:

One pathway, demonstrated in hypercholesterolemia, involves monocyte and possibly platelet interactions, which may stimulate fibrous-plaque formation by growth-factor release from the different cells. The second pathway involves direct stimulation of endothelium, which may release growth factors that can induce smooth-muscle migration and proliferation, and possibly autogenous growth-factor release by the stimulated smooth-muscle cells. This pathway or variants of it may be important in diabetes, hypertension, cigarette smoking, or other circumstances associated with an increased incidence of atherosclerosis.

The specific manner by which chronically elevated blood pressure is translated into vascular damage involves three interrelated mechanisms: pulsatile flow, endothelial denudation, and the replication of smooth muscle cells. It should be noted that the higher systolic pressures are likely more involved in these processes than are the lower diastolic levels, providing an explanation for the closer approximation of cardiovascular risk to systolic pressure as noted in Chapter 1.

*Pulsatile Flow.* O'Rourke (1985) has summarized the evidence concerning the importance of pulsatile phenomena:

The physiologically important changes in contour of the arterial pressure wave in hypertension are summarized [in Fig. 4.7]. These include rise in mean pressure, increase in pulse pressure, increase in maximal $dP/dt$, increase in mean systolic pressure, and

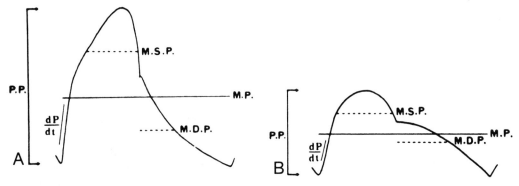

**Figure 4.7.** Diagrammatic representation of the effects of hypertension on the ascending aortic pressure wave. (*A*) hypertensive subject. (*B*) normotensive subject. *PP*, pulse pressure; *MSP*, mean systolic pressure; *MDP*, mean diastolic pressure; *MP*, mean pressure throughout the whole cardiac cycle; *dP/dt*, the maximum rate of rise of pressure. In hypertension, MP is increased as a result of increased peripheral resistance; dP/dt is increased as a result of increased characteristic impedance; and PP is increased as a result of this and early return of wave reflection during late systole. (From O'Rourke MF: *J Cardiovasc Pharmacol* 7:S14, 1985.)

variable change in mean diastolic pressure. Principally because of the earlier return of wave reflection during systole, there is a greater difference between mean systolic and mean diastolic pressure. The primary change in hypertension is in mean pressure; the other consequences follow. Ill effects of hypertension are attributable to these secondary consequences. . . .

Tension in the arterial wall is dependent on arterial pressure and caliber according to the law of Laplace. Such tension is placed on lamellar units of collagen and elastin in the wall. These are the units that are damaged in the complications of hypertension—medionecrosis, aneurysm formation, atherosclerosis, rupture, and hemorrhage. The stresses that cause such damage can be related to mean arterial pressure, pulse pressure, and maximal *dP/dt*.

Applying these principles [of stress on physical materials] to the arterial wall, one would expect that pulse pressure and maximal *dP/dt* would be more important in causing arterial degeneration and damage, and ultimately rupture, than mean arterial pressure. In other words, and as for the heart, hypertension per se is probably not as important a factor in causing arterial complications as is the resulting altered distensibility and accelerated reflection that leads to increased pulse pressure and maximal *dP/dt*, with resulting fatigue, degeneration, and ultimate rupture.

The critical importance of pulsatile flow in causing damage to vessel walls has been shown by Palmer (1981) in studies on turkeys who are hypertensive and susceptible to dissecting aneurysms. When given small amounts of propranolol, not enough to lower their blood pressure or pulse rate but enough to lower *dP/dt*, these animals are protected from dissection. Palmer has also demonstrated the importance of distensibility or compliance: When a segment of the femoral artery of a dog is wrapped to make it

stiffer, thereby increasing steepness of the pulsatile wave-form, fragmentation of elastic tissue and lipid deposition are noted only in the wrapped segment. The lesser compliance of resistance arterioles would create "a steeper, more energetic wave configuration" that would transfer to them "the brunt of the wave-form energy and therefore [cause them to] suffer more injury" (Palmer, 1981).

*Endothelial Denudation.* The manner by which the stresses of heightened pulsatile pressure leads to vascular damage likely involves denudation of the endothelial lining of vessels. Such denudation may invoke both functional and structural changes that lead to contraction and fibrosis, respectively. As to functional changes, a number of circulating and locally acting factors either constrict or relax arterial smooth muscle (Miller et al, 1989). For example, the normal endothelium produces endothelium-derived relaxing factor, which induces relaxation in response to numerous stimuli. With damage to endothelium, less of the relaxing factor is available, enhancing vascular contraction.

The structural changes may involve adherence of platelets to the denuded areas and the release of platelet-derived growth factor that accelerates the replication of both intimal and medial smooth muscle cells, resulting in the hyperplasia and fibrosis of chronic hypertensive vascular disease (Schwartz and Reidy, 1987).

*Smooth Muscle Proliferation.* An intriguing connection between these mechanical factors, causing injury to the vessel wall, and the reaction by the arterial wall that may lead to atherosclerosis has been demonstrated. The connection is based upon two premises that have experimental support: (1) The in vitro life span of diploid cells is related inversely to the number of previous replications in vivo, and (2) the process of atherogenesis is directly related to the rate and number of cell replications. Bierman et al (1981) cultured arterial smooth muscle cells from tissue both proximal to and distal from aortic coarctations resected from patients. Cells from the proximal area had a shorter in vitro life span (fewer replications) and a slower growth rate. These findings suggest that the accelerated rate of atherosclerosis typically found in the aorta proximal to the coarctation is secondary to an increased number of previous replications of smooth muscle cells in response to high arterial pressure. Such stimulation of arterial smooth muscle migration and proliferation by hypertension has been demonstrated (Grünwald et al, 1987). Therefore, hypertension may accelerate atherosclerosis by stimulating arterial smooth muscle cell replications in response to the injury induced by heightened pulsatile flow and endothelial denudation. A number of stimuli are likely involved in smooth muscle proliferation, some arising from platelets and other circulating cells, some arising from the endothelium, and some from the smooth muscle cells themselves (Schwartz and Reidy, 1987).

### Types of Arterial Lesions

Aggravation of atherosclerosis is only one of the pathological consequences of hypertension. None is specific: Charcot-Bouchard cerebral aneurysms, which were believed to be relatively specific for hypertension, are found in normotensive older people. The more common vascular lesions found in hypertension are described below:

—Hyperplastic or proliferative arteriolosclerosis (Fig. 4.6), a proliferative reaction of the vessel wall to injury, is seen most commonly with diastolic blood pressure levels above 120 mm Hg.
—Hyaline arteriolosclerosis (Fig. 4.6) with thickening and hyalinization of the intima and media results in narrowing of the lumen.
—Miliary aneurysms in small cerebral penetration arterioles, usually at their first branching, represent poststenotic dilations beyond areas of intimal thickening. When they rupture, they cause the cerebral hemorrhages so typical of hypertension.
—Atherosclerosis or nodular arteriosclerosis

produces plaques where thrombi form that are likely responsible for the ischemia and infarction of heart, brain, kidney, and other organs that occur more frequently among hypertensives.
—Other defects in the media of arteries—such as those at the circle of Willis causing subarachnoid hemorrhages—may be accentuated by hypertension but are probably congenital in origin. Medial damage in the wall of the aorta may lead to the formation of large plaques with eventual aneurysmal dilation and rupture. The process of cystic medial necrosis that is responsible for some aortic dissections also occurs more frequently in hypertensives.

## Causes of Death

These arterial lesions either rupture or become occluded enough to cause ischemia or infarction of the tissues they supply. One way to determine their effect is simply to look at the causes of death in patients with hypertension. The overall increase in mortality associated with hypertension was examined in Chapter 1; a more detailed look at the causes of death in hypertensives is provided in Table 4.6. The series in the table include different types of patients, so comparisons between them should be made with caution. The following conclusions can be drawn from these data, however:

—As shown in the data from Smith et al (1950), cardiovascular diseases are responsible for more deaths as the severity of the hypertension worsens.
—Heart disease remains the leading cause of death.
—Considerable data not included here show that, since the use of effective antihypertensive therapy, the nature of the heart disease has changed from congestive heart failure to coronary artery disease. As Doyle (1988) stated:

> Data indicate that antihypertensive treatment has greatly reduced the incidence of complications of hypertension that are directly due to the raised blood pressure, most notably congestive heart failure. By contrast, the percentage of deaths due to coronary events has risen since the introduction of antihypertensive drug treatment, leaving it as the major cause of death in treated hypertension. Presumably the removal of other causes of death, and the lengthened survival time in hypertensive patients, allows the development of coronary artery disease, which is apparently

**Table 4.6. Causes of Death in Primary Hypertension**

| | Year | No. of Deaths | Percentage of Deaths | | | |
|---|---|---|---|---|---|---|
| | | | Heart Disease[a] | Stroke | Renal Failure | Nonvascular Causes |
| UNTREATED | | | | | | |
| Janeway, 1913 | 1903–1912 | 212 | 33 | 14 | 23 | 30 |
| Hodge and Smirk, 1967 | 1959–1964 | 173 | 48 | 22 | 10 | 20 |
| Bechgaard, 1976 | 1932–1938 | 293 | 45 | 16 | 10 | 29 |
| Smith et al, 1950 | 1924–1948 | 376 | | | | |
| Group 1[b] | | 100 | 28 | 9 | 3 | 60 |
| Group 2 | | 100 | 46 | 17 | 2 | 35 |
| Group 3 | | 76 | 52 | 18 | 16 | 14 |
| Group 4 | | 100 | 22 | 16 | 59 | 3 |
| Bauer, 1976b | 1955–1974 | 144 | 41 | 34 | 15 | 10 |
| TREATED | | | | | | |
| Breckenridge 1966 | 1952–1959 | 87 | 18 | 28 | 44 | 10 |
| Breckenridge et al, 1970 | 1960–1967 | 203 | 38 | 21 | 29 | 11 |
| Dollery et al, 1984 | 1962–1966 | 79 | 58 | 19 | 2 | 20 |
| Strate et al, 1986 | 1970–1980 | 132 | 42 | 7 | 7 | 44 |
| Bulpitt et al, 1986 | 1971–1981 | 410 | 51 | 18 | 3 | 28 |
| Isles et al, 1986 | 1968–1983 | 750 | 52 | 23 | ? | 25 |

[a]Includes ischemic heart disease and congestive failure.
[b]Grouping according to Keith-Wagener classification of hypertensive retinopathy.

little affected if at all by control of blood pressure.

—As noted in Chapter 1, stroke mortality has impressively fallen, even before the advent of effective and widespread antihypertensive therapy but more so since then.

—A general pattern of mortality seems to accompany various types of hypertension: Patients with severe, resistant disease die of strokes; those presenting with advanced retinopathy and renal damage die of renal failure; the majority, with moderately high pressure, die of the complications of ischemic heart disease.

From the opposite side, the probability of surviving over an average 9.5 year interval was determined for the persons aged 50 years and older who were selected as a representative sample of the adult United States population for the 1971 to 1975 National Health and Nutrition Examination Survey I (Cornoni-Huntley et al, 1989) (Fig. 4.8). It is obvious that more hypertensive women but fewer blacks survive, further pointing out the need to consider the makeup of the population in examining the consequences of hypertension.

## SPECIFIC ORGAN INVOLVEMENT

Having tabulated the major causes of death resulting from the arterial pathology related to hypertension, let us examine in more detail the pathophysiology of these various complications. The clinical and laboratory manifestations of these various target organ damages were described in Chapter 2 as part of the evaluation of the hypertensive patient. The following will consider the pathogenesis and consequences of these damages.

In general, the complications of hypertension can be considered to be either "hypertensive" or "atherosclerotic" (Table 4.7). Those listed as hypertensive are more directly caused by the increased level of the blood pressure per se, whereas the atherosclerotic complications have more multiple causes. However, the major contribution of hypertension to the atherosclerotic diseases is clearly shown by the epidemiological data (Figs. 1.1 and 1.5).

### Hypertensive Heart Disease

Hypertension accelerates the development of atherosclerosis within the coronary vessels and puts increased tension on the myocardium, which causes it to hypertrophy. These in turn may result in myocardial ischemia, and this ischemia coupled with hypertrophy may lead to congestive heart failure, arrhythmias, and sudden death (Massie et al, 1989) (Fig. 4.9). Each of these will now be covered in more detail.

#### Coronary Artery Disease

As described in Chapter 1, hypertension is quantitatively the largest risk factor for coronary artery disease (CAD). The development of myocardial ischemia reflects an imbalance between myocardial oxygen supply and demand. Hy-

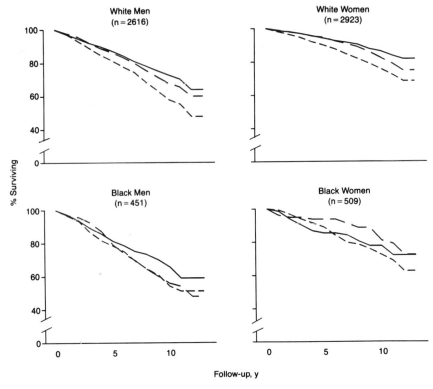

**Figure 4.8.** Probability of survival for up to 12 years according to blood pressure category [normal (*solid line*), borderline hypertension (*long dashes*), and definite hypertension (*short dashes*)] among persons aged 50 years and over. [National Health Epidemiologic Follow-up Study (NHEFS)]. (From Cornoni-Huntley J, LaCroix AZ, Havlik RJ: *Arch Intern Med* 149:780, 1989.)

**Table 4.7.  Complications of Hypertension[a]**

Hypertensive
  Accelerated-malignant hypertension (grades III and IV retinopathy)
  Encephalopathy
  Cerebral hemorrhage
  Left ventricular hypertrophy
  Congestive heart failure
  Renal insufficiency
  Aortic dissection
Atherosclerotic
  Cerebral thrombosis
  Myocardial infarction
  Coronary artery disease
  Claudication syndromes

[a]From Smith WM: Treatment of mild hypertension: Results of a ten-year intervention trial. *Circ Res* 40(Suppl 1):I-98, 1977, and by permission of the American Heart Association.

pertension, by reducing the supply and increasing the demand, can easily tip the balance.

*Myocardial Infarction.*  In a 30-year follow-up of the Framingham cohort, the incidence of myocardial infarction (MI) among those with hypertension was more than twice that of normotensive persons (Kannel et al, 1985) (Fig. 4.10). Moreover, the proportion of MIs that was

unrecognized was significantly higher, about 3-fold, among those with hypertension than among those who were normotensive. Hypertensives are thus at an increased risk both for sustaining an MI and for the MI to be unrecognized.

Hypertension may play an even greater role in the pathogenesis of CAD than is commonly realized, since preexisting hypertension may go unrecognized in patients first seen after a myocardial infarction. In some, the blood pressure falls immediately after the infarct and may never return to its prior high level. Of 58 hypertensives having a MI, 37 showed a transient normalization of their BP although most redeveloped hypertension by 3 months (Astrup et al, 1978).

Once a MI occurs, the prognosis is affected both by the preexisting and the subsequent BP. In prospective studies done in Manitoba (Rabkin et al, 1977), Framingham (Kannel et al, 1980), and throughout the United States (Coronary Drug Project, 1984), patients with prior hypertension who experienced a MI had greater mortality rates. Among the Framingham and Coronary Drug Project patients, an increase in post-MI mortal-

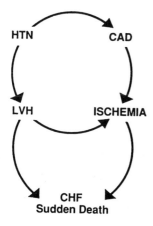

**Figure 4.9.** Schematic representation of the probable interrelationships between hypertension, left ventricular hypertrophy (*LVH*), and the various manifestations of hypertensive heart disease. The probable synergism between LVH and myocardial ischemia related to coronary artery disease is emphasized and is likely to be responsible for many of the cases of congestive heart failure (*CHF*) and sudden death. (From Massie BM, Tubau JF, Szlachcic J, et al: *J Cardiovasc Pharmacol* 13(Suppl 1):S18, 1989.)

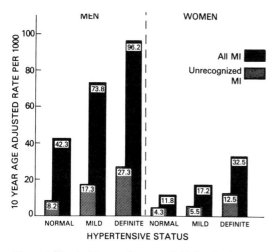

**Figure 4.10.** Incidence of myocardial infarction by sex and hypertensive status in a 30-year follow-up of Framingham cohort subjects (ages 33 to 90) free of coronary heart disease at examination 1. (From Kannel WB, Dannenberg AL, Abbott RD: *Am Heart J* 109:581, 1985.)

ity occurred among those whose BP fell significantly, presumably a reflection of poor pump function. On the other hand, among the Framingham subjects, if the BP remained elevated, the prognosis was even worse (Kannel et al, 1980), presumably representing a severe load on a damaged myocardium, so that care must be taken with patients having either lower or high BP after an infarction.

Acute rises in BP may follow the onset of myocardial ischemic pain (Figueras and Cinca, 1981), most likely as a consequence of the release of catecholamines and other "stress" hormones. Though caution is needed not to treat truly transient rises in BP too aggressively, if the hypertension persists, antihypertensive therapy may prove useful (Renard et al, 1983).

## Myocardial Ischemia

*Mechanisms.* The presence of hypertension is associated with multiple factors that accelerate CAD, including:

—acceleration of atherosclerotic narrowing of larger coronary arteries;
—abnormally high resistance of the coronary microvasculature, identified by an enhanced vasoconstrictor response to ergonovine (Brush et al, 1988);
—"limited coronary reserve," i.e., a reduced capacity for an impairment of the coronary bed to vasodilate, which reduces the expected increase in coronary blood flow in response to various stimuli (Klocke, 1987). This impairment is ordinarily related to three events: (1) myocardial hypertrophy that outstrips the vascular bed; (2) thickened coronary arteries that are less able to dilate and; (3) the higher cavitary pressures within the left ventricle that impede flow through these vessels (Dellsperger and Marcus, 1988).

*Clinical Manifestations.* These multiple mechanisms render hypertensives more susceptible to silent ischemia (Szlachcic et al, 1989), unrecognized myocardial infarction and sudden death (Kannel et al, 1985) (Fig. 4.10). The increased prevalence of sudden death among hypertensives (Kannel et al, 1984a) likely involves left ventricular hypertrophy, possibly mediated through an increased frequency of high-grade ventricular ectopy (Messerli et al, 1984). Unfortunately, the diagnosis of CAD in hypertensives may be difficult even with various noninvasive procedures (Prisant et al, 1987).

*Relationship to Therapy.* As will be noted in detail in the next chapter, the treatment of hypertension has not been found to reduce the incidence of coronary disease in most controlled trials. Beyond other possible reasons, Cruickshank (1988) has presented evidence that a treatment-induced reduction in perfusion pressures through coronary vessels either narrowed or having impaired vasodilatory reserve may invoke ischemic events. Therefore, the presence of coronary artery disease may present additional difficulties in the treatment of hypertension.

## Left Ventricular Hypertrophy

One of the mechanisms for myocardial ischemia is the increased demand for blood supply from an hypertrophied left ventricle. Hypertrophy as a response to the increased afterload of elevated systemic vascular resistance can be viewed as protective up to a certain point. Beyond that point, a variety of dysfunctions accompany left ventricular hypertrophy (LVH) (Strauer, 1987).

*Prevalence.* Whereas LVH is identified by electrocardiography in only 5 to 10% of hypertensives, it has been reported in 19 to 80% of hypertensives by echocardiography (Savage et al, 1979; Devereux, 1989). Its prevalence is closely correlated with systolic blood pressure (Levy et al, 1988) (Fig. 4.11). In addition, independent correlations are seen with increasing body weight and age (Hammond et al, 1988).

Some increase in left ventricular wall thickness can be seen among children with minimally elevated pressures (Burke et al, 1987) and even in normotensive adolescents with at least one hypertensive parent (Radice et al, 1986), suggesting that cardiac involvement may precede the elevation of blood pressure or that both may have a genetic basis.

Along with LVH, left atrial enlargement (Miller et al, 1988) and right ventricular hypertrophy (Nunez et al, 1987) may also be identified by echocardiography.

*Pathogenesis.* Beyond the effect of blood pressure, i.e., pressure load, a number of other variables influence the degree of left ventricular mass. One of these is volume load as reflected by a higher cardiac output and wider pulse pressure (Pannier et al, 1989), which likely serves as the explanation of the strong correlation noted with dietary sodium intake (Schmieder et al, 1988). Other determinants are obesity, levels of sympathetic nervous system and renin-angiotensin activity, and whole blood viscosity, presumably by way of its influence on peripheral resistance (Devereux, 1989). The correlation is much closer between LVH and pressures taken during the stresses of work by ambulatory monitoring than between LVH and casual pressures (Devereux, 1989). Similarly, there is a closer correlation of LVH to systolic blood pressure during or at the end of exercise than during rest (Papademetriou et al, 1989).

The basic signals that initiate and maintain myocardial hypertrophy likely include a number of growth factors whose effects may be transmitted via the alpha$_1$-adrenergic receptor to activate intracellular transducing proteins and ribonucleic acid (RNA) transcription factors (Long et al, 1989). Increased concentration of a specific beta-myosin heavy chain has been found in the myocardium of hypertensive baboons (Henkel et al, 1989).

*Consequences.* Hypertensives with LVH have a greater likelihood of experiencing cardiovascular morbidity than do those without LVH (Casale et al, 1986). The risk for a coronary event was 60% higher among elderly people in the Framingham cohort who had LVH by echocardiography after adjustment for other major risk factors (Levy et al, 1989).

Before these late events, changes in both sys-

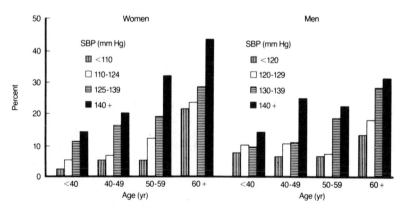

**Figure 4.11.** Age-specific prevalence (rate/100) of left ventricular hypertrophy using left ventricular mass/height criteria by approximate quartiles of systolic blood pressure (*SBP*) from the Framingham study. (Reproduced, with permission, from: Levy D, Anderson K, Savage D, et al: Echocardiographically detected left ventricular hypertrophy: Prevalence and risk factors. *Ann Intern Med* 1988; 108:7.)

tolic and diastolic function accompany LVH (Devereux, 1989). Those with minimally increased left ventricular muscle mass may have supernormal contractility reflecting an increased inotropic state with a high percentage of fractional shortening and increased wall stress (de Simone et al, 1988). Those with substantial concentric LVH may have high ejection fractions, reflecting small left ventricular end-diastolic cavity dimensions. A group of such patients with "hypertensive hypertrophic cardiomyopathy," all elderly and mostly female and black, has been described who presented with chest pain or dyspnea suggesting heart failure (Topol et al, 1985; Karam et al, 1989). Their status was worsened by vasodilator medications that reduced afterload and caused hypotension by further increasing the already excessive left ventricular emptying and reducing diastolic filling.

Those with eccentric LVH are often obese, which apparently presents a volume load to the left ventricle. Such patients have normal cardiac output but increased left ventricular wall stresses especially during exercise.

In a minority of hypertensives with LVH, subtle abnormalities of systolic functional reserve may be identified by either a borderline resting ejection fraction or a minimal response to exercise (Massie et al, 1989).

*Diastolic Dysfunction.* The earliest functional cardiac changes in hypertension are in left ventricular diastolic relaxation shown first as abnormally slow diastolic filling (Fouad et al, 1980; Harizi et al, 1988). With Doppler echo (Spirito and Maron, 1988), M mode echo (Shapiro and Gibson, 1988) or radionuclide angiography (Caruana et al, 1988), the following abnormalities are frequently noted, sometimes in the absence of significant LVH or systolic dysfunction: prolongation and incoordination of isovolumic relaxation; reduced rate of rapid filling; and increase in the relative amplitude of the "a" wave, likely caused by increased passive stiffness. In general, abnormalities in diastolic function are correlated with the degree of LVH but low peak filling rates have been found in a third of hypertensives without LVH by echo (Harizi et al, 1988). The effects of hypertension may mirror those of aging so separating the roles of each may not be possible in hypertensives after age 55 (White et al, 1989).

Doppler echo in normotensive adolescents may reveal subtle alterations in diastolic function that are related to the level of DBP within the normal range and that may represent very early prehypertensive changes in left ventricular function (Graettinger et al, 1988). The alterations, mainly in peak early diastolic flow velocity, were seen mostly in those with bimodal P waves in lead $V_1$ of the electrocardiogram.

*Regression of LVH.* Since the presence of LVH may connote a number of deleterious effects of hypertension on cardiac function, a great deal of effort has been expended in showing that treatment of hypertension will cause LVH to regress. This will be explored further in Chapter 7 when various agents are covered. It should be noted that treatment with all antihypertensive drugs except those that further activate sympathetic nervous activity, i.e., diuretics and direct vasodilators such as hydralazine when used alone, has been shown to regress LVH (Massie et al, 1989). With regression, left ventricular function usually improves (Muiesan et al, 1988) and the risk of cardiovascular events is reduced (Kannel et al, 1988).

## Congestive Heart Failure

The various alterations of systolic and diastolic function seen with LVH could obviously progress into left ventricular pump failure or congestive heart failure (CHF). Hypertension is responsible for a large portion of CHF episodes, as noted in Framingham (Kannel et al, 1972) and more recently in Gothenburg (Eriksson et al, 1988). Although its contribution to CHF may be receding with more widespread therapy, hypertension remains the major preventable factor in the disease that is involved in over 200,000 deaths and almost 2 million events each year in the United States (Gillum, 1987). Data suggest that antihypertensive treatment does not completely prevent CHF but postpones its development by several decades (Yusuf et al, 1989). Angiotensin-converting enzyme inhibitors have been found to prolong survival of normotensive patients with CHF and these agents may be even more beneficial in hypertensive patients with CHF.

Most episodes of CHF in hypertensive patients are associated with dilated cardiomyopathy and a reduced ejection fraction. Recall, however, the presence of pulmonary congestion with intact or even supernormal systolic function but marked diastolic dysfunction associated with severe concentric LVH seen particularly among elderly hypertensive women (Topol et al, 1985).

## Arrhythmias

The last feature of hypertensive heart disease with LVH is an increased propensity to ventricular ectopy, which is a major risk factor for sudden death (Messerli et al, 1984). As confirmed in Framingham (Levy et al, 1987) and Glasgow (McLenachan et al, 1987), these serious complex ventricular arrhythmias are seen increasingly with increasing degrees of LVH. However, in a study of 50 never treated hypertensives, the prevalence of ventricular arrhythmias was significantly *lower* in those with ECG evidence of LVH but the presence of LVH appeared to sensitize the hypertrophied myocardium to the arrhythmogenic effect of low potassium levels (James and Jones, 1989).

## Large Vessel Disease

Hypertension is a risk factor in the development of peripheral vascular disease. The relationship is less than with coronary heart disease and much less than with atherothrombotic brain infarction. With noninvasive Doppler and other techniques to examine peripheral vessels, abnormalities are found more frequently (Maarek et al, 1987). Moreover, hypertension is present in about half of patients with Takayasu's arteriopathy, a chronic inflammatory disease of large arteries reported most frequently from Japan (Ishikawa, 1988).

### Abdominal Aortic Aneurysms

The incidence of abdominal aortic aneurysms appears to be increasing, at least in England and Wales (Fowkes et al, 1989), and a large majority of patients with aortic aneurysm are hypertensive (Silver and Roberts, 1983). Among 201 hypertensive men over age 60, 9% were found to have an aortic aneurysm by ultrasound with the size varying from 3.6 to 5.9 cm (Lederle et al, 1988). Since abdominal palpation detected only half of these, primarily among those who were thin, the wider use of abdominal ultrasound among older hypertensive men with evidence of atherosclerosis seems appropriate, particularly if they are obese.

### Aortic Dissection

From 70 to 90% of patients with aortic dissection have hypertension (DeSanctis et al, 1987). The mechanism of dissection likely involves the combination of high pulsative wave stress and accelerated atherosclerosis described under Arterial Pathology, since the higher the pressure, the greater the likelihood of dissection.

Aortic dissection may occur either in the ascending aorta (proximal or Type A) or in the descending aorta (distal or Type B). Hypertension is more frequently a factor with distal dissections, whereas Marfan's syndrome and cystic medial necrosis are seen more frequently with the proximal lesion (DeSanctis et al, 1987). Echocardiography will almost always make the diagnosis (Erbel et al, 1989). Treatment is covered in Chapter 8.

## Cerebral Vascular Disease

Each year over 400,000 people in the United States have a stroke, and about one-third of them die, making stroke the third most common cause of death after heart disease and cancer. Stroke death rate is even higher, by about 50%, among United States blacks, a rate similar to that noted in numerous other groups with low per capita income (Gillum, 1988). Mortality rates from stroke have fallen markedly over the past 35 years in most industrialized countries throughout the world (Kesteloot et al, 1988). However, incidence has risen, likely because of the larger number of elderly people (Alfredsson et al, 1986) and the introduction of computed tomography that increases the detection of smaller strokes (Broderick et al, 1989). However, in the Framingham cohort, a higher incidence has been noted in subjects aged 55 to 64 in 3 successive decades beginning in 1953 (Wolf et al, 1989) so that other factors are likely involved.

About 75% of strokes are caused by cerebral infarction due to either arterial thrombosis or embolism, 10% to 15% are caused by intraparenchymal hemorrhage, another 5% by subarachnoid hemorrhage, and 5% are of unknown cause (Bogousslavsky et al, 1988). In Japan (Omae and Ueda, 1988) and among South African blacks (Rosman, 1986), a larger proportion, about one-third, are caused by hemorrhage, likely reflecting a larger contribution from hypertension. Reports of a higher proportion of intracerebral hemorrhages may also reflect the increased use of computed tomography, which makes their identification much easier (Rowe et al, 1988). Transient ischemic attacks, mainly related to atherothrombotic disease of the larger arteries, including the carotids, add about 10 to 25% to the total of completed strokes (Sandercock et al, 1989).

## Role of Hypertension

Even more than with heart disease, hypertension is the major cause of stroke. The following statement by a committee of the Stroke Council of the American Heart Association provides an appraisal of the role of hypertension:

Hypertension is the dominant predisposing factor for stroke and is as strongly related to atherothrombotic brain infarction as it is to intraparenchymal hemorrhage. . . . The risk of stroke is directly related to the elevation of blood pressure. For stroke generally and for atherothrombotic brain infarction specifically, there is no evidence that women tolerate hypertension better than men, nor is there a waning of the effect of hypertension in the elderly in whom most strokes occur. The Framingham data strongly suggest that control of hypertension is as important for stroke prevention in the eighth and ninth decades of life as it is at younger ages. When all of the components of blood pressure are studied in relation to the incidence of brain infarction, systolic pressure is most closely linked to stroke (Dyken et al, 1984).

As noted in Chapter 1, isolated systolic hypertension in the elderly is associated with a 2 to 4 times greater incidence of strokes than seen in normotensive people of the same age (Kannel et al, 1981). Mortality after a stroke is increased among those with preexisting hypertension (Rabkin et al, 1978).

Whether hypertensive or normotensive before their stroke, the majority of stroke patients at the time they are first seen will have a transient elevation of blood pressure that spontaneously falls within a few days, with the overall fall averaging 20/10 mm Hg in 334 consecutive admissions (Wallace and Levy, 1981). These findings document the need for caution in lowering the blood pressure in the immediate poststroke period.

## Pathology

The following pathological features in the brain are found at a higher rate among patients with hypertension (Graham, 1989):

—increased formation of atheroma, both in larger arteries and in smaller penetrating vessels;
—hyaline arteriosclerosis;
—microaneurysms of Charcot-Bouchard;
—lacunae, small 0.5- to 1.5-cm cavities that are found in 10% of normotensive elderly people but 90% of hypertensive patients. They likely represent multiple infarcts;
—multi-infarct dementia;
—subcortical arteriosclerotic encephalopathy (Binswanger's disease);
—hypertensive encephalopathy (see Chapter 8).

The development of these pathological features reflects a balance between protective mechanisms, mainly vascular hypertrophy, and factors that predispose to stroke (Baumbach and Heistad, 1988) (Fig. 4.12). Chronic hypertension appears to impair both endothelium-dependent relaxation of cerebral arterioles and responses of collateral blood vessels.

### Extracranial Vascular Disease

Perhaps of greatest importance because more can be done to prevent progression of the disease to stroke is the recognition of extracranial vascular disease, which is also more common in hypertensives (Lusiani et al, 1987). Atherosclerotic disease in extracranial arteries is responsible for asymptomatic carotid bruits, transient ischemic attacks (TIAs), and other clinical syndromes (Table 4.8).

The value of treatment of coexisting hypertension in all of these cerebrovascular diseases seems well documented, as will be described in Chapter 5. There may also be a special place for calcium entry blockers, e.g., nimodipine, in countering vasospasm after subarachnoid hemorrhage or acute ischemic stroke (Langley and Sorkin, 1989). On the other hand, overly aggressive treatment of elderly hypertensives may lead to cerebral ischemia (Jansen et al, 1986).

### Renal Damage

As noted in Chapter 3, renal dysfunction, both structural and functional, is almost always demonstrable in hypertensive patients, even those with minimally elevated pressures. Pathologically, the changes of milder degrees of hypertension are mainly hyalinization and sclerosis of the walls of the afferent arterioles, referred to as arteriolar nephrosclerosis. As noted earlier in this chapter, renal involvement may be asymptomatic and not demonstrable by usual clinical testing. The earliest usual symptom is nocturia and the earliest abnormal lab test is microalbuminuria, reflecting intraglomerular hypertension (Giaconi et al, 1989). Even with severe nephrosclerosis, daily proteinuria rarely exceeds 2 g (Morduchowicz et al, 1986), but any degree of proteinuria poses a risk for mortality (Kannel et al, 1984b). The elevated serum uric acid level present in one-third of untreated hypertensives likely reflects nephrosclerosis (Messerli et al, 1980).

The loss of renal function is progressively greater the higher the blood pressure (Lindeman et al, 1987), but only a minority of hyperten-

## Chronic Hypertension

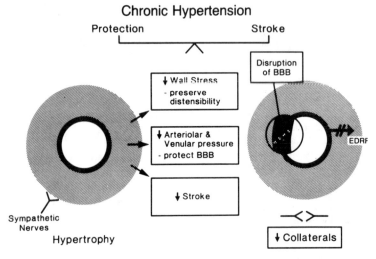

**Figure 4.12.** Balance of protective mechanisms and factors that predispose to encephalopathy and stroke in chronic hypertension. *BBB*, blood-brain barrier; *EDRF*, endothelium-derived relaxing factor. (From Baumbach GL, Heistad DD: Cerebral circulation in chronic arterial hypertension. *Hypertension* 12:89, 1988, and by permission of the American Heart Association.)

**Table 4.8. Clinical Features of Extracranial Vascular Disease**

Recurrent transient ischemic attacks
  Weakness or paresthesias in arms
  Unilateral blindness
Reduced pulsation in carotid arteries
  Localized bruit
  Murmur on either side
Involvement of central retinal artery
  Decreased intraocular pressure by
    ophthalmodynamometry
  Retinal emboli
Dilated collateral vessels over forehead
Unilateral headache

sives die as a result of renal failure (Table 4.6). Nonetheless, hypertension remains a leading risk for end stage renal disease, being largely responsible for the twice higher incidence in blacks than in whites in the eastern United States (Sugimoto and Rosansky, 1984). Blacks suffer greater renal damage than whites with equal degrees of hypertension (Levy et al, 1978). Despite good control of the hypertension, renal function may deteriorate and this, too, is more common among blacks (Rostand et al, 1989). Among the 10,940 patients in the Hypertension Detection and Follow-up Program, mortality rates increased progressively with increasing levels of serum creatinine at baseline (Shulman et al, 1989) (Fig. 4.13). Despite better overall control of hypertension, the incidence of end stage renal disease as a consequence of hypertensive nephrosclerosis seems to be increasing (Whelton and Klag, 1989).

## ALTERING THE NATURAL HISTORY

Now that the possible mechanisms, natural history, and major consequences of untreated primary hypertension have been covered, an additional word about prognosis is in order. As shown in Chapter 1, mortality and morbidity from various cardiovascular diseases have been decreasing in the United States, and the improved management of hypertension almost certainly is responsible for some of this decrease. We will examine in Chapter 5 the evidence that effective treatment of hypertension will protect patients from the various complications described in this chapter.

Therapy, however, is difficult for many patients to receive and for most to take. Millions of patients remain at risk because they have uncontrolled hypertension. Therefore, hypertension remains among the leading causes of disease and death. A great deal more is yet to be accomplished through wider application of both nondrug and drug therapy.

However, attempts to *prevent* hypertension must also be more widely promoted and followed. Without knowledge of the specific cause(s), no single preventive measure can be promoted with the assurance that it will work. However, to insist that specific causes be known before prevention is attempted is akin to saying

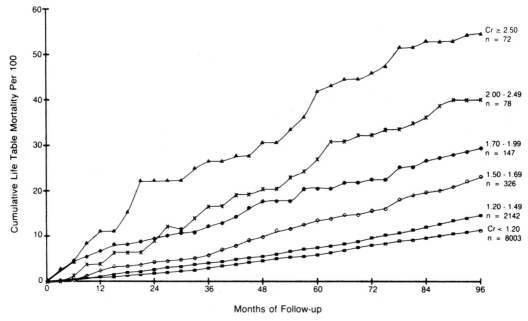

**Figure 4.13.** Cumulative 8-year life table mortality curves (percentage at months of follow-up) for selected strata of baseline serum creatinine. The sample size (*n*) and the creatinine stratum limits (mg/dl) are noted to the right of each curve. (From Shulman NB, Ford CE, Hall WD, et al: Prognostic value of serum creatinine and effect of treatment of hypertension on renal function: Results from the Hypertension Detection and Follow-up Program. *Hypertension* 23(Suppl I):I-80, 1989, and by permission of the American Heart Association.)

that water purification was unjustified before *Salmonella* was shown to be the cause of typhoid fever. The preventive measures likely to help—moderation in sodium, reduction of obesity, maintenance of physical conditioning, avoidance of stress, and greater attention to the other coexisting risk factors for premature cardiovascular disease—will do no harm and may do a great deal of good. More about those measures will be covered in Chapter 6.

## References

Abbott RD, Donahue RP, MacMahon SW, et al: *JAMA* 257:949, 1987.

Alfredsson L, von Arbin M, Faire U de: *Br Med J* 292:1299, 1986.

Amery A, Birkenhäger W, Brixko P, et al: *Lancet* 1:1349, 1985.

Anderson F, Cowan NR: *Br J Prev Soc Med* 30:231, 1976.

Astrup J, Bisgaard-Frantzen HO, Kvetny J: *Dan Med Bull* 25:260, 1978.

Barrett-Connor E, Khaw K: *Circulation* 72:53, 1985.

Bauer GE: *Aust NZ J Med* 6:492, 1976a.

Bauer GE: *Drugs* 11(Suppl 1):39, 1976b.

Baumbach GL, Heistad DD: *Hypertension* 12:89, 1988.

Bechgaard P: In: Stamler J, Stamer R, Pullman TN (eds). *The Epidemiology of Hypertension.* New York: Grune & Stratton, 1967:357.

Bechgaard P: *Clin Sci Mol Med* 51:673, 1976.

Bechgaard P: *Acta Med Scand* 676(Suppl):9, 1983.

Bierman EL, Brewer C, Baum D: *Proc Soc Exp Biol Med* 166:335, 1981.

Birkenhäger W, de Leeuw PW: *J Hypertension* 6(Suppl 1):S21, 1988.

Bogousslavsky J, Van Melle G, Regli F: *Stroke* 19:1083, 1988.

Breckenridge A: *Lancet* 1:15, 1966.

Breckenridge A, Dollery CT, Parry EHO: *Q J Med* 39:411, 1970.

Broderick JP, Phillips SJ, Whisnant JP, et al: *Stroke* 20:577, 1989.

Brush JE Jr, Cannon RO III, Schenke WH, et al: *N Engl J Med* 319:1302, 1988.

Buck C, Baker P, Bass M, et al: *Hypertension* 9:204, 1987.

Bulpitt CJ, Beevers G, Butler A, et al: *J Hypertension* 4:93, 1986.

Bulpitt CJ, Breckenridge A: *Br Heart J* 38:689, 1976.

Burke GL, Arcilla RA, Culpepper WS, et al: *Circulation* 75:106, 1987.

Caruana M, Al-Khawaja I, Lahiri A, et al: *Br Heart J* 59:218, 1988.

Casale PN, Devereux RB, Milner M, et al: *Ann Intern Med* 105:173, 1986.

Celentano A, Galderisi G, Garofalo M, et al: *J Hypertension* 6(Suppl 4):S107, 1988.

Charcot JM, Bouchard C: *Arch Physiol* 1:110, 1868.

Chobanian A: *Am Heart J* 116:319, 1988.

Colwell JA, Lopes-Virella M: *Am J Med* 85(Suppl 5A):113, 1988.

Coope J, Warrender TS: *Br Med J* 293:1145, 1986.

Cooper WD, Glover DR, Hormbrey JM, et al: *J Human Hypertens* 3:41, 1989.

Cornoni-Huntley J, LaCroix AZ, Havlik RJ: *Arch Intern Med* 149:780, 1989.

Coronary Drug Project Research Group: *JACC* 4:1135, 1984.

Cruickshank JM: *Br Med J* 297:1277, 1988.

Cumes-Rayner DP, Price J: *J Psychosomat Res* 33:63, 1989.

Danner SA, De Beaumont J-J, Dunning AJ: *Br Med J* 2:663, 1978.

de Biase L, Amorosi C, Sulpizii L, et al: *J Hypertension* 6 (Suppl 1):S63, 1988.

Dellsperger KC, Marcus ML: *Am J Hypertens* 1:200, 1988.

DeSanctis RW, Doroghazi RM, Austen WG, et al: *N Engl J Med* 317:1060, 1987.

De Simone G, Di Lorenzo L, Costantino G, et al: *Hypertension* 11:457, 1988.

Devereux RB: *Am J Hypertens* 2:186S, 1989.

Dollery CT, Hartley K, Bulpitt PF, et al: *Hypertension* 6(Suppl II):II-82, 1984.

Doyle AE: *Am J Hypertens* 1:319, 1988.

Dyken ML, Wolf PA, Barnett HJM, et al: *Stroke* 15:1105, 1984.

Erbel R, Daniel W, Visser C, et al: *Lancet* 1:457, 1989.

Eriksson H, Svärdsudd K, Caidahl K, et al: *Acta Med Scand* 223:197, 1988.

Figueras J, Cinca J: *Circulation* 64:60, 1981.

Fishberg AM: *Arch Intern Med* 34:503, 1924.

Fontbonne A, Tchobroutsky G, Eschwege E, et al: *Int J Obesity* 12:557, 1988.

Fouad RM, Tarazi RC, Gallagher JH, et al: *Clin Sci* 54:411s, 1980.

Fowkes FGR, Macintyre CCA, Ruckley CV: *Br Med J* 298:33, 1989.

Francis GS, Goldsmith SR, Levine TB, et al: *Ann Intern Med* 101:370, 1984.

Garrison RJ, Kannel WB, Stokes J III, et al: *Prevent Med* 16:235, 1987.

Giaconi S, Levanti C, Fommei E, et al: *Am J Hypertens* 2:259, 1989.

Gillum RF: *Am Heart J* 113:1043, 1987.

Gillum RF: *Stroke* 19:1, 1988.

Graettinger WF, Longfellow JV, Klein RC, et al: *Am J Hypertens* 1:100S, 1988.

Graham DI: *Am J Cardiol* 63:6C, 1989.

Grünwald J, Chobanian AV, Haudenschild CC: *Atherosclerosis* 67:215, 1987.

Hammond IW, Devereux RB, Alderman MH, et al: *JACC* 12:996, 1988.

Harizi RC, Bianco JA, Alpert JS: *Arch Intern Med* 148:99, 1988.

Helgeland A: *Am J Med* 69:725, 1980.

Henkel RD, VandeBerg JL, Shade RE, et al: *J Clin Invest* 83:1487, 1989.

Hennerici M, Bürrig K-F, Daffertshofer M: *Hypertension* 13:315, 1989.

Hjermann I, Helgeland A, Holme I, et al: *J Epidemiol Comm Health* 32:117, 1978.

Hodge JV, Smirk FH: *Am Heart J* 73:441, 1967.

Hofman A, Feinleib M, Garrison RJ, et al: *Br Med J* 287:267, 1983.

Ishikawa K: *J Am Coll Cardiol* 12:964, 1988.

Isles CG, Walker LM, Beevers GD, et al: *J Hypertension* 4:141, 1986.

James MA, Jones JV: *J Hypertension* 7:409, 1989.

Janeway TC: *Arch Intern Med* 12:755, 1913.

Jansen PAF, Gribnau FWJ, Schulte BPM, et al: *Br Med J* 293:914, 1986.

Jensen T, Borch-Johnsen K, Kofoed-Enevoldsen A, et al: *Diabetologia* 30:144, 1987.

Julius S, Li Y, Brant D, et al: *Hypertension* 13:422, 1989.

Kannel WB: *J Cardiovasc Pharmacol* 13(Suppl 1):S4, 1989.

Kannel WB, Castelli WP, McNamara PM, et al: *N Engl J Med* 287:781, 1972.

Kannel WB, D'Agostino RB, Levy D, et al: *Circulation* 78(Suppl II):II-89, 1988 (abst).

Kannel WB, Dannenberg AL, Abbott RD: *Am Heart J* 109:581, 1985.

Kannel WB, McGee DL, Schatzkin A: *Drugs* 28(Suppl 1):1, 1984a.

Kannel WB, Sorlie P, Castelli WP, et al: *Am J Cardiol* 45:326, 1980.

Kannel WB, Stampfer MJ, Castelli WP, et al: *Am Heart J* 108:1347, 1984b.

Kannel WB, Wolf PA, McGee DL, et al: *JAMA* 245:1225, 1981.

Karam R, Lever HM, Healy BP: *J Am Coll Cardiol* 13:580, 1989.

Kesteloot H, Yuan XY, Joossens JV: *12th International Society Hypertension Meeting*, Kyoto, Japan, June 1988:0007 (abst).

Klocke FJ: *Circulation* 76:1183, 1987.

Knowler WC, Bennett PH, Ballintine EJ: *N Engl J Med* 302:645, 1980.

Kotchen JM, McKean HE, Kotchen TA: *Hypertension* 4(Suppl III):III-128, 1982.

Labarthe DR: *Scand J Clin Lab Invest* 49(Suppl 192):13, 1989.

Landahl S, Lernfelt B, Sundh V: *J Hypertension* 4:745, 1987.

Langer RD, Ganiats TG, Barrett-Connor E: *Br Med J* 298:1356, 1989.

Langley MS, Sorkin EM: *Drugs* 37:669, 1989.

Lederle FA, Walker JM, Reinke DB: *Arch Intern Med* 148:1753, 1988.

Leitschuh M, Chobanian A: *Med Clin North Am* 71:827, 1987.

Lerner DJ, Kannel WB: *Am Heart J* 111:383, 1986.

Levy D, Anderson KM, Plehn J, et al: *Am J Cardiol* 159:836, 1987.

Levy D, Anderson KM, Savage DD, et al: *Ann Intern Med* 108:7, 1988.

Levy D, Garrison RJ, Savage DD, et al: *Ann Intern Med* 110:101, 1989.

Levy SB, Talner LB, Coel MN, et al: *Ann Intern Med* 88:12, 1978.

Lindeman RD, Tobin JD, Shock NW: *Nephron* 47(Suppl 1):62, 1987.

Lipsitz LA, Nyquist RP Jr, Wei JY, et al: *N Engl J Med* 309:81, 1983.

Long CS, Ordahl CP, Simpson PC: *J Clin Invest* 83:1078, 1989.

Losito A, Fortunati F, Zampi I, et al: *Br Med J* 296:1562, 1988.

Lusiani L, Visona A, Castellani V, et al: *Int J Cardiol* 17:51, 1987.

Maarek B, Simon ACh, Levenson J, et al: *Am J Cardiol* 59:414, 1987.

Mahoney LT, Schieken RM, Clarke WR, et al: *Hypertension* 12:206, 1988.

Management Committee: *Lancet* 1:1261, 1980.

Management Committee: *Lancet* 1:184, 1982.

Massie BM, Tubau JF, Szlachcic J, et al: *J Cardiovasc Pharmacol* 13(Suppl 1):S18, 1989.

Mattila K, Haavisto M, Rajala S, et al: *Br Med J* 296:887, 1988.

Maxwell MH: *Kidney Int* 8(Suppl 5):1533, 1975.

McLenachan JM, Henderson E, Morris KI, et al: *N Engl J Med* 317:787, 1987.

Messerli FH, Frohlich ED, Dreslinski GR, et al: *Ann Intern Med* 93:817, 1980.

Messerli FH, Ventura HO, Elizardi DJ, et al: *Am J Med* 77:18, 1984.

Miller JT, O'Rourke RA, Crawford MH: *Am Heart J* 116:1048, 1988.

Miller WL, Redfield MM, Burnett JC Jr: *J Clin Invest* 83:317, 1989.

Mogensen CE, Christensen CK: *Hypertension* 7(Suppl II):II-64, 1985.

Morduchowicz G, Boner G, Ben-Bassat M, et al: *Arch Intern Med* 146:1513, 1986.

Muiesan ML, Agabiti-Rosei E, Romanelli G, et al: *J Hypertension* 6(Suppl 4):S97, 1988.

Munger RG, Prineas RJ, Gomer-Marin O: *J Hypertension* 6:647, 1988.

Nunez BD, Messerli FH, Amodeo C, et al: *Am Heart J* 114:813, 1987.

Omae T, Ueda K: *J Hypertension* 6:343, 1988.

Opsahl JA, Abraham PA, Halstenson CE, et al: *Am J Hypertens* 1:117S, 1988.

O'Rourke MF: *J Cardiovasc Pharmacol* 7:S14, 1985.

Palmer RF: In: Laragh JH, Buhler FR, Seldin DW (eds). *Frontiers in Hypertension Research*. New York: Springer-Verlag, 1981.

Pannier B, Brunel P, El Aroussy W, et al: *J Hypertension* 7:127, 1989.

Papademetriou V, Notargiacomo A, Sethi E, et al: *Am J Hypertens* 2:114, 1989.

Parving H-H, Mogensen CE, Jensen HA, et al: *Lancet* 1:1190, 1974.

Pearson AC, Gudipati CV, Labovitz AJ: *JACC* 12:989, 1988.

Perera GA: *J Chronic Dis* 1:33, 1955.

Perry HM Jr, McFate Smith W, McDonald RH, et al: *Stroke* 20:4, 1989.

Phillips A, Shaper AG: *Lancet* 1:1005, 1989.

Prisant LM, Frank MJ, Carr AA, et al: *Hypertension* 10:467, 1987.

Rabkin SW, Mathewson FAL, Tate RB: *Am J Cardiol* 40:604, 1977.

Rabkin SW, Mathewson FAL, Tate RB: *Ann Intern Med* 89:15, 1978.

Radice M, Alli C, Avanzini F, et al: *Am Heart J* 111:115, 1986.

Ranges HA: *Med Clin North Am* (May):611, 1949.

Renard M, Riviere A, Jacobs P, et al: *Br Heart J* 49:522, 1983.

Rinaldi GJ, Cattaneo EA, Cingolani HE: *J Mol Cell Cardiol* 19:773, 1987.

Ross R: *N Engl J Med* 314:488, 1986.

Rostand SG, Brown G, Kirk KA, et al: *N Engl J Med* 320:684, 1989.

Rowlands DB, Stallard TJ, Littler WA: *J Hypertension* 1 (Suppl 2):71, 1983.

Rowe CC, Donnan GA, Bladin PF: *Br Med J* 297:1177, 1988.

Saltzberg S, Stroh JA, Frishman WH: *Med Clin North Am* 72:523, 1988.

Savage DD, Drayer JIM, Henry WL, et al: *Circulation* 59:623, 1979.

Schmieder RE, Messerli FH, Garavaglia GE, et al: *Circulation* 78:951, 1988.

Schwartz SM, Reidy MA: *Hum Pathol* 18:240, 1987.

Schwartz SM, Ross R: *Prog Cardiovasc Dis* 26:366, 1984.

Schweitzer MD, Gearing FR, Perera GA: *J Chronic Dis* 18:847, 1965.

Shapiro LM, Gibson DG: *Br Heart J* 59:438, 1988.

Shulman NB, Ford CE, Hall WD, et al: *Hypertension* 13(Suppl I):I-80, 1989.

Siegel D, Kuller L, Lazarus NB, et al: *Am J Epidemiol* 126:385, 1987.

Silver MA, Roberts WC: *Circulation* 68(Suppl III):III-92, 1983.

Simon A, Levenson J: *Int J Cardiol* 16:1, 1987.

Simonson DC: *Diabetes Care* 11:821, 1988.

Smith DE, Odel HM, Kernohan JW: *Am J Med* 9:516,1950.

Smith WM: *Circ Res* 40(Suppl 1):I-98, 1977.

Spirito P, Maron BJ: *Ann Intern Med* 109:122, 1988.

Stamler R, Stamler J, Gosch FC, et al: *JAMA* 262:1801, 1989.

Stewart IMcDG: *Lancet* 1:1261, 1953.

Stewart IMcDG: *Lancet* 1:355, 1971.

Stokes J III, Kannel WB, Wolf PA, et al: *Hypertension* 13(Suppl I):I-13, 1989.

Stout RW: *Atherosclerosis* 27:1, 1977.

Strate M, Thygesen K, Ringsted C, et al: *Acta Med Scand* 219:153, 1986.

Strauer BE: *Am Heart J* 114:948, 1987.

Sugimoto T, Rosansky SJ: *Am J Public Health* 74:14, 1984.

Szlachcic J, London M, Tubau JF, et al: *JACC* 13:105A, 1989 (abst).

Szlachcic J, O'Kelly B, Tubau JF, et al: *Am J Hypertension* 2:77A, 1989 (abst).

Thomas GW, Mann JI, Beilin LJ, et al: *Br Med J* 2:805, 1977.

Topol EJ, Traill TA, Fortuin NJ: *N Engl J Med* 312:277, 1985.

Ueda K, Omae T, Hasuo Y, et al: *J Hypertension* 6:991, 1988.

Veterans Administration Cooperative Study Group on Antihypertensive Agents: *JAMA* 202:116, 1967.

Veterans Administration Cooperative Study Group on Antihypertensive Agents: *JAMA* 213:1143, 1970.

Veterans Administration Cooperative Study Group on Antihypertensive Agents: *Circulation* 45:991, 1972.

Wallace JD, Levy LL: *JAMA* 246:2177, 1981.

Weiss NS: *N Engl J Med* 287:631, 1973.

Whelton PK, Klag MJ: *Hypertension* 13(Suppl I):I-19, 1989.

White WB, Schulman P, Dey HM, et al: *Am J Cardiol* 63:1343, 1989.

Wolf PA, O'Neil A, D'Agostino RB, et al: *Stroke* 20:158, 1989 (abst).

Wollner L, McCarthy ST, Soper NDW, et al: *Br Med J* 1:1117, 1979.

Yusuf S, Thom T, Abbott RD: *Hypertension* 13(Suppl I):I-74, 1989.

Zavaroni I, Bonora E, Pagliara M, et al: *N Engl J Med* 320:702, 1989.

# 5 Treatment of Hypertension: Rationale and Goals

In the preceding four chapters, the epidemiology, natural history, and pathophysiology of primary (essential) hypertension were reviewed. We will now turn to its treatment, examining the benefits and costs of therapy in this chapter and the use of both nondrug and drug modalities in the following two chapters.

This chapter addresses a question that many have simply answered "on faith"—Is the treatment of hypertension beneficial? The answer is clearly "yes" for those people with more severe degrees of hypertension, severity defined both by the level of blood pressure and the extent of target organ damage. The answer, I believe, is much less certain for those with milder degrees of hypertension and for some, the answer is clearly "no." As we shall see, practitioners and experts in the United States have been much more willing to pursue therapy aggressively, whereas those in England and elsewhere in Europe tend to be much more cautious.

## CHANGING ATTITUDE TOWARD DRUG THERAPY

We have witnessed a major therapeutic revolution, matched in this century only by the advent of antibiotics. Spurred by the recognition of the major role played by uncontrolled hypertension in accelerating premature cardiovascular disease and encouraged by the success in treating the more severe forms of the disease, physicians have begun drug therapy for millions of patients with milder degrees of hypertension. A mounting, almost unbridled enthusiasm for "early and aggressive" drug therapy of mild hypertension began in the late 1970s, so that in the United States the treatment of hypertension is now the major reason for office visits to physicians (Fig. 5.1) and for the use of prescription drugs (Gross et al, 1989). Surveys show that from a third to a half of United States physicians customarily begin drug therapy when diastolic blood pressure is between 90 and 94 mm Hg (Cutler et al, 1984; Cloher and Whelton, 1986). As a result of this unbridled enthusiasm, antihypertensive medication was being taken by over 30% of all Americans aged 55 to 64 and by over 40% of those aged 65 to 74 in 1982 to 1984 (Havlik et al, 1989). Since then, the proportions of those being treated has likely risen further.

It is of historical interest that not too long ago, the situation was far different, with two leading clinicians writing in 1966 that "Our attitude is one of skepticism and restraint in accepting drugs that lower blood pressure as even a partial answer to the management of hypertensive disease" (Goldring and Chasis, 1966).

As will be noted at the end of this chapter, most of the rest of the world is less aggressive in treating hypertension than are physicians in the United States.

## RATIONALE FOR DRUG THERAPY

Let us examine in detail the reasons for this major change in attitude about the need to reduce the blood pressure with antihypertensive agents. Part of this comes from epidemiological and experimental sources, but the most important comes from the results of large scale therapeutic trials.

### Relation of Disease and Death to Blood Pressure Levels

This evidence, covered in Chapter 1, provides a clear conclusion: The risks for cardiovascular

% Change

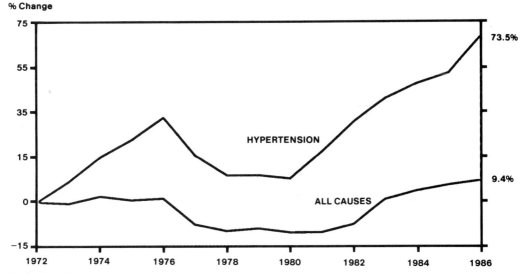

**Figure 5.1.** Percentage of change in numbers of visits to physicians in the United States for all causes and for hypertension from 1972 to 1986. (From National Disease and Therapeutic Index, IMS America, Ambler, PA, 1986.)

morbidity and mortality rise progressively with increasing blood pressure levels (MacMahon et al, 1990).

## Progressive Nature of Hypertension

The 15- to 17-year longitudinal study among Welshmen by Miall and Chinn (1973) and the 24-year follow-up of American aviators by Oberman et al (1967) strongly support the concept that hypertension begets further hypertension. In both of these studies, the higher the pressure, the greater was the rate of change of pressure. These data point to an obvious conclusion: Further hypertension can be prevented by keeping the pressure down. This conclusion is further supported by the results of the five major placebo-controlled trials of the therapy of hypertension (Table 4.4). Whereas 10 to 17% of those on placebo progressed beyond the respective threshold levels of diastolic pressure above 110 mm Hg, only a small handful of those on drug treatment did so.

## Natural Experiments in Humans

There are three situations wherein vascular damage and the level of blood pressure can be closely correlated: unilateral renal vascular disease, coarctation, and pulmonary hypertension. These three experiments of nature provide evidence that what is important is the level of the pressure flowing through a vascular bed and not some other deleterious effect associated with systemic hypertension. Tissues with lower pressure are protected; those with higher pressure are damaged.

### Unilateral Renal Vascular Disease

The kidney with a renal artery stenosis is exposed to a lower pressure than the contralateral kidney without a stenosis. Arteriolar nephrosclerosis develops in the nonstenotic kidney, occasionally to such a degree that hypertension can be relieved only by removal of the nonstenotic kidney, along with repair of the stenosis (Thal et al, 1963).

### Coarctation of the Aorta

The vessels exposed to the high pressure above the coarctation develop atherosclerosis clinically and accumulate mucopolysaccharides, sodium, and water experimentally, whereas these changes do not occur in the vessels below the coarctation, where the pressure is low (Hollander et al, 1976).

### Pulmonary Hypertension

The low pressure within the pulmonary artery ordinarily protects these vessels from damage. When patients develop pulmonary hypertension secondary to mitral stenosis or certain types of congenital heart disease, both arteriosclerosis and arteriolar necrosis often develop within the vessels (Heath and Edwards, 1958).

### Experimental Evidence

Just as hypertension accelerates and worsens atherosclerosis in man, animals made hypertensive develop more atherosclerosis than normotensive animals fed the same high cholesterol diet (Bronte-Stewart and Heptinstall, 1954). The lesions caused by hypertension, including accelerated atherosclerosis, can be prevented by lowering the pressure with antihypertensive agents (Masson et al, 1958; Hollander et al, 1976).

The evidence for reversal of structural damage by reduction of the blood pressure in humans revolves mainly around the decrease in vascular events observed during the therapeutic trials that will soon be described. More specific evidence for reversal of cardiac hypertrophy has been reported (Agabiti-Rosei et al, 1988; Motz and Strauer, 1989). In addition, most of the functional hemodynamic changes of primary hypertension and at least some of the structural changes in resistance arterioles have been shown to be reversed after successful antihypertensive treatment (Hartford et al, 1988; Heagerty et al, 1988; Aalkjaer et al, 1989).

## BENEFITS OF ANTIHYPERTENSIVE THERAPY: CLINICAL TRIALS

The last piece of evidence—that there is benefit from lowering an elevated blood pressure—is the most important. Evidence accumulated over the past 30 years, since easy-to-use antihypertensive therapy has become available, shows that protection has been demonstrated at progressively lower levels of blood pressure, originally for patients with diastolics above 140 mm Hg, but more recently down to levels of 95 mm Hg. The benefits of drug therapy in malignant hypertension were easy to demonstrate in view of its predictable, relatively brief, and almost uniformly fatal course in untreated patients. Starting in 1958, a number of studies appeared showing a significant effect of medical therapy in reducing mortality in malignant hypertension (see Chapter 8).

The demonstration that therapy made a difference in nonmalignant, essential hypertension took a great deal longer. However, during the late 1950s and early 1960s, reports began to appear that suggested that therapy did make a difference (Leishman, 1959; Hodge et al, 1961; Hood et al, 1963). These and other series reported during the early 1960s suffered from various defects—often being retrospective, comparing dissimilar patients, and being poorly controlled. Not until 1964 did a properly controlled, albeit small, study appear. This first controlled study, by Hamilton et al (1964), showed a marked decrease in complications over

a 2- to 6-year interval between 31 untreated and 26 effectively treated patients.

## Veterans Administrative Cooperative Study (1967, 1970)

The first definitive proof of the protection provided by antihypertensive therapy in nonmalignant hypertension came from the Veterans Administration (VA) Cooperative Study, begun in 1963. The value of therapy in the 73 men with diastolic blood pressures (DBPs) of 115 to 129 mm Hg given hydrochlorothiazide, reserpine, and hydralazine became obvious after less than 1 1/2 years (Table 5.1).

Along with these men with DBP of 115 to 129, another 380 with DBP between 90 and 114 were also randomly assigned to either placebo or active therapy. It took a longer time—up to 5.5 years with an average of 3.3 years—to demonstrate a statistically clear advantage of therapy in this group with more moderate hypertension. A total of 19 of the placebo group but only eight of the treated group died of hypertensive complications, and serious morbidity occurred more among the placebo group (Table 5.2). Overall, major complications occurred in 29% of the placebo group and 12% of the treated group.

Further analysis showed that the difference in morbidity was highly significant for those 210 men with diastolic pressures between 105 and 114 mm Hg but only suggestively so for those 170 with initial diastolic pressures between 90 and 104 (Veterans Administration Cooperative Study Group on Antihypertensive Agents, 1972).

It should be noted that the VA study involved only men whose blood pressures were determined after 6 days of hospital bed rest. Therefore, it may not be applicable to women or to

**Table 5.1. VA Cooperative Study: Mortality and Morbidity in Patients with Diastolic Blood Pressure Between 115 and 129 mm Hg[a]**

|  | Placebo | Antihypertensive Drug |
|---|---|---|
| No. in study | 70 | 73 |
| Deaths | 4 | 0 |
| Complications | 23 | 2 |
|    Accelerated hypertension | 12 | 0 |
|    Cerebrovascular accident | 4 | 1 |
|    Coronary artery disease | 2 | 0 |
|    Congestive heart failure | 2 | 0 |
|    Renal damage | 2 | 0 |
|    Treatment failure | 1 | 1 |

[a]From Veterans Administration Cooperative Study Group on Antihypertensive Agents: *JAMA* 202:116, December 11, 1967.

**Table 5.2.  VA Cooperative Study: Mortality and Morbidity in Patients with Diastolic Blood Pressure between 90 and 114 mm Hg[a]**

| | Placebo | | Antihypertensive Drugs[b] | |
|---|---|---|---|---|
| | Fatal | Nonfatal | Fatal | Nonfatal |
| Cerebrovascular accident | 7 | 13 | 1 | 4 |
| Coronary artery disease | 11[c] | 2 | 6 | 5 |
| Congestive heart failure | 0 | 11 | 0 | 0 |
| Accelerated hypertension | 0 | 4 | 0 | 0 |
| Renal damage | 0 | 3 | 0 | 0 |
| Aortic aneurysm rupture | 1 | 1 | 1 | 0 |
| Other | 0 | 3 | 0 | 5 |
| Total | 19 | 37 | 8 | 14 |

[a]From Veterans Administration Cooperative Study Group on Antihypertensive Agents: *JAMA* 213:1143–1152, August 17, 1970.
[b]There were 194 patients treated with placebo, 186 by antihypertensive drug.
[c]Includes sudden deaths.

the many patients whose initially elevated pressures would come down to below 90 after a period of bed rest. Beyond these exceptions, the VA study documented significant protection only in those men with DBP between 90 and 104 who were over age 50 or who had a preexisting cardiovascular abnormality (Alderman and Madhavan, 1981).

## Controlled Trials in Mild Hypertension With NonTreated Controls

The promising results of the VA study prompted the initiation of a number of additional controlled trials of therapy of hypertension. A meta-analysis has been performed on the data from all 14 randomized trials of therapy of patients with any degree of hypertension that were not confounded by additional interventions for other risk factors, e.g., Multiple Risk Factor Intervention Trial (Collins et al, 1990). The combined results of these 14 trials of all degrees of hypertension show clear evidence of protection against strokes and vascular death (Fig. 5.2). The reduction in all coronary heart disease (CHD) events was less (12%) but still statistically significant. However, the reduction in CHD mortality was only 7%, which was statistically insignificant.

The analysis that follows will exclude those trials of the treatment of moderate and severe hypertension, i.e., DBP > 110, since the evidence about them is so straightforward and obvious. Since the overwhelming majority of hypertensive patients are in the mild category, the evidence about treatment of mild hypertension is of particular interest. Considering that almost 60% of the excess mortality associated with hypertension occurs among those with DBP between 90 and 104 mm Hg (Fig. 1.12), the importance of proving that protection could be

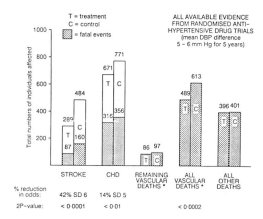

**Figure 5.2.** Combined results of the 14 unconfounded randomized trials of antihypertensive drug therapy in patients with all degrees of hypertension (total subjects = 37,000, mean DBP at entry = 99 mm Hg, mean DBP difference during follow-up = 6 mm Hg, mean time from entry to vascular event = 3 years). (From Collins R, Peto R, MacMahon S, et al: *Lancet* 335:827, 1990).

provided such patients by therapy is obvious. However, considering the slow progression of such mild hypertension, the methodological problems of keeping enough patients under observation for a long enough time to document the benefits are also obvious.

As of early 1990, 10 trials of the treatment of mild hypertension (DBP < 110 mm Hg) have been completed, six with untreated controls (Table 5.3) and four with treated controls (Table 5.4). One more trial involving elderly patients with more severe hypertension (DBP 105 to 120 mm Hg) has also been completed (Coope and Warrender, 1986) and will be covered later along with the MAPHY portion of the HAPPHY trial (Wikstrand et al, 1988a). It is likely, consid-

**Table 5.3.** Randomized Trials in Less Severe Hypertension with Untreated Controls: Design and Blood Pressure Results[a]

| | Study and Year Reported | | | | | | |
|---|---|---|---|---|---|---|---|
| | VA, 1970 | PHS, 1977 | VA-NHLBI, 1978 | ANBP, 1980 | Oslo, 1980 | MRC, 1985 | EWPHE, 1985 |
| Population Age (yr) | Mean 52 | 21–55 | 21–50 | 30–69 | 40–49 | 35–64 | ≥60 (mean 72) |
| % Male | 100 | 80 | 81 | 80 | 100 | 52 | 30 |
| Entry DBP (mm Hg) | 90–114 | 90–114 | 85–105 | 95–109 | <110 and DBP ≥95 or SBP ≥150 | 90–109 | 90–119 |
| EOD | Severe EOD excluded | Excluded | Excluded | Excluded | Excluded | Severe EOD excluded | Severe EOD excluded |
| Total Sample Size (½ in each group) | 380 | 389 | 1,012 | 3,427 | 785 | 17,354 | 840 |
| Follow-up (yr) | 3.8 | 6.5–9.0 | 1.5 | 4.0 | 5.5 | 5.5 | 4.7 |
| Controls | DB, plbo | DB, plbo | DB, plbo | SB, plbo | Open, no treatment | SB, plbo | DB, plbo |
| Drugs (mg/d) I | HCTZ (100) RES (0.2) HRDZ (75) | CTZ (1,000) RAUW (200) | CTLD (50) | CTZ (500–1,000) | HCTZ (50) | BDFZ (10) or PROP (80–240) | CTZ (25–50) TMTR (50–100) |
| II | HDRZ (150) | — | CTLD (100) | AMD PROP PIND | AMD (500–1,000) PROP (80–320) | AMD GUAN | |
| III | — | — | RES (0.25) | HDRZ CLON | — | | |
| Withdrawn from randomized treatment or dropouts | | | | | | | |
| Treatment | 16 | 33 | 19 | 34 | 1 | 40 | 36 |
| Control | 14 | 35 | 21 | 37 | 20 | 44 | 37 |
| DBP (mm Hg) Baseline | 104 | 99 | 93 | 100 | 97 | 98 | 101 |
| Change, treated group | –18 | –11 | –12 | –12 | –10 | — | –16 |
| Change, control group | +1 | –1 | –5 | –6 | –0 | — | –6 |
| Net change | –19 | –10 | –7 | –6 | –10 | –6 | –10 |

[a]Abbreviations: EOD, end-organ damage; DB, double-blind; plbo, placebo; SB, single-blind; HCTZ, hydrochlorothiazide; RES, reserpine; HDRZ, hydralazine; CTZ, chlorothiazide; RAWU, *Rauwolfia*; CTLD, chlorthalidone; TMTR, triametrene; BDFZ, bendrofluazide; PROP, propranolol; AMD, alpha methyldopa; PIND, pindolol; GUAN, guanethidine; CLON, clonidine. (From MacMahon SW, Cutler JA, Furberg CD, et al: *Prog Cardiovasc Dis* 29(3 Suppl 1):99, 1986).

ering the difficulty and expense of such trials, that these are all that will be done, with the exception of trials on systolic hypertension in the elderly, one of which was started in the United States in early 1985 (Perry et al, 1989) and another planned to start in Europe in 1990 (European Working Party on High Blood Pressure in the Elderly, 1989). In addition to the details shown in Tables 5.3 and 5.4, additional consideration will be given to the larger and more recent trials.

The major end points in all of the trials were deaths from strokes and heart attacks (coronary heart disease). In most of the trials, nonfatal strokes and heart attacks were also tabulated. As shown in Figure 5.3, MacMahon et al (1986) and Cutler et al (1989) have presented the overall mortality (and morbidity) data from all of

**Table 5.4. Treatment Trials in Less Severe Hypertension With Treated Controls: Design and Blood Pressure Results**[a]

| | Study and Year Reported | | | |
| --- | --- | --- | --- | --- |
| | HDFP, 1979 | MRFIT, 1982 | IPPPSH, 1985 | HAPPHY, 1987 |
| Population | | | | |
| Age (yr) | 30–69 | 35–57 | 40–64 | 40–64 |
| % Male | 54 | 100 | 50 | 100 |
| % Black | 45 | 7 | — | — |
| Entry DBP (mm Hg) | I 90–104 | ≤115 | 100–125 | 100–130 |
| | II 105–114 | Hypertensives: 90– | | |
| | III ≥115 | 114 or on drugs at entry | | |
| EOD | Included | Excluded | Excluded | Excluded |
| Total sample size | 10,940 | 12,866 | 6,357 | 6,569 |
| ½ in each group | | Hypertensives: 8,012 | | |
| Follow-up (yr) | 5 | 6–8 | 3–5 | 3.7 (mean) |
| Controls | Referred care | Usual Care | Placebo + nonbeta-blocker drugs | Diuretic + nonbeta-blocker drugs |
| Drugs (mg/d) | | | | |
| I | CTLD (25–100) | CTLD (25–100) or HCTZ (25–100) | OXPR (≥160) | Atenolol (100) or Metoprolol (200) |
| II | RES (0.1–0.25) or AMD (500–2,000) | RES (0.1–0.25) or AMD (500–2,000) or PROP (80–480) | AMIL, SPIR, TMTR, AMD, CLON, RES, GUAN, RESC, HDRZ, PRAZ, NFDP | Hydralazine (75–100) |
| III | HDRZ (30–200) | HDRZ (30–200) | | SPIR (750–100) |
| DBP (mm Hg) | | | | |
| Baseline | 101 | 96 | 108 | 107 |
| Change, study treated | − 17 | − 14 | − 19 | − 19 |
| Change, study control | − 12 | − 10 | − 18 | − 18 |
| Net change | − 5 | − 4 | − 1 | − 1 |

[a]Abbreviations: EOD, end-organ damage; CTLD, chlorthalidone; HCTZ, hydrochlorothiazide; OXPR, oxprenolol; RES, reserpine; AMD, alpha methyldopa; PROP, propranolol; AMIL, amiloride; SPIR, spironolactone; TMTR, triamterene; CLON, clonidine; GUAN, guanethidine; RESC, rescinnamide; HDRZ, hydralazine; PRAZ, prazosin; NFDP, nifedipine. (From MacMahon SW, Cutler JA, Furberg CD, et al: *Prog Cardiovasc Dis* 29(3 Suppl 1):99, 1986).

the 7 trials with nontreated controls plus the two trials (HDFP and MRFIT) with treated controls who were given less intensive therapy and, therefore, ended up with higher pressures than the intervention groups. These overall results are identified as *All Trials* at the bottom of Figure 5.3.

**United States Public Health Service Trial**

The first trial specifically designed to examine the effects of therapy of mild hypertension involved 389 patients, aged 21 to 55, with an average blood pressure of 148/99 and no target organ damage at the onset (Smith, 1977). Therapy consisted of chlorothiazide, plus rauwolfia.

The results show that therapy, which lowered the mean blood pressure by 16/10 mm Hg, was over 50% protective against hypertensive complications but did not significantly reduce atherosclerotic complications. There were no differences in mortality rates, which were very low, a total of two in each group. Most of the

protection was in electrocardiographic and x-ray indicators of left ventricular hypertrophy.

**Veterans Administration-National Heart, Lung, and Blood Institute (VA-NHLBI) Trial**

This was a feasibility trial involving 1000 asymptomatic mild hypertensive men ages 35 to 55 (Perry et al, 1978). It was discontinued after a follow-up of only 1.5 years because of an apparent lack of resources to follow the estimated 10,000 patients for at least 7.5 years that would be needed to obtain definitive data. The number of deaths was two in the treated half and none in the control half.

**Australian Trial in Mild Hypertension**

The 3427 men and women included in this trial had a diastolic blood pressure between 95 and 109 mm Hg on the second set of blood pressure readings and were free of clinical evidence of cardiovascular disease (Management Committee of the Australian National Blood

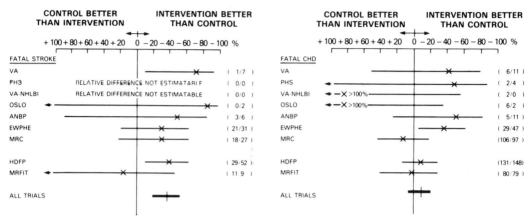

**Figure 5.3.** The results of nine clinical trials of the treatment of mild hypertension, portraying the effects of antihypertensive therapy (intervention) versus placebo (control) in the top seven trials and more therapy versus less therapy in the bottom two. The effects are shown for fatalities from strokes (*left*) and coronary heart disease (*right*). The X on each line represents the mean difference; the length of the line represents the 95% percent confidence interval. The actual number of events (intervention/control) is given on the *right* of each line. (From MacMahon SW, Cutler JA, Furberg CD, et al: *Prog Cardiovasc Dis* 29(3 Suppl 1):99, 1986.)

Pressure Study, 1980, 1982) (Table 5.3). One-half were given placebo, and the trial was constantly monitored so that when a clear difference between the two groups appeared, the trial was stopped. It took 3 years to show a significant 30% difference in trial end points [i.e., death, stroke, myocardial infarction, angina, congestive heart failure (CHF), dissecting aneurysm, grade 3 or 4 retinopathy, renal damage with serum creatinine > 2 mg/dl, or hypertensive encephalopathy].

These results appear to be strong affirmation of the value of active drug therapy for hypertensives with diastolic levels between 95 and 109 mm Hg, particularly if they are thin and smoke (Management Committee of the Australian National Blood Pressure Study, 1984). However, a closer look at the Australian data shows that the excess in morbidity among the placebo-treated half was limited to those whose DBP averaged above 100, and 80% of the entire placebo-treated group with initial DBP between 95 and 109 had an average DBP below 100 during the 4 years of the trial. In fact, for those whose average DBP was 100 or below, there was less morbidity among those on placebo than among those on drug therapy (Doyle, 1982) (Fig. 5.4). Moreover, there were more nonfatal MIs in the treated half of the study population.

Despite statistical pitfalls in such retrospective subgroup analysis (Abernathy, 1986) and the differences in the numbers of patients in the two groups, the data shown in Figure 5.4 are somewhat disturbing. There were no apparent

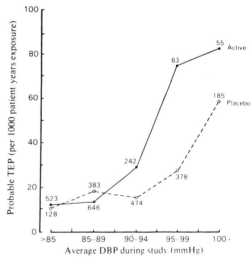

**Figure 5.4.** Relationship between average diastolic blood pressure (*DBP*) during the 3 years of the Australian Therapeutic Trial and trial end points (*TEP*) in the groups treated with active drug or given placebo. The numbers of patients in each group at each range of blood pressure are given. (Reprinted by permission from Doyle AE: *Clin Sci* 63:431s, copyright 1982, The Biochemical Society, London.)

differences between the two groups in weight loss or smoking cessation to explain why the placebo-treated group with end DBP below 100 had fewer cardiovascular complications. These data suggest that uncomplicated patients whose DBP stay below 100 and certainly below 95 may be better off if they are not on drug therapy. As we shall see, antihypertensive drugs may have adverse effects on various cardiovascular risk factors, thereby diminishing, ablating, or out-weighing the benefits of a reduction in blood pressure in those whose hypertension is quite mild.

Regardless, this trial shows an overall reduction in morbidity and mortality in patients with DBP between 95 and 109 mm Hg. It does not shed light on the issue of whether therapy is useful for those with DBP below 95 mm Hg.

## Oslo Trial

This trial was similar to the Australian one in that it included only uncomplicated patients free of target organ damage with DBP below 110 and randomly divided them into no therapy and drug groups (Helgeland, 1980). It differed in being smaller in size and involving only men, all of whom were below 50 years of age (Table 5.3).

For those with an initial DBP below 100, there was no difference in either mortality or cardiovascular events between the nontreated and drug-treated groups. However, among those with an initial DBP above 100, the incidence of cardiovascular disease was 16.4% in those not treated and only 7.6% in those given drug therapy. This difference in cardiovascular morbidity among those with an initial DBP above 100 was accompanied by a 10-mm Hg lower DBP in the drug-treated group.

Thus, both the Australian and the Oslo trials document the relative, short-term benignity of DBP below 100 and the relative danger of DBP above 100.

## Medical Research Council Trial

In many ways similar in design to the Australian and Oslo trials, the Medical Research Council (MRC) trial was much larger and utilized two types of drug therapy for the half assigned to active treatment, either a diuretic or a beta-blocker (Medical Research Council Working Party, 1985, 1988). The results are similar to those observed in the other placebo-controlled trials: Strokes were decreased, but coronary disease and total mortality were not significantly reduced by therapy (Fig. 5.3).

The total mortality rate was little affected by therapy overall or by either specific drug. However, strokes were reduced more in those on diuretic therapy, likely because they achieved a greater fall in blood pressure since more of them were given a second drug as well. Among men who did not smoke, beta-blocker therapy reduced the incidence of coronary events (Medical

Research Council Working Party, 1988). The interaction between the type of drug and smoking status was important: Smokers treated with propranolol had no reduction in stroke or MI, whereas nonsmokers had a significant fall in both. The possibility that smoking reduced the effectiveness of beta-blocker therapy by increasing the rate of propranolol degradation in the liver suggests that a nonlipid soluble beta-blocker may be a better choice among smokers.

The conclusions of the MRC investigators (1985) were as follows:

The trial has shown that if 850 mildly hypertensive patients are given active antihypertensive drugs for one year about one stroke will be prevented. This is an important but an infrequent benefit. Its achievement subjected a substantial percentage of the patients to chronic side effects, mostly but not all minor. Treatment did not appear to save lives or substantially alter the overall risk of coronary heart disease. More than 95% of the control patients remained free of any cardiovascular event during the trial.

Neither of the two drug regimens had any clear overall advantage over the other. The diuretic was perhaps better than the beta-blocker in preventing stroke, but the beta-blocker may have prevented coronary events in non-smokers.

## European Working Party on High Blood Pressure in the Elderly (EWPHE) Trial

This is the only one of the seven trials with untreated controls to show a statistically significant decrease in deaths from CHD (Fig. 5.3) (Amery et al, 1985, 1986). However, nonfatal MIs were more frequent in the treated group and the overall effect on strokes was not significant.

Two features differentiate this study from the remainder: First, it involved only elderly hypertensives over age 60, average age of 72; and, second, therapy included a potassium-sparing agent, triamterene, so that diuretic-induced hypokalemia (and hypercholesterolemia) were avoided.

As to the first point, elderly patients included in other controlled trials fared as well (or poorly) as did younger patients (Hypertension Detection and Follow-up Program, 1979b). However, no benefit was seen in the patients over 80 in the EWPHE trial, most of whom were women with intrinsically lower rates of complications (Amery, 1986). The issue of isolated systolic hypertension in the elderly remains unsettled: Protection was shown in the EWPHE trial (O'Malley et al, 1988) but not in the other trial involving only elderly patients, that of Coope and Warrender (1986) wherein the levels of blood pressure were beyond the "mild" category being considered in this section.

As to the second point, the EWPHE trial is the only one of all of the diuretic-based trials to carefully avoid diuretic-induced hypokalemia by use of a small dose of a diuretic and a potassium-sparing agent. Those given just the diuretic plus triamterene did equally as well as those also given methyldopa, and the average serum potassium level in the actively treated group (4.05 mmol/l) was minimally less than that seen in the placebo-treated (4.25 mmol/l) (Amery et al, 1988). There is no way to be certain, but the protection against the biochemical alterations of the usually higher doses of naked diuretic used in the other trials (Tables 5.3 and 5.4) could be an important reason why CHD deaths were reduced in the EWPHE but not in the other trials (Fig. 5.3).

In concert with data from other trials to be described later in this chapter, mortality rates had a J-shaped relation with diastolic pressure, both among those treated with drugs and those on placebo (Staessen et al, 1989).

### Elderly Patients in Primary Care

This is the only other published study on treatment of an elderly population (Coope and Warrender, 1986), but the patients in this study had more severe hypertension—a diastolic between 105 to 120 mm Hg—than in those covered in the preceding section. Treatment, largely with bendrofluazide and atenolol, was provided half of the 884 patients aged 60 to 79 years at entry. Over a mean follow-up of 4.4 years, the treated group had an average fall of 18/11 mm Hg in blood pressure, a 30% reduction in fatal strokes, a 58% decrease in all strokes, but no decrease in the incidence of MI or total mortality compared with the non-treated group.

Among these subjects, 23% had isolated systolic hypertension above 170 mm Hg with diastolics below 90. In those with isolated systolic hypertension who received drug therapy, the cardiovascular death rate was almost 50% higher than in those who did not (30.0 versus 20.3 per 1000).

### Trials With Treated Controls

Although the data are more difficult to interpret as being purely related to either an overall difference in blood pressure or a specific difference of one mode of therapy versus another, we will now consider the large studies involving different forms and degrees of therapy in mild hypertension. Data are provided in Table 5.4.

### Hypertension Detection and Follow-up Program

The HDFP was designed to test the value of antihypertensive therapy for all degrees of hypertension among a representative sample of the American population aged 30 to 69 (HDFP, 1979a,b; 1982a,b; 1984a,b; 1985; 1986; 1988). Of the 10,940 patients, over 7,800 had DBP between 90 and 104. Because patients with more severe hypertension were also included, it was considered inappropriate to leave any on placebo, so all patients were offered therapy. Half were referred to usual sources of medical care (i.e., Referred Care, or RC); the other half were given more intensive therapy using the stepped care drug regimen (i.e., Stepped Care, or SC). The SC patients received free medication, free transportation to the special centers, and advice on smoking, diet, and weight reduction.

Over the 5 years of the study, more of the SC group received medication and reached the goal of therapy. Overall, 5-year mortality was reduced by 17% in the SC group (6.4 versus 7.7 per 100). Even more impressively, the SC half of the 7800 with "mild" hypertension (DBP of 90 to 104) achieved a 20% reduction in mortality. This was presumably a reflection of the higher proportion of the SC group who received medication and achieved the goal of therapy— a DBP below 90 or a level 10 mm Hg below the initial DBP. They ended the trial with an average DBP some 5 mm Hg lower than did the RC group, 83 compared with 88 mm Hg. Equally impressive, the degree of protection was even greater among those with mildest hypertension: Among the 5300 with DBP between 90 and 104 who were not taking antihypertensive drugs and were free of end organ damage on entry, 5-year mortality was reduced 28.6% for the SC group (HDFP, 1982a). When this population was subdivided further, the greatest degree of protection was found in those with entry DBP of 90 to 94. This has been taken as evidence that any patient with DBP above 90 mm Hg needs active drug therapy, particularly in view of the almost 4-fold higher rate of mortality among those with target organ damage on entry, compared to those without such damage.

*Questions about the HDFP Data.* The 20% reduction in overall mortality among the mild hypertensives (5.9 versus 7.4 per 100) is highly significant statistically and has been accepted as strong evidence for the benefit of treating mild hypertension to achieve a DBP below the 90 mm Hg level (HDFP, 1986). The persistence of a lower mortality in the SC group even 2 years after the trial was stopped has been taken as evidence that the more effective SC treatment provided regression of hypertensive end organ damage (HDFP, 1988).

However, the meaning of the HDFP results is not entirely clear, and doubts have been expressed about their having conclusively proven the benefit of active drug therapy for mild hypertension (Alderman and Madhavan, 1981; Guttmacher et al, 1981; Kaplan, 1981). Some of the reservations about the HDFP data for those with mild hypertension are:

1. The reduction in overall mortality included both a 20% decrease in cardiovascular deaths and a 13% decrease in noncardiovascular deaths. The former are likely attributable to the lowering of the blood pressure, but the latter likely reflect the more intensive overall medical care provided the SC group. Thus, the results may represent "as much a trial of medical care as of antihypertensive drugs" (Peart and Miall, 1980).

   However, statistical analyses suggest that more than one-half of the lower mortality in the SC group is attributable to their greater use of antihypertensive therapy (Hardy and Hawkins, 1983). Moreover, the SC group had a lower incidence of strokes (HDFP, 1982b) as well as a greater degree of both prevention and reversal of left ventricular hypertrophy (HDFP, 1985), both of which seem likely related to more effective antihypertensive therapy and not to overall medical care.

2. Neither white women nor patients under age 50 in the SC group had decreased mortality. Explanations for the lack of benefit in these two groups have been offered. As for the white women, those in the RC group were so frequently treated that they differed little from the SC group; differences in their mortality would hardly be expected. The lack of benefit for the patients under age 50 likely reflects their relatively small number and low rate of mortality.

3. The mortality data include a nebulous category called "ischemic heart disease," and there were 9% *more* deaths from this cause in the SC group than in the RC group.

## Multiple Risk Factor Intervention Trial

Unlike the other trials, MRFIT was designed to test the value of reductions of all three major risk factors for coronary disease—cigarette smoking, hypercholesterolemia, and hypertension in special intervention (SI) clinics (MRFIT, 1982, 1985). As with HDFP, the inclusion of patients with DBP up to 114 mm Hg led the investigators to offer therapy to the other half through usual sources of care in the community (Usual Care, or UC). Of the total of 12,866 enrollees, 8012 were hypertensive. Those given SI care ended with a 7/4-mm Hg greater fall in blood pressure at the end of the 6 years than did those given UC care.

The difference in coronary mortality, 7.1% lower in the SI group than in the UC group, was not statistically significant, most likely because the UC patients received so much care that they had a much lower mortality than expected. When the effects of the three special intervention programs were examined separately, the treatment of hypertension was the one that failed to result in any improvement and, in fact, was of apparent harm to some of the 62% of the total group who had hypertension. As shown in Table 5.5, those with initial DBP of 90 to 94 mm Hg who were more intensively treated with drugs (the SI group) had higher coronary and total mortality rates than did those less intensively treated (the UC group). No difference was observed in those with DBP of 95 to 99 mm Hg, and protection was demonstrated by more intensive therapy in those whose DBP were at or above 100 mm Hg. Of additional concern was the higher coronary death rate in the more intensively treated SI hypertensives who had an abnormal baseline resting ECG.

Despite the overall lack of coronary protection, those given SI care developed less new left ventricular hypertrophy (LVH) and more often experienced regression of existing LVH than did the UC group (MacMahon et al, 1989).

Subsequent analysis of these data showed an association between ECG abnormalities at entry and diuretic therapy, with the relative risk of coronary heart disease mortality for those prescribed diuretics compared with those not prescribed diuretics estimated as 3.34 among those with baseline ECG abnormalities at rest and as 0.95 among those without such abnormalities (MRFIT, 1985). This surprising finding prompted the Oslo and HDFP investigators to look at their participants in the same manner. Both found

**Table 5.5. MRFIT: Mortality in Hypertensive Patients Given Therapy[a]**

| Initial BP (mm Hg) | No. of Patients | | CHD Deaths per 1000 Patients | | Total Deaths per 1000 Patients | |
|---|---|---|---|---|---|---|
| | SI | UC | SI | UC | SI | UC |
| 90–94 | 1157 | 1181 | 14.7 | 10.2 | 40.6 | 26.2 |
| 95–99 | 830 | 846 | 22.9 | 22.5 | 51.8 | 46.1 |
| ≥100 | 771 | 739 | 20.8 | 29.8 | 32.4 | 60.9 |
| Normal ECG | 2785 | 2808 | 15.8 | 20.7 | 35.9 | 43.4 |
| Abnormal ECG | 1233 | 1185 | 29.2 | 17.7 | 60.0 | 39.7 |

[a]Data from Multiple Risk Factor Intervention Trial Research Group: *JAMA* 248:1465, September 24, 1982.
MRFIT, Multiple Risk Factor Intervention Trial; SI, special intervention; UC, usual sources of care; CHD, coronary heart disease.

similar results: Coronary morbidity in the Oslo trial (Holme et al, 1984) and coronary mortality in the HDFP trial (HDFP, 1984b) were higher in those who entered with an abnormal ECG and who received therapy, in the Oslo trial, or more therapy, in the HDFP (Table 5.6). Though in neither trial did these results reach statistical significance, the uniformity of the data strongly suggest that therapy *as it was given in these trials* could increase the likelihood of coronary events in patients with mild hypertension. These findings will be considered further in the subsequent discussion as to the appropriate goal of therapy since they obviously suggest that there is danger from either the specific drugs used or the magnitude of reduction of the pressure, at least in patients with preexisting CHD.

## Trials Comparing Two Forms of Therapy

The remaining controlled studies in Table 5.4 differ from the others listed in Tables 5.3 and 5.4 in that their purpose was not to determine the benefit of a reduction in blood pressure but rather to compare the benefits of two forms of therapy. The first, the IPPPSH trial, compared

therapy with or without a specific beta-blocker; the second, the HAPPHY trial, compared therapy with one of two beta-blockers versus therapy with a diuretic. Together with the MRC trial wherein the half of the patients given therapy were equally divided between a diuretic and a beta-blocker, these trials can be used to examine the benefits of therapy with a beta-blocker against therapy without a beta-blocker.

## International Prospective Primary Prevention Study in Hypertension (IPPPSH)

This study was designed to examine the value of inclusion of a specific beta-blocker, oxyprenolol, in the regimen to lower the pressure (IPPPSH Collaborative Group, 1985). Half of the 6357 patients were given oxyprenolol in a randomized, double-blind fashion; the other received a placebo. Both groups could then be given as many of a variety of other drugs as needed to control the hypertension, but no other beta-blocker. To achieve control, 70% of the oxyprenolol half and 85% of the placebo half were given other drugs, predominately diuretics. Care was taken to prevent a fall in the serum

**Table 5.6. Coronary Event Rates per 1000 Person-Years with or without ECG Abnormalities at Entry**

| Trial | No. of Subjects | Coronary Heart Disease Rate per 1000 Person-Years | | | End Point |
|---|---|---|---|---|---|
| | | Less Therapy | More Therapy | Difference (%) | |
| MRFIT, 1982 | | | | | |
| Normal ECG | 5593 | 3.4 | 2.6 | −24 | Death |
| Abnormal ECG | 2418 | 2.9 | 4.9 | +70 | |
| HDFP, 1984b | | | | | |
| Normal ECG | 3210 | 3.1 | 2.0 | −35 | Death |
| Abnormal ECG | 1963 | 3.5 | 4.3 | +23 | |
| | | No Therapy | Therapy | Difference (%) | |
| Oslo (Holme et al, 1984) | | | | | |
| Normal ECG | 498 | 7.2 | 8.8 | +22 | Event |
| Abnormal ECG | 287 | 6.4 | 12.0 | +88 | |

potassium level with potassium sparers and supplements.

After 3 to 5 years, there was only a 1-mm Hg difference in the degree of fall in diastolic blood pressure between the two groups. Total mortality and CHD mortality were insignificantly lower (108 versus 114 and 40 versus 46, respectively) in those given the beta-blocker but neither nonfatal MI nor the combination of nonfatal and fatal CHD were different between the two groups.

### Heart Attack Primary Prevention in Hypertension (HAPPHY) Trial

This study was designed to determine whether a beta-blocker based regimen differs from a thiazide diuretic-based regimen with regard to the prevention of coronary heart disease events and death (Wilhelmsen et al, 1987). The 6569 40- to 64-year-old men were divided into two groups, half receiving a beta-blocker, either metoprolol or atenolol, the other half a diuretic, either bendrofluazide or hydrochlorothiazide. When the multicenter study was begun in March 1976, only metoprolol was used; in the third year of the trial, atenolol was added and eventually an equal number of patients took either beta-blocker (Fig. 5.5). The HAPPHY trial was discontinued at the end of 1985, but the half of the patients who were in the metoprolol versus diuretic limb were followed for another 14 months. The slightly prolonged metoprolol limb was then analyzed separately and published as the Metoprolol Atherosclerosis Prevention in Hypertensives Study in April 1988.

The overall HAPPHY data show no difference in the incidence of CHD or mortality between the diuretic and the beta-blocker (metoprolol or atenolol) treatment groups (Fig. 5.6, *right*). The two forms of therapy were equally well tolerated and had similar antihypertensive efficacy although additional drugs had to be given more often in the diuretic group to achieve adequate control. The authors concluded that "Antihypertensive treatment based on a β-blocker or on a thiazide diuretic could not be shown to affect the prevention of hypertensive complications, including CHD, to a different extent."

### Metoprolol Atherosclerosis Prevention in Hypertensives (MAPHY) Study

As noted above, the half of the patients enrolled in the HAPPHY trial who were on the metoprolol limb were continued for another 14 months and their data published as the MAPHY study (Wikstrand et al, 1988a). The authors state their decision to continue the metoprolol half was not based upon information about the results of the larger HAPPHY trial but rather upon other evidence that metoprolol might have special cardioprotective properties.

The author's hunch was correct: The metoprolol half of the MAPHY group had significantly lower total mortality than did those on diuretics, with fewer deaths from both CHD and stroke (Fig. 5.6, *left*). The authors chose the median follow-up time of 4.2 years to demonstrate the greatest difference between the two groups because there was some admixture of the two forms of therapy toward the end of the 11 years of the study. The difference in total mortality was 48% at 4.2 years, but by the end of the study, the difference had shrunken to a statistically insignificant 22%.

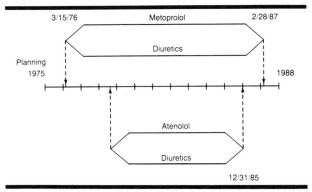

**Figure 5.5.** Design of the overall HAPPHY trial completed on 12/31/85 and the MAPHY limb, which proceeded until 2/28/87. (From Wikstrand J, Warnold I, Olsson G, et al: *JAMA* 260:1715, 1988b, copyright 1988, American Medical Association.)

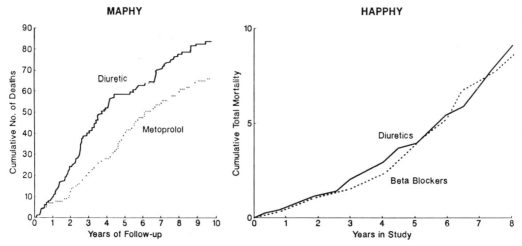

**Figure 5.6.** *Left*: Total cumulative mortality in the two groups in the MAPHY trial. *Solid line*, diuretic therapy (n = 1625); *broken line*, metoprolol (n = 1609) (P = .028). (From Wikstrand J, Warnold I, Olsson G, et al: *JAMA* 259:1976, 1988a, copyright 1988, American Medical Association.) *Right*: Cumulative total mortality in the two groups in the HAPPHY trial. (From Wilhelmsen L, Berglund G, Elmfeldt D, et al: *J Hypertens* 5:561, 1987.)

Beyond the questionable use of the median time rather than the end of the study, as is the usual practice, numerous questions have been raised about the disparate data from the HAP-PHY and MAPHY trials. Although the investigators defend their decision to consider the two as separate studies (Wilhelmsen, 1988), others have questioned the legitimacy of the split (Gifford, 1988) as well as the use of different statistical techniques to analyze the data (Kaplan, 1988).

Regardless, the MAPHY data have been defended as the first documentation of primary protection against coronary disease by one type of drug (metoprolol) compared with another (thiazide diuretic) (Wikstrand, 1988). Since there was no placebo group, the data cannot be used as evidence that metoprolol lowered the incidence of CHD below that of an untreated population, but only that it was superior to a diuretic. Most of the reduction in total mortality in the metoprolol-treated group was attributable to a much greater protection found among the one-third of the patients who were cigarette smokers (Tuomilehto et al, 1989). They had a 33% reduction in total mortality at the end of the study compared with only a 10% reduction among the nonsmokers who received metoprolol.

The MAPHY investigators (Wikstrand et al, 1988a) offer a number of "speculations" as to their positive results compared with the negative or nonconclusive results of the other three primary preventive studies comparing a beta-blocker

against a diuretic (Table 5.7). These include: (1) fewer technical problems, including a lower dropout rate, better compliance, and, most strikingly, a virtual completeness of follow-up, with only one patient lost; (2) the inclusion only of men, compared with the approximately half of the patients who were women in both the MRC and IPPPSH studies, since men's higher rates of coronary events would increase the likelihood of detecting a reduction in the event rate attributable to the treatment; (3) the stratification of coronary risks, not performed in the MRC and IPPPSH studies, which presumably would better match patients assigned to the two treatments; and (4) the type of beta-blocker used with metoprolol being a relatively beta$_1$-selective agent that presumably would not cause as much peripheral beta-blockade and thereby not expose the vasculature to unopposed alpha-constriction from smoking-induced epinephrine surges.

Whatever the reasons for the differences between the MAPHY data and the other beta-blocker based trials, the data shown in Table 5.7 indicate that the differences are not related to *lower* coronary or total mortality in those who received metoprolol in MAPHY compared with those who received either metoprolol or atenolol in HAPPHY. In fact, coronary and total mortality rates were just a tiny bit higher in the metoprolol treated MAPHY patients than in the metoprolol- or atenolol-treated HAPPHY patients (Steering Committee of the HAPPHY Trial, 1989).

The differences in the two trials are related

**Table 5.7. Characteristics of the Trial Therapies for Hypertension, Including Mortality Rates for the Half of Subjects Receiving Beta-Blockers (BB) and the Half of the Subjects Not Receiving Beta-Blockers (Non-BB)**

| Trial | N | Age range | Sex | Beta-blocker | Coronary BB | Coronary Non-BB | Stroke BB | Stroke Non-BB | Total BB | Total Non-BB |
|---|---|---|---|---|---|---|---|---|---|---|
| MRC[a] | 8700 | 35–64 | M, W | propranolol | 2.3 | 2.7 | 0.7 | 0.5 | 5.5 | 6.0 |
| IPPPSH[b] | 6357 | 40–64 | M, W | oxyprenolol | 3.2 | 3.2 | 0.4 | 0.6 | 8.3 | 8.8 |
| HAPPHY[c] | 6569 | 40–64 | M | atenolol or metoprolol | 4.4 | 4.1 | 0.2 | 0.8 | 7.7 | 8.3 |
| MAPHY[d] | 3234 | 40–64 | M | metoprolol | 4.5 | 5.4 | 0.2 | 1.1 | 8.0 | 10.3 |

Cumulative Mortality Rates per 1000 Patient Years

[a]Medical Research Council (MRC): Br Med J 1985;291:97.
[b]International Prospective Primary Prevention Study in Hypertension (IPPPSH): J Hypertens 1985;3:379.
[c]Heart Attack Primary Prevention in Hypertensives (HAPPHY): J Hypertens 1987;5:561.
[d]Metoprolol Atherosclerosis Prevention in Hypertension (MAPHY): JAMA 1988;259:1976.

to *higher* coronary and total mortality in the diuretic-treated half of MAPHY than in the diuretic-treated half of HAPPHY shown under the non-BB columns in Table 5.7. When the influence of smoking status in the four beta-blocker versus non-beta-blocker trials is examined, the adverse experience of the diuretic-treated MAPHY patients is seen to be particularly striking (Table 5.8). In all four trials, about one-third of the patients were smokers. In both the MRC and IPPPSH trials, those smokers who took a beta-blocker had higher mortality or morbidity rates than did those who took a diuretic, whereas in the overall HAPPHY experience, those smokers who took a beta-blocker had a slightly lower mortality rate. In the MAPHY group, the total mortality rate was slightly higher in the smokers on metoprolol than in the HAPPHY smokers on a beta-blocker. However, the most striking difference is a considerably higher mortality rate among the smokers in MAPHY who took a diuretic. That difference is, in turn, responsible for the apparent protection by metoprolol in MAPHY, which makes this trial the only one to find a significant reduction in coronary and total mortality with a beta-blocker compared with a diuretic.

**Table 5.8. Total Mortality by Smoking Status, with and without a Beta-Blocker (BB)**

| | MRC | IPPPSH[a] | HAPPHY | MAPHY |
|---|---|---|---|---|
| *Nonsmokers* | | | | |
| Without BB | 5.3 | (11.6) | 5.1 | 6.3 |
| With BB | 4.2 | (5.4) | 5.5 | 5.7 |
| *Smokers* | | | | |
| Without BB | 7.7 | (14.5) | 14.0 | 19.7 |
| With BB | 9.1 | (18.1) | 12.1 | 13.2 |

[a]IPPPSH data are for men only and show both fatal and non-fatal CHD in parentheses.

## Overall Impact of Beta-Blocker Therapy

The data from the three trials, which only compared beta-blocker therapy with non-beta-blocker therapy, can be combined with that from the MRC trial wherein the half of the subjects who received drug therapy were randomly allocated to either a diuretic (bendrofluazide) or a beta-blocker (propranolol). A meta-analysis of these four sets of data has been performed, computing the differences between the beta-blocker- and non-beta-blocker-based therapies for each trial and for the two sexes separately (Staessen et al, 1988) (Fig. 5.7). The meta-analysis shows that therapy with a beta-blocker tended to decrease mortality in men but tended to increase mortality in women. When the total follow-up (end) data of the MAPHY trial that involved only men are compared with those of the other three, the findings are seen to be quite similar.

All in all, beta-blocker-based therapy appears to offer better protection than does diuretic or non-beta-blocker-based therapy in men but not in women. In two of three trials, the beta-blocker was more cardioprotective in those who did not smoke, whereas in the MAPHY trial the beta-blocker was more protective in those who did smoke.

## Other Forms of Therapy

Unfortunately, the preceding data on the treatment of mild to moderate hypertension examine only diuretic and beta-blocker-based therapies. There are simply no long-term large-scale trials on the effects of any other classes of agents.

## Overview of Therapeutic Trials

The overall results of these 11 large-scale controlled trials, as shown in Figures 5.3 and

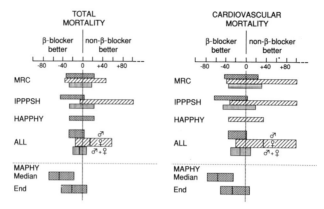

**Figure 5.7.** Percentage of differences (means and 95% confidence intervals) in total (*left*) and cardiovascular (*right*) mortality between beta-blocker- and non-beta-blocker-based antihypertensive treatment in various trials and two sexes. For Metoprolol Atherosclerosis Prevention in Hypertensives (MAPHY) Study, statistics refer to median and total (end of study) follow-up. In meta-analysis (ALL), results of three trials were combined [MRC, International Prospective Primary Prevention Study in Hypertension (IPPPSH), and Heart Attack Primary Prevention in Hypertensives (HAPPHY)]. (From Staessen J, Fagard R, Amery A: *JAMA* 260:1713, 1988, copyright 1988, American Medical Association.)

5.7, indicate that the treatment of mild to moderate hypertension with either diuretic or beta-blocker-based therapy will clearly reduce morbidity and mortality from strokes but not heart attacks. Despite an overall lack of protection against heart attacks, a significant decrease in CHD mortality was observed in the EWPHE trial with therapy based on a diuretic plus a potassium sparer compared with a placebo and in the MAPHY half of the HAPPHY trial with metoprolol compared with a naked diuretic. Since there were no untreated patients in the MAPHY trial, the apparent protection noted in the beta-blocker treated half could simply reflect a higher than expected mortality rate in the diuretic-treated half. This possibility receives some support from the markedly higher mortality in diuretic-treated smokers in the MAPHY trial than in the other trials (Table 5.8).

These data have been analyzed by numerous epidemiologists and statisticians including Geoffrey Rose (1987), Ingar Holme (1988), and Hebert et al (1988). All have come to the same conclusion—strokes have been significantly reduced, heart attacks have not.

A similar lack of protection against heart attacks has also been noted in numerous smaller or uncontrolled studies, most also based on naked diuretic therapy (Stewart, 1979; Morgan et al, 1984; Callcott et al, 1984; Kannel et al, 1988a). In the Framingham study, the risk of sudden death was almost doubled among those patients who were receiving antihypertensive therapy compared with those who were untreated, whether or not they had prior manifes-

tations of coronary heart disease (Table 5.9). The authors state that "These data suggest that some feature of antihypertensive treatment as practiced in the general population may contribute to sudden death incidence" (Kannel et al, 1988a).

## Unresolved Risks of Treated Hypertension

Beyond these formidable data documenting a failure to protect against coronary disease, an even more ominous fact emerges from studies involving relatively larger groups of patients who have been treated with antihypertensive medications for prolonged periods: The mortality rate of patients whose pressures have been "successfully" treated remained higher than that seen among untreated people with similar levels of blood pressure. From multiple sources, it is clear that antihypertensive therapy, as it has been practiced, does not reduce the risk of coronary disease to normal (Samuelsson et al, 1985; Strate

**Table 5.9. Risk of Sudden Death by Antihypertensive Treatment Among Hypertensive Subjects**[a]

| Anti-HBP Treatment Status | Age-Adjusted Rate per 1000 | | | |
|---|---|---|---|---|
| | No CHD | | With CHD | |
| | Men | Women | Men | Women |
| Untreated | 4.3 | 1.6 | 25.6 | 9.1 |
| Treated | 7.1[b] | 3.1[c] | 48.8[b] | 15.9[c] |

[a]From Kannel WB, Cupples LA, D'Agostino RB, Stokes J: *Hypertension* 11(Suppl II):II-45, 1988b.
[b]p<.0.05.
[c]Not significant.
HBP, high blood pressure; CHD, coronary heart disease.

et al, 1986; Bulpitt et al, 1986; Isles et al, 1986; Hansson, 1988).

Perhaps the clearest demonstration of this failure of therapy to reduce risk of cardiovascular disease to that seen in untreated people with similar levels of blood pressure is the experience of the Glasgow Blood Pressure Clinic where 3783 patients were treated between 1968 and 1983, for an average of 6.5 years. The mortality rates for those patients whose diastolic blood pressure was reduced to less than 90 mm Hg were compared with the rates for age- and sex-matched populations in two nearby communities, Renfrew and Paisley (Isles et al, 1986) (Fig. 5.8). It is obvious that mortality rates remained higher in the treated groups.

Why are the excess risks associated with elevated blood pressure not removed by prolonged reduction of the pressure to the levels seen in untreated people? A number of possibilities exist.

### Multifactorial Origin of CHD

CHD, much more than stroke, is causally related to multiple factors. Although hypertension may be the quantitatively dominant risk, age, cholesterol, smoking, diabetes, and numerous others are involved. It may not be possible, then, to reduce CHD risk significantly by attacking only one risk factor. Most trials have done just that. Moreover, the extent of silent but significant coronary artery disease may have been more advanced among many participants than was generally recognized (O'Kelly et al, 1989).

### Short Duration of Intervention

Even when multiple risks are attacked, as in the MRFIT trial, the intervention may not have been begun early enough or continued long enough to have a meaningful impact on the atherosclerotic process.

Both of these reasons suggest that the expectation of success in relatively short-term trials of therapy may have been wishful and naive.

### Hazards of Therapy

As will be delineated in Chapter 7, every antihypertensive drug induces adverse effects. The two drugs almost exclusively used in the majority of patients in most of the trials—diuretics and beta-blockers—are particularly prone to induce various metabolic changes that may adversely affect coronary risk. The high doses of diuretics used in most trials are particularly suspect since they may raise total and LDL cholesterol, worsen glucose tolerance, lower serum potassium and, at the same time, fail to reduce the burden of left ventricular hypertrophy.

The potential impact of one of the adverse effects of diuretic and beta-blocker therapy, the rise in serum cholesterol, is suggested by data from a 12-year study of 686 men in Gothenberg, Sweden, who were treated for up to 12 years with one or both antihypertensive agents without concomitant attempts to alter their lipid status. Their pressures fell to varying degrees and, simultaneously, their serum cholesterol levels rose or fell variably. The coronary heart disease morbidity that developed during the 4th to 12th year

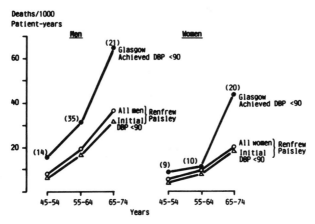

**Figure 5.8.** Age- and sex-specific mortality rates (deaths/1000 patient-years) in Glasgow Clinic patients whose diastolic blood pressures (DBPs) were reduced to less than 90 mm Hg by treatment at their last clinic visit, compared with subjects in the Renfrew/Paisley control population. Deaths in the Glasgow Clinic are given in parentheses. (From Isles CG, Walker LM, Beevers GD, et al: *J Hypertens* 4:141, 1986.)

of therapy was closely predicated on the combined effects of therapy on the blood pressure and the serum cholesterol level (Samuelsson et al, 1987) (Fig. 5.9). Even with the maximal degree of blood pressure reduction ($-20\%$), little impact on CHD morbidity was noted among those whose cholesterol levels rose by an average of 7%. Those whose cholesterol levels fell by an average of 11% achieved the maximal degree of protection.

### Lack of Adequate Control

In many trials, a significant portion of the study population was not successfully treated to the usual goal of a DBP below 90 mm Hg. As again well documented in the patients treated in the Glasgow Clinic, the mortality rates of treated patients are determined not by their initial blood pressure but by the level of pressure achieved during therapy (Isles et al, 1986) (Fig. 5.10). Thus, inadequate or poorly sustained reductions in pressure may have been responsible for the persistence of higher risk during therapy.

### Overtreatment of Susceptible Patients

Conversely, overtreatment may have also contributed, at least among the sizeable portion of the hypertensive population susceptible to ischemic injury, by a reduction in perfusion pressure. An association between reduction of blood pressure and ischemic injury was first suggested by Stewart (1979) who reported a 5-fold increase in myocardial infarction among patients whose DBP was reduced to below 90 mm Hg. Stewart's report was largely neglected but when Cruickshank et al (1987) reported the same phenomenon, interest immediately focused on the problem and has intensified progressively. As

Cruickshank (1988) reported, six separate trials have demonstrated a "J-curve" relation between coronary morbidity or mortality and the extent of diastolic blood pressure reduction (Table 5.10 and Fig. 5.11). Similar data have more recently been reported in a 2 year follow up of over 1000 patients, with a similar "J-curve" of coronary morbidity, higher in those with the least and the most reduction in blood pressure (Alderman et al, 1989). In addition to these seven trials, data from both HDFP (Cooper et al, 1988) and the MRFIT studies (Kuller et al, 1986) have shown a higher rate of coronary mortality in those patients with ECG abnormalities whose pressure was reduced the most, the relation again displaying a J-curve.

Increased cardiovascular mortality has also been reported among nontreated people whose natural diastolic blood pressure is below 90 mm Hg. This was reported in an analysis of the Framingham data by Anderson (1978) and among elderly hypertensives who served as controls in the trials of Coope and Warrender (1986) and the European Working Party on High Blood Pressure in the Elderly (Staessen et al, 1989). Such a higher mortality with lower blood pressure could reflect the presence of serious, debilitating illness at the time of blood pressure ascertainment, but that seems unlikely in these populations, as well as in the others reported by Cruickshank, in view of the long follow-up period. Nonetheless, among the elderly in the EWPHE trial, deaths from noncardiovascular causes also followed a J-curve, suggesting some deterioration of general health among those with the lowest pressures.

Cruickshank (1988) postulates that the probable mechanism for the increase in coronary

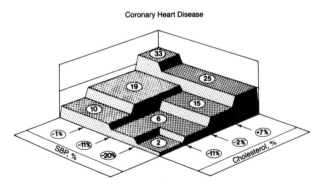

**Figure 5.9.** Coronary heart disease morbidity during the 4th to 12th year of antihypertensive treatment in relationship to relative change (during initial 4 years of follow-up) of both systolic blood pressure (*SBP*) and serum cholesterol levels divided into quartiles. Rates adjusted for risk at entry. (From Samuelsson O, Wilhelmsen L, Andersson OK, et al: *JAMA* 258:1768, 1987, copyright 1989, American Medical Association.)

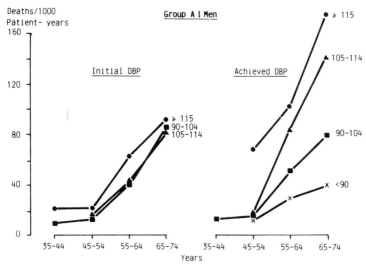

**Figure 5.10.** Age-specific mortality rates (death/1000 patient-years) for a subset of 1162 men not initially on therapy whose blood pressures were measured both at entry to the clinic and thereafter during treatment. At all ages the influence of achieved blood pressure on mortality was greater than that of initial blood pressure. *DBP*, diastolic blood pressure. (From Isles CG, Walker LM, Beevers GD, et al: *J Hypertens* 4:141, 1986.)

ischemia is an inability to maintain coronary blood flow as perfusion pressure falls due to impairment of autoregulation within atherosclerotic vessels, i.e., a fall in coronary flow reserve. As Strandgaard and Haunsø (1987) have demonstrated, the coronary circulation has poor autoregulatory reserve and, since oxygen extraction is nearly maximal at rest, lowering of perfusion pressure can lead to myocardial ischemia. The problem is obviously compounded in the presence of myocardial hypertrophy and high heart rates.

As noted in Chapter 2, nocturnal falls in blood pressure may be profound and further accentuated by inadvertent overtreatment. Floras (1988) has suggested that unrecognized nocturnal hypotension may contribute to the increase in coronary ischemia seen with more intensive therapy.

Cruickshank's presentation and concept have not gone unchallenged, with a steady stream of disclaimers published as letters to the *Lancet* in 1987 and to the *British Medical Journal* in late 1988 and early 1989. In particular, questions have been raised as to the inexactness of the critical level where the break in the curve appears (Hansson, 1989) and the relatively few events that make up the curves (Waller et al, 1988a). Nonetheless, I am persuaded that, beyond a certain degree of blood pressure reduction, coronary ischemia can be incited and that this break point in the J-curve can be at a considerably higher level than most think to be safe.

The issue clearly has an impact on the level of pressure that is the appropriate goal for therapy.

Simply stated, inadvertent overtreatment, particularly but not exclusively among patients with preexisting coronary disease, likely contributes to the failure to demonstrate a reduction in heart attacks in patients treated for mild to moderate hypertension.

There are, then, multiple reasons why antihypertensive therapy, as previously and currently provided, has not fulfilled the promise of protection against coronary disease.

## Other Data on the Benefits of Antihypertensive Therapy

In addition to the large controlled trials that have looked primarily at the effects of therapy on CHD and stroke, a goodly number of smaller studies have examined the influence of antihypertensive therapy on various end points. These end points include total mortality and the distribution of specific causes of death as well as both morbidity and mortality from the damage induced by hypertension on the major end organs as described in Chapter 4, the heart, brain, kidneys, and large arteries.

### Overall Mortality and Specific Causes of Death

Total mortality rates have fallen over the past 20 years, both for hypertensive and normotensive people in the United States and in most

**Table 5.10. Details of Studies of Hypertension That Showed a J Curve Relation Between Diastolic Blood Pressure and Morbidity or Mortality, or Both, from Myocardial Infarction[a]**

| | Design | No. and Sex of Patients | Age Range (Years) | Degree of Hypertension | Treatment | Length of Follow-Up | |
|---|---|---|---|---|---|---|---|
| Cruickshank et al, 1987 | Open | 932 (585 men, 347 women) | 17–77 | Moderate to severe | Atenolol ± diuretic ± vasodilator ± other | Up to 10-2 years (mean 6.1) | J curve only in patients with ischaemia (mortality) |
| Wilhelmsen et al, 1987 | Randomised, controlled, open | 6569 men | 40–64 | Mild to moderate | Atenolol, metoprolol, or diuretic | Mean 3.8 years | |
| Samuelsson et al, 1987 | Open | 686 men | 47–54 | Mild to moderate | β-Blocker ± diuretic ± vasodilator ± other | 12 Years | |
| Coope and Warrender, 1987 | Randomised, open | 884 (273 men, 611 women) | 60–79 | Mild to moderate | Atenolol ± diuretic or no treatment | Up to 10 years (mean 4.4) | J curve in both treated and untreated groups (mortality) |
| Waller et al 1988a | Open | 3350 (1660 men, 1690 women) | 25–84 | Mild to severe | Not stated | Up to 15 years (mean 6.5) | J curve in both men and women with and without ischaemia; independent of treatment with specific drug (mortality) |
| Fletcher et al 1988 | Open | 2145 (1075 men, 1070 women) | 13–89 | Mild to severe | β-Blockers, diuretics, methyldopa, hydralazine, etc | Up to 10.5 years (mean 4.3) | J curve in both men and women (mortality) |

[a]From Cruickshank JM: *Br Med J* 297:1227, 1988.

industrialized societies. Most of this fall is attributable to a decrease in deaths caused by cardiovascular diseases, stroke more than coronary disease. In the 14 major controlled trials, total mortality was significantly reduced in those given antihypertensive therapy compared with those left untreated (Collins et al, 1990).

However, the contribution made by such therapy per se is uncertain. In the controlled trials, it seems likely that treatment is the major, if not exclusive, mechanism with its predominant effect on stroke mortality. In the larger population, the control of hypertension is given much less credit for the fall in stroke (Bonita and Beaglehole, 1989) and in overall and coronary mortality, with a larger role attributed to decreases in cholesterol and smoking (Goldman and Cook, 1984). Similarly, the role of improved therapy of hypertension is uncertain in the improvement of long-term survival in patients who have had a myocardial infarction (Gomez-Marin et al, 1987).

As shown in Table 4.6, a major shift in the causes of death among hypertensive patients has occurred over the past 30 years, the time during which effective antihypertensive therapy has been available. Whereas congestive heart failure was responsible for over half of the deaths in hypertensive patients before 1950, its role has diminished dramatically (Doyle, 1988). At the same time, the deaths attributed to CHD have risen from less than 15% to over 40% of the total.

## Coronary Heart Disease

This increased proportion of deaths from CHD likely reflects the failure of antihypertensive therapy to reduce CHD mortality while it has reduced mortality from other cardiovascular causes, e.g., congestive failure and stroke. As summarized by Doyle (1988), "Presumably the removal of other causes of death and the lengthened survival time in hypertensive patients allows the development of coronary artery disease, which is apparently little affected if at all by control of blood pressure."

As noted earlier, there is increasing suspicion

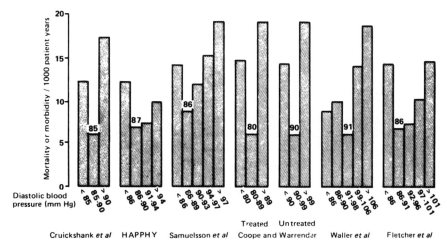

**Figure 5.11.** Relation of diastolic blood pressure (phase V) during treatment to mortality or morbidity from coronary heart disease. The six studies included 14,536 patients as shown in Table 5.11. Information on Heart Attack Primary Prevention in Hypertension trial (HAPPHY) is by personal communication (L. Wilhelmsen). The numbers within histograms indicate diastolic blood pressure in millimeters of mercury at which *J* point (lowest incidence of myocardial infarction) occurred. (From Cruickshank JM: *Br Med J* 297:1227, 1988.)

that inadvertent overtreatment of hypertension has been responsible for an increase in coronary ischemic events in patients whose diastolic pressures have been lowered to less than 85 mm Hg (Cruickshank, 1988). However, this increase is not to levels beyond that seen in untreated or poorly controlled hypertension so the contribution of the J-curve should not be overestimated. It may be responsible for less protection but it is not responsible for actual increases in CHD mortality.

## Left Ventricular Hypertrophy and Function

LVH is a major marker for mortality, and hypertension clearly is a major mechanism for LVH (Massie et al, 1989). Reduction of the blood pressure can cause regression of LVH, as demonstrated as long ago as 1945 after sympathectomy (White et al, 1945) and amply documented since then with various antihypertensive agents excluding diuretics and direct vasodilators used alone (Messerli et al, 1988). The reversal of LVH has been associated with a 25% reduction in the risk of cardiovascular events in the Framingham cohort (Kannel et al, 1988b). On the other hand, reversal of LVH was not accompanied by a significant decrease in cardiovascular mortality in the MRFIT study (MacMahon et al, 1989). Perhaps the protection appears only after many years.

In keeping with the evidence that overtreatment may induce myocardial ischemia, the rapid

reduction of blood pressure may elicit electrocardiographic repolarization abnormalities (Pepi et al, 1988). Furthermore, thiazide diuretic-based therapy may neither regress LVH nor suppress the risk of arrhythmias (Messerli et al, 1988; Levy et al, 1988).

## Cerebrovascular Disease

In the large clinical trials, the treatment of hypertension was associated with a striking fall in stroke morbidity and mortality, to about the same degree as seen in the overall population. Data from the population of Rochester, Minnesota, show a progressive fall in the incidence of stroke from 1950 to 1980, which is closely mirrored by the rise in the number of patients successfully treated for hypertension (Garraway and Whisnant, 1987). However, in the same population over the same interval, stroke recurrences were not reduced (Meissner et al, 1988). Moreover, in the entire United States population, only between 16 and 25% of the overall reduction in stroke mortality can be attributed to the treatment of hypertension (Bonita and Beaglehole, 1989). As small a contribution as this is, it is somewhat more than would be assumed from the clinical trial data, which would suggest only between 6 and 16% was due to the increased treatment of hypertension (Bonita and Beaglehole, 1989). Moreover, as with coronary disease, overzealous treatment may induce cerebral ischemia and stroke, particularly in the elderly (Jansen et al, 1986).

### Renal

It has been difficult to demonstrate a protective effect of antihypertensive therapy on renal function save in small numbers of patients with diabetic nephropathy (Dworkin and Benstein, 1989). Since progressive glomerulosclerosis is the likely consequence of the direct transmission of high systemic pressures (Baldwin and Neugarten, 1986), the lowering of systemic pressure ought to slow the progression of hypertensive renal damage. This has been seen in some patients (Brazy et al, 1989) but not in others (Ruilope et al, 1988). With or without good control of the blood pressure, renal function may deteriorate in perhaps 15% over a 5-year interval, more frequently in black patients than in white (Rostand et al, 1989).

### Large Arteries

After prolonged periods of antihypertensive therapy, remodeling of the hypertrophic changes within resistance vessels has been measured both directly (Heagerty et al, 1988) and indirectly (Hartford et al, 1988). This improvement does not restore all of the abnormal structural or functional responses seen within these vessels (Aalkjaer et al, 1989) but is likely responsible for the significant decrease in total peripheral resistance that accompanies successful reduction in blood pressure (Agabiti-Rosei et al, 1989).

### Overall Impact of Antihypertensive Therapy

As a last point in this discussion, it should be noted that the analyses of the effect of antihypertensive therapy on the overall rates of cardiovascular disease in the population have shown that the more extensive treatment and control of hypertension have had a relatively small impact. As noted at the end of Chapter 1, only 8 to 12% of the fall in coronary and stroke mortality over the past 15 years can be attributed to improved control of hypertension (Goldman and Cook, 1984; Beaglehole, 1986). Furthermore, cost-effectiveness calculations have concluded that the pharmacological therapy of hypertension is an extremely expensive way to prevent strokes, much less coronary disease. For the population of New Zealand in 1988, the estimated cost of preventing a single death from stroke was between approximately $200,000 and $1,000,000 United States dollars (Malcolm et al, 1988). These same

investigators have analyzed the benefits of therapy of mild to moderate hypertension (DBP 90 to 114 mm Hg) in patients aged 30- to 60-years, based on the results of the nine major clinical trials described in Figure 5.3 (Kawachi and Malcolm, 1989). Their analysis shows only very small gains in "quality-adjusted life-years" for men (Fig. 5.12) and even smaller gains for women.

## CURRENT ATTITUDE TOWARD DRUG THERAPY

### Advocates of Universal Therapy

Despite the various concerns expressed in the preceding analysis of the uncontrolled clinical trials of the treatment of mild hypertension, these trials have been widely accepted in the United States as providing definitive proof of the benefits of antihypertensive drug therapy for those with DBP above 90 mm Hg (Gifford, 1989). The 1988 JNC-4 report is more conservative than its predecessors, but it concludes that many, if not most, people with diastolic pressures over 90 should be given drug therapy after a "vigorous" use of nonpharmacological approaches.

United States physicians are more "therapeutic activists" than are physicians elsewhere. One English practitioner wrote, "According to at least 90% of clinicians I have met in the United States, the threshold for diagnosis is the threshold for treatment. The question 'to treat or not to treat' need no longer be asked. A free-fire zone has been created

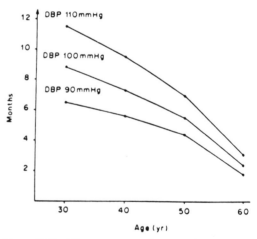

**Figure 5.12.** Life expectancy gains, assuming mean reduction in mortality and morbidity as observed in 9 major clinical trials, for males from age 30 to 60 with DBP levels of 90, 100, or 110 millimeters of mecury. (From Kawachi I and Malcolm LA: *J Clin Epidemiol* 42:905, 1989.)

above diastolic 90, in which we simply shoot everything that moves'' (Hart, 1983). Further evidence for the difference in attitude and practice is found in the treatment of patients over age 70 with isolated systolic hypertension: In England, only about 12% treat if the systolic pressure is at 170 mm Hg (Bucknall et al, 1986); in the United States over half of physicians surveyed said they treat if the systolic is at 170 (Breckenridge and Kostis, 1989).

In a fascinating book, *Medicine and Culture*, on differences in medical attitudes and practices in the United States, England, West Germany, and France, Lynn Payer (1988) points out that ''This medical aggressiveness [of United States physicians] reflects an aggressiveness of the American character that has often been attributed to the effect the vast frontier had on the people who came to settle it. . . . Disease could be conquered, but only by aggressively ferreting it out diagnostically and just as aggressively treating it.''

In an incisive essay, Guttmacher and associates (1981) provide two major reasons for the widespread acceptance of active drug therapy for mild hypertension, even in advance of evidence of its benefits. The first is that it is *preventive*, again based on the demonstrated evidence for the benefit of therapy for more severe hypertension. The second is *sociological*, related to two widely held attitudes: (1) ''technological optimism—the disposition to employ technologies in the belief that the benefits that flow from them will outweigh whatever unforeseen and undesirable effects that might ensue, and that these effects will themselves be manageable by existing or potential technological means,'' and (2) ''therapeutic activism—physicians prefer to take the risk of treating when intervention may not be called for to the potential error of not treating when treatment is needed'' (Guttmacher et al, 1981).

## Advocates of More Limited Therapy

### Outside the United States

In most of the world outside the United States, the treatment of hypertension is less aggressively pursued, mainly as to the level of blood pressure deemed to mandate institution of active drug therapy. No better example can be provided than the 1989 report of the British Hypertension Society Working Party (1989) composed of seven major English clinicians and epidemiologists in the hyper-

tension area. Their conclusions are: Treat patients under age 80 with diastolic pressures over 100 mm Hg after repeated measurements for 3 to 4 months; observe patients with pressures of 95 to 99 mm Hg every 3 to 6 months, measure the blood pressure yearly of patients whose blood pressure is initially raised but falls below 95 mm Hg.

This more conservative view reflects, in part, ethical concerns that have been voiced about the use of drug intervention among large numbers of asymptomatic people with mild hypertension in an attempt to reduce the risk for a small portion of the entire group. One of the more eloquent has been that of Geoffrey Rose (1981), who wrote:

In reality the care of the symptomless hypertensive person is preventive medicine, not therapeutics. . . . If a preventive measure exposes many people to a small risk, then the harm it does may readily . . . outweigh the benefits, since these are received by relatively few. . . . We may thus be unable to identify that small level of harm to individuals from long-term intervention that would be sufficient to make that line of prevention unprofitable or even harmful. Consequently we cannot accept long-term mass preventive medication.

### Within the United States

Despite the general enthusiasm of United States physicians to treat early and at low levels of hypertension, voices have been heard in the United States for caution. As far back as 1977, doubt was expressed about the wisdom of accepting the VA Cooperative Study to validate the treatment of all hypertensives with diastolic pressure greater than 105 mm Hg (Alderman, 1977; Ingelfinger and Goldman, 1977). Subsequently, others have questioned the practice of routine therapy for all with diastolics above 90 mm Hg (Kaplan, 1981; Madhavan and Alderman, 1981; Freis, 1982).

Beyond the concerns expressed by Guttmacher et al (1981), others have questioned the ethics of treating mild hypertension, such as Dr. Allan Brett (1984) who wrote:

In medical practice, the duty to inflict no harm (nonmaleficence) continuously competes with the duty to benefit the patient (beneficence). It follows that equivocal data on interventional efficacy may be sufficient to justify a recommendation to change some habits, since the risk of doing harm is small. Conversely, reasonably certain data is necessary to justify pharmacologic interventions, since the risk of doing harm is relatively greater. This argument assumes importance for a medicalized society in which unbridled enthusiasm to medicate often precedes reasonable proof of efficacy. (Reproduced with permission from Brett AS: *Am J Med* 76:557, 1984.)

## Development of a Consensus

As a result of the somewhat more cautious attitude arising in the United States and the definitely more conservative views expressed by most English and European authorities, a consensus seems to have developed for institution of therapy at a level of diastolic pressure persistently above 95 mm Hg. Thus, the guidelines published by participants in a conference sponsored jointly by the World Health Organization (WHO) and the International Society of Hypertension (ISH) indicated that, after 3 to 6 months of observation, 95 mm Hg should be the level at which treatment should be started (WHO/ISH, 1989) (Fig. 5.13).

The report of the United States Fourth Joint National Committee (JNC) on Detection, Evaluation, and Treatment of High Blood Pressure (JNC IV, 1988) states:

The benefits of drug therapy appear to outweigh any known risks to individuals with a persistently elevated DBP greater than 94 mm Hg and to those with lesser elevations who are otherwise at high risk, e.g., men, smokers, or patients with target organ damage, diabetes mellitus, hyperlipidemia, or other major risk factors for cardiovascular disease.

Patients whose DBPs fall between 90 and 94 mm Hg and who are otherwise at relatively low risk of developing cardiovascular disease should be treated with nonpharmacologic approaches.

Initially, nonpharmacologic therapy is the preferred treatment approach for most patients with isolated systolic hypertension. However, when the SBP is consistently 160 mm Hg or greater and the DBP is less than 90 mm Hg despite nonpharmacologic therapy, antihypertensive drug treatment should be considered.

## Current Recommendations

The consensus, therefore, seems to have settled on 95 mm Hg. Selectivity is advocated for the very sizeable number with DBP between 90 and 95 mm Hg, who make up 40% of the entire population with DBP above 90 (Fig. 1.11). That is, drugs should be provided more quickly to those at high risk, but only after a period of observation plus nondrug therapy for the majority. Hopefully, such selectivity in using drug therapy will protect those in immediate need while at the same time postponing or perhaps removing the need for such therapy in many more patients (Browner and Hulley, 1989).

This approach is based upon these premises:

1. All patients should be kept under surveillance. In all of the trials for mild hypertension, a certain percentage of patients, varying from 10

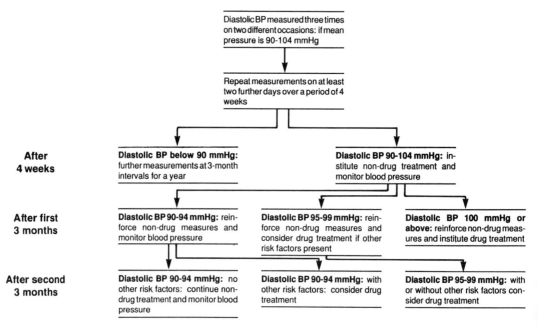

**Figure 5.13.** Recommendations for the definition and management of mild hypertension by participants at the Third Mild Hypertension Conference of the World Health Organization and the International Society of Hypertension. (From World Health Organization/International Society of Hypertension. *J Hypertens* 7:689, 1989.)

to 17%, have had a rapid progression of their blood pressure to levels where risk is imminent (Table 1.5). There is no sure way to identify those susceptible to this rapid progression; therefore, all need to be watched.

2. Those at relatively low risk will likely not suffer from deferral of active drug therapy. Recall the experience of the placebo-treated half of the patients in the Australian Trial: Over 4 years, the average blood pressure fell below 95 mm Hg in 47.5% of those who started between 95 and 109 mm Hg, and excess mortality and morbidity were increased significantly only in those whose average DBP remained above 100 mm Hg.

3. Patients at relatively high risk can be identified. As described in Chapter 2, the Framingham data can be used to determine an individual's cardiovascular risk at various levels of blood pressure, based upon age, gender, and the coexistence of other known risk factors, utilizing the Coronary Risk Handbook provided by the American Heart Association.

4. The recognition that the decision to use drug therapy is based on a balance between risk and benefit may mandate even more aggressive use of drugs in some patients, such as hypertensive diabetics with evidence of early renal damage. The poor prognosis of such patients if they are left untreated and the evidence that reduction of their hypertension will slow the inexorable progress of renal damage (Parving et al, 1987) may be used in the future as justification for therapy in those with DBP well below 90 mm Hg if proof of the benefit from such a course becomes available.

5. All patients, regardless of risk status, should be offered and strongly encouraged to follow those nondrug therapies that are likely to help: weight reduction, moderate sodium restriction, regular isotonic exercise, relief of stress, and moderation of alcohol intake.

The final line comes down to this: The majority of hypertensive people have fairly mild, asymptomatic hypertension and the effectiveness of treatment, measured as the reduction in complications, progressively falls, the milder the degree of hypertension. This translates into the need to treat a larger and larger group of patients to prevent complications. These patients, while receiving relatively little benefit, are, nonetheless, exposed both to the risks of adverse effects and to the fairly large financial costs of therapy.

The overall dilemma is accurately described by the Swedish investigator, G. Berglund (1989), who wrote:

According to the major trials, 300 patients with mild hypertension have to be treated one year to postpone one complication one year. Out of these 300 patients, 10 will develop severe side effects leading to withdrawal of the drug, around 50 will get subjective complaints decreasing their quality of life and 75 will have worsened biochemical risk indicators like decreased serum potassium, increased blood sugar, LDL-cholesterol and uric acid. Thus, 135 out of 300 will have some form of negative effect from the given treatment. The cost of the drugs given to these 300 patients will vary from $5,000 US/year (thiazide diuretic) to $105,000 US/year (ACE inhibitors or Ca-channel blockers) depending on the choice of first line drug.

The dilemma is clear and the results of massive clinical trials simply have not provided a simple solution. We hoped that these trials would do so but that was a false hope. Thus, each patient and practitioner must end up making the decision to treat milder degrees of hypertension by weighing the multiple benefits and costs of either action or inaction (Table 1.1). Increasingly, economic considerations will influence the decision and there will be increasing demands to document the value of mass therapy of mild hypertension (Harlan, 1989).

Now that the rationale for the institution of therapy has been analyzed, let us turn to the issue of how far to lower the pressure.

## GOAL OF THERAPY

Until recently, the goal of therapy was simply to reduce the diastolic blood pressure to lower than 90 mm Hg and then to "the lowest diastolic blood pressure consistent with safety and tolerance" (JNC-3, 1984), a level below 85 based on the results of the HDFP wherein fewer complications were seen in the SI group whose average diastolic BP was 83 mm Hg compared with the UC group who averaged 88 mm Hg. The premise has been the lower the achieved blood pressure, the greater the protection from cardiovascular complications. This is described as line *A* in Figure 5.14 (Safar, 1988).

However, the results of the multiple clinical trials, as described in the preceding pages, have suggested that the consequences of therapy are better portrayed as either line *B*, wherein little if any additional benefit is derived from increasingly greater reduction in pressure, or line *C*, wherein additional risks arise as the pressure is reduced further, i.e., a J-curve. The J-curve has been noted mainly in patients with preexisting CHD.

The situation is in a state of flux: Some do

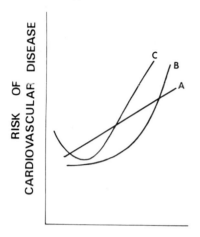

**Figure 5.14.** Three models representing hypothetical relationships between levels of blood pressure and risk of cardiovascular disease. (From Epstein FH: Proceedings of the XVth International Congress of Therapeutics, September 5–9, 1979. Brussels: *Excerpta Medica*, 1980.)

not believe it is desirable to alter the goal of reducing DBP below 85 mm Hg (Waller et al, 1988b; Hansson, 1989). Others believe the wiser course is to bring the DBP only down to 90, particularly in those with known CHD, and then perhaps to 85 but no lower (Beevers, 1988; Cruickshank, 1989). Concern has also been raised about the potential for inadvertent overtreatment, particularly during the hours of sleep when pressures tend to fall even more, unless ambulatory monitoring is done to learn what the course of the blood pressure is throughout the 24 hours (O'Brien and O'Malley, 1988).

There is less certainty about the appropriate goal of therapy in regard to the systolic level, particularly in the elderly with predominantly systolic hypertension. Until the Systolic Hypertension in the Elderly Program (SHEP) trial data are reported, a level of 160 would appear to be a reasonable and safe goal.

Despite these concerns, we should not lose sight of the fact that the reason for the lesser protection found among treated hypertensives could reflect not overtreatment, but undertreatment (Hansson, 1988). Clearly it is essential that all patients have

their DBP brought down to the 85- to 90-mm Hg range in order to provide the demonstrated benefits of therapy. In order to be sure about the adequacy of therapy, all patients who are willing should monitor their own pressures, using one of the inexpensive, semiautomatic, accurate devices now available (Evans et al, 1989).

As I have written:

> The bottom line regarding the J-curve is the need for greater caution in lowering the blood pressure of patients with preexisting CHD, with the goal of therapy being a slowly reached diastolic level of 90 and, if no harm has been noted at that level, perhaps down toward but seldom below 85. Some caution is probably advisable for all middle-aged and older hypertensives, considering the virtual ubiquity of coronary atherosclerosis. There is a need to be particularly cautious in treating the elderly with predominant systolic hypertension (Kaplan, 1989).

As we focus on the blood pressure as the primary goal of therapy, we must not lose sight of the need, often greater than that of lowering the blood pressure, of reducing other known cardiovascular risk factors. These obviously include cigarette smoking, hyperlipidemia, glucose intolerance, and upper body obesity. To neglect these by focusing only on the blood pressure is to lose sight of the only reason for all of our efforts, the protection of the patient from premature disability and death while preserving the best possible quality of life.

## Importance of Population Strategies

Most of our current efforts are directed at the individual patient with existing hypertension. Clearly we need to also advise the larger population to do those things that may protect against the development of hypertension, the approach directed toward "sick populations" rather than only "sick individuals" (Rose, 1985). Such population strategies cannot include medications but rather utilize totally safe and easily applied nondrug therapies.

The next chapter describes these nondrug therapies. Though they are described mainly for those with hypertension, they clearly should be utilized as well by the larger population at risk in hopes of prevention.

## References

Aalkjaer C, Eiskjaer H, Mulvany MJ: *J Hypertens* 7:305, 1989.
Abernathy JD: *JAMA* 256:3134, 1986.
Agabiti-Rosei E, Muiesan ML, Geri A, et al: *J Hypertens* 6(Suppl 4):S94, 1988.
Agabiti-Rosei E, Muiesan ML, Muiesan G, et al: *Am J Hypertens* 2:70S, 1989.
Alderman MH: *N Engl J Med* 296:753, 1977.

Alderman MH, Madhavan S: *Hypertension* 3:192, 1981.
Alderman MH, Ooi WL, Madhavan S, et al: *JAMA* 262:920, 1989.
Amery A, Birkenhager W, Brixko P, et al: *Lancet* 1:1349, 1985.
Amery A, Birkenhager W, Brixko P, et al: *Lancet* 2:589, 1986.

Amery A, Birkenhager W, Bulpitt C, et al: *J Hypertens* 6:925, 1988.
Anderson TW: *Lancet* 2:1139, 1978.
Baldwin DS, Neugarten J: In: Mitch WE, Brenner BM, Stein JH, (eds): *The Progressive Nature of Renal Disease*. New York: Churchill Livingstone, 1986:81.
Barsky AJ: *N Engl J Med* 318:414, 1988.

Beaglehole R: *Br Med J* 292:33, 1986.

Beevers DG: *Br Med J* 297:1212, 1988.

Berglund G: *Future directions in hypertension* [Abstract]. Paris, April 12, 1989.

Bonita R and Beaglehole R: *Hypertension* 13(Suppl 1):I-69, 1989.

Brazy PC, Stead WW, Fitzwilliam JF: *Kidney Int* 35:670, 1989

Breckenridge MB, Kostis JB: *Am J Med* 86:370, 1989.

Brett AS: *Am J Med* 76:557, 1984.

Bronte-Stewart B, Heptinstall RH: *J Pathol Bacteriol* 68:407, 1954.

Browner WS, Hulley SB: *Hypertension* 13(Suppl I):I-51, 1989.

Bucknall CA, Morris GK, Mitchell JRA: *Br Med J* 293:739, 1986.

Bulpitt CJ, Beevers DG, Butler A, et al: *J Hypertens* 4:93, 1986.

Callcott R, Dobson AJ, Gibberd RW, et al: *Med J Aust* 141:419, 1984.

Chasis H: *J Chron Dis* 39:933, 1986.

Cloher TP, Whelton PK: *Arch Intern Med* 146:529, 1986.

Collins R, Peto R, MacMahon S, et al: *Lancet* 335:827, 1990.

Coope J, Warrender TS: *Br Med J* 293:1145, 1986.

Cooper SP, Hardy RJ, Labarthe DR, et al: *Am J Epidemiol* 127:387, 1988.

Cruickshank JM, Thorp JM, Zacharias FJ: *Lancet* 1:581, 1987.

Cruickshank JM: *Br Med J* 297:1227, 1988.

Cruickshank JM: *Br Med J* 298:458, 1989.

Cutler JA, MacMahon SW, Furberg CD: *Hypertension* 13(Suppl I):I-36, 1989.

Cutler J, Mattson M, Goor R, et al: *Circulation* 70(Suppl II):II-281, 1984.

Doyle AE: *Clin Sci* 63:431s, 1982.

Doyle AE: *Am J Hypertens* 1:319, 1988.

Dworkin LD, Benstein JA: *Am J Hypertension* 2:162S, 1989.

Ehrhart LA, Ferrario CM: *Hypertension* 3:479, 1981.

European Working Party on High Blood Pressure in the Elderly: In: *Proceedings of Fourth European Meeting on Hypertension*, Milan, 18-21 June 1989 [Abstract].

Evans CE, Haynes RB, Goldsmith CH, et al: *J Hypertens* 7:133, 1989.

Floras JS: *Lancet* 2:994, 1988.

Forrow L, Wartman SA, Brock DW: *JAMA* 259:3161, 1988.

Freis ED: *N Engl J Med* 307:306, 1982.

Garraway WM, Whisnant JP: *JAMA* 258:214, 1987.

Gelmers HJ, Gorter K, de Weerdt CJ, et al: *N Engl J Med* 318:203, 1988.

Gifford RW: *JAMA* 260:1714, 1988.

Gifford RW: *Am J Cardiol* 63:8B, 1989.

Goldman L, Cook EF: *Ann Intern Med* 101:825, 1984.

Goldring W, Chasis H: In: Ingelfinger FJ, Relman AS, Finland M, eds. *Controversy in International Medicine*. Philadelphia: WB Saunders, 1966:83.

Gomez-Marin O, Folsom AR, Kottke TE, et al: *N Engl J Med* 316:1353, 1987.

Gross TP, Wise RP, Knapp DE: *Hypertension* 13(Suppl 1):I-113, 1989.

Guttmacher S, Teitelman M, Chapin G, et al: *Hastings Center Report*, February, 1981:12.

Hamilton M, Thompson EN, Wisniewski TKM: *Lancet* 1:235, 1964.

Hansson L: *Am J Hypertens* 1:414, 1988.

Hansson L: *Br Med J* 298:52, 1989.

Hardy RJ, Hawkins CM: *Am J Epidemiol* 117:566, 1983.

Harlan WR: *Hypertension* 13(Suppl I):I-158, 1989.

Hart JT: In: Gross FK, Strasser T, (eds). *Mild Hypertension: Recent Advances*. New York: Raven Press, 1983:365.

Hartford M, Wendelhag I, Berglund G, et al: *JAMA* 259:2553, 1988.

Havlik RJ, LaCroix AZ, Kleinman JC, et al: *Hypertension* 13(Suppl I):I-28, 1989.

Heagerty AM, Bund SJ, Aalkjaer C: *Lancet* 2:1209, 1988.

Heath D, Edwards JE: *Circulation* 18:533, 1958.

Heart Attack Primary Prevention in Hypertensives (HAPPHY): *J Clin Hypertens* 5:561, 1987.

Hebert PR, Fiebach NH, Eberlein KA, et al: *Am J Epidemiol* 127:581, 1988.

Helgeland A: *Am J Med* 69:725, 1980.

Hodge JVG, McQueen EG, Smirk FH: *Br Med J* 1:1, 1961.

Hollander W, Madoff I, Paddock J, et al: *Circ Res* 38(Suppl 2):II-63, 1976.

Hood B, Bjork S, Sannerstedt R, et al: *Acta Med Scand* 174:393, 1963.

Holme I, Helgeland A, Hjermann I, et al: *JAMA* 251:1298, 1984.

Holme I: *Stat Med* 7:1109, 1988.

Hypertension Detection and Follow-Up Program (HDFP): *JAMA* 252:2562, 1979a.

Hypertension Detection and Follow-Up Program (HDFP): *JAMA* 252:2572, 1979b.

Hypertension Detection and Follow-Up Program (HDFP): *N Engl J Med* 307:976, 1982a.

Hypertension Detection and Follow-Up Program (HDFP): *JAMA* 247:633, 1982b.

Hypertension Detection and Follow-Up Program (HDFP): *Hypertension* 6(Suppl I):I-198, 1984a.

Hypertension Detection and Follow-Up Program (HDFP): *Circulation* 70:996, 1984b.

Hypertension Detection and Follow-Up Program (HDFP): *Hypertension* 7:105, 1985.

Hypertension Detection and Follow-Up Program (HDFP): *Prog Cardiovasc Dis* 29:(3 Suppl 1):1, 1986.

Hypertension Detection and Follow-Up Program (HDFP): *JAMA* 259:2113, 1988.

Ingelfinger JA, Goldman P: *JAMA* 238:1369, 1977.

International Prospective Primary Prevention Study in Hypertension (IPPPSH): *J Hypertens* 3:379, 1985.

Isles CG, Walker LM, Beevers GD, et al: *J Hypertens* 4:141, 1986.

Jansen PAF, Gribnau FWJ, Schulte BPM, et al: *Br Med J* 293:914, 1986.

Joint National Committee on Detection, Evaluation, and Treatment of High Blood Pressure (JNC 3): *Arch Intern Med* 144:1045, 1984.

Joint National Committee on Detection, Evaluation, and Treatment of High Blood Pressure (JNC IV): *Arch Intern Med* 148:1023, 1988.

Kannel WB, D'Agostino RB, Levy D, et al: *Circ* 78 (4 Suppl II):II-89, 1988b.

Kannel WB, Cupples LA, D'Agostino RB, et al: *Hypertension* 11(Suppl II):II-45, 1988a.

Kaplan NM: *Am Heart J* 101:867, 1981.

Kaplan NM: *Am J Hypertens* 1(4 pt 1):428, 1988.

Kaplan NM: *Am J Hypertens* 2:132, 1989.

Kawachi I, Malcolm LA: *J Clin Epidemiol* 42:905, 1989.

Khatri I, Gottdiener J, Notargiacomo A, et al: *Clin Sci* 59:435s, 1980.

Kuller LH, Hulley SB, Cohen JD, et al: *Circulation* 73:114, 1986.

Leishman AWD: *Br Med J* 2:1361, 1959.

Levy D, Anderson KM, Christiansen JC, et al: *Am J Cardiol* 62:147, 1988.

Madhavan S, Alderman MH: *Arch Intern Med* 141:1583, 1981.

MacMahon SW, Cutler JA, Furberg CD, et al: *Prog Cardiovasc Dis* 29(3 Suppl 1):99, 1986.

MacMahon S, Collins G, Rautaharju P, et al: *Am J Cardiol* 63:202, 1989.

MacMahon S, Peto R, Cutler J, et al: *Lancet* 335:765, 1990.

Malcolm LA, Kawachi I, Jackson R, et al: *NZ Med J* 101:167, 1988.

Management Committee of the Australian National Blood Pressure Study: *Lancet* 1:1261, 1980.

Management Committee of the Australian National Blood Pressure Study: *Lancet* 1:185, 1982.

Management Committee of the Australian National Blood Pressure Study: *Circ* 69:668, 1984.

Massie BM, Tubau JF, Szlachcic J, et al: *J Cardiovasc Pharmac* 13(Suppl 1):S18, 1989.

Masson GMC, McCormack LJ, Dustan HP, et al: *Am J Pathol* 34:817, 1958.

Medical Research Council (MRC) Working Party: *Br Med J* 291:97, 1985.

Medical Research Council (MRC) Working Party: *Br Med J* 296:1565, 1988.

Meissner I, Whisnant JP, Garraway WM: *Stroke* 19:459, 1988.

Messerli FH, Oren S, Grossman E: *Drugs* 35(Suppl 5):27, 1988.

Metoprolol Atherosclerosis Prevention in Hypertension (MAPHY): *JAMA* 259:1976, 1988.

Miall WE, Chinn S: *Clin Sci Mol Med* 45:235, 1973.

Morgan T, Adam W, Hodgson M: *J Cardiovasc Pharmacol* 6:S269, 1984.

Motz W, Strauer BE: *Hypertension* 13:43, 1989.

Multiple Risk Factor Intervention Trial Research Group: *JAMA* 248:1465, 1982.

Multiple Risk Factor Intervention Trial Research Group: *Am J Cardiol* 55:1, 1985.

Oberman A, Lane NE, Harlan WR, et al: *Circulation* 36:812, 1967.

O'Brien E, O'Malley K: *Br Med J* 297:1607, 1988.

O'Kelly BF, Massie BM, Tubau JF, et al: *Ann Intern Med* 110:1017, 1989.

O'Malley K, McCormack P, O'Brien ET: *J Hypertens* 6(Suppl 1):S105, 1988.

Parving H-H, Andersen AR, Smidt UM, et al: *Br Med J* 294:1443, 1987.

Payer L: In: *Medicine & Culture*. New York: Henry Holt and Company, 1988.

Peart WS, Miall WE: *Lancet* 1:104, 1980.

Pepi M, Alimento M, Maltagliati A, et al: *Hypertension* 11:84, 1988.

Perry HM Jr, Goldman AI, Lavin MA, et al: *Ann NY Acad Sci* 304:266, 1978.

Perry HM, Smith WM, McDonald RH, et al: *Stroke* 20:4, 1989.

Report of the British Hypertension Society Working Party: *Br Med J* 298:694, 1989.

Rose G: *Br Med J* 282:1847, 1981.

Rose G: *Int J Epidemiol* 14:32, 1985.

Rose G: *Am Heart J* 114:1013, 1987.

Rose G: In: Mathias CJ, Sever PS, (eds): *Concepts in Hypertension*. New York: Springer-Verlag, 1989:39.

Rostand SG, Brown G, Kirk KA, et al: *N Engl J Med* 320:684, 1989.

Ruilope LM, Miranda B, Oliet A, et al: *J Hypertens* 6(Suppl 4):S744, 1988.

Safar M: *Am Heart J* 115:702, 1988.

Samuelsson O, Wilhelmsen L, Pennert K, et al: *J Hypertens* 3(Suppl 3):S497, 1985.

Samuelsson O, Wilhelmsen L, Andersson OK, et al: *JAMA* 258:1768, 1987.

Smith WM: *Circ Res* 40(Suppl 1):1, 1977.

Staessen J, Bulpitt C, Clement D, et al: *Br Med J* 298:1552, 1989.

Staessen J, Fagard R, Amery A: *JAMA* 260:1713, 1988.

Steering Committee of the HAPPHY Trial: *JAMA* 262:3273, 1989.

Stewart IMG: *Lancet* 1:861, 1979.

Strandgaard S, Haunsø S. *Lancet* 2.658, 1987.

Strate M, Thygesen K, Ringsted C, et al: *Acta Med Scand* 219:153, 1986.

Thal HP, Grage TB, Vernier RL: *Circulation* 27:36, 1963.

Tuomilehto J, Wikstrand J, Olsson G, et al: *Hypertension* 13:773, 1989.

Veterans Administration Cooperative Study Group on Antihypertensive Agents: *JAMA* 202:1028, 1967.

Veterans Administration Cooperative Study Group on Antihypertensive Agents: *JAMA* 213:1143-1152, 1970.

Veterans Administration Cooperative Study Group on Antihypertensive Agents: *Circulation* 45:991, 1972.

Waller PC, Isles CG, McInnes GT: *Br Med J* 297:1606, 1988a.

Waller PC, Isles CG, Lever AF, et al: *J Human Hypertens* 2:7, 1988b.

White PD, Smithwick RH, Mathews MW, et al: *Am Heart J* 30:165, 1945.

White WB, Schulman P, Karimeddini MK, et al: *Am Heart J* 117:145, 1989.

Wikstrand J: *Am Heart J* 116:338, 1988.

Wikstrand J, Warnold I, Olsson G, et al: *JAMA* 259:1976, 1988a.

Wikstrand J, Warnold I, Olsson G, et al: *JAMA* 260:1715, 1988b

Wilhelmsen L, Berglund G, Elmfeldt D, et al: *J Hypertens* 5:561, 1987.

Wilhelmsen L: *JAMA* 260:1713, 1988.

World Health Organization/International Society of Hypertension: *J Hypertens* 7:689, 1989.

# 6 Treatment of Hypertension: Nondrug Therapy

With an appreciation of the benefits and costs of antihypertensive therapy, we now will consider the practical aspects of accomplishing a reduction in blood pressure. First, the use of nondrugs will be examined. In the next chapter the use of drugs will be covered.

The use of nondrug therapies as initial therapy for most patients, at least for the first 3 to 6 months after recognition of their hypertension, is being more widely advocated (Joint National Committee on Detection, Evaluation, and Treatment of High Blood Pressure, 1988; Report of the British Hypertension Society Working Party, 1989). Such therapy may lower pressure to a level considered safe for many of the 40% of patients with diastolic levels between 90 and 94 mm Hg. For the remainder, nondrug therapy may not be enough, but it can aid in reducing the pressure without risk, so that less drug therapy will be needed.

The following nondrug "prescription" should be practical for most hypertensives:

—If body weight is excessive, weight reduction should be the primary goal.
—Dietary sodium intake should be restricted to 2 g/day (88 mmol/day), with caution not to reduce the intake of calcium-rich foods, i.e., low-fat milk and cheese products.
—Dietary potassium intake need not be specifically increased because it will rise when sodium intake is reduced.
—Until their antihypertensive efficacy is established, supplemental calcium and magnesium should only be given to those who are deficient.
—More fiber and less saturated fat are beneficial for other reasons and may also lower the blood pressure.
—Caffeine-containing beverages need not be limited unless the patient is highly sensitive to their effects.
—Smoking should obviously be discouraged, not to lower the blood pressure but to lower the overall risks for heart disease more than any other possible single action.
—Alcohol should be limited to 1 ounce per day, as contained in two usual portions of wine, beer, or spirits.
—Regular isotonic exercise should be encouraged.
—Some type of relaxation therapy should be encouraged. Sedatives and tranquilizers will not lower the blood pressure.

## ISSUE OF EFFICACY

Many practitioners, though they recognize the potential benefits of these nondrug treatments, do not use them. There are two main reasons: First it is too much trouble and, second, many patients do not respond. The time and effort needed to instruct and motivate patients to use these therapies is undoubtedly greater than that needed to write out a prescription. However, various nonphysician practitioners—nurses, dieticians, psychologists—are available in most places to help in the effort.

Although it is true that many patients do not adhere to these nondrug therapies, poor compliance is also a major problem with drug treatment as well. The same type of aids to improve patient adherence to drug therapy that will be described in the next chapter should help with both.

### Nonspecific Effects

An antihypertensive effect has been claimed for virtually everything that has been tried, including some remedies as dilute hydrochloric acid (Ayman, 1930) or cholecystectomy (Volini and Flaxman, 1939), that almost certainly are worthless. In view of the repeated observations that blood pressures tend to fall spontaneously for the first 6 to 12 weeks of observation, as noted in Chapter 2, studies must obviously be properly designed with adequate run-in periods or parallel observations on groups randomly allocated to the nondrug therapy or left untreated.

## Protection Against the Risks

The larger issue of whether these nondrug therapies will, in fact, reduce the risks from hypertension—which some may demand before they will accept their use—may never be settled. The difficulty of demonstrating such protection in the various therapeutic trials using antihypertensive drugs was described in Chapter 5. There is likely no way to document the efficacy of nondrug therapies, which are less potent and more difficult to monitor than drug treatment. Nondrug therapies must be accepted on the evidence they will lower the blood pressure without risk, and with a reasonable chance of adherence by most patients.

Attempts to better document the long-term antihypertensive effect of nondrug therapies are in progress. Small-scale studies indicate that even modest degrees of either weight reduction or sodium restriction will maintain lower levels of blood pressure in patients previously treated with antihypertensive drugs (Oberman et al, 1990; Stamler et al, 1987). Even more impressively, a modest nutritional-exercise program was shown to reduce the 5-year incidence of hypertension from 19.2% in the control group to 8.8% in the group who followed the program (Stamler et al, 1989).

## COMBINED THERAPIES

In addition to the study of Stamler et al, others have shown a significant antihypertensive effect of multiple nondrug therapies utilized simultaneously. Dodson et al (1985) followed 32 patients being treated with antihypertensive drugs for 3.9 years on a dietary regimen of high-fiber, low-fat, and low-sodium intake. They observed a significant decrease in blood pressure (12/14 mm Hg) that was accomplished while at the same time the number of antihypertensive drugs was reduced by half. Vertes et al (1988) accomplished similar effects with 46 hypertensives who were placed on a very low calorie, 1-g sodium diet with increased physical activity and relaxation therapy.

Unlike these studies, most of the trials of nondrug therapy examine the effect of only one modality at a time. We will examine the data on each modality in sequence, recognizing that relatively few well-controlled studies with clear-cut results and low risk of error have been performed (Sackett, 1986). The evidence has been expanding rapidly, as seen in the overall conclusions about the effectiveness of various nondrug modalities provided by Andrews et al, 1982 and by Beilin 6 years later. Andrews et al (1982) found that only weight loss, yoga, and muscle relaxation had been found to accomplish significant reductions in blood pressure. Beilin (1988) concluded that a number of modalities had been shown to lower either blood pressure or coronary risk or both (Table 6.1).

Along with the paucity of large scale, long-term trials of any nondrug therapy, there are even fewer that have compared one form of nondrug therapy with another or with a drug. Kostis et al (1989) performed a randomized placebo-controlled study comparing nondrug with beta-blocker therapy of 86 hypertensive men. The nondrug regimen consisted of reductions in calories, sodium and alcohol intake, and exercise and stress management. After 3 months, the patients assigned to the nondrug regimen had greater improvements in blood pressure and various other cardiovascular risk factors than did those assigned to the beta-blocker. On the other hand, Berglund et al (1989) found that beta-blocker-based drug therapy was considerably more effective in reducing blood pressure but worsened lipid levels, which were improved by the diet lower in calories and sodium (Table 6.2).

Preliminary results have been presented of two large scale comparative studies. In one, the Trial of Antihypertensive Intervention and Management (TAIM), 878 patients with mild hypertension were randomly assigned to one of

**Table 6.1. Dietary and Related Measures Which Reduce Blood Pressure and/or Cardiovascular Risk[a]**

| | Blood Pressure ↓ | Coronary Risk ↓ |
|---|---|---|
| Exercise | Yes | Yes |
| Weight control | Yes | Yes |
| Decrease in total and saturated fat | ? | Yes |
| Increase of fish consumption | ? | Yes |
| Increase in vegetables and fruit | Yes | Yes |
| Decrease in sodium intake | Yes | Yes |
| Cessation of smoking | No | Yes |
| Alcohol reduced to 10-20 g/day | Yes | Yes |

[a]From Beilin LJ: *J Hypertens* 6:85, 1988.

**Table 6.2. Comparison Between Diet and Drug Therapy for 12 Months in Obese Men With Mild Hypertension**[a]

|  | Diet | Drug (Atenolol +) |
|---|---|---|
| Weight (kg) | −7.6 | +0.9 |
| Urine Na$^+$ (mmol/d) | −42 | −10 |
| Blood Pressure (mm Hg) | −4/−3 | −16/−11 |
| % DBP < 90 | 29% | 73% |
| Serum Cholesterol (mg/dl) | −13 | +2 |
| Triglycerides (mg/dl) | −20 | +37 |

[a]From Berglund et al: *Br Med J* 299:480, 1989.

three agents (placebo, chlorthalidone, or atenolol) plus one of three diets (usual, lower calorie, or lower sodium + higher potassium) (Blaufox et al, 1989). At the end of 6 months, those on either chlorthalidone or atenolol and the lower calorie diet, who lost an average of 10.4 pounds, had the greatest fall in blood pressure. Weight reduction per se provided a significant fall in pressure and at the same time did not cause changes in the patients' quality of life (Smoller et al, 1989).

In the second, the Treatment of Mild Hypertension Study (TOMHS), all 468 patients were first placed on a program of weight, sodium, and alcohol reduction plus exercise and then on either a placebo or one of five different antihypertensive drugs (Grimm et al, 1989). After 18 months, blood pressure fell from 140/90 to 131/82 for the placebo + nutritional-exercise group and to 123/78 for those on a drug as well. The study is ongoing, with the hope of documenting long-term benefits of the various drugs compared with the nondrug regimen.

We will now examine the effects of individual nondrug modalities.

## WEIGHT REDUCTION

As noted in Chapter 3, obesity, in particular that located in the upper body, is commonly associated with hypertension, and the combination may, in turn, be related to hyperinsulinemia secondary to insulin resistance (Kaplan, 1989). Obese hypertensives have as much coronary disease as the lean (Kannel et al, 1989; Phillips and Shaper, 1989). Beyond their analysis of 10 other prospective studies that show an almost equal overall degree of risk, Phillips and Shaper add their data on 7735 middle-aged men followed for an average of 7.5 years wherein risk was 30% greater for the obese. As described further in Chapter 16, children who lose weight tend to have a fall in their blood pressure (Clarke et al, 1986), so that weight reduction may be a way to prevent the development of hyperten-

sion. Moreover, a significant fall in blood pressure will usually be noted even with only modest weight reduction (Eliahou et al, 1981; Sonne-Holm et al, 1989).

### Clinical Experience

Only a relatively few well-controlled studies have documented an antihypertensive effect of weight reduction (Staessen et al, 1989). A few have compared groups that were randomly assigned to either a diet or similar follow-up without a diet: Some observed an effect of weight loss (Reisin et al, 1978) (MacMahon et al, 1985); the others found no effect, perhaps because their subjects lost a smaller amount of weight (Haynes et al, 1984). The data of MacMahon et al are particularly impressive. Over a 21-week period, those randomly assigned to weight reduction lost an average of 7.4 kg and, compared with those on placebo or a beta-blocker, they had a greater fall in blood pressure that was accompanied by improvements in blood lipids.

Staessen et al (1989) have plotted the effect of varying degrees of weight loss on the systolic and diastolic blood pressures in 11 studies published from 1954 to 1985 involving almost 650 patients (Fig. 6.1). When only the adequately controlled studies (Tyroler et al, 1975; Reisin et al, 1978; Fagerberg et al, 1984; MacMahon et al, 1985) were considered, the mean effect of a 1-kg fall in body weight was a 1.6/1.3-mm Hg fall in systolic and diastolic pressures.

There may be a need to consider the composition of the weight reduction diet. With most lower calorie diets, fat intake is markedly reduced and carbohydrate is increased. This mixture, by potentiating hyperinsulinemia, may reduce the effectiveness of weight loss in reducing the blood pressure and the metabolic disturbances of obesity (Parillo et al, 1988).

In the last few years, a major increase in the use of 400- to 600-calorie liquid formula diets, e.g., Optifast, has occurred in the United States. Although many patients regain considerable portions of the lost weight (Hovell et al, 1988), those who are able to maintain the weight loss usually achieve significant falls in blood pressure (Dornfeld et al, 1985; Vertes et al, 1988).

The issue as to whether weight loss will lower the blood pressure in the absence of sodium restriction is unsettled: Some find little effect without concomitant sodium restriction (Fagerberg et al, 1984); others find weight loss to lower the blood pressure with or without sodium restriction (Reisin et al, 1983; Maxwell et al,

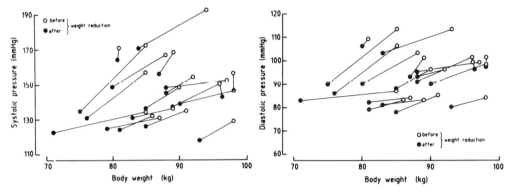

**Figure 6.1.** Systolic and diastolic blood pressure before and after body weight reduction in 11 studies published from 1954 to 1985. (From Staessen J, Fagard R, Lijnen P, et al: *J Hypertens* 7(Suppl 1):S19, 1989.)

1984). In clinical practice it is likely that the two will work together to achieve a greater fall in blood pressure than either could achieve alone (Gillum et al, 1983).

## Mechanisms

With very low calorie intake, a massive natriuresis initially causes significant weight loss (Krieger and Landsberg, 1989). Thereafter, two factors appear to be responsible for the continued fall in blood pressure, a fall in sympathetic nervous activity (Fagerberg et al, 1985) and a fall in plasma insulin (Rocchini et al, 1987).

In view of the apparent critical importance of the distribution rather than the total amount of excess fat, there is evidence that weight loss will accomplish a decrease in upper body obesity with concomitant improvements in blood glucose and lipids (den Besten et al, 1988).

Weight loss likely lowers the blood pressure, how ever it is accomplished. Very low calorie formulas are effective and safe (Amatruda et al, 1988) and may be the most practical way to manage markedly obese patients. Less stringent diets will also work, particularly when accompanied by appropriate behavioral modification and exercise (Rocchini et al, 1988). Caution is needed in the use of sympathomimetic agents to reduce the appetite since they may raise the blood pressure (Weintraub and Bray, 1989), but either serotonin blockers, e.g., fluoxetine (Harto et al, 1988), or thermogenic beta-agonists (Connacher et al, 1988) may prove to be safe and helpful.

## SODIUM RESTRICTION

The considerable circumstantial evidence that incriminates the excessive intake of sodium in most modern diets as being a necessary though not sufficient cause of primary hypertension is reviewed in Chapter 3. Almost all of us ingest amounts of sodium far in excess of any possible physiological need. Even if it does not cause hypertension, such high sodium intake may make it more difficult to treat the disease, and a reduced sodium intake may improve the effectiveness of most antihypertensive drugs with the possible exception of calcium entry blockers (Luft and Weinberger, 1988).

The viewpoint that follows is in favor of moderate sodium restriction and is shared by most authorities but not by all. Some believe moderate sodium restriction is unlikely to provide any benefit (Brown et al, 1984), and a few warn of potential hazards (Laragh and Pecker, 1983). After review of available data, more and more researchers have called for proper large-scale studies to settle the issue (Brown et al, 1984; Nicholls, 1984; Beard and Heller, 1987).

Although dietary sodium restriction had been shown to lower blood pressure by Ambard in 1906 and Allen in 1920, it was Kempner (1944) who popularized rigid sodium restriction at a time when little else was available for therapy. Kempner's rice diet was shown to be effective because it was so low in sodium (Watkin et al, 1950). However, Watkin et al concluded that "protracted effective maintenance of the Kempner regimen. . .imposes such hardship upon the patient and so much difficulty in control as to make it virtually impractical for general use."

After thiazides were introduced during the late 1950s and their mode of action was shown to involve a mild state of sodium depletion, both physicians and patients eagerly adopted this form of therapy in place of dietary sodium restriction.

In discarding rigid salt restriction, physicians disregarded the benefits of modest restriction both for its inherent antihypertensive effect and for its potential of reducing diuretic-induced hypokalemia. Moreover, many fail to realize that the amount of salt ingested by some patients, 15 to 20 g per day, may completely overcome the antihypertensive effectiveness of diuretics (Winer, 1961).

## Clinical Experience

### Antihypertensive Effect

Modest restriction of dietary sodium intake, to about one-half of the usual intake down to a level of 70 to 100 mmol/day, has been shown in most of the recently reported controlled studies to lower the blood pressure 4 to 8 mm Hg below levels seen with higher sodium intake (Staessen et al, 1989) (Fig. 6.2). These lines are taken from 16 studies published from 1973 to 1987 involving 24 groups with slightly over 400 subjects altogether. When data from only the 11 of these 16 studies that were considered to have been adequately controlled were analyzed, the average effect of a 100 mmol/day reduction in sodium intake was a 5.4/6.5-mm Hg fall in systolic and diastolic pressures.

Subsequently, in an attempt to ascertain the level of sodium restriction needed for an antihypertensive effect, MacGregor et al (1989) gave three levels of sodium—50, 100, or 200 mmol/day each for 4 weeks—to 20 mild hypertensives in a double-blind, randomized, crossover study. Compared with the level on 200 mmol/day, the average supine blood pressure fell 8/5 mm Hg on the 100-mmol/day intake and 16/9 mm Hg on the 50-mmol/day intake. The authors conclude:

The study showed an apparently linear dose response to sodium restriction in this group of patients. This graded response suggests that at least over the range of sodium intakes studied, there is no threshold value below which sodium intake needs to be reduced. Therefore, to obtain the maximum effect, sodium intake should be reduced as far as is practicable.

As seen in Figure 6.2 and confirmed in the analysis of more than 50 studies of altered sodium intake on blood pressure by Morgan and Nowson (1986), the higher the initial level of blood pressure, the greater the fall after sodium restriction. This, of course, holds true for all antihypertensive remedies. Normotensive subjects should not be expected to experience much effect from short-term interventions.

More recently, the antihypertensive efficacy of moderate (60 to 100 mmol/day) restriction in sodium intake has been additionally confirmed in studies each involving over 100 subjects (Weinberger et al, 1988; Australian National Committee, 1989). These studies not only document the efficacy of moderate sodium restriction, but they also demonstrate the ability of most people to adhere to such a regimen. An additional benefit of moderate sodium restriction by 60 mmol/day has been seen in a randomized controlled 3-month study in 34 patients with type II diabetes who experienced an average fall of 20 mm Hg in systolic pressure (Dodson et al, 1989). Elderly subjects with isolated systolic hypertension may respond particularly well, perhaps because their hypertension is more volume dependent, in keeping with their lower plasma renin levels (Niarchos et al, 1984).

Not all patients will have a fall in blood pressure with such modest reductions in sodium intake (Longworth et al, 1980; Watt et al, 1983). The response tends to be greater in those with

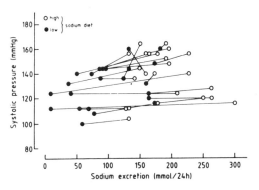
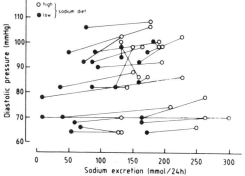

**Figure 6.2.** Systolic and diastolic blood pressure on a high and low sodium intake in 16 studies published from 1973 to 1987 involving 24 groups. (From Staessen J, Fagard R, Lijnen P, et al: *J Hypertens* 7(Suppl 1):S19, 1989.)

low plasma renin levels that do not rise much during sodium restriction (Oshima et al, 1989). Such patients may be the "nonmodulators" described in Chapter 3 (Burgess et al, 1988). Beyond the influence of the renin-aldosterone mechanism, sodium sensitivity may also be related to variable responses in sympathetic nervous activity and calcium regulation. Responsiveness may also be familial but independent of age and weight (Miller et al, 1986).

## Protection from Diuretic-Induced Potassium Loss

Unlimited access to dietary sodium and the daily intake of a diuretic make every patient vulnerable to the major side effect of diuretic therapy—hypokalemia. The diuretic inhibits sodium reabsorption at the cortical diluting segment of the nephron, proximal to that part of the distal convoluted tubule wherein exchange of potassium ion ($K^+$) for sodium ion ($Na^+$) occurs. Consider what happens when thiazides are given daily while the patient ingests large amounts of sodium (Fig. 6.3).

1. The initial diuretic-induced sodium depletion shrinks plasma volume, activating renin release and secondarily increasing aldosterone secretion.
2. The thiazide continues to inhibit sodium reabsorption proximal to the $K^+$-$Na^+$ exchange site. More $Na^+$ is delivered to this distal site.
3. The increased amounts of aldosterone act to increase sodium reabsorption at the distal exchange site, thereby increasing potassium secretion, and the potassium is swept into the urine.

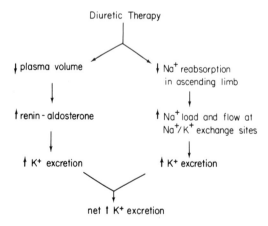

Diuretic Therapy

↓ plasma volume

↓ $Na^+$ reabsorption in ascending limb

↑ renin - aldosterone

↑ $Na^+$ load and flow at $Na^+/K^+$ exchange sites

↑ $K^+$ excretion

↑ $K^+$ excretion

net ↑ $K^+$ excretion

**Figure 6.3.** The manner by which continuous diuretic therapy will cause an increase in urinary potassium excretion.

With modest sodium restriction (50 to 100 mmol/day), less sodium would be delivered to the distal exchange site, and therefore less potassium would be swept into the urine. This modest restriction should not further activate the renin-angiotensin-aldosterone (RAA) mechanism to cause more distal tubular sodium-for-potassium exchange since that usually occurs only with more rigid sodium restriction. More rigid sodium restriction, impractical as it is, could be counterproductive: By inducing further secondary aldosteronism, more potassium would be wasted as the diuretic continues to deliver sodium to the distal exchange site (Landmann-Suter and Struyvenberg, 1978).

When this postulate was tested in 12 hypertensive patients, the results were confirmatory (Ram et al, 1981). The patients were given one of three diuretics for 4-week intervals while ingesting a diet with either 72 or 195 mmol per day of sodium. While on the modestly restricted diet, total body potassium levels fell only half as much.

## Mechanisms

Most of the detailed studies on the responses to sodium restriction have used much more rigid deprivation (usually 10 mmol/day) over short intervals. Though these may amplify what happens with more modest sodium restriction, caution is advised in interpolating the data from rigid to modest sodium restriction as noted in relation to potassium wastage.

With that caveat in mind, the effects of fairly rigid sodium restriction have been shown to include: (1) a fall in cardiac output but no change in peripheral resistance (Omvik and Lund-Johansen, 1986); (2) a reduction in left ventricular wall thickness (Schmieder et al, 1988); (3) a transient rise in plasma norepinephrine, which is related to a decrease in clearance of the hormone (Linares et al, 1988), but a subsequent fall in plasma catecholamine levels (Kjeldsen et al, 1986); (4) an increase in beta-adrenergic responsiveness in lymphocytes (Feldman et al, 1987); and (5) activation of the renin-aldosterone mechanism (Luft et al, 1986).

It is possible that the antihypertensive effect of sodium restriction may be mediated by a decrease in the circulating sodium transport inhibitor postulated to be involved in the induction of hypertension (Chapter 3). A reduced intracellular sodium concentration (Ambrosioni et al, 1982; Krzesinski and Rorive, 1985) has been measured in blood cells after dietary sodium restriction, but no change in red cell sodium efflux was noted (El Ashry et al, 1987). On the other hand, the limited effectiveness of sodium restriction is likely due to the compensatory rises in the RAA system.

Considering the probable benefits, the question remains: Why are such modestly restricted diets not more widely followed? Dahl (1972) provided the following four reasons:

1. To palates accustomed since infancy to saltiness, the absence of salt is at first distressing.
2. Most low-sodium diets are prescribed haphazardly and unenthusiastically.
3. Even when prepared by knowledgeable sources, these diets may be so complex as to discourage all but the most persistent.
4. Most patients are unaware of the naturally high sodium content of cow's milk and the added sodium in cheese and in most processed foods.

The major problem is in processed foods to which salt is added as a taste enhancer, tenderizer, color preserver, or leavener (Table 6.3). From 60 to 80% of the sodium ingested by people in the United States (Altschul and Grommet, 1982), Canada (Shah and Belonje, 1983), and England (Sanchez-Castillo et al, 1984) comes from processed foods and is, in that sense, nondiscretionary. Hopefully, more food processors will put the sodium content on the labels so that at least some can be avoided but, in 1989, only about 40% of processed foods sold in the United States were so labeled. Despite requests from various public and professional groups, the United States Food and Drug Administration has been unwilling to mandate sodium labeling, although it will require the sodium content to be added to those labels already listing other ingredients.

Therefore, the unknowing consumer will continue to be assaulted with salt. As more than 20% of all meals eaten in the United States are from "fast food" restaurants, we are exposed to an additional source of unsuspected sodium (Table 6.3).

In response to the demand from various sources, the processors of baby foods have stopped adding sodium to these products. However, mothers accustomed to a high-salt diet may continue to add extra sodium to their baby's food by habit or to satisfy their own taste (Kerr et al, 1978).

Additional problems may make even modest sodium restriction difficult to achieve:

—Sodium is present in large amounts in many antacids (Drake and Hollander, 1981): Alka-Seltzer, Bromo Seltzer, and Biosodol have 500 to 1540 mg per tablet. Lower-sodium preparations are available: One Rolaids has 53 mg, Tums, Titralac, and Maalox Plus have only 1 to 2 mg per tablet.
—The high sodium content of some injectable antibiotics may be a problem for hospitalized patients, adding as much as 140 mmol/day to their intake (Baron et al, 1984).
—Hypertensives may have an increased preference for salt (Schechter et al, 1974).
—The elderly may lose some of their perception of the saltiness of food and therefore add even more to satisfy their taste (Schiffman, 1977).
—Some beverages (e.g., Vichy water, V8 vegetable juice) are high in sodium content. Most tap and bottled waters are quite low, but the sodium content of some tap water, particularly if obtained from wells, may be quite high.

Help is increasingly available to enable more

**Table 6.3. Sodium Content of Some American Foods (1000 mg Sodium–44 MEq Sodium)**

*Comparable foods with either low or high sodium content*

| Low | | High | |
|---|---|---|---|
| Shredded wheat: | 1 mg/cup | Corn flakes: | 305 mg/oz |
| Green beans, fresh: | 5 mg/cup | Green beans, canned: | 686 mg/cup |
| Orange juice: | 2 mg/cup | Tomato juice: | 640 mg/cup |
| Turkey, roasted: | 70 mg/3 oz | Turkey dinner: | 1735 mg |
| Ground beef: | 57 mg/3 oz | Frankfurter, beef: | 425 mg each |
| Pork, uncooked: | 65 mg/3 oz | Bacon, uncooked: | 1400 mg/3 oz |

| *Fast foods* | | *Frozen Foods* | |
|---|---|---|---|
| Kentucky Fried Chicken (dinner with | | Swanson's Macaroni & Cheese: | 1815 mg |
| potatoes and coleslaw): | 2285 mg | Morton's Chicken Pot Pie: | 1246 mg |
| McDonald's Big Mac: | 1010 mg | Weight Watcher's Pizza: | 750 mg |
| Jack in the Box Cheeseburger: | 875 mg | Stouffer's Lean Cuisine | |
| Arby's Roast Beef Sandwich: | 880 mg | Spaghetti with Beef: | 1140 mg |
| Pizza Hut Pan Pizza, 1 slice: | 820 mg | Armour Lite Beef with Broccoli: | 2120 mg |
| Burger King Whopper: | 975 mg | | |

patients to achieve a moderate degree of sodium restriction. Some of the helpful techniques include:

—the availability of a larger number of processed foods with lower sodium content;
—the recognition that the taste preference for sodium diminishes after a few months on a lower sodium intake (Beauchamp et al, 1983), so that table salt usage does not increase when less sodium is in the diet (Beauchamp et al, 1987);
—the demonstration that adherence to a lower sodium diet can be improved by the positive feedback provided by immediate monitoring techniques for urinary sodium content, either in the office (Kaplan et al, 1982) or at home (Luft et al, 1984);
—the use of sodium substitutes with less (e.g., Morton Lite-Salt) or no sodium (e.g., Co-Salt) that are available on the market. Caution is advised in using these preparations that substitute potassium for sodium in patients with renal damage, particularly if they are also taking potassium-sparing diuretics; they may develop hyperkalemia from the additional load of potassium. One-half teaspoonful of Co-Salt provides 35 mmol of potassium.

In various trials involving relatively small groups of either normotensive (Jeffery et al, 1984) or hypertensive (Weinberger et al, 1988; Australian National Committee, 1989) people, the majority have followed diets moderately restricted in sodium. Less success has been reported in less well controlled studies of dietary counseling (Evers et al, 1987) or community wide mass media campaigns (Pietinen et al, 1987; Staessen et al, 1988). On the other hand, Rose (1989) has described a successful community intervention trial among people in rural Portugal who were previously on a very high salt intake. Ellison et al (1989) have shown that a 15 to 20% reduction in sodium intake can easily be achieved by changes in food purchasing and preparation with a resultant significant fall in overall blood pressure levels.

Beyond the bother of having to give up highly salted food, there is virtually no danger of moderate sodium restriction. The possibility of reducing other necessary dietary nutrients, e.g., calcium, does not appear to happen (Nowson and Morgan, 1988). A short-term very rigid low-sodium diet will raise plasma uric acid and lipid levels, the former by renal retention, the latter likely by hemoconcentration (Masugi et al, 1988).

As discussed further in Chapter 9, a few hypertensives with renal disease, particularly those with analgesic nephropathy, will waste considerable amounts of sodium. In such patients, too rigid sodium restriction may worsen renal function and, by activating renin release, could aggravate hypertension. However, for the overwhelming majority of hypertensives, moderate sodium restriction is worthwhile and feasible. The reduction of the overall level of blood pressure by as little as 4 mm Hg, which likely could be achieved by moderate sodium restriction, has been calculated to provide a 10.8% reduction in the overall population risk for coronary heart disease (Blackburn, 1984). The real potential for benefit, with the very remote possibility of harm, makes moderate sodium restriction a desirable goal both for the individual hypertensive patient and for the population at large.

## POTASSIUM SUPPLEMENTS

Many of the benefits of reduced sodium intake could reflect an increased potassium intake. To achieve even modest sodium restriction, high sodium-low potassium processed foods are usually replaced with low sodium-high potassium natural foods. The high ratio of sodium to potassium in the modern diet has been held responsible for the development of hypertension, and the reversal of this ratio back to that consumed by our ancestors has been offered as a way to prevent and relieve hypertension (Meneely and Battarbee, 1976). In various populations, higher blood pressure is correlated more closely to low potassium intake than to high sodium intake (Dai et al, 1984; Reed et al, 1985). The lower blood pressure of vegetarians has been ascribed to their large potassium intake (Ophir et al, 1983). Hypertensives have been found to have lower plasma and total body potassium levels and there are multiple hemodynamic effects of potassium that could explain a hypotensive effect (Ullian and Linas, 1987).

### Clinical Experience

An expanding number of carefully performed studies have documented a hypotensive effect of potassium supplements given to mild hypertensives on regular sodium intake. In the early 1980s, open, non-placebo-controlled short-term studies reported an even more impressive fall in blood pressure, averaging about 10 mm Hg for both systolic and diastolic (Iimura et al, 1981; Morgan, 1982; Smith et al, 1983; Overlack et al, 1983). More recently, randomized, placebo-controlled, and often double-blinded studies have shown a more modest but consistent effect, comparable to that reported with moderate sodium restriction (Table 6.4).

The combination of potassium supplements and sodium restriction has been examined and generally found to offer little additional effect to that provided by sodium restriction alone (Smith et al, 1985; Valori et al, 1987; Grobbee et al, 1987). However, the use of a potassium-containing salt substitute has been shown to enhance the antihypertensive effect of a beta-blocker (Suppa et al, 1988; Salvetti et al, 1988).

Beyond the effect on blood pressure, a very dramatic protective effect of increased dietary potassium intake on the mortality from stroke has been reported in a 12-year prospective study of 859 older people (Khaw and Barrett-Conner, 1987). They found a 40% reduction in the risk of stroke with a 10 mmol/day increase in potassium intake, an effect that was independent of other known cardiovascular risk factors. Similar protection against thromboembolic stroke mortality has been noted among Japanese men in Honolulu (Lee et al, 1987). These striking effects receive experimental support from the protection shown by increased dietary potassium against endothelial damage (Sugimoto et al, 1988) and atherosclerotic cholesterol ester deposition in the aortas of stroke-prone spontaneously hypertensive rats (Tobian et al, 1989).

## Mechanisms

The major obvious effect of the short-term addition of potassium is a natriuresis (Fujita and Sato, 1983; Smith et al, 1983). Other effects include a dampening of vasoconstriction induced either by ouabain-like inhibitors of the $Na^+$, $K^+$-ATPase pump (Glanzer et al, 1983) or by norepinephrine (Bianchetti et al, 1984). Beyond these, potassium exerts numerous ef-

fects on cardiovascular and endocrine mechanisms, some raising, others lowering the blood pressure (Ullian and Linas, 1987). Dietary potassium restriction for 9 days caused a 4.1-mm Hg rise in mean blood pressure in normotensive men (Krishna et al, 1989). The infusion of saline further increased their blood pressure but had no effect in potassium replete subjects.

## Practical Aspects

Even though potassium supplements may lower the blood pressure, they are too costly and potentially hazardous for routine use in the treatment of hypertension. They may be indicated to prevent or treat diuretic-induced hypokalemia (Kohvakka, 1988), and a microencapsulated formulation seems less irritating to the gastrointestinal tract than a wax matrix one (McLoughlin, 1985). For the larger population, a reduction of high sodium-low potassium processed foods with an increase of low sodium-high potassium natural foods is all that is needed to achieve the potential benefits. Fruits and beans provide the largest quantity of potassium per serving. The use of potassium-containing salt substitutes, e.g., Co-Salt, will be of further help and will add little expense.

## CALCIUM SUPPLEMENTS

Calcium intake may be lower among hypertensive patients than normotensive people (McCarron, 1982), and calcium supplements may lower the blood pressure of normotensive young adults (Belizan et al, 1983), normal pregnant women (Repke et al, 1989), and perhaps one-third of hypertensive patients (McCarron and Morris, 1985) (Fig. 6.4).

## Mechanisms

The report by McCarron and Morris has provoked a steady stream of studies on the antihypertensive efficacy of calcium supplements.

**Table 6.4. Randomized, Placebo-Controlled Trials of Supplemental Potassium in Hypertensive Patients**

| Reference | No. of Patients | KCl Supplement | | Urinary Potassium Excretion | | Blood Pressure (mm Hg) | | |
|---|---|---|---|---|---|---|---|---|
| | | mmol/day | weeks | Placebo | +KCl | Control | Δ Placebo | Δ +KCl |
| MacGregor et al, 1982 | 23 | 60 | 4 | 62 | 118 | 154/99 | +1/0 | −6/4 |
| Richards et al, 1984 | 12 | 200 | 4 | @60 | @200 | 150/92 | | −2/1 |
| Kaplan et al, 1985[a] | 16 | 60 | 6 | 36 | 82 | 131/96 | +2/1 | −4/4 |
| Matlou et al, 1986 | 32 | 65 | 6 | 52 | 114 | 154/105 | −3/2 | −10/5 |
| Siani et al, 1987 | 37 | 48 | 15 | 57 | 87 | 145/92 | +1/1 | −14/10 |
| Svetkey et al, 1987 | 101 | 120 | 8 | — | — | 147/95 | −0/2 | −6/4 |

[a]Patients were hypokalemic and on diuretic therapy.

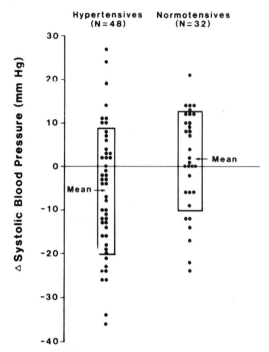

**Figure 6.4.** Distribution of the change in standing systolic blood pressure after 8 weeks of calcium supplementation. (Reproduced, with permission, from: McCarron DA and Morris CD: *Ann Intern Med* 103(6 Part 1):825, 1985.)

Volume
expansion ---> ↑$U_{Ca}$ ---> ↓plasma $_{Ca}$ ---> ↑PTH ---> ↑BP

↑Ca
intake ---> $\begin{bmatrix} \text{further} \\ \text{↑}U_{Ca} \end{bmatrix}$ ---> ↑plasma $_{Ca}$ ---> ↓PTH ---> ↓BP

**Figure 6.5.** A potential explanation for a hypotensive action of increased dietary calcium intake. The postulated mechanism by which volume expansion leads to hypercalciuria, low plasma $Ca^{2+}$ and high PTH is shown to be ameliorated by increased $Ca^{2+}$ intake. (From Kaplan NM: *Semin Nephrol* 8:176, 1988.)

As summarized by McCarron (1989), about half of them show a significant effect, the other half do not. Although McCarron attributes the lack of effect to various methodological faults, my interpretation is that the effect is seen in only a portion of the entire hypertensive population (Kaplan, 1988). That portion appears to be those who have a mild degree of secondary hyperparathyroidism that arises to compensate for increased urinary calcium excretion that, in turn, reduces plasma ionized calcium levels. The entire sequence may very well begin with high sodium intake which causes volume expansion in sodium-sensitive, low-renin patients and leads to increased urinary calcium excretion (Fig. 6.5).

Support for this concept comes from the finding of lower ionized calcium and elevated serum parathyroid hormone (PTH) levels in some hypertensive patients (Hvarfner et al, 1988). Moreover, those who respond to supplemental calcium tend to be those with low calcium and high PTH levels (Grobbee and Hofman, 1986; Lyle et al, 1988; Resnick, 1989).

Beyond what is shown in Figure 6.5, there is no logical explanation for a hypotensive effect of additional calcium intake since a rise in extracellular calcium should, if anything, tend to raise intracellular calcium levels and raise the blood pressure further (Kaplan and Meese, 1986).

In addition to dampening mild secondary PTH excess, supplemental calcium may lower blood pressure by a natriuretic action, an action supported by some (Lasaridis et al, 1989) but not by others (Luft et al, 1989).

## Practical Aspects

As shown in Figure 6.4 and in virtually every study published since, calcium supplements may raise the blood pressure in some patients and lower the pressure in others. Moreover, as shown in Figure 6.5, calcium supplements may raise further the hypercalcuria responsible for the development of "calcium sensitivity" and thereby lead to kidney stones.

Until there is a simple way to determine calcium sensitivity, the best course seems to be to ensure a reasonable dietary calcium intake but not to give calcium supplements to either prevent or treat hypertension. There may be other reasons to ensure adequate dietary intake since it may protect against colon cancer (Slattery et al, 1988). A possible lipid-lowering effect of calcium supplementation has not been corroborated (Karanja et al, 1987). After thorough review of the evidence, the use of calcium supplements to prevent or treat osteoporosis was found to be "not justified" by present evidence (Kanis and Passmore, 1989).

## MAGNESIUM SUPPLEMENTS

The same advice seems to be appropriate in regard to magnesium. The theoretical connection between magnesium deficiency and hypertension is more direct and logical than that for calcium (Ryan and Brady, 1984), but serum and intracellular magnesium levels are normal in most untreated hypertensives (Kjeldsen et al, 1989).

The antihypertensive effect of supplemental magnesium has been less well studied than potassium or calcium. In an open study the administration of 15 mmol/day of magnesium as aspartate hydrochloride for 6 months resulted in an average fall in blood pressure of 12/8 mm Hg in 20 patients, whereas the 19 controls had an average fall of 0/4 mm Hg (Dyckner and Wester, 1983). However, in a double-blind randomized crossover study, the same amount of magnesium for 1 month caused no fall in blood pressure compared with placebo or pretreatment values in 17 hypertensive patients (Cappuccio et al, 1985).

Similarly, the effect of magnesium supplements in patients on long-term diuretic therapy is uncertain: In an open trial, 600 mg of magnesium per day for 4 weeks lowered the blood pressure by 7.5/3.0 mm Hg (Saito et al, 1988) whereas no significant effect was noted in two randomized, placebo-controlled, double-blind studies, one with 300 mg of magnesium per day for 6 months (Henderson et al, 1986), the other with 600 mg/day for 3 months (Murphy et al, 1989).

## MACRONUTRIENTS

The blood pressure may fall in response to the type of macronutrients in the diet. As noted previously, vegetarians tend to have low blood pressure, which may be attributable to the high potassium content of their diet (Ophir et al, 1983). When hypertensives consume a vegetarian diet under controlled conditions for 6 weeks, an average 5-mm Hg fall in systolic blood pressure has been observed (Margetts et al, 1988). The effect is not attributable to any specific component of the diet (Sacks and Kass, 1988).

### Fiber

One feature of a vegetarian diet is the increased amount of fiber. Plant fiber has been given, either alone (Anderson, 1983; Schlamowitz et al, 1987) or with a low-fat, low-sodium diet (Pacy et al, 1984), and has been found to lower the blood pressure by 5 to 10 mm Hg. A persistent antihypertensive effect of a similar high-fiber, low-fat, low-sodium diet over a 4-year interval has been observed in the 19 of 32 patients with primary hypertension who continued the regimen (Dodson et al, 1985).

### Fat and Fish Oil

#### Dietary Fats

The rather confusing literature on dietary fats and blood pressure has been carefully reviewed by FM Sacks (1989). He concludes that:

Comparisons of blood pressure patterns among populations suggest that low-fat diets or consumption of unsaturated fatty acids decrease blood pressure. However, in most single populations dietary fatty acids and total fat, as determined by diet history, are not significantly correlated with blood pressure. Dietary fatty acids, quantitated by levels in adipose tissue or plasma lipoproteins, had no consistent association with blood pressure. Dietary fatty acids and total fat were not predictive of the development of hypertension over four years in a large cohort of nurses in the United States (Wittemann et al, 1989). Although several dietary trials lacking randomized controls suggested effects of dietary fats on blood pressure, 11 of 12 controlled trials showed no significant effects. All seven double-blind trials, and the two trials of longest duration (one and five years), showed no effect of either varying the content of total fat or of exchanging polyunsaturated for saturated fatty acids. In summary, there is little convincing evidence that the amount or type of dietary fat, varied within customary dietary patterns, affects blood pressure levels in persons with normal or mildly elevated blood pressure.

#### Increases in Fish Oil

The omega-3 polyunsaturated fatty acids found in highest concentration in cold water fish, eicosapentaenoic and docosahexaenoic acids, are being widely touted for their ability to decrease platelet aggregation, reduce vascular occlusive disease, inhibit inflammation, and lower blood pressure, presumably by their influence on the production of endogenous eicosanoids, mainly prostaglandins. Radack and Deck (1989) found only six randomized controlled studies in the 22 reports published from 1970 to 1988 on the effects of omega-3 fatty acids on blood pressure. Of these, only one (Norris et al, 1986) examined hypertensives and it reported the greatest reduction of blood pressure (-8/-1 compared with the control group) in those who ingested 16.5 g/day of encapsulated fish oil for 6 weeks.

In a more recent study not included in Radack and Deck's review, Knapp and FitzGerald (1989) examined the effects of small (3 g) and large (15 g) amounts of n-3 fatty acids from fish oil versus that of n-6 fatty acids from safflower oil and a mixture of oils that approximated the fats present in the American diet each in eight men with mild hypertension. They noted a fall of blood pressure of 6.5/4.4 mm Hg in those given the high dose of fish oil but not in the other groups.

### Protein

Little is known about the effects of protein on the blood pressure of people other than a lack of difference between meat and nonmeat protein (Prescott et al, 1988). Protein intake was inversely related to blood pressure levels among 8000 Japanese men in Hawaii (Reed et al, 1985).

## Carbohydrate

High carbohydrate intake for brief periods causes sodium retention but no increase in blood pressure (Affarah et al, 1986). However, plasma insulin levels, already high in hypertensives, are driven even higher by such diets and may interfere with the antihypertensive effect of weight reduction if it involves the use of high carbohydrate-low fat diets (Parillo et al, 1988).

## Other Dietary Changes

Claims of a blood pressure lowering effect have been made for crude onion extract in hypertensive people (Louria et al, 1985) and for garlic in hypertensive rats (Foushee et al, 1982). A Chinese herbal preparation consisting of a mixture of 12 herbs had no antihypertensive effect (Black et al, 1986).

## CAFFEINE

Although the blood pressure often rises by 5 to 15 mm Hg within 15 minutes after consumption of 250 mg of caffeine (the amount in two to three cups of brewed coffee) and may stay up for 2 hours, chronic caffeine ingestion (as much as 500 mg/day for 4 weeks) was not accompanied by significant rises in blood pressure (Robertson et al, 1984). This tolerance to the hemodynamic effects of caffeine may explain why most epidemiological surveys do not display a relation between coffee consumption and prevalence of hypertension (van Dusseldorp et al, 1989).

## SMOKING

Smoking, in a manner similar to caffeine, acutely raises blood pressure, but tolerance to the nicotine-induced hemodynamic effects develops so that chronic smoking is not associated with higher levels of blood pressure or a higher frequency of hypertension (Ballantyne et al, 1978). In fact, when smokers quit, the blood pressure may rise a bit, probably because they usually gain weight (Friedman and Siegelaub, 1980). Nonetheless, the marked increased risk of stroke from cigarette smoking (Shinton and Beevers, 1989) is another reason to insist that hypertensives quit.

## ALCOHOL

As detailed in Chapter 3, the consumption of more than 1 to 2 ounces of ethanol per day is associated with a higher prevalence of hypertension and has been shown to produce an acute pressor action in controlled studies (Potter et al, 1986). On the other hand, most large-scale surveys find no higher blood pressures among those who consume less than three drinks per day (MacMahon, 1987; Shaper et al, 1988). Since consumption of that amount has clearly been associated with a lower mortality and morbidity rate from coronary disease than either abstinence or higher amounts (Burr, 1988), the following guidelines seem appropriate:

—Carefully assess alcohol intake.
—If intake is more than three drinks, equivalent to about 1.5 ounces of ethanol per day, advise a reduction at least to that level.
—If a significant pressor effect seems likely from even that amount, advise abstinence.
—For most of those who consume less than three drinks per day, no change seems necessary.

A reduction in weekly alcohol intake from 537 ml to 57 ml was associated with a 6.9/4.0-mm Hg fall in pressure (Pudley et al, 1989). Physicians should always advise those who drink too much to reduce consumption since a significant number will follow that advice (Wallace et al, 1988).

## EXERCISE

During isotonic (aerobic) exercise—jogging, walking, swimming—the systolic and, to a lesser degree, the diastolic blood pressure rises in a linear manner along with cardiac output and heart rate until the anaerobic threshold is reached when the rise in systolic pressure tends to accelerate in a nonlinear manner (Spence et al, 1987). A rise of systolic pressure to 200 mm Hg or higher may be predictive of the subsequent development of hypertension (Davidoff et al, 1982). The rise in mean arterial pressure is greater in hypertensives but, after a period of training, the rise in arterial pressure and heart rate is less marked (Sannerstedt et al, 1973).

After regularly repeated aerobic exercise, the resting blood pressure is usually lowered. In a study of 13 untreated middle-aged hypertensives, after 6 weeks of three or seven per week 45-minute bicycling exercises at 60 to 70% of maximal capacity, the resting supine pressures 48 hours after exercise fell by 11/9 mm Hg with three times per week exercise and by 16/11 mm Hg with seven times per week exercise (Nelson et al, 1986) (Fig. 6.6). Similar effects have been observed in most other controlled studies using either parallel groups of nonexercising subjects (Bonanno and Lies, 1974; Kukkonen et al, 1982; Duncan et al, 1985; Urata et al, 1987) or a cross-over design (Roman et al, 1981; Hagberg et al, 1983).

## Mechanisms

There are inadequate data to know whether the effect of exercise on blood pressure is related to or dependent upon an increase in maximal oxygen uptake or any other cardiovascular adaptation. After strenuous dynamic exercise, vasodilation persists, and the systolic blood pressure remains about 25% below the preexercise level for at least 90 minutes (Bennett et al, 1984). Those who perform enough isotonic exercise repetitively to reach the "trained" or "conditioned" state usually have a slower heart rate at rest. These short- and long-term effects may reflect a reduction in sympathetic nervous activity (Duncan et al, 1985; Jennings et al, 1986). Other changes after repetitive dynamic exercise that could have lasting effects upon the blood pressure include increased levels of vasodilatory prostaglandins (Rauramaa et al, 1984), decreased levels of plasma renin activity (Kiyonaga et al, 1985), decreased plasma volume (Urata et al, 1987), reduced plasma viscosity (Letcher

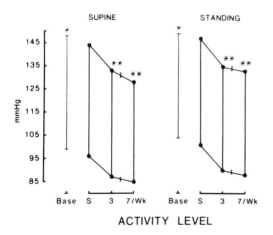

**Figure 6.6.** Resting, supine, and standing blood-pressure at three levels of physical activity that were sequenced in a random fashion by a Latin square design. Baseline measurement (*Base*), sedentary activity (*S*), 3 times/week exercise (3), and 7 times/week exercise (7). *p <0.05, difference from sedentary value for both systolic and diastolic blood-pressure; **p <0.01. (From Nelson L, Jennings GL, Esler MD, et al: *Lancet* 2:473, 1986.)

et al, 1981), and changes in the baroreceptor reflex mechanisms (Pagani et al, 1988).

## Potential for Prevention

Among a large group of Harvard alumni, Paffenbarger et al (1983) found that those who did not engage in vigorous physical activity were at 35% greater risk of developing hypertension, whether they had higher blood pressures while at Harvard, a family history of hypertension, or obesity, all of which increased further the risk of hypertension. Similarly, in a 1- to 12-year follow-up of 6039 men and women, those who had low levels of physical fitness at the initial examination had a 1.52 greater relative risk for the development of hypertension than did those with higher levels of physical fitness after appropriate adjustment for age, sex, baseline blood pressure, and body mass index (Blair et al, 1984). Even among schoolchildren, lower levels of blood pressure are found among those who maintain high levels of leisure time physical activity (Strazzullo et al, 1988). After aerobic exercise training, dampening of cardiovascular reactivity was greatest among Type A men with borderline hypertension (Sherwood et al, 1989), so the potential for benefit may be greatest in those most in need.

These studies, as hopeful as they are, obviously do not prove that regular performance of exercise or the attainment of high levels of physical fitness will prevent the development of hypertension. Those who exercise and become physically fit may also follow a healthier life style that includes less dietary sodium, fat, and alcohol as well as more relaxation and less reaction to stress, all of which may protect against the development of hypertension.

Regardless, among multiple populations, maintenance of physical fitness clearly has been associated with a lower rate of cardiovascular disease (Kannel et al, 1985) (Fig. 6.7). This protection has been demonstrated in groups as diverse as Harvard graduates (Paffenbarger et al, 1986), United States railroad workers (Slattery and Jacobs, 1988), middle-aged Finnish men (Pekkanen et al, 1987), and Belgian factory workers (Sobolski et al, 1987). Beyond the blood pressure-lowering effect, regular aerobic exercise may also increase the amount of weight lost with any given level of caloric restriction (Katch et al, 1988), favorably alter plasma lipids (Hespel et al, 1988), and improve insulin sensitivity (Rodnick et al, 1987), thereby lowering plasma insulin levels (Bjorntorp et al, 1973) that may,

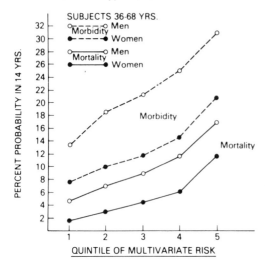

**Figure 6.7.** The risk of cardiovascular morbidity and mortality by quintile of multivariate risk of physical fitness indicators in the Framingham cohort in subjects aged 36 to 68. The indicators were physical activity index, relative weight, vital capacity, and heart rate. (From Kannel WB, Wilson P, Blair SN, et al: *Am Heart J* 109:876, 1985.)

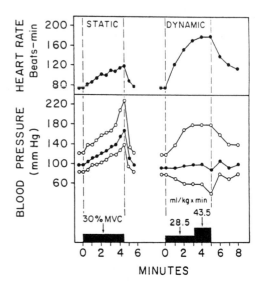

**Figure 6.8.** Changes in blood pressure (systolic, mean, and diastolic) and heart rate during static (isometric) exercise to 30% of maximal (*left*) and dynamic (isotonic) exercise to levels of 28.5 and 43.5 ml/kg X min oxygen consumption (*right*) in normotensive subjects. (From Riendl et al: *Proc Soc Exp Biol Med* 154:171, 1977.)

in turn, contribute to the blood pressure reduction.

There seems no reason, then, to curtail reasonable aerobic exercise in patients with mild or moderate hypertension. On the other hand, isometric exercise may need to be curtailed, at least until the pressure is under control. During isometric or static exercise—pushing, pulling, lifting—both the diastolic and systolic pressures and heart rate increase, in response to reflexes that abruptly withdraw vagal tone and increase peripheral resistance (Riendl et al, 1977) (Fig. 6.8). In untreated hypertensives, the blood pressure may rise to very high levels (Ewing et al, 1973). However, the pressor response is attenuated in resistance-trained athletes (Fleck, 1988) and they do not have higher resting blood pressure levels (Colliander and Tesch, 1988).

Sexual intercourse may also cause significant rises in pulse and blood pressure (Nemec et al, 1976) (Table 6.5). The responses in these 10 normal young men were the same whether the man was on the top or bottom, despite the presumably greater amount of isometric contractions with the man-on-top position.

### Effects of Antihypertensive Therapy

As more patients with hypertension exercise, they may experience problems with various antihypertensive drugs: Diuretic-induced hypokalemia may reduce muscle blood flow (Knochel,

1982); beta-blockers blunt exercise-mediated increases in heart rate and cardiac output and may reduce performance (Wilcox et al, 1984). Nonetheless, the hemodynamic responses to both static and dynamic exercise can break through beta-blockade, and a training effect can be achieved (Madden et al, 1988). The rise in blood pressure during exercise may be better blunted by use of alpha-blockers (Hamada et al, 1987) or calcium entry blockers (Garavaglia et al, 1988) than beta-blockers.

### RELAXATION

Relaxation of skeletal muscles has been known for a long time to lower the blood pressure (Jacobson, 1939). More recently, a variety of relaxation therapies—including transcendental meditation (TM), yoga, biofeedback, and psychotherapy—have been shown to reduce the blood pressure of hypertensive patients at least transiently. Though each has its advocates, none has been conclusively shown to be either practical for the majority of hypertensives or effective in maintaining a significant long-term effect.

#### Biofeedback

A review of biofeedback in the treatment of hypertension, after examining the results of almost 60 published series, concluded:

Biofeedback cannot be recommended as a first-line treatment for essential hypertension. . . . For pa-

**Table 6.5. Blood Pressure and Pulse Responses During Sexual Intercourse in Ten Normal Men[a]**

|  | Rest | Intromission | Orgasm | 2 Minutes Later |
|---|---|---|---|---|
| Blood pressure |  |  |  |  |
| Man on top | 112/66 | 148/79 | 163/81 | 118/69 |
| Man on bottom | 113/70 | 143/74 | 161/77 | 121/71 |
| Heart rate |  |  |  |  |
| Man on top | 67 | 136 | 189 | 82 |
| Man on bottom | 65 | 125 | 183 | 77 |

[a]From Nemec ED, Mansfield L, Kennedy JW: *Am Heart J* 92:274, 1976.

tients with mild hypertension or adverse reactions to medications, biofeedback may be useful adjunctively to reduce medication requirements. . . . Current studies indicate that biofeedback is no more effective than various other relaxation therapies, such as yoga, meditation, and autogenic relaxation. (Reprinted with permission from Health and Public Policy Committee, American College of Physicians: *Ann Intern Med* 102:709, 1985.)

The report documents the average fall in blood pressure reported in patients with either mild or moderate hypertension, 8 and 6 mm Hg, respectively, but emphasizes the large variability and the need for additional controlled trials.

One of the better trials is that of Patel et al (1985), who identified over 200 hypertensives in a screening program at an English industrial firm and randomly assigned half to a biofeedback-aided relaxation program for 8 weeks while the other half served as controls. At the end of the active relaxation program, 6 months, and 4 years later (during which time the subjects had been asked to continue to practice relaxation and stress management but had not been seen), the blood pressures of the treated group were significantly lower. These patients who underwent relaxation and stress management training also had experienced fewer cardiovascular complications while maintaining a higher quality of life (Patel and Marmot, 1987). These investigators have also reported successful use of these techniques by general practitioners (Patel and Marmot, 1988).

**Relaxation Response**

The "relaxation response" described by Herbert Benson has been shown to reduce sympathetic nervous system responsivity: Subjects practicing relaxation who underwent orthostatic and isometric stress had higher levels of plasma norepinephrine but no higher heart rate or blood pressure than did control subjects (Hoffman et al, 1982). The technique is simple and easily used at home (Benson and Caudill, 1984) and likely provides as much effect as does biofeed-

back (Goldstein et al, 1984). Relaxation with or without biofeedback was found to reduce the level of blood pressure and the need for hospitalization in a group of women with hypertension during pregnancy (Little et al, 1984).

**Progressive Muscle Relaxation**

In a carefully controlled study, 22 weeks of progressive muscle relaxation was shown to have little antihypertensive effect other than in some of the "young, anxious patients with mild hypertension who have a high resting sympathetic tone" (Cottier et al, 1984).

**Other Techniques**

Transcendental meditation (Wallace et al, 1983) and group psychotherapy (Peled-Ney et al, 1984) have also been found to lower blood pressure. Stress management using patient-generated training has been successfully used among hypertensive employees at worksite (Charlesworth et al, 1984).

The results of all of these trials must be recognized to reflect, at least in part, the expectations of the subjects. Agras et al (1982) told one group preparing to undergo relaxation training to expect a delayed blood pressure lowering, the other to expect immediate lowering. The systolic blood pressure decrease during the training period was 17.0 mm Hg for the immediate group but only 2.4 mm Hg for the delayed group.

Whereas some report modest antihypertensive effects of relaxation therapy (Chesney et al, 1987; Lee et al, 1988; Glasgow et al, 1989), others do not find it to be helpful (Jacob et al, 1986; Haynes et al, 1989).

My conclusion about all of this is that if it is available and acceptable to the patient, one or another form of relaxation therapy should be tried. There seems little to lose and perhaps a great deal to gain, although patients should be forewarned that short-term effects may not be maintained, so continued surveillance is needed.

## Hospital and Bed Rest

When patients are hospitalized, their blood pressure almost always comes down, mainly because the sympathetic nervous system becomes less active (Hossman et al, 1981). Long term hospital care is hardly indicated to treat hypertension, but such effects certainly may confound the analysis of whatever is being studied when patients are admitted. Patients difficult to control as outpatients may be easily managed in the hospital for a variety of reasons, including better adherence to diet and drug therapy.

## Miscellaneous

The blood pressure falls about 20% during sleep (Littler et al, 1975). Some believe they can reduce the blood pressure chronically by overcoming fatigue with increased sleep, less arousal, and the use of diazepam (Valium) (Nixon and Dighton, 1976). However, there are no well-controlled therapeutic trials verifying the antihypertensive action of diazepam or any other sedative or tranquilizer. Monoamine oxidase (MAO) inhibitors, an entirely different class of drugs used as antidepressants, will lower the blood pressure, but their use is limited by the potential for bad pressor reactions with tyramine-containing foods.

Even acupuncture has its advocates (Tam and Yiu, 1975), but no controlled studies have been done. Paranormal healing by laying on of hands was not found to have an effect beyond that of simply repeated measurement of the blood pressure (Beutler et al, 1988).

## Surgical Procedures

From about 1935 through the 1950s, surgical sympathectomy, along with the rigid low-salt diet, was about all that was available for treating hypertension. It was shown to be beneficial for those with severe disease (Thorpe et al, 1950). With current medical therapy, there seems no place for sympathectomy. Similarly, implantation of an electric stimulator on the carotid sinus nerve has been shown to lower the blood pressure (Brest et al, 1972), but modern medical therapy has made the procedure unnecessary.

A totally uncontrolled study has reported remarkable success by decompression of one or another intracranial artery supposedly compressing the left lateral medulla oblongata (Jannetta et al, 1985).

## CONCLUSIONS: THE POTENTIAL FOR PREVENTION

These various nondrug therapies will reduce the blood pressure of most hypertensives, in some to a level that is safe enough to obviate drug therapy. As discussed earlier, the use of one or more of these nondrug therapies should be tried in all patients. Those with mild hypertension may thereby be able to stay off drugs; those with more severe hypertension may need less medication.

Caution is obviously needed in accepting the short- and long-term efficacy of the various nondrug therapies. Part of their antihypertensive effect may be attributable to the "natural" fall in blood pressure seen when repeated readings are taken. Such falls may reflect a statistical regression toward the mean, a placebo effect, or a relief of anxiety and stress with time. The same phenomenon is likely responsible for much of the initial response to drug therapy as well, so both drugs and nondrugs may be given credit not deserved by either.

An even greater possible value for nondrug therapies is their potential for lowering the blood pressure even a small amount in the broader community and thereby delaying if not preventing the development of hypertension as shown in the controlled trial reported by Stamler et al (1989). Beilin (1988) has concluded that:

. . .in subjects aged 20–45 years, appropriate changes in diet, alcohol consumption and physical activity could produce a fall in population mean systolic blood pressure of between 10 and 20 mm Hg, with an 80–90% reduction in the prevalence of so-called essential hypertension (>140 mm Hg systolic or 90 mm Hg diastolic blood pressure). Such changes could be expected if average levels of body fat and alcohol consumption fell to within the current lower quartiles, were accompanied by increased levels of physical activity and fitness and were combined with a change to some of the dietary habits thought to prevent blood pressure elevation. Presumably the knowledge of how to cope better with day-to-day "stress" would add to these effects by minimizing acute rises in pressure.

Beilin is likely overenthusiastic over the potential preventive benefit of multiple nondrug therapies. Nonetheless as Watt (1989) has stated:

A mass strategy for the prevention of high blood pressure and its complications is likely to be more effective than high-risk strategies for several reasons: there is no practicable way of identifying in advance a large proportion of future hypertensives; a minority of hypertensive complications occur in individuals with pressures high enough to warrant [drug] treatment; and treatment has little or no effect on the incidence of the major hypertensive complication, coronary heart attacks. The effect of a broad-based dietary prevention programme is not proven, but such a strategy offers a reasonable prospect of a broad range of benefits, and is likely to prove acceptable to the general public.

Nondrug therapies then should be enthusiastically promoted for everyone. However, they will not be enough for most with significant hypertension who will likely need one or more of the drugs described in the next chapter.

## References

Affarah HB, Hall WD, Heymsfield SB, et al: *Am J Clin Nutr* 44:341, 1986.

Agras WS, Horne M, Taylor DB: *Psychosom Med* 44:398, 1982.

Allen FM: *JAMA* 74:652, 1920.

Altschul AM, Grommet JK: *Hypertension* 4(Suppl III):III-116, 1982.

Amatruda JM, Richeson JF, Welle SL, et al: *Arch Intern Med* 148:873, 1988.

Ambard L: *Semaine Med* 26:361, 1906.

Ambrosioni E, Costa FV, Borghi C, et al: *Hypertension* 4:789, 1982.

Anderson JW: *Ann Intern Med* 98:842, 1983.

Andrews G, MacMahon SW, Austin A, et al: *Br Med J* 284:1523, 1982.

Australian National Health and Medical Research Council Dietary Salt Study Management Committee: *Lancet* 1:399, 1989.

Ayman D: *JAMA* 95:246, 1930.

Ballantyne D, Devine BL, Fife R: *Br Med J* 1:880, 1978.

Baron DN, Hamilton-Miller JMT, Brumfitt W: *Lancet* 1:1113, 1984.

Barrett-Connor E, Khaw KT: *Circulation* 72:53, 1985.

Beard TC, Heller RF: *Med J Aust* 147:29, 1987.

Beauchamp GK, Bertino M, Engelman K: *Ann Intern Med* 98:763, 1983.

Beauchamp GK, Bertino M, Engelman K: *JAMA* 258:3275, 1987.

Beilin LJ: *J Hypertension* 5(Suppl 5):S447, 1987.

Beilin LJ: *J Hypertension* 6:85, 1988.

Belizan JM, Villar J, Pineda O, et al: *JAMA* 249:1161, 1983.

Bennett E, Wilcox RG, MacDonald IA: *Clin Sci* 67:97, 1984.

Benson H, Caudill MA: *Prim Cardiol* 137: September 1984.

Berglund A, Andersson OK, Berglund G, et al: *Br Med J* 299:480, 1989.

Beutler JJ, Attevelt JTM, Schouten SA, et al: *Br Med J* 296:1491, 1988.

Bianchetti MG, Beretta-Piccoli C, Weidmann P, et al: *J Hypertension* 2(Suppl 3):445, 1984.

Bjorntorp P, De Jounge K, Sjostrom L, et al: *Scand J Clin Lab Invest* 32:41, 1973.

Black HR, Ming S, Poll DS, et al: *J Clin Hypertens* 4:371, 1986.

Blackburn H: *Ann Clin Res* 16(Suppl 43):11, 1984.

Blair SN, Goodyear NN, Gibbons LW, et al: *JAMA* 252:487, 1984.

Blaufox MD, Oberman H, Langford H, et al: *Am J Hypertens* 2:42A, 1989 (abst).

Bonanno JA, Lies JE: *Am J Cardiol* 33:760, 1974.

Brest AN, Wiener L, Bachrach B: *Am J Cardiol* 29:821, 1972.

Brown JJ, Lever AF, Robertson JIS, et al: *Q J Med* 53:427, 1984.

Burgess ED, Keane PM, Watanabe M: *J Hypertension* 6(Suppl 4):S85, 1988.

Burr ML: *Proc Nutr Soc* 47:129, 1988.

Cappuccio FP, Markandu ND, Beynon GW, et al: *Br Med J* 291:235, 1985.

Charlesworth ED, Williams BJ, Baer PE: *Psychosom Med* 46:387, 1984.

Chesney MA, Black GW, Swan GE, et al: *Psychosom Med* 49:250, 1987.

Clarke WR, Woolson RF, Lauer RM: *Am J Epidemiol* 124:195, 1986.

Colliander EB, Tesch PA: *Can J Spt Sci* 13:31, 1988.

Connacher AA, Jung RT, Mitchell PEG: *Br Med J* 296:1217, 1988.

Cottier C, Shapiro K, Julius S: *Arch Intern Med* 144:1954, 1984.

Dahl LK: *Am J Clin Nutr* 25:231, 1972.

Dai WS, Kuller LH, Miller G: *J Chron Dis* 37:75, 1984.

Davidoff R, Schamroth CL, Goldman AP, et al: *Aviat Space Environ Med* 53:591, 1982.

den Besten C, Vansant G, Weststrate JA, et al: *Am J Clin Nutr* 47:840, 1988.

Dodson PM, Beevers M, Hallworth R, et al: *Br Med J* 298:227, 1989.

Dodson PM, Pacy PJ, Cox EV: *Human Nutr: Clin Nutr* 39C:213, 1985.

Dornfeld LP, Maxwell MH, Waks AU, et al: *Int J Obesity* 9:381, 1985.

Drake D, Hollander D: *Ann Intern Med* 94:215, 1981.

Duncan JJ, Farr JE, Upton SJ, et al: *JAMA* 254:2609, 1985.

Dyckner T, Wester PO: *Br Med J* 286:1847, 1983.

El Ashry A, Heagerty AM, Alton SM, et al: *J Hum Hypertens* 1:105, 1987.

Eliahou HE, Ianina A, Gaon T, et al: *Int J Obesity* 5:157, 1981.

Ellison RC, Capper AL, Stephenson WP, et al: *J Clin Epidemiol* 42:201, 1989.

Evers SE, Bass M, Donner A, et al: *Prev Med* 16:213, 1987.

Ewing DJ, Irving JB, Kerr F, et al: *Br Heart J* 35:413, 1973.

Fagerberg B, Andersson O, Isaksson B, et al: *Br Med J* 288:11, 1984.

Fagerberg B, Andersson OK, Persson B, et al: *Hypertension* 7:586, 1985.

Feldman RD, Lawton WJ, McArdle WL: *J Clin Invest* 79:290, 1987.

Fleck SJ: *Med Sci Sports Exerc* 20:S146, 1988.

Foushee DB, Ruffin J, Banerjee U: *Cytobios* 34:145, 1982.

Friedman GD, Siegelaub AB: *Circulation* 61:716, 1980.

Fujita T, Sato Y: *Kidney Int* 24:731, 1983.

Garavaglia GE, Messerli FH, Schmieder RE, et al: *J Hum Hypertens* 2:247, 1988.

Gillum RF, Prineas RJ, Jeffery RW, et al: *Am Heart J* 105:128, 1983.

Glanzer K, Kramer HJ, Adams O, et al: *J Hypertension* 1(Suppl 2):214, 1983.

Glasgow MS, Engel BT, D'Lugoff BC: *Psychosom Med* 51:10, 1989.

Goldstein IG, Shapiro D, Thananopavaran C: *Psychosom Med* 46:398, 1984.

Grimm R, Neaton J, Elmer P, et al: *Circulation* 80(Suppl II):II-302, 1989 (abst).

Grobbee DE, Hofman A: *Lancet* 2:703, 1986.

Grobbee DE, Hofman A, Roelandt JT, et al: *J Hypertension* 5:115, 1987.

Hagberg JM, Goldring D, Ehsani AA, et al: *Am J Cardiol* 52:763, 1983.

Hamada M, Kazatani Y, Shigematsu Y, et al: *J Hypertension* 5:305, 1987.

Harto NE, Spera KF, Branconnier RJ: *Psychopharmacol Bull* 24:220, 1988.

Haynes RB, Adsett CA, Bellissimo A: *Clin Res* 37:313A, 1989.

Haynes RB, Harper AC, Costley SR, et al: *J Hypertension* 2:535, 1984.

Health and Public Policy Committee, American College of Physicians: *Ann Intern Med* 102:709, 1985.

Henderson DG, Schierup J, Schodt T: *Br Med J* 293:664, 1986.

Hespel P, Lijnen P, Faagard R, et al: *J Hypertension* 6:159, 1988.

Hoffman JW, Benson H, Arns PA, et al: *Science* (Wash DC) 215:190, 1982.

Hossman V, FitzGerald GA, Dollery CT: *Hypertension* 3:113, 1981.

Hovell MF, Koch A, Hofstetter CR, et al: *Am J Public Health* 78:663, 1988.

Hvarfner A, Bergstrom R, Lithell H, et al: *Clin Sci* 75:543, 1988.

Iimura O, Kijima T, Kikuchi K, et al: *Clin Sci* 61:77s, 1981.

Jacob RG, Shapiro AP, Reeves RA, et al: *Arch Intern Med* 146:2335, 1986.

Jacobson E: *Ann Intern Med* 12:1194, 1939.

Jannetta PJ, Segal R, Wolfson SK Jr: *Ann Surg* 201:391, 1985.

Jeffery RW, Pirie PL, Elmer PJ, et al: *Am J Public Health* 74:492, 1984.

Jennings GL, Nelson L, Nestel P, et al: *Circulation* 73:30, 1986.

1988 Joint National Committee: *Arch Intern Med* 148:1023, 1988.

Kanis JA, Passmore R: *Br Med J* 298:137, 1989.

Kannel WB, Garrison RJ, Zhang T: *JACC* 13:104A, 1989 (abst).

Kannel WB, Wilson P, Blair SN, et al: *Am Heart J* 109:876, 1985.

Kaplan NM: *Arch Intern Med* 149:1514, 1989.

Kaplan NM: *Semin Nephrol* 8:176, 1988.

Kaplan NM, Carnegie A, Raskin P, et al: *N Engl J Med* 312:746, 1985.

Kaplan NM, Meese RB: *Ann Intern Med* 105:947, 1986.

Kaplan NM, Simmons M, McPhee C, et al: *Arch Intern Med* 142:1638, 1982.

Karanja N, Morris CD, Illingworth DR, et al: *Am J Clin Nutr* 45:60, 1987.

Katch V, Becque MD, Marks C, et al: *Am J Clin Nutr* 47:26, 1988.

Kempner W: *JAMA* 125:48, 1944.

Kerr CM Jr, Reisinger KS, Plankey FW: *Pediatrics* 62:331, 1978.

Kiyonaga A, Arakawa K, Tanaka H, et al: *Hypertension* 7:125, 1985.

Kjeldsen SE, Os I, Beckmann SL, et al: *J Hypertension* 4(Suppl 6):S200, 1986.

Kjeldsen SE, Sejersted OM, Frederichsen P, et al: *J Hypertension* 7(Suppl 6):S156, 1989.

Khaw K-T, Barrett-Connor E: *N Engl J Med* 316:235, 1987.

Knapp HR, FitzGerald GA: *N Engl J Med* 320:1037, 1989.

Knochel JP: *Am J Med* 72:521, 1982.

Kohvakka A: *Int J Clin Pharmacol Ther Toxicol* 26:273, 1988.

Kostis JB, Rosen R, Taska LS, et al: *JACC* 13:104A, 1989 (abst).

Krezesinski JM, Rorive GL: *Klin Wochenschr* 63(Suppl III):45, 1985.

Krieger DR, Landsberg L: In: Laragh JH, Brenner BM, Kaplan NM (eds). *Perspectives in Hypertension*, vol 2: *Endocrine Mechanisms in Hypertension*. New York: Raven Press, 1989:105.

Krishna GG, Miller E, Kapoor S: *N Engl J Med* 320:1177, 1989.

Kukkonen K, Rauramaa R, Voutilainen E, et al: *Ann Clin Res* 14(Suppl 34):139, 1982.

Landmann-Suter R, Struyvenberg A: *Eur J Clin Invest* 8:155, 1978.

Laragh JH, Pecker MS: *Ann Intern Med* 98:735, 1983.

Lasaridis AN, Kaisis CN, Zananiri KI, et al: *Nephron* 51:517, 1989.

Lee CN, Reed DM, MacLean CJ, et al: *N Engl J Med* 318:995, 1987.

Lee DD-P, DeQuattro V, Allen J, et al: *Am Heart J* 116:637, 1988.

Letcher RL, Pickering TG, Chien S, et al: *Clin Cardiol* 4:172, 1981.

Linares OA, Zech LA, Jacquez JA, et al: *Am J Physiol* 254:E222, 1988.

Little BC, Benson P, Beard RW, et al: *Lancet* 1:865, 1984.

Littler WA, Honour AJ, Carter RD, et al: *Br Med J* 3:346, 1975.

Longworth DL, Drayer JIM, Weber MA, et al: *Clin Pharmacol Ther* 27:544, 1980.

Louria DB, McAnally JF, Lasser N, et al: *Curr Ther Res* 37:127, 1985.

Luft FC, Aronoff GR, Fineberg NS, et al: *Am J Hypertens* 2:14, 1989.

Luft FC, Sloan RS, Lang CL, et al: *Arch Intern Med* 144:1963, 1984.

Luft FC, Weinberger MH: *Hypertension* 11(Suppl I):I-229, 1988.

Luft FC, Weinberger MH, Grim CE, et al: *J Hypertension* 4(Suppl 5):S198, 1986.

Lyle RM, Melby CL, Hyner GC: *Am J Clin Nutr* 47:1030, 1988.

MacGregor GA, Markandu ND, Sagnella GA, et al: *Lancet* 2:1244, 1989.

MacGregor GA, Smith SJ, Markandu ND, et al: *Lancet* 2:567, 1982.

MacMahon S: *Hypertension* 9:111, 1987.

MacMahon SW, Macdonald GJ, Bernstein L, et al: *Lancet* 1:1233, 1985.

Madden DJ, Blumenthal JA, Ekelund L-G: *Hypertension* 11:470, 1988.

Margetts BM, Beilin LJ, Armstrong BK, et al: *Am J Clin Nutr* 48:801, 1988.

Matlou SM, Isles CG, Higgs A, et al: *J Hypertension* 4:61, 1986.

Masugi F, Ogihara T, Hashizume K, et al: *J Hypertens* 1:293, 1988.

Maxwell MH, Kushiro T, Dornfeld LP, et al: *Arch Intern Med* 144:1581, 1984.

McCarron DA: *Hypertension* 4(Suppl III):III-27, 1982.

McCarron DA: *Kidney Int* 35:717, 1989.

McCarron DA, Morris CD: *Ann Intern Med* 103:825, 1985.

McLoughlin JC: *Lancet* 1:581, 1985.

Meneely GR, Battarbee HD: *Am J Cardiol* 38:768, 1976.

Miller JZ, Weinberger MH, Christian JC: *26th Conference on Cardiovascular Disease Epidemiology, March 3-5, 1986*. Dallas, American Heart Association, 1986.

Morgan T, Nowson C: *Can J Physiol Pharmacol* 64:786, 1986.

Morgan TO: *Clin Sci* 63(Suppl):407S, 1982.

Murphy MB, Zebrauskas D, Schutte S, et al: *Am J Hypertens* 2:43A, 1989 (abst).

Nelson L, Jennings GL, Esler MD, et al: *Lancet* 2:473, 1986.

Nemec ED, Mansfield L, Kennedy JW: *Am Heart J* 92:174, 1976.

Niarchos AP, Weinstein DL, Laragh JH: *Am J Med* 77:1061, 1984.

Nicholls MG: *Hypertension* 6:795, 1984.

Nixon PGF, Dighton DH: *Br Med J* 2:525, 1976.

Norris PJ, Jones CJH, Weston MJ: *Lancet* 2:104, 1986.

Nowson CA, Morgan TO: *Clin Exp Pharmacol Physiol* 15:225, 1988.

Oberman A, Wassertheil-Smoller S, Langford HG, et al: *Ann Intern Med* 112:89, 1990.

Omvik P, Lund-Johansen P: *J Hypertension* 4:535, 1986.

Ophir O, Peer G, Gilad J, et al: *Am J Clin Nutr* 37:755, 1983.

Oshima T, Matsuura H, Kido K, et al: *J Hypertension* 7:223, 1989.

Overlack A, Muller H-M, Kolloch R, et al: *J Hypertension* 1(Suppl 2):165, 1983.

Pacy PJ, Dodson PM, Kubicki AJ, et al: *J Hypertension* 2:215, 1984.

Paffenbarger RS Jr, Hyde RT, Wing AL, et al: *N Engl J Med* 314:605, 1986.

Paffenbarger RS JR, Wing AL, Hyde RT, et al: *Am J Epidemiol* 117:245, 1983.

Pagani M, Somers V, Furlan R, et al: *Hypertension* 12:600, 1988.

Patel C, Marmot M: *Br Med J* 296:21, 1988.

Patel C, Marmot MG: *J Hypertension* 5(Suppl 1):S21, 1987.

Patel C, Marmot MG, Terry DJ, et al: *Br Med J* 290:1103, 1985.

Pekkanen J, Marti B, Nissinen A, et al: *Lancet* 1:1473, 1987.

Peled-Ney R, Silverberg DS, Rosenfeld JB: *Israel J Med Sci* 20:12, 1984.

Phillips JA, Shaper AG: *Lancet* 1:1005, 1989.

Pietinen P, Huttunen JK: *Eur Heart J* 8(Suppl B):9, 1987.

Potter JF, Macdonald IA, Beevers DG: *J Hypertension* 4:435, 1986.

Prescott SL, Jenner DA, Beilin LJ, et al: *Clin Sci* 74:665, 1988.

Pudley IB, Parker M, Vandongen R, et al: *J Hypertens* 7(Suppl 6):S393, 1989.

Radack K, Deck C: *J Am Coll Nutr* 8:376, 1989.

Ram CVS, Garrett BN, Kaplan NM: *Arch Intern Med* 141:1015, 1981.

Rauramaa R, Salonen JT, Kukkonen-Harjula K, et al: *Br Med J* 288:603, 1984.

Reed D, McGee D, Yano K, et al: *Hypertension* 7:405, 1985.

Repke JT, Villar J, Anderson C, et al: *Am J Obstet Gynecol* 160:684, 1989.

Reisin E, Abel R, Modan M, et al: *N Engl J Med* 298:1, 1978.

Reisin E, Frohlich ED, Messerli FH, et al: *Ann Intern Med* 98:315, 1983.

Report of the British Hypertension Society Working Party: *Br Med J* 298:694, 1989.

Resnick LM: *Am J Hypertens* 2:179S, 1989.

Richards AM, Nicholls MG, Espiner EA, et al: *Lancet* 1:757, 1984.

Riendl AM, Gotshall RW, Reinke JA, et al: *Proc Soc Exp Biol Med* 154:171, 1977.

Robertson D, Hollister AS, Kincaid D, et al: *Am J Med* 77:54, 1984.

Rocchini AP, Katch V, Anderson J, et al: *Pediatrics* 82:16, 1988.

Rocchini AP, Katch V, Schork A, et al: *Hypertension* 10:267, 1987.

Rodnick KG, Haskell WL, Swislocki ALM, et al: *Am J Physiol* 253:E489, 1987.

Roman O, Camuzzi AL, Villalon E, et al: *Cardiology* 67:230, 1981.

Rose G: In: Mathias CJ, Sever PS (eds). *Concepts in Hypertension*. New York: Springer-Verlag, 1989:39.

Ryan MP, Brady HR: *Ann Clin Res* 16(Suppl 43):6, 1984.

Sackett DL: *Can J Physiol Pharm* 64:871, 1986.

Sacks FM: *Nutr Rev* 47:291, 1989.

Sacks FM, Kass EH: *Am J Clin Nutr* 48:795, 1988.

Saito K, Hattori K, Omatsu T, et al: *Am J Hypertension* 1:71S, 1988.

Salvetti A, Bichisao E, Caiazza A, et al: *Am J Hypertens* 1:201S, 1988.

Sanchez-Castillo CP, Warrender S, Whitehead T, et al: *Ann Clin Res* 16(Suppl 43):44, 1984.

Sannerstedt R, Wasir H, Henning R, et al: *Clin Sci* 45:145S, 1973.

Schechter PJ, Horwitz D, Henkin RI: *Am J Med Sci* 267:320, 1974.

Schiffman S: *J Gerontol* 32:586, 1977.

Schlamowitz P, Halberg T, Warnoe O, et al: *Lancet* 2:622, 1987.

Schmieder RE, Messerli FH, Ruddel H, et al: *J Hypertension* 6(Suppl 4):S148, 1988.

Shah BG, Belonje B: *Nutr Res* 3:629, 1983.

Shaper AG, Wannamethee G, Whincup P: *J Human Hypertens* 2:71, 1988.

Sherwood A, Light KC, Blumenthal JA: *Psychosom Med* 51:123, 1989.

Shinton R, Beevers G: *Br Med J* 298:789, 1989.

Siani A, Strazzullo P, Russo L, et al: *Br Med J* 294:1453, 1987.

Slattery ML, Jacobs DR Jr: *Am J Epidemiol* 127:571, 1988.

Slattery ML, Sorenson AW, Ford MH: *Am J Epidemiol* 128:504, 1988.

Smith SJ, Markandu ND, Sagnella GA, et al: *J Hypertension* 1(Suppl 2):27, 1983.

Smith SJ, Markandu ND, Sagnella GA, et al: *Br Med J* 290:110, 1985.

Smoller SW, Blaufox MD, David B, et al: *Am J Hypertension* 2:16A, 1989 (abst).

Sobolski J, Kornitzer M, De Backer G, et al: *Am J Epidemiol* 125:601, 1987.

Sonne-Holm S, Sørensen TIA, Jensen G, et al: *Br Med J* 299:767, 1989.

Spence DW, Peterson LH, Friedewald VE Jr: *Am J Cardiol* 59:1342, 1987.

Staessen J, Bulpitt CJ, Fagard R, et al: *J Hypertension* 6:965, 1988.

Staessen J, Fagard R, Lijnen P, et al: *J Hypertension* 7(Suppl 1):S19, 1989.

Stamer R, Stamler J, Gosch FC, et al: *JAMA* 262:1801, 1989.

Stamler R, Stamler J, Grimm R, et al: *JAMA* 257:1484, 1987.

Strazzullo P, Cappuccio FP, Trevisan M, et al: *Am J Epidemiol* 127:726, 1988.

Sugimoto T, Tobian L, Ganguli MC: *Hypertension* 11:579, 1988.

Suppa G, Pollavini G, Alberti D, et al: *J Hypertension* 6:787, 1988.

Svetkey LP, Yarger WE, Feussner JR, et al: *Hypertension* 9:444, 1987.

Tam KC, Yiu HH: *Am J Chin Med* 3:369, 1975.

Thorpe JJ, Welch WJ, Poindexter CA: *Am J Med* 9:500, 1950.

Tobian L, Jahner T, Johnson MA: *Clin Res* 37:604A, 1989 (abst).

Tyroler HA, Heyden S, Hames CG: In: Paul O (ed). *Epidemiology and Control of Hypertension*. Miami: Symposia Specialist, 1975:p 177.

Ullian ME, Linas SL: *Semin Nephrol* 7:239, 1987.

Urata H, Tanabe Y, Kiyonage A, et al: *Hypertension* 9:245, 1987.

Valori C, Bentivoglio M, Corea L, et al: *J Hypertension* 5(Suppl 5):S315, 1987.

van Dusseldorp M, Smits P, Thien T, et al: *Hypertension* 14:563, 1989.

Vertes V, Frolkis JP, Martin PJ: *Mt Sinai J Med* 55:296, 1988.

Volini IF, Flaxman N: *JAMA* 112:2126, 1939.

Wallace P, Cutler S, Haines A: *Br Med J* 297:663, 1988.

Wallace RK, Silver J, Mills PJ, et al: *Psychosom Med* 45:41, 1983.

Watkin DM, Froeb HF, Hatch FT, et al: *Am J Med* 9:441, 1950.

Watt G: *J Hypertension* 7(Suppl 1):S29, 1989.

Watt GCM, Edwards C, Hart JT, et al: *Br Med J* 296:432, 1983.

Weinberger MH, Cohen SJ, Miller JZ, et al: *JAMA* 259:2561, 1988.

Weintraub M, Bray GA: *Med Clin N Amer* 73:237, 1989.

Wilcox RG, Bennett T, MacDonald IA, et al: *Br J Clin Pharmacol* 17:273, 1984.

Winer BM: *Circulation* 24:788, 1961.

Wittemann JC, Willett WC, Stampfer MJ, et al: *Circulation* 80:1320, 1989.

# 7 Treatment of Hypertension: Drug Therapy

The treatment of hypertension is now the leading indication for the use of drugs in the United States (National Prescription Audit, IMS America, Ambler, PA, 1989, personal communication). Worldwide, sales of antihypertensive drugs increased more than 4-fold from 1970 to 1982 (Bauer et al, 1985). As impressive as has been the recent growth in the use of antihypertensive drugs, even greater use is foreseen as more patients are identified and deemed to be in need of therapy.

In the previous two chapters, I review the evidence for the need for blood pressure reduction and the use of a variety of nondrug therapies to lower the blood pressure. This chapter first provides general guidelines for the drug treatment of hypertension with emphasis upon achieving adherence to therapy. Then each drug currently available is described. An analysis of the issues of which drug to use first and of the subsequent order of additional therapy follows, along with considerations of a number of special management problems, including the elderly, the resistant, and the impotent patient.

## GENERAL GUIDELINES

In keeping with the proliferation of new therapeutic agents in this field, the treatment of hypertension has been the subject of a massive amount of clinical research. The proliferation of the medical literature makes it almost im-

possible for the practicing physician to be aware of important advances in the area, and it becomes increasingly difficult to put many of these studies into an overall perspective which can be translated into improved patient care. I have constantly attempted to maintain an objective view, both about the use of drugs overall and about the relative value of individual agents. While I certainly advocate certain approaches, the coverage in this chapter is based as much as possible on hard data which will allow the individual clinician the opportunity to develop his or her own approach.

### Comparisons Between Drugs: Efficacy

The individual practitioner's choice of drug is often based on perceived differences in efficacy and the likelihood of side effects. In fact, there is relatively little difference in efficacy between the various available drugs; in order to gain FDA approval for marketing in the United States, the drug must have been shown to be effective in reducing the blood pressure in a large portion of the 1500 or more patients given the drug during its clinical investigation. Moreover, the dose and formulation of drug is chosen so as not to precipitously lower the pressure too much or too fast so as to avoid hypotensive side effects. Virtually all drugs, save the few intended for parenteral use in patients with hypertensive emergencies, are designed to do the same: lower the blood pressure about 10% in the majority of patients with mild to moderate hypertension (Gomez and Cirillo, 1985).

Not only is each approved drug then known to be effective in large populations of hypertensive patients, but also the drug must have been tested against currently available agents to show at least equal efficacy (Temple, 1989). When comparisons between various drugs, e.g., diuretic versus beta-blocker, angiotensin-converting enzyme (ACE) inhibitor versus calcium entry blocker (CEB), are made, they almost always come out very close to one another (Helgeland et al, 1986).

### Individual Patient Trials

Despite the fairly equal overall efficacy of various antihypertensive drugs, individual patients may vary considerably in their response to different drugs. Some of this variability can be accounted for by patient characteristics. Perhaps the most clearly defined factor is race: Black hypertensives tend to respond better than do nonblacks to diuretics but less well to beta-blockers [Veterans Administration (VA) Cooperative Study Group, 1982a] or ACE inhibitors (Pool et al, 1987). Age has also been claimed to affect drug responsiveness (Bühler et al, 1984). However, the large body of more recent data from properly performed clinical trials does not support a significantly greater or lesser effectiveness of these various agents in the elderly (Kaplan, 1989a).

When fairly homogeneous groups of patients are tested with different drugs in random order, some are found to respond well to one agent, others to another (Bidiville et al, 1988). Unfortunately not enough such intraindividual trials have been done to ascertain what characterizes patients who are more or less responsive to any particular class of drug.

A rather obvious solution to this problem has been provided: individual patient, randomized clinical trials (Guyatt et al, 1988). The idea is simple: The patient undergoes multiple treatment periods, each providing an active drug and a matched placebo assigned at random with both the patient and the physician blinded to the choice, which is made by the pharmacist. The process can go on as long as needed until an effective and well-tolerated agent is found for each individual patient.

Although the concept is simple, I doubt whether many practitioners (or their patients) will go to that much trouble. Fortunately, the physician can make a fairly exact ascertainment, if not of the "best" drug, certainly of an effective and well-tolerated one. This simply requires an open mind, a willingness to try one drug after another, each chosen from the seven classes of available antihypertensive agents, with careful monitoring of the patient, preferably by using home blood pressure readings, and a thorough ascertainment of side effects. This approach—the individualized choice of therapy with substitution for drugs found to be ineffectual or bothersome—is preferable to the rigid "diuretic-first step-care" approach so widely advocated and practiced. More about this will follow the description of the various choices now available.

### Comparisons Between Drugs: Side Effects

As to the issue of differences in side effects between different agents, two points are obvious: First, no drug that causes dangerous side effects beyond a rare idiosyncratic reaction when given in usual doses will remain on the market even if it slips by the approval process, as witnessed by the uricosuric diuretic ticrynafen; second, drugs that cause frequent, bothersome, though not dangerous side effects, such as guanethidine, will likely no longer by utilized now that so many choices are available.

There are significant differences between various antihypertensive agents both in the frequency of side effects and, even more so, in their nature. There are no carefully conducted trials comparing members of all major classes with each other, although one is now in process (Grimm et al, 1989). Multiple comparisons of two or three agents are available. Perhaps the most widely quoted study comparing different drugs is that of Croog et al (1986). In this multicenter double-blind trial, 626 men with mild to moderate hypertension were randomly treated with one of three drugs each given twice daily in these doses: captopril, 50 mg; methyldopa, 500 mg; or propranolol, 80 mg. If the DBP was not below 95 mm Hg after 8 weeks, HCTZ, 25 mg twice daily, was added for the remaining 16 weeks. Thorough questionnaires were completed by the patients before and at the end of the 24-week study.

The results clearly indicate an advantage of the ACE inhibitor over the beta-blocker and the central alpha-agonist (Table 7.1). This study clearly defines a number of important issues regarding differences between different drugs.

**Table 7.1. Effects of Three Antihypertensive Drugs on Quality of Life[a]**

| | Captopril | Methyldopa | Propranolol |
|---|---|---|---|
| Number of patients treated | 213 | 201 | 212 |
| Quality of life measurements | | | |
| General well-being | | | |
| Improvement (%) | 51 | 39 | 39 |
| Worsening (%) | 31 | 51 | 45 |
| Physical symptoms | | | |
| Improvement (%) | 29 | 20 | 17 |
| Worsening (%) | 25 | 37 | 37 |
| Sexual dysfunction | | | |
| Improvement (%) | 18 | 9 | 9 |
| Worsening (%) | 19 | 24 | 26 |
| Number of adverse reactions | 30 | 89 | 51 |
| Number of withdrawals due to adverse reactions | 17 | 39 | 27 |
| Percentage requiring diuretic to control blood pressure | 33 | 28 | 22 |

[a]Data from Croog et al: *N Engl J Med* 314:1657, 1986.

First, the assessment of changes in the "quality of life" or well-being are important guidelines for the selection of drugs that are fairly comparable in efficacy. Many more studies such as that of Croog et al are clearly needed. Second, even though the effects of drugs on various aspects of the "quality of life" can be fairly easily ascertained, it may not be possible to determine whether changes in symptoms reflect the nonspecific lowering of blood pressure with any drug or the specific side effects of individual drugs.

Further analysis by Croog et al (1988) of their data has provided a third important point: Side effects of one drug may be altered considerably when a second drug is added to achieve adequate antihypertensive control. As seen in Table 7.1, more of those given captopril needed to have HCTZ added at week 8 to achieve a DBP below 95 than those given either of the other two agents. The addition of HCTZ rather strikingly worsened the overall "physical sexual symptoms distress index." Whether this reflects a nonspecific effect of the further reduction in blood pressure (which seems likely) or a specific action of HCTZ is uncertain. The major point is that the comparisons between the side effects of drugs should be determined at a point of equal degrees of antihypertensive action.

A fourth point is that untreated hypertensives have a fairly high prevalence of various symptoms. Of the 196 hypertensive men who had been on no therapy, 44% noted some problem with sexual performance during the previous month (Croog et al, 1988). No side effect should be ascribed to a drug unless it was known not to be present in the absence of the drug.

The fifth point made by Croog and coworkers' data is that, even with the "best" drug of the three compared, side effects ascribable to therapy are fairly common. Of the patients who started with one or another agent, treatment was discontinued, usually because of side effects, in 15% of those on captopril, 23% on propranolol, and 27% on methyldopa.

**Problems in Ascertainment**

In most large-scale trials lasting for as long as 5 years, from 20 to 40% of patients will drop out, mostly because of adverse side effects (Curb et al, 1985). However, the frequency of milder but yet still bothersome side effects—bothersome enough to cause patients in ordinary clinical practice to stop taking the drug and even worse, to drop out of all blood pressure management—may be much higher. The fact that fewer than half of patients known to be hypertensive are taking medication is perhaps the most telling indictment of the troubles experienced. Hopefully, the situation can be improved, using techniques to be covered in a following section of this chapter.

**Dose-Response Relationships**

The major reasons that most antihypertensive drugs have equal efficacy in clinical practice is, first, the choice of equivalent doses that provide the desired effect and, second, the generally fairly flat dose-response curve of most of these agents, so that, even if considerably more drug is given, relatively little additional effect will be noted (Fig. 7.1). For a few drugs, e.g., guanethidine, a progressively increased effect occurs throughout the therapeutic range so that the more drug given, the greater the effect, up to a point. Care is needed in regulating the dose of such a drug. For most antihypertensive agents,

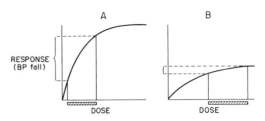

**Figure 7.1.** Idealized dose-response relationships. *A*, a steep curve as with guanethidine; *B*, a flat curve as with thiazide diuretics.

however, the dose-response curve is fairly flat, so that once a certain fixed dose is reached, little if any benefit is seen with larger doses although side effects may be more bothersome.

## Height of the Pretreatment Pressure

Many reports of the efficacy of various antihypertensive drugs correlate the change in blood pressure that occurs with their use to the pretreatment level of the blood pressure. When the correlation has been strongly positive, as with recent trials with calcium antagonists (Erne et al, 1984), the results have been taken as evidence of an effect of the drug on a basic mechanism responsible for the pathogenesis of hypertension. However, as pointed out by Gill et al (1985) and reiterated by Sumner et al (1988), such conclusions may not be valid since the change in blood pressure depends directly upon the pretreatment level, so "There is consequently a logical and mathematical relation between the change in blood pressure and the pretreatment blood pressure which is not attributable to any treatment effect" (Gill et al, 1985). The failure to recognize this fact is likely responsible for the widely held view that the elderly respond more to various drugs. Most of this apparent superresponsiveness can be attributed to the almost universally higher systolic and mean pressures in the elderly than in the younger hypertensive population (Murray and Lesaffre, 1988).

The clinical lesson is simple: the higher the pretreatment blood pressure, the greater the fall with any drug (or nondrug).

## Problem of Compliance

More attention must be given to the major problem of keeping patients on therapy. The prescription of therapy is the easiest part of the process of treating hypertension, but, of those who start, as many as 50% will have dropped out within 1 year (Hollenberg, 1987) and only about 30% of patients who know themselves to be hypertensive are under adequate control. This is largely a reflection of the multiple factors that combine to impede compliance to antihypertensive therapy (Table 7.2) (Vetter et al, 1985; Horan and Page, 1988).

### Patient and Disease Characteristics

Hypertensives have special problems related to the nature of their disease. Many are largely unaware of the definition, possible causes, sequelae, and therapeutic needs of hypertension.

**Table 7.2.   Factors That Reduce Compliance to Therapy**

Patient and disease characteristics
   Asymptomatic
   Chronic condition
   Social isolation
   Disrupted home situation
   Psychiatric illness

Treatment characteristics
   Lack of specific appointment times
   Long waiting time in office
   Long duration of therapy
   Complicated regimens
   Expensive medications
   Side effects of medications
   Multiple behavioral modifications

Being asymptomatic, there is little motivation to seek or follow treatment. Many are found to have high blood pressure at an age, in their late 30s and early 40s, when the threat of a loss of vigor and vitality is insidiously beginning and the recognition of hypertension often provokes a strong denial reaction (McClellan et al, 1988). Moreover, the diagnosis carries considerable economic and social threats—loss of job, insurance, and sexual potency—that may further inhibit people from accepting the diagnosis and dealing with the problem.

### Treatment Characteristics

The therapy of hypertension has all the wrong characteristics for adherence as described by Blackwell (1973): "Patients with prolonged conditions are clearly prone to lapses in compliance, especially when the treatment is prophylactic or suppressive, when the condition is mild or asymptomatic or when the consequences of stopping therapy may be delayed."

It is little wonder that hypertensives are slow in seeking and sloppy in following therapy. Unfortunately both the physician and his/her therapy often make the situation worse (Table 7.2).

Although it is widely believed that a once-a-day regimen will be more closely followed than multiple doses, two careful studies have shown equal adherence to one or two doses a day (but less to three) (Pullar et al, 1988) and almost equal adherence to one, two, or three doses a day (but much less to four) (Cramer et al, 1989). Nonetheless, those regimens that involve large numbers of pills, often adding up to considerable expense, will pose a burden for many people.

Side effects discourage compliance, and side effects are common. In the Hypertension Detection and Follow-up Program, 32.7% of the

5485 patients in stepped care discontinued therapy because of definite or probable side effects (Curb et al, 1985). In particular, sexual dysfunctions with or without drug therapy may happen more frequently than most physicians realize since many are reticent to ask about them. Using a questionnaire given to 761 employed white males aged 21 to 65, Croog et al (1988) identified some problem in sexual performance during the previous month in 44% of those not on antihypertensive therapy at the time and in 59% on therapy.

Similar to the occurrence of impotence with diuretics, the symptoms that follow institution of drug therapy may not be expected from the the known pharmacological effects of the drug. Weakness, slowing of the walking pace, vivid dreams, dry mouth, and diarrhea each appeared in a significant number of hypertensive patients treated with a variety of drugs (Bulpitt and Fletcher, 1988).

**Assessment of Compliance**

Before the problem can be dealt with, it must be recognized. Unfortunately, most physicians, though confident that they can predict the compliance of their patients with therapy, make predictions no more accurate than obtained by the toss of a coin (Haynes, 1983). However, there are simple ways to assess patients' compliance, including these:

—monitoring of attendance at scheduled appointments;
—monitoring of blood pressure response (effects of drugs on biochemical or physiological measurements are not very helpful);
—asking if the patient is taking the medication regularly, remembering that patients tend to overestimate the amount of medication they take: "If patients say yes, they may or may not be telling the truth; however, if they say no they are virtually always telling the truth" (Sackett, 1979).
—asking the patient to describe the regimen;
—counting the patient's pills;
—monitoring the frequency of medication refills;
—determining blood or urine levels of medications (Prinoth et al, 1986).

**Ways to Improve Compliance**

Reviews of techniques that improve compliance to therapy in general and to antihypertensive therapy specifically are available (Haynes, 1983; Eraker et al, 1984; Greenfield et al, 1985;

Vetter et al, 1985; Horan and Page, 1988). Haynes (1983) summarized "the two outstanding features of most successful compliance interventions [are] the level of supervision of, or attention paid to, the patient and the extent to which compliance is reinforced, rewarded or encouraged."

Guidelines to improve patient compliance are given in Table 7.3. A few of these deserve more emphasis.

*Maintain Contact with the Patient.* Pharmacists, nurses, and paraprofessional aides have all been shown to be effective in keeping more patients under treatment (Gillum et al, 1978).

*Keep Care Inexpensive and Simple.* The evidence that little laboratory work is needed for most patients was presented in Chapter 2, and much of Chapter 5 described the use of nondrug therapies. To further reduce the cost of therapy, generic brands may be used (Nightingale and Morrison, 1987) or pills may be broken in half, with awareness that some may not break easily

**Table 7.3. General Guidelines to Improve Patient Adherence to Antihypertensive Therapy**

1. Be aware of the problem and be alert to signs of patient nonadherence.
2. Establish the goal of therapy: to reduce blood pressure to near normotensive levels with minimal or no side effects.
3. Educate the patient about the disease and its treatment.
   a. Involve the patient in decision making.
   b. Encourage family support.
4. Maintain contact with the patient.
   a. Encourage visits and calls to allied health personnel.
   b. Allow the pharmacist to monitor therapy.
   c. Give feedback to the patient via home BP readings.
   d. Make contact with patients who do not return.
5. Keep care inexpensive and simple.
   a. Do the least workup needed to rule out secondary causes.
   b. Obtain follow-up laboratory data only yearly unless indicated more often.
   c. Use home blood pressure readings.
   d. Use nondrug, no-cost therapies.
   e. Use the fewest daily doses of drugs needed.
   f. If appropriate, use combination tablets.
   g. Tailor medication to daily routines.
6. Prescribe according to pharmacological principles.
   a. Add one drug at a time.
   b. Start with small doses, aiming for 5- to 10-mm Hg reductions at each step.
   c. Prevent volume overload with adequate diuretic and sodium restriction.
   d. Be willing to stop unsuccessful therapy and try a different approach.
   e. Anticipate side effects.
   f. Adjust therapy to ameliorate side effects that do not spontaneously disappear.
   g. Continue to add effective and tolerated drugs, stepwise, in sufficient doses to achieve the goal of therapy.

or equally (Stimple et al, 1985). Fortunately, with improved delivery systems, such as an osmotic pump within a tablet (McInnes and Brodie, 1988), more and more once-a-day formulations will be available.

*Reduce the Pressure Slowly.* The need to reduce the blood pressure slowly, by 5- to 10-mm Hg steps, should be emphasized. The rationale for such a gentle, gradual approach is based upon what is known about the autoregulation of cerebral and coronary blood flow (Strandgaard and Haunso, 1987) (Fig. 7.2).

Normally, cerebral blood flow (CBF) remains relatively constant at about 50 ml/minute/100 g of brain (Strandgaard and Paulson, 1989). When the systemic blood pressure falls, the vessels dilate; when the pressure rises, the vessels constrict. The limits of cerebral autoregulation in normal people are between mean arterial pressure of about 60 and 120 mm Hg, e.g., 80/50 to 160/100.

In hypertensives without neurological deficits, the CBF is not different from that found in normotensives. This constancy of the CBF reflects a shift in the range of autoregulation to the right to a range of mean pressure from about 100 to 180 mm Hg, e.g., 130/85 to 240/150 (Fig. 7.2). This shift maintains a normal CBF despite the higher pressure but makes the hypertensive vulnerable to cerebral ischemia when the pressure falls to a level that is well tolerated by normotensives (Barry, 1985).

Note that the lower limit of autoregulation capable of preserving CBF in hypertensive patients is at a mean blood pressure around 110 mm Hg. Thus, acutely lowering the pressure from 160/100 (mean = 127) to 140/85 (mean = 102) may induce cerebral hypoperfusion, though hypotension in the usual sense has not been induced. This likely explains why many patients experience symptoms of weakness, easy fatigability, and postural dizziness at the start of antihypertensive therapy, i.e., manifestations of cerebral hypoperfusion, even though blood pressure levels do not seem inordinately low.

Fortunately, with effective control of the blood

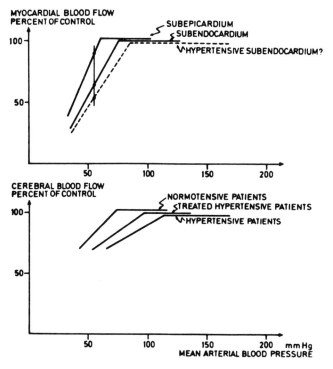

**Figure 7.2.** Autoregulation of myocardial (*above*) and cerebral (*below*) blood flow. Mean myocardial blood flow autoregulation curves are shown for subepicardium and corresponding subendocardial layers of the left ventricle in canine hearts, modified from Haunsø (*Acta Physiol Scand* 112:349, 1981). The autoregulatory curve of subendocardial blood flow in hypertensive hearts is suggested. During low arterial pressure (*vertical line*), when autoregulation is exhausted in both myocardial layers, subendocardial blood flow is lower than in the more superficial layers of the left ventricle. Mean cerebral blood flow autoregulation curves from normotensive, severely hypertensive, and effectively treated hypertensive patients are shown. Modified from Strandgaard (*Circulation* 53:720, 1976). (From Strandgaard S, Haunsø: *Lancet* 2:658, 1987.)

pressure by medication, the curve drifts back toward normal (Strandgaard and Haunsø, 1987). This may explain the eventual ability of hypertensive patients to tolerate falls in pressure to levels that initially produced symptoms of cerebral ischemia. Not all patients show a readaptation toward normal; presumably their structural changes are not reversible. Thus, older patients with more cerebral atherosclerosis may remain susceptible to cerebral ischemia when their blood pressure is lowered even gently (Jansen et al, 1986).

The coronary circulation, particularly in those with extensive atherosclerosis, may also autoregulate very poorly, and patients with preexisting coronary artery disease may be particularly prone to subendocardial ischemia as their pressures are lowered (Strandgaard and Haunsø, 1987; Cruickshank, 1988). Since the hypertrophied myocardium often found in chronic hypertensives can extract little additional oxygen beyond what is removed under normal conditions, the vulnerability of patients to myocardial infarction when their pressure is lowered below the critical level needed to maintain adequate perfusion is easily understood. This issue is examined more completely in Chapter 5. Clearly caution is needed when lowering the pressure so as not to induce either cerebral or coronary hypoperfusion.

Now that the general principles about therapy have been considered, let us turn to the specifics about antihypertensive drugs.

## SPECIFICS ABOUT ANTIHYPERTENSIVE DRUGS

Orally effective drugs that could be taken without major side effects have been available only since the early 1950s (Gross et al, 1989). Some used extensively elsewhere are still not available in the United States and they are also covered, along with some of the newer agents that are on the horizon (Taylor and Kaplan, 1989). Those drugs that have outlived their usefulness are disregarded. In view of the potentially lethal consequences of pressor reactions with monoamine oxidase (MAO) inhibitors, they are also excluded.

We will consider the drugs in the order shown in Table 7.4. It is of interest to notice the changes in their relative frequency of usage in the United States over the years 1984 through 1988 (Fig. 7.3). Clearly, diuretics remain the most popular but their use is falling; beta-blockers are the second most popular but their use, too, is likely diminishing, whereas the newer classes—ACE inhibitors and calcium entry blockers—are rising rapidly. The reasons for these changes should become obvious in the remainder of this chapter.

After a description of some of the basic pharmacology and clinical usefulness of each agent, we will consider the choice of first and second drugs, the selection of specific drugs for various types of hypertensive patients, the use of combinations, and conditions wherein special care is advised in the choice of drugs. The use of drugs in various secondary forms of hypertension, e.g., ACE inhibitors in renovascular hypertension and spironolactone in primary aldosteronism, is considered in the respective chapters on these secondary states.

## DIURETICS

Diuretics are still the most frequently prescribed drugs used to treat hypertension. Hydrochlorothiazide (HCTZ) has been the most commonly used drug in the United States during the 1980s with over 90 million prescriptions for diuretics dispensed in 1988 for the treatment of hypertension (Fig. 7.3). As an example of their continued popularity, a 1988 survey of New Jersey physicians found that 65% chose a diuretic as the initial drug to treat elderly patients with isolated systolic hypertension (Kostis and Breckenridge, 1989). Their continued use has been stoutly defended as the easiest, least expensive, and most effective drug therapy for most patients (Freis, 1989; Gifford and Borazanian, 1989). However, the increasing recognition of biochemical changes that could increase cardiovascular risk and the lack of protection against coronary mortality in trials using diuretics as first agent have caused others to question the wisdom of their widespread use (Kaplan, 1983; Zusman, 1988).

Diuretics can be classified in numerous ways. They differ in structure and major site of action within the nephron (Fig 7.4), which in turn determines their relative efficacy, as expressed in the maximal percentage of filtered sodium chloride excreted when they are given (Lant, 1986).

Agents acting in the proximal tubule (Site I) are seldom used to treat hypertension. For the majority of patients who have mild to moderate hypertension, treatment is usually initiated with a thiazide-type diuretic, acting at Site III in Figure 7.4. If renal function is severely impaired (i.e., serum creatinine above 2.5 mg/dl), a loop diuretic, acting at Site II, or metolazone (Zaroxolyn, Diulo) may be required. A potassium-sparing agent, acting at Site IV, either spiron-

**Table 7.4.  Antihypertensive Drugs Available In The United States**

| Volume Depleters | Adrenergic Inhibitors | | Vasodilators |
|---|---|---|---|
| Diuretics | Peripheral | Beta-Receptor | Direct |
| Thiazides | Bethanidine | Acebutolol | Hydralazine |
| Chlorthalidone | Guanadrel | Atenolol | Minoxidil |
| Indapamide | Guanethidine | Betaxolol | |
| Metolazone | Reserpine | Carteolol | Calcium Blockers |
| | | Metoprolol | Diltiazem |
| Loop Diuretics | Central | Nadolol | Isradipine |
| Bumetanide | Clonidine | Penbutolol | Nicardipine |
| Furosemide | Guanabenz | Pindolol | Nifedipine |
| | Guanfacine | Propranolol | Verapamil |
| K+Savers | Methyldopa | Timolol | |
| Amiloride | | | Converting Enzyme |
| Spironolactone | Alpha-Receptor | Combined alpha and beta | Inhibitors |
| Triamterene | Doxazosin | Labetalol | Captopril |
| | Prazosin | | Enalapril |
| | Terazosin | | Lisinopril |

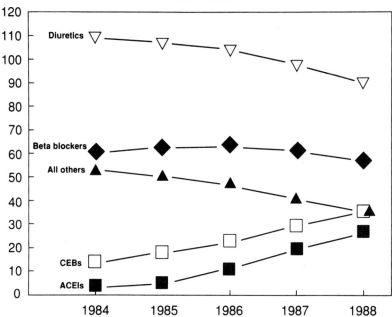

**Figure 7.3.**  Numbers of prescriptions written for antihypertensive drugs in millions in the United States from 1984 to 1988 (National Prescription Audit. Ambler, Pennsylvania: *IMS*, 1989.)

olactone (Aldactone), triamterene (Dyrenium), or amiloride (Midamor), may be given with the diuretic to reduce the likelihood of hypokalemia. By themselves, they are relatively weak antihypertensives.

Chlorthalidone and indapamide are structurally different, though still related to the thiazides and will be covered with them. Metolazone is more potent and will work in patients with renal insufficiency. Although it is also a thiazide de-

rivative, it will be considered with the loop diuretics. Potassium sparers will be covered separately. The specific agents now available in the United States are listed in Table 7.5.

## THIAZIDE DIURETICS

### Mode of Action

The thiazide diuretics act by inhibiting sodium and chloride cotransport across the luminal

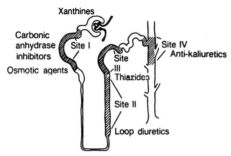

**Figure 7.4.** Diagrammatic representation of the nephron showing the four main tubular sites where diuretics interfere with sodium reabsorption. The main action of xanthines on the kidney is upon vascular perfusion of the glomerulus though some effect on sodium reabsorption at site I is also likely. [From Lant A: *Drugs* 31(Suppl 4):40, 1986.]

membrane of the early segment of the distal tubule (Shimizu et al, 1988) (Site III, Fig. 7.4). Plasma and extracellular fluid (ECF) volume are thereby shrunken, and cardiac output falls (Fig 7.5). With chronic use, plasma volume returns partially toward normal but at the same time peripheral resistance decreases (Conway and Louwers, 1960; Tarazi et al, 1970). The decrease in peripheral resistance may involve a decrease in intracellular sodium as seen in white blood cells (Hilton, 1985), which may be accompanied by decreases in intracellular calcium

(Zidek et al, 1984). Whether these changes in blood cells reflect changes within vessel walls remains to be seen.

**Accompanying Changes**

A number of interrelated hemodynamic changes may influence the degree of blood pressure (BP) reduction with continued diuretic therapy. Those who respond less well with a fall in mean BP of less than 10% were found to have a greater degree of plasma volume depletion and greater stimulation of renin and aldosterone, which likely contributed to a persistently high peripheral resistance (van Brummelen et al, 1980). In those whose BP responds better, the renin levels may rise equally, but the responders may have a lesser response of aldosterone secretion to the same degree of renin-angiotensin stimulation (Weber et al, 1977). Blockage of the reactive rise in renin-angiotensin-aldosterone by addition of an angiotensin-converting enzyme inhibitor will potentiate the antihypertensive action even though there is little additional fluid volume loss (van Schaik et al, 1987).

In addition to causing variable degrees of secondary aldosteronism, diuretics cause a modest rise in plasma norepinephrine levels (Lake et al, 1979). The fall in resistance could be secondary to activation of vasodepressor mechanisms: Both plasma prostacyclin levels (Wilson, 1986) and

**Table 7.5.  Diuretics and Potassium-Sparing Agents**

|  | Daily Dosage (*mg*) | Duration of Action (*hr*) |
|---|---|---|
| **Thiazides** | | |
| Bendroflumethiazide (Naturetin) | 2.5–5.0 | More than 18 |
| Benzthiazide (Aquatag, Exna) | 12.5–50 | 12–18 |
| Chlorothiazide (Diuril) | 125–500 | 6–12 |
| Cyclothiazide (Anhydron) | 0.5–2 | 18–24 |
| Hydrochlorothiazide (Esidrix, HydroDIURIL, Oretic) | 12.5–50 | 12–18 |
| Hydroflumethiazide (Saluron) | 12.5–50 | 18–24 |
| Methyclothiazide (Enduron) | 2.5–5.0 | More than 24 |
| Polythiazide (Renese) | 1–4 | 24–48 |
| Trichlormethiazide (Metahydrin, Naqua) | 1–4 | More than 24 |
| **Related sulfonamide compounds** | | |
| Chlorthalidone (Hygroton) | 12.5–50 | 24–72 |
| Indapamide (Lozol) | 2.5 | 24 |
| Metolazone (Zaroxolyn, Diulo) | 1–10 | 24 |
| Quinethazone (Hydromox) | 25–100 | 18–24 |
| **Loop diuretics** | | |
| Bumetanide (Bumex) | 0.5–5 | 4–6 |
| Ethacrynic acid (Edecrin) | 25–100 | 12 |
| Furosemide (Lasix) | 40–480 | 4–6 |
| **Potassium-sparing agents** | | |
| Amiloride (Midamor) | 5–10 | 24 |
| Spironolactone (Aldactone) | 25–100 | 8–12 |
| Triamterene (Dyrenium) | 50–150 | 12 |

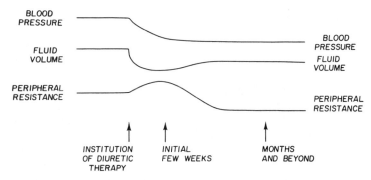

**Figure 7.5.**  Scheme of the hemodynamic changes responsible for the antihypertensive effects of diuretic therapy.

urine kallikrein activity (O'Connor et al, 1981) have been found to be raised in those whose blood pressure responds to diuretics. Moreover, the concomitant intake of inhibitors of prostaglandin synthesis will blunt the effect of most diuretics (Wilson, 1986).

### Special Features of Indapamide

Indapamide (Lozol) is a sulfamoyl chlorobenzamide compound that differs in having no thiazide ring but a methylindoline moiety, which may provide additional antihypertensive actions beyond its diuretic effect (Carretta et al, 1988). It may decrease vascular reactivity and resistance in some special way, perhaps as a weak calcium antagonist (Mironneau, 1988), but the evidence overall is unconvincing that it acts much differently than other thiazides (Chaffman et al, 1984).

It is equally effective in reducing the BP as are thiazides. However, it may not adversely alter serum lipids as do other diuretics. Some report no significant changes in lipids (Gerber et al, 1985); others, rises in total and falls in high-density lipoprotein (HDL)-cholesterol (Osei et al, 1986); yet others, rises in both total and HDL-cholesterol with no change in the ratio between them (Yoshino et al, 1987; Prisant et al, 1989). Lipid problems, then, may be less with indapamide, but hypokalemia can appear with its use (Gerber et al, 1985).

### Clinical Use

After 3 to 4 weeks, when used alone, thiazides achieved a BP decrease that varied from 8/4 to 19/11 mm Hg in two large, controlled clinical studies (VA Cooperative Study, 1962; Smith et al, 1964). In more recent studies comparing the long-term effectiveness of a diuretic with members of other classes of drugs when each is used alone, the antihypertensive effect is quite similar. This includes comparisons with alpha-blockers (Stamler et al, 1988), beta-blockers (Berglund and Andersson, 1981), calcium entry blockers (Frishman et al, 1987), and ACE inhibitors (Woo et al, 1987). Blacks and the elderly may respond better to diuretics than do nonblacks and younger patients (VA Cooperative Study, 1982a; Freis et al, 1988).

Diuretics potentiate the effect of all other antihypertensive agents with the possible exception of calcium entry blockers (Nicholson et al, 1989), perhaps because the CEBs provide their own natriuretic action. This potentiation depends upon the contraction of fluid volume by the diuretic (Finnerty et al, 1970) and the prevention of fluid accumulation that frequently follows the use of other antihypertensive drugs. Due to the altered pressure-natriuresis curve of essential hypertension described in Chapter 3, whenever the blood pressure is lowered, fluid retention is expected (Fig. 7.6). The data from Finnerty et al and from the Cleveland Clinic (Dustan et al, 1972) show the dependence of the continued antihyperten-

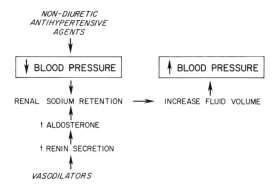

**Figure 7.6.**  Manner by which nondiuretic antihypertensive agents may lose their effectiveness by reactive renal sodium retention.

sive action by various drugs upon the maintenance of a shrunken intravascular volume. Fortunately, more recently introduced therapies, including converting enzyme inhibitors and calcium antagonists, may continue to work without a diuretic, so the need to start or to add a diuretic may no longer be present with their use.

## Dosage

### Monotherapy

The recommended dose of thiazide diuretics has been progressively falling from as high as 200 mg/day of hydrochlorothiazide or equivalent doses of other thiazides in the early 1960s to as little as 10 to 12.5 mg/day in the late 1980s.

In hypertensives with good renal function, most of the antihypertensive effect will be obtained from such small doses with less hypokalemia and other side effects (McVeigh et al, 1988) (Fig. 7.7). McVeigh et al used cyclopenthiazide, which is somewhat longer acting than HCTZ and approximately 70 times more potent milligram for milligram. The one-quarter dose, equivalent to about 9 mg of HCTZ, provided an antihypertensive effect equal to that of the full 500-μg dose equivalent to 35 mg of HCTZ. Rather surprisingly, the 125 μg lowered the BP without raising plasma renin activity, which runs counter to the prevailing opinion that an effective dose of a diuretic, by shrinking fluid volume and lowering blood pressure, would inherently raise PRA.

Beyond questioning the mechanism of action

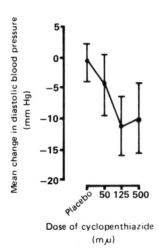

**Figure 7.7.** Antihypertensive effect of a placebo and varying doses of the thiazide diuretic cyclopenthiazide, each given for 8-week intervals to 12 to 15 hypertensives. (From McVeigh G, Galloway D, Johnston D: *Br Med J* 297:95, 1988.)

of diuretics, the data of McVeigh et al bring up two issues: First, what is the least effective dose of a thiazide in the usual hypertensive patient; second, what additional effect will be provided by doses above the least effective dose. As to the first issue, a dose of 12.5 mg of HCTZ will lower the BP by at least 10 mm Hg in perhaps half of patients with mild hypertension, the effect usually somewhat greater on systolic than on diastolic levels (Multicenter Study Group, 1984; McKenney et al, 1986). With the long-acting thiazide derivative chlorthalidone, 15 mg/day provided a 12.6/6.7-mm Hg fall in standing and a 9.0/7.2-mm Hg fall in supine blood pressure in a 12-week study of 71 patients whereas placebo lowered the pressure only a few mm Hg in a parallel group (Vardan et al, 1987). An even larger body of data document an effect from 25 mg of HCTZ or an equivalent dose of other thiazides (Degnbol et al, 1973; Medical Research Council Working Party, 1987).

As to the second issue, larger doses of HCTZ or other thiazides seem to provide some additional antihypertensive effect but the degree is limited, i.e., the dose-response curve with HCTZ is fairly flat. In the Medical Research Council trials (Medical Research Council Working Party, 1987), 5.0 mg of bendrofluazide or 25 mg of HCTZ provided equal antihypertensive efficacy as did twice larger doses. With chlorthalidone, 15 mg provided almost the same effect as 25 (Vardan et al, 1987).

Even though the data confirm a good response to such small doses, some patients will respond more to larger doses. Freis et al (1988) gave HCTZ alone twice a day to 343 patients with mild to moderate hypertension, starting with 50 mg (25 mg twice a day) and doubling the dose every 2 weeks if needed to reduce the DBP to below 90 mm Hg. Of the 65% who responded to diuretic alone, 52% did so with 50 mg/day; an additional 29% required 100 mg/day and 17% more required 200 mg/day.

Whereas others have also found additional effect from larger and larger doses (Henning et al, 1980; Andersson et al, 1984), the majority do not (McKenney et al, 1986; Medical Research Council Working Party, 1987; Wyndham et al, 1987; McVeigh et al, 1988). The overall evidence clearly documents that many will respond to very small doses of thiazide diuretic, i.e., 12.5 mg of HCTZ, and that relatively little additional effect will be achieved by raising the daily dose beyond 50 mg/day.

Parenthetically, the most widely prescribed

diuretic in the United States for many years has been the combination of HCTZ with triamterene, marketed as Dyazide. The capsule contains 25 mg of HCTZ but only about 40% is absorbed, providing the patient with only about 10 mg of the diuretic (Tannenbaum et al, 1968). Dyazide has been most widely prescribed on a one capsule, once-a-day dosage (Baum et al, 1985) that, with only 10 mg of bioavailable HCTZ, presumably has provided all of the antihypertensive effect desired by the majority of practitioners.

## Combination Therapy

Even more convincing data confirm a significant effect of small doses, even below 12.5 mg/day of HCTZ, when diuretics are added to a variety of other drugs to enhance their antihypertensive efficacy. MacGregor et al (1983) reported that 12.5 mg of HCTZ provided an additional effect equivalent to 25 or 50 mg/day when added to 400 mg of acebutolol. Andren et al (1983) and Dahlöf et al (1988) found equivalent additive effects of 6.25, 12.5, and 25 mg of HCTZ added to 10 or 20 mg/day of the ACE inhibitor enalapril.

Again, to be sure, not all agree: MaGee and Freis (1986) found no effect of 12.5 mg of HCTZ added to 80 mg of the beta-blocker nadolol; 25 mg lowered the systolic but it took 50 mg to significantly lower both the systolic and diastolic pressures beyond that seen with nadolol alone.

The logical approach when diuretics are used either alone or in combination for patients with usual hypertension is to use the lowest effective dose. There is no hurry and therefore doses of 12.5 mg/day seem an appropriate starting dose.

## Resistant Patients

In those who respond poorly to small or moderate doses of a thiazide but who have good renal function, excessive dietary sodium intake may overwhelm the diuretic's ability to maintain a shrunken fluid volume (Winer, 1961). For those with renal impairment (i.e., serum creatinine above 2.5 mg/dl or creatinine clearance below 30 ml/minute) thiazides will likely not work, though some find they continue to do so (Jones and Nanra, 1979). Since these drugs must get into the renal tubules to work and since endogenous organic acids that build up in renal insufficiency compete with diuretics for transport into the proximal tubule, the renal response progressively falls with increasing renal damage. The usual choice is to turn to two or three

doses of furosemide or a daily dose of metolazone, which remain effective even in the presence of significant renal insufficiency (Paton and Kane, 1977), since, in large enough doses, adequate amounts of them can reach their site of action. The combination of thiazide with one of these will often work when neither works alone (Wollam et al, 1982).

Food affects the absorption and bioavailability of different diuretics to variable degrees (Neuvonen and Kivistø, 1989), so the drugs should be taken in a uniform pattern as to the time of day and food ingestion.

Nonsteroidal antiinflammatory drugs (NSAIDs) will blunt the effect of most diuretics (Wilson, 1986) mainly by their prevention of diuretic-induced changes in renal hemodynamics, through their inhibition of prostaglandin synthesis (Nies et al, 1983).

## Relation to Renin Levels

As noted previously, the degree of response to diuretics has long been predicated on their capacity to activate the counterregulatory defenses to a lower blood pressure and shrunken fluid volume, in particular, a reactive rise in renin levels. Those who start with low, suppressed plasma renin activity (PRA) levels and who are capable of mounting only a weak rise after diuretics are begun have been assumed to be more "diuretic responsive." Data, mainly from John Laragh's unit, have supported that view: Their patients with low PRA levels had greater falls in BP with diuretic therapy than did those with normal or high PRA (Niarchos and Laragh, 1984).

As logical as this finding seems to be, others have failed to find a relation between response to either HCTZ (Wyndham et al, 1987) or chlorthalidone (Salvetti et al, 1987) with pretreatment PRA levels or to their rise after therapy.

## Side Effects (Fig. 7.8)

The likely pathogenesis for most of the more common complications related to diuretic use arise from the intrinsic activity of the drugs and most are therefore related to the dose and duration of diuretic use. Logically they occur with about the same frequency and severity with equipotent doses of all diuretics, and their occurrence will diminish with lower doses.

In general, the longer lasting the diuretic action, the more the various complications: More hypokalemia occurs when two doses of 50 mg of hydrochlorothiazide are given 12 hours apart

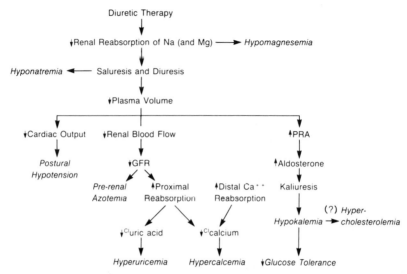

**MECHANISMS BY WHICH CHRONIC DIURETIC THERAPY MAY LEAD TO VARIOUS COMPLICATIONS**

**Figure 7.8.** Mechanisms by which chronic diuretic therapy may lead to various complications. The mechanism for hypercholesterolemia remains in question, although it is shown as arising via hypokalemia.

than when a single dose of 100 mg is given once a day (McInnes et al, 1982).

### Hypokalemia

Urinary potassium wasting occurs with diuretics because they increase delivery of sodium and water to the distal nephron where high levels of aldosterone stimulate potassium secretion (Nader et al, 1988). In a review of published series, the fall in serum potassium with diuretic therapy of hypertension was found to average 0.67 mmol/L (Morgan and Davidson, 1980) (Fig. 7.9). The incidence of hypokalemia, defined as a serum potassium below 3.5 mmol/L or a plasma potassium below 3.3 mmol/L (Hyman and Kaplan, 1985), depends in part upon the height of the pretreatment level: With an average 0.7-mmol/L fall, a patient starting at 3.7 would become hypokalemic; a patient starting at 4.7 would not. It may be more appropriate to consider a fall of greater than 0.5 mmol/L as significant and worthy of correction.

In various series, the percentage of diuretic-treated patients who develop hypokalemia varies from zero to as many as 40%. The differences may reflect variable dietary sodium and potassium intakes, the degree of secondary aldosteronism invoked by the diuretic, the concomitant use of laxatives or other $K^+$-wasting mechanisms, and the unveiling of hypokalemia by intracellular shifts in the presence of acidosis.

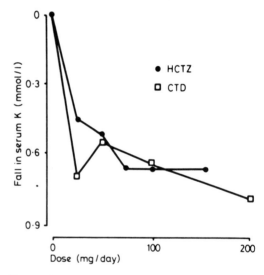

**Figure 7.9.** Mean fall in serum potassium concentration (*mmol/l*) according to dose (*mg*) after chronic hydrochlorothiazide (*HCTZ*) or chlorthalidone (*CTD*) therapy of patients with hypertension. (From Morgan DB, Davidson C: *Br Med J* 280:905, 1980.)

Those who eat more sodium will waste more potassium (Ram et al, 1981); those who eat less potassium, particularly the elderly poor, will be more susceptible (Abdulla et al, 1975).

The plasma contains less than 1% of total body potassium (TBK), most of the remainder being within cells. The majority of isotopic measurements of TBK in hypertensive patients receiving diuretics find only about a 200- to 300-mmol decrease, somewhat less than 10% of body stores, though almost all show a more significant fall in plasma $K^+$ (Nader et al, 1988). Moreover, significant decreases in skeletal muscle $K^+$ may occur after chronic diuretic use despite the maintenance of normal serum $K^+$ levels with potassium supplements (Dørup et al, 1988).

Potassium loss may be partially compensated in time: Both the degree of hypokalemia (Lemieux et al, 1980) and the fall in TBK (Leemhuis et al, 1976) are lessened after a few months, despite continued therapy. This may reflect a decrease in the secretion of potassium after the higher initial fluid flow rate down the nephron has caused more to be swept into the urine (Good and Wright, 1979) as well as a depression of distal nephron $K^+$ excretion and of aldosterone secretion by the lower serum $K^+$ levels.

The degree of hypokalemia is related both to the dose and duration of action of the diuretic (Fig. 7.9). Small doses of long-acting diuretics such as chlorthalidone may cause more hypokalemia since there is no time when the patient is not under the influence of the drug.

Obviously, the physician should always check the blood potassium level before starting diuretic therapy. Hypokalemia unprovoked by diuretics often turns out to be primary aldosteronism (Chapter 13), whereas hypokalemia induced by diuretics very rarely represents that disease (Kaplan, 1967).

*The Dangers of Hypokalemia.* Most of the hazards of diuretic-induced hypokalemia have been seen only with fairly marked $K^+$ depletion (Knochel, 1984). For the typical hypertensive with relatively mild hypokalemia, muscle weakness, polyuria, and a propensity toward arrhythmias might appear. Those on digitalis may develop toxicity (Packer et al, 1986), perhaps because both digitalis and hypokalemia inhibit the sodium-potassium pump, whose activity is essential to normal intracellular electrolyte balance and membrane potential (Cumberbatch and Morgan, 1981).

*Ventricular Arrhythmias and Stress.* A controversy has arisen about whether diuretic-induced hypokalemia can give rise to ventricular ectopic activity that, in turn, could incite fatal arrhythmias. As noted in Chapter 5, the controversy has been incited by the findings of higher rates of coronary mortality, mainly sudden death, in three major trials of the therapy of mild hypertension among patients who had abnormal

electrocardiograms (ECGs) at entry to the trials and who were given high doses of diuretic (see Table 5.6). In addition, a number of small, less well controlled studies have shown a higher rate of serious ventricular arrhythmias among patients who have an acute myocardial infarction (MI) if they are hypokalemic at the time of admission (Duke, 1978; Solomon, 1984; Cooper et al, 1984; Johansson and Dziamski, 1984; Nordrehaug and von der Lippe, 1983) (Fig. 7.10).

The development of hypokalemia in the immediate postinfarct period likely reflects stress-induced falls in blood potassium levels. Blood potassium levels fall significantly within minutes of the infusion of just enough adrenaline to bring the plasma concentration to "stress levels" (Struthers et al, 1983; Brown et al, 1983) (Fig. 7.11). The absolute fall in serum potassium, as much as 1.0 mmol/l, was equally as great after the subjects had received a thiazide diuretic during the prior week, which led to a preinfusion lowering of their serum potassium levels from 3.7 to 3.2 mmol/l.

Therefore, the presence of prior diuretic-induced hypokalemia will obviously increase the likelihood of more serious hypokalemia appearing after stress. This adrenaline-mediated fall in serum potassium represents a $beta_2$-receptor-mediated activation of the $Na^+$, $K^+$-ATPase pump that causes potassium to enter cells in exchange for sodium. Prevention of such $beta_2$-receptor-mediated shifts of potassium could explain much of the protection against mortality in patients given beta-blocker drugs immediately after an acute myocardial infarction (Johansson, 1986).

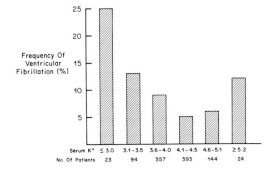

**Figure 7.10.** Number and percentage of patients with acute myocardial infarction developing ventricular fibrillation over the next 2 days in relation to serum potassium concentration on admission. Of the 117 patients with hypokalemia, 17.2% developed ventricular fibrillation, as compared with 7.5% of the 918 normokalaemic patients (p < 0.01). (From Nordrehaug JE, von der Lippe G: *Br Heart J* 50:525, 1983.)

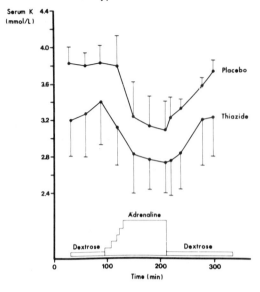

**Figure 7.11.** Serum potassium (mean ± SD) during infusion of 5% dextrose, 0.06 μg/kg/minute of adrenaline, and 5% dextrose again in six healthy subjects after pretreatment with placebo or bendrofluazide (5 mg) for 7 days. (From Struthers AD, Whitesmith R, Reid JL: *Lancet* 1:1358, 1983.)

*Ventricular Ectopic Activity.* The increased likelihood of ventricular arrhythmias noted in multiple series suggests a hazard from diuretic-induced hypokalemia. They likely interact with the increasingly recognized hazard for sudden death in the large portion of hypertensives who have left ventricular hypertrophy (Messerli et al, 1984; Levy et al, 1987). That portion, perhaps half of the hypertensive population, have an increased frequency of complex ventricular arrhythmias that may contribute to their higher risk of sudden death (McLenachan et al, 1987).

With diuretics, extracellular potassium concentration tends to fall more than intracellular levels, thereby hyperpolarizing the cell membrane and leading to an increased threshold for excitation. Although this may reduce the likelihood of arrhythmias due to reentrant phenomena, hypokalemia, by delaying conduction and prolonging the duration of the action potential, may lower the threshold for ventricular fibrillation (Hohnloser et al, 1986). This may develop most commonly in the presence of Q-T prolongation (Khan et al, 1981), which may lead to the bizarre form of ventricular tachycardia known as torsade de pointe (McKibbin et al, 1984).

The issue has been examined by simply observing asymptomatic hypertensives before and after they are made hypokalemic with diuretics. The first study (Holland et al, 1981) gave strong

evidence for increased VEA with diuretic-induced hypokalemia; subsequent studies have both confirmed and denied the association (Table 7.6). In addition, Hollifield (1984) and Bause et al (1987) have reported higher frequencies of exercise-related VEA after diuretic therapy. Moreover, diuretic therapy and hypokalemia were associated with the development of a significantly greater frequency of ventricular premature beats on routine ECGS in over 12,000 men enrolled in the MRFIT study (Cohen et al, 1987). On the other hand, diuretic-induced hypokalemia was not a risk factor for coronary mortality among 3783 treated hypertensives in Glasgow (Robertson et al, 1986).

The issue is not settled. As Freis (1986; 1989) argues, most of the studies shown in Table 7.6 to be associated with a higher incidence of VEA can be faulted for various reasons. Some did not have a prediuretic monitor and others used only 24 hours of monitoring, which may preclude the ability to distinguish the natural marked variability in VEA from an induced change. Others found the problem among patients with preexisting coronary disease, a group that differs from the larger population of uncomplicated hypertensives. Nonetheless, the evidence, both circumstantial and direct, strongly suggests the need for caution. I believe that significant falls in serum potassium of more than 0.5 mmol/l should be corrected (Kaplan, 1984). Others believe that more harm than good will likely follow the wider use of potassium sparers and supplements that such a course would entail (Kassirer and Harrington, 1985).

*Effect on Blood Pressure.* Hypokalemia can set off various processes that can affect the blood pressure (Ullian and Linas, 1987). Dietary potassium depletion has been found to raise the blood pressure (Krishna et al, 1989). The correction of diuretic-induced hypokalemia has been shown to result in a lowering of the mean blood pressure by an average of 5.5 mm Hg in a group of 16 hypertensives on a constant dose of diuretic (Kaplan et al, 1985).

## Management of Diuretic-Induced Hypokalemia

Prevention is preferable. By lowering dietary sodium, increasing dietary potassium, and using the least amount of diuretic needed, potassium depletion may be avoided. A lower dietary sodium intake (72 mmol/day) reduced diuretic-induced $K^+$ loss by half of that observed on a higher sodium intake (195 mmol/day) (Ram et

**Table 7.6. Ventricular Ectopic Activity with Diuretic-Induced Hypokalemia**

| Reference | Known Coronary Disease | Length of Monitoring (hr) | Duration of Diuretic Therapy | Average Fall in Serum $K^+$ | Incidence of Lown Grades 3–5 VEA per Number of Subjects |
|---|---|---|---|---|---|
| Holland et al, 1981 | – | 24 | 4 wk | 4.0 → 3.0 | 4/21 |
| Madias et al, 1984 | – | 24 | 4 wk | 4.4 → 3.0 | 0/20 |
| Caralis et al, 1984[a,b] | + | 24 | 4–6 wk | 4.1 → 3.4 | 5/8 |
| Whelton, 1984[c] | – | | 2 mo | 4.1 → 3.8 | 0/39 |
| Whelton, 1984[b,c] | – | 24 | 6+ mo | 4.1 → 3.6 | 27/82 |
| Lief et al, 1984 (abstract) | – | 48 | 1–6 mo | 4.0 → 3.0 | 0/13 |
| Stewart et al, 1985 | + | 24 | 8 wk | 4.3 → 3.3 | 5/9 |
| Ragnarsson et al, 1987[c] | – | 24 | ? | 4.0 → 3.7 | 19/42 |
| Holland et al, 1988[b] | – | 48 | 4 wk | 4.1 → 3.2 | 6/21 |
| Papademetriou et al, 1988 | – | 48 | 4 wk | 4.1 → 3.4 | 10/27 (11/27 before diuretic) |

[a]At baseline, six of the eight had some Grade 3 VEA; after diuretic-induced hypokalemia, seven of eight had significantly more Grade 3 VEA and five of eight had Grade 4A VEA.
[b]These studies also demonstrated decreases in VEA after correction of hypokalemia.
[c]No baseline monitoring.

al, 1981). Dietary sources of extra $K^+$ may be higher in calories as well, but fresh vegetables may provide a moderate amount of $K^+$ without excessive calories. A $K^+$-sparing agent with the diuretic will reduce the degree of $K^+$ loss (Nader et al, 1988) but may not prevent the development of hypokalemia (Sawyer and Gabriel, 1988). A beta-blocker or converting enzyme inhibitor may blunt diuretic-induced $K^+$ loss; one either may be added to the diuretic if two drugs are needed or may be used in its place.

If prevention does not work, the $K^+$ deficiency can be replaced with supplemental $K^+$ preferably given as the chloride; other anions will not correct the alkalosis or correct the intracellular $K^+$ deficiency as well (Schwartz et al, 1968). However, K citrate may be used, particularly in patients given a thiazide to reduce urinary calcium excretion in order to prevent renal stones (Nicar et al, 1984). The KCl may be given as a potassium-containing salt substitute; a number are available, and they are less expensive than potassium supplements (Sopko and Freeman, 1977).

If additional potassium is needed, potassium chloride in a microencapsulated form can be safely used and is much more acceptable to patients than the various liquid preparations. The microencapsulated form causes fewer upper gastrointestinal (GI) mucosal lesions (Hutcheon et al, 1988) and less upper GI bleeding (Strom et al, 1987) than the wax-matrix form.

The amount of supplemental potassium needed to overcome thiazide-induced hypokalemia, if the patient is continued on the thiazide, was found to be 40 to 60 mEq per day (Schwartz

and Swartz, 1974). In those who need continued diuretic therapy, the combination with a $K^+$-sparing agent may be safer and more physiological than the administration of supplemental KCl (Krishna et al, 1988): (1) The $K^+$-sparer will diminish additional $K^+$ wastage, whereas most of the KCl will be excreted; (2) The $K^+$-sparer will reduce acid excretion, helping overcome the accompanying metabolic alkalosis; and (3) The $K^+$-sparer will help prevent further diuretic-induced magnesium wastage.

In addition to the rare occurrence of GI bleeding, adverse reactions to KCl supplements were noted in 5.8% of almost 5000 patients, the most common being hyperkalemia (Lawson, 1974). Most of these adverse effects were seen in elderly patients, those with renal insufficiency, and those given both oral and parenteral potassium, and most of the seven fatalities were related to inappropriate use of KCl.

**Hypomagnesemia**

Many of the problems attributed to hypokalemia may be caused by hypomagnesemia instead, and potassium repletion may not be possible in the presence of magnesium depletion.

Serum magnesium levels below 0.6 mmol/l (1.2 mEq/l) have been found in about 7% of hospitalized patients (Whang, 1984) and in 19% of those receiving digitalis (Whang et al, 1985b). In another survey, 41% of patients found to have hypokalemia also had hypomagnesemia (Whang et al, 1984). The importance of magnesium— the second most prevalent intracellular cation— has been more widely recognized as ''nature's physiologic calcium blocker'' (Iseri and French,

1984). Evidence of the potentially serious consequences of magnesium depletion keeps growing (Altura and Altura, 1984; Whang et al, 1985a,b).

*Features of Magnesium Depletion.* The symptoms and signs tend to progress from weakness, nausea, and neuromuscular irritability to tetany, mental changes and convulsions and, finally, to stupor and coma. An important feature is the appearance of ventricular arrhythmias, particularly on the background of digitalis therapy, which are resistant to repletion of concomitant hypokalemia (Whang et al, 1985a).

The arrhythmias may arise from the inhibiting effect of magnesium deficiency on cell membrane $Na^+$, $K^+$-ATPase pump activity, with resultant partial depolarization causing hyperirritability of excitable tissues. Since the impaired pump is less able to transfer extracellular potassium into cells, attempts to correct intracellular potassium depletion by raising blood potassium levels may be unsuccessful. Such pump inhibition may lead not only to cardiac irritability but also, by increasing intracellular free calcium, to increased tone and reactivity of vascular smooth muscle (Altura and Altura, 1984).

*Role of Diuretics.* Although loop diuretics tend to cause more urinary magnesium loss than do thiazides, hypomagnesemia and significant cellular depletion may occur with either (Dørup et al, 1988). The urinary loss of magnesium may reflect both inhibition of tubular magnesium reabsorption (which is mainly in the thick ascending portion of the loop of Henle, where the loop diuretics work) as well as interactions between diuretic-induced changes in calcium handling and magnesium excretion (Leary and Reyes, 1984).

Relatively few uncomplicated hypertensives on reasonable doses of diuretic will develop clinically important Mg deficiency although the frequency may be higher in the elderly (Martin and Milligan, 1987). Hypomagnesemia was rare with doses of thiazide below 100 mg/day but was seen in 12% of those on that dose (Kroenke et al, 1987). In a portion of the participants in the MRFIT trial, low serum Mg levels were found in about 15% of those having taken a diuretic for 6 to 7 years (Kuller et al, 1985). In that trial and elsewhere, chlorthalidone use has been associated with more Mg deficiency (Cocco et al, 1987).

Magnesium wastage is lessened by use of smaller doses of diuretics. Concomitant use of a potassium-sparing agent may also decrease Mg wastage (Martin and Milligan, 1987). Oral magnesium oxide, 200 to 400 mg/day (10 to 20 mmol) may be tolerated without GI distress (Reinhart, 1988).

## Hyperuricemia

High plasma uric acid levels are seen in as many as 30% of untreated hypertensives and may reflect early renal vascular damage (Messerli et al, 1980). Thiazide therapy increases the incidence of hyperuricemia and may provoke gout, with an annual incidence of 4.9% at levels above 9 mg/dl (Campion et al, 1987). Since the thiazides induce hyperuricemia by decreasing renal uric acid excretion as a result of the shrinkage in plasma volume (Weinman et al, 1975), the fear was voiced that slowly progressive urate deposition in the kidneys would occur and contribute to a deterioration in renal function (Cannon et al, 1966). Despite their continuous use for over 12 years, evidence of overt renal damage attributable to thiazides was not observed (Beevers et al, 1971). Moreover in 524 gouty subjects followed for up to 12 years, hyperuricemia alone had no deleterious effect on renal function (Berger and Yu, 1975).

Therefore, the opinion of most experts is that thiazide-induced hyperuricemia need not be treated (Campion et al, 1987). However, hyperuricemia has been noted to be associated with higher mortality independent of all other known risk factors in a 12-year follow-up of Swedish women (Bengtsson et al, 1988). If the plasma uric acid level is above 9 mg/dl in women or 10 mg/dl in men, therapy to reduce the level may be indicated, mainly to prevent gout and perhaps to reduce cardiovascular risk as well, although most would wait for the first kidney stone or other evidence of trouble before commencing therapy (Dykman et al, 1987). If therapy is to be given, the logical choice is probenecid to increase renal excretion of uric acid. Only in patients who are hyperuricemic from excessive uric acid production, unrelated to diuretic use, should allopurinol be used since it may cause serious toxicity (Dykman et al, 1987).

For a short time, a uricosuric diuretic, ticrynafen, was available, but the appearance of hepatic toxicity caused it to be removed from clinical use (Yu et al, 1981). Other uricosuric diuretics, including indacrinone (Brooks et al, 1984) and traxanox (Fujimura et al, 1989), are under investigation.

## Hypercalcemia

Along with the increase in renal uric acid reabsorption, calcium reabsorption is also increased with chronic thiazide therapy, and urinary calcium excretion is decreased by 40 to 50% (Nader et al, 1988). A slight rise in serum calcium, i.e., 0.1 to 0.2 mg/dl, is usual, but hypercalcemia in previously normocalcemic patients occurs rarely (Duarte et al, 1971). Hypercalcemia is much more frequently provoked in patients with preexisting hyperparathyroidism or vitamin D-treated hypoparathyroidism. The fact that serum calcium levels do not continue to rise in the face of reduced calcium excretion likely reflects the combination of reduced intestinal absorption of calcium (Sakhaee et al, 1984; Bushinsky et al, 1984) and retention of calcium in bone (Lemann et al, 1985). The former effect likely reflects a suppression of parathyroid hormone and vitamin D synthesis from the slight hypercalcemia and makes thiazide therapy a practical way to treat patients with renal stones caused by hypercalciuria from increased calcium absorption. The latter effect may offer protection from osteoporosis (Ray et al, 1989) and fractures (La Croix et al, 1990).

## Hyperlipidemia

Although thiazide-induced hypercholesterolemia was reported in 1964 (Schoenfeld and Goldberger, 1964), the problem was not widely recognized until the report by Ames and Hill in 1976 of a rise in serum cholesterol of 12 mg/dl and in serum triglyceride of 26 mg/dl in 32 hypertensives treated for 1 year with chlorthalidone. Since then, multiple reports have documented the adverse effects on serum lipids of various diuretics (Lardinois and Neuman, 1988; Pollare et al, 1989). Total serum cholesterol, low density lipoprotein (LDL)-cholesterol, and triglyceride levels rise, whereas high density lipoprotein (HDL)-cholesterol levels tend not to change (Weidmann et al, 1985) (Fig 7.12). Fewer lipid changes have been noted with indapamide (Gerber et al, 1985).

The question has been raised as to the duration of the lipid-altering effects of diuretics (Freis, 1989). The majority of the studies in Weidmann and associates' survey were of short duration. In two studies, the lipid-raising effect of diuretics appeared to disappear after 1 year (Veterans Administration Cooperative Study Group, 1982a) or 2 years (Williams et al, 1986) of con-

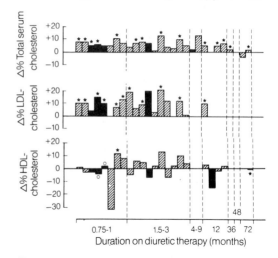

**Figure 7.12.** Percentage of changes in serum lipoprotein-cholesterol fractions as related to the duration of a monotherapy with thiazide-type (*hatched bars*) or loop diuretics (*solid bars*). The data shown are from published studies with a minimum number of 10 subjects and a minimum duration of 4 weeks. *Asterisks* (*) denote statistically significant changes as compared with pretreatment conditions, p < 0.05. *Open circles* (○) denote measurements by electrophoresis. (From Weidmann P, Uehlinger DE, Gerber A: *J Hypertension* 3:297, 1985.)

tinued therapy. In the analysis by Williams et al (1986) of part of the HDFP trial population who received chlorthalidone, the initial rise in serum cholesterol was noted only in those with baseline levels below 250 mg/dl; those with initially higher levels tended to show a progressive fall. This may reflect a regression toward the mean or changes in weight or diet.

On the other hand, persistent hyperlipidemic effects of diuretic therapy have been observed in small groups (Middeke et al, 1987) and in the large population of the MRFIT trial (Lasser et al, 1984). In the latter trial, in the presence of diuretic therapy, the fall in plasma cholesterol accomplished with an intensive dietary program was significantly less, as compared with that achieved by the same cholesterol-lowering regimen in the absence of diuretics (Lasser et al, 1984). Those taking a diuretic had cholesterol higher by 4 mg/dl, HDL-cholesterol lower by 0.8 mg/dl, and triglyceride higher by 35 mg/dl at the end of 6 years than did those not taking a diuretic. With the large number of patients involved (more than 3200), these differences are statistically highly significant.

Although some downplay the potential hazard and emphasize the transient nature of these changes, diuretic therapy may adversely alter lipids. According to estimates from Framingham data, the adverse lipid changes could largely negate the benefits of the lower blood pressure achieved by diuretic therapy (Ames, 1988).

The mechanism for the effect is unknown. Since the change in cholesterol was correlated to decreases in glucose tolerance, Ames has postulated that the same mechanism is responsible for both (Ames, 1984). Though these are both shown to result from hypokalemia in Figure 7.8, the mechanism has not been identified. It can occur with as little as 12.5 mg of HCTZ a day (McKenney et al, 1986) and in the absence of a significant fall in serum potassium (Anderson et al, 1985). When a potassium sparer was given with HCTZ (average daily dose of 50 mg of each) to 44 hypertensives for 3 months, the lipid abnormalities and glucose intolerance developed despite no change in plasma potassium levels (Ames, 1989).

Regardless of how it comes about and even if it is only transient, adverse lipid changes can occur with diuretic use. Lipid levels should be monitored; a low-saturated fat diet should be encouraged; and, if necessary, other agents, such as spironolactone or other classes of antihypertensive drugs, should be chosen (Ames and Peacock, 1984). Caution is even more important in view of the evidence that hypertension and hyperlipidemia frequently coexist (Williams et al, 1988).

### Hyperglycemia

Impairment of glucose tolerance, a decrease in insulin sensitivity, worsening of diabetic control, and, rarely, precipitation of overt diabetes have been observed in patients taking thiazides (Wilkins, 1959; Goldner et al, 1960; Pollare et al, 1989). Very rarely, diuretics may precipitate hyperosmolar nonketotic diabetic coma, particularly in elderly patients (Fonseca and Phear, 1982).

In a prospective study involving 137 hypertensives who started with normal glucose tolerance, 1 year of therapy with various diuretics did not significantly alter mean levels of blood sugar, insulin, or free fatty acids (Kohner et al, 1971). Further observation of 51 of these patients showed a significant deterioration of glucose tolerance after 6 years of diuretic therapy (Lewis et al, 1976). After 14 years, the 34 of these patients still being followed had higher glucose levels, both fasting and after an oral glucose load (Murphy et al, 1982) (Fig. 7.13).

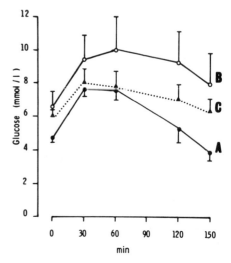

**Figure 7.13.** Results of oral glucose tolerance tests before (*A*) and after (*B*) 14 years of thiazide treatment, and 7 months after withdrawal of therapy (*C*) (n = 10). (From Murphy MB, Kohner E, Lewis PJ, et al: *Lancet* 2:1293, 1982.)

Note that glucose levels fell significantly 7 months after withdrawal of thiazide therapy (curve C in Fig. 7.13). In another study, increased risk of developing diabetes over a 12-year follow-up was noted in patients taking diuretics, as compared with those not taking antihypertensive drugs (Bengtsson et al, 1984). Not all report a worsening of glucose tolerance with chronic diuretic therapy: 2.5 mg of bendroflumethazide given to 37 men for 10 years did not (Berglund et al, 1986).

As with rises in plasma lipids, these adverse effects on glucose metabolism may pose additional risks for cardiovascular disease (Fuller et al, 1983; Pollare et al, 1989). The decrease in insulin sensitivity, reflected in higher plasma insulin levels (Swislocki et al, 1989) may turn out to be a major problem since hyperinsulinemia appears to be a factor in the cardiovascular risks associated with upper body obesity and a pressor mechanism in the pathogenesis of primary hypertension, as delineated in Chapter 3.

### Hyponatremia

This occurs less commonly in edema-free hypertensives than in edematous patients given thiazides for diuresis. With chronic diuretic use, the contraction of effective blood volume will decrease the ability of the kidney to excrete water, and slight, asymptomatic falls in serum sodium concentration may be noted (Nader et al, 1988).

Rarely, severe, symptomatic hyponatremia develops, usually soon after diuretics are started
in elderly female patients who appear to have
an expanded fluid volume from increased water
intake in the face of a decreased ability to excrete free water (Friedman et al, 1989).

## Miscellaneous

Fever and chills (Hoss and Nierenberg, 1988),
blood dyscrasias, pancreatitis, necrotizing vasculitis, acute interstitial nephritis (Magil et al,
1980), and noncardiogenic pulmonary edema
(Bowden, 1989) have been seen rarely. A 2-
fold increase in the risk of acute cholecystitis
was noted in two case-control studies (Rosenberg et al, 1980; Van der Linden et al, 1984)
but not in another (Porter et al, 1981). Allergic
skin rashes occur in 0.28% of patients (Arndt
and Jick, 1976) and a few cases of cutaneous
lupus erythematosus have been reported (Reed
et al, 1985). As with all other antihypertensive
agents, impotence has been reported with diuretic therapy: In the large randomized MRC
trial, impotence was complained about by 22.6%
of the men on bendrofluazide, as compared with
a rate of 10.1% among those on placebo and
13.2% among those on propranolol (Medical
Research Council Working Party, 1981).

## Loop Diuretics

The other class of diuretics used to treat hypertension primarily block chloride reabsorption
by inhibition of the $Na^+/K^+/Cl^-$ cotransport
system of the luminal membrane of the thick
ascending limb of Henle's loop and thereby cause
a marked sodium chloride diuresis (Hendry and
Ellory, 1988). The loop diuretics are more potent and have a more rapid onset of action than
the thiazides. However, they are no more effective in lowering the blood pressure or less
likely to cause side effects if given in equipotent
amounts. They are effective in the presence of
renal insufficiency, as is metolazone, a thiazide
derivative that also blocks sodium reabsorption
in the proximal tubule (Paton and Kane, 1977).

### Furosemide (Lasix)

Used intravenously, this potent diuretic is very
helpful in the treatment of acute hypertensive
crises (see Chapter 8). Given orally, it may be
especially useful in the control of the volume-
dependent hypertension commonly accompanying chronic renal disease (see Chapter 9) and
in patients with severe hypertension (Mroczek
et al, 1974).

Furosemide is being widely used in the treatment of uncomplicated primary hypertension,
but when given twice daily in 40-mg doses it
was less effective than 50 mg of hydrochlorothiazide twice daily, while producing similar
hyperuricemia and hypokalemia (Anderson et
al, 1971). Although some report good antihypertensive effects from once daily 40- to 80-mg
doses of furosemide (Mroczek et al, 1978), most
agree with the findings of Anderson et al that
even twice daily furosemide is less effective
than twice daily hydrochlorothiazide (Araoye et
al, 1978; Holland et al, 1979) or once daily
chlorthalidone (Healy et al, 1970). The need to
maintain a slightly shrunken body fluid volume
that is critical for an antihypertensive action from
diuretic therapy is not met by the short duration
of furosemide action, less than 6 hours for an
oral dose; during the remaining hours, sodium
is retained so that fluid balance is left unaltered
(Wilcox et al, 1983). There thus seems little
reason to favor it over thiazides in the majority
of patients with uncomplicated hypertension. If
furosemide is used twice daily, the first dose
should be given early in the morning and, the
second in the midafternoon both to provide diuretic action at the time of sodium intake and
to avoid nocturia.

One indication for the use of a loop diuretic
is in patients on lithium who may have a rise
in serum levels when given a thiazide, presumably from enhanced proximal reabsorption of
lithium. With furosemide, no increase was seen,
perhaps because lithium reabsorption in the loop
of Henle was blocked (Jefferson and Kalin, 1979).

Loop diuretics may cause fewer metabolic
problems than longer-acting agents because of
their shorter duration of action (Nader et al,
1988). With similar durations of action, the side
effects are similar, including the hyperlipidemic
effect (Fig. 7.12). Pancreatitis (Stenvinkel et al,
1988) and inhibition of insulin release (Sandström and Sehlin, 1988) are two more of the
thiazide-associated problems also seen with furosemide.

Probenecid prolongs the duration of furosemide's action (Chennavasin et al, 1979) whereas
prostaglandin inhibitors block the immediate hemodynamic effects and some of the diuretic and
antihypertensive effect of furosemide (Brater,
1985).

### Bumetanide (Bumex)

This agent, though 40 times more potent than
furosemide on a weight basis, is identical in its

actions when given in an equivalent dose (Ramsay et al, 1978).

### Ethacrynic Acid (Edecrin)

Though structurally different from furosemide, this drug also works primarily in the ascending limb of Henle and has an equal potency. It is used much less than furosemide, mainly because of its greater propensity to cause permanent hearing loss (Cooperman and Rubin, 1973).

### Metolazone (Diulo, Microx, Zaroxolyn)

This long-acting thiazide derivative also has the ability to maintain its effect in the presence of renal insufficiency (Paton and Kane, 1977). Small doses (0.5 to 1.0 mg/day) of a new formulation (Microx) (Miller et al, 1988) may be equal to ordinary long-acting thiazide diuretics, and the agent may be particularly useful in patients with azotemia and resistant hypertension.

### Loop Diuretics under Investigation

A number of loop diuretics are currently under investigation and may become available in the United States (Beermann and Grind, 1987). These include a number that are similar to furosemide: azosemide, etozoline, muzolimine, piretanide, and torasemide. None seems to offer any advantage over furosemide except muzolimine, which is considerably longer acting.

In addition, two other agents, mefruside (Henningsen et al, 1980) and xipamide (Ramsay and Freestone, 1984), share some properties: They structurally are a cross between the thiazides and furosemide and are similar to the thiazides in action.

## Potassium-Sparing Agents

These drugs act in the distal tubule to prevent potassium loss, one (spironolactone) as an aldosterone antagonist, the others (triamterene and amiloride) as direct inhibitors of potassium secretion (Krishna et al, 1988). All three are effective in reducing diuretic-induced $K^+$ wastage, but progressive hypokalemia may still occur with their use (Sawyer and Gabriel, 1988). With less hypokalemia, less hypercholesterolemia may develop with their use but adequate controlled comparisons are not available.

### Spironolactone (Aldactone)

The similarities in the structure of spironolactone to that of the mineralocorticoid hormones enable this drug, when given in relatively large amounts, to inhibit competitively the binding of those steroids to their intracellular receptors, thereby antagonizing their physiological effects (Krishna et al, 1988). Three clinical uses for this antagonism are:

—as a diagnostic test and relatively specific therapy for the hypertension associated with primary aldosteronism (see Chapter 13);
—as a diuretic in edematous states such as nephrosis and cirrhosis with ascites, wherein very high levels of aldosterone play a major role;
—as an inhibitor of the aldosterone-mediated exchange of $Na^+$ and $K^+$ in the distal tubule to prevent potassium wastage.

This latter action provides the major place for spironolactone in the treatment of primary hypertension although the drug will provide significant antihypertensive effect on its own if given in modest doses. When used alone in average doses of 100 mg once per day, it produced a 18/10-mm Hg fall in blood pressure over a mean follow-up of 20 months (Jeunemaitre et al, 1987). With that dose, gynecomastia was noted in 37 of 222 men. With doses of 25 to 50 mg/day, gynecomastia was seen in 30 of 431 men, but the blood pressure fell only half as much. When spironolactone alone was compared with the combinations of a thiazide with either triamterene or amiloride, all three provided comparable antihypertensive efficacy but the plasma $K^+$ rose 0.7 mmol/L with spironolactone and only 0.1 to 0.2 mmol/L with the combinations (Jeunemaitre et al, 1988). When used in smaller doses in combination with HCTZ (Aldactazide tablets with 25 mg of spironolactone and 25 mg of HCTZ), less hypokalemia develops than with the thiazide alone, and side effects seen with higher doses of spironolactone—gynecomastia and amenorrhea—rarely occur.

As with the other $K^+$ sparers caution is advised in the presence of renal insufficiency, wherein hyperkalemia may appear because of the decreased ability to excrete potassium. The natriuresis induced by spironolactone is antagonized by aspirin (Tweeddale and Ogilvie, 1973).

A disturbing association with breast cancer was suggested in a letter to the editor of *Lancet* (Loube and Quirk, 1975). No documentation has followed, and no association was found in a careful study (Jick and Armstrong, 1975). However, spironolactone has been shown to be a tumorigen in chronic toxicity studies in rats.

## Triamterene (Dyrenium)

Though this drug has less intrinsic antihypertensive action than spironolactone (McKenna et al, 1971), it acts to inhibit potassium wasting with no hormonal side effects. It enhances the natriuretic effect of thiazides while minimizing their kaliuretic effect (Krishna et al, 1988) and preserves serum and muscle potassium and magnesium levels (Widmann et al, 1988).

For many years a combination of HCTZ, 25 mg, plus triamterene, 50 mg, marketed as Dyazide, was the most widely prescribed antihypertensive drug in the United States. The capsule formulation of Dyazide in some way reduced the absorption of both ingredients to about 30 to 40% (Tannenbaum et al, 1968).

A new tablet formulation of the combination of HCTZ and triamterene has been marketed under the trade name Maxzide, which allows 60 to 80% of both ingredients to be absorbed (Williams et al, 1987a). Maxzide was first marketed in a dose of 50 mg of HCTZ plus 75 mg of triamterene. The larger amount of HCTZ—actually some 3 to 4 times more than that provided in Dyazide—may be more diuretic than needed and could lead to more of the various thiazide-related side effects. Fortunately, a lower-dose formulation with 25 mg of HCTZ and 37.5 mg of triamterene is now available. Even with that lower dose, the logical starting dose is one-half tablet per day.

Triamterene may be excreted into the urine and may find its way into renal stones (Sörgel et al, 1985). However, no higher frequency of hospitalization for renal stones was found among users of triamterene than among users of HCTZ alone or with other drugs (Jick et al, 1982). The simultaneous use of triamterene and the prostaglandin inhibitor indomethacin has been reported to induce reversible acute renal failure (Sica and Gehr, 1989).

## Amiloride (Midamor)

Amiloride is structurally different from both spironolactone and triamterene. It inhibits a number of transport proteins that facilitate the movement of sodium ions either alone or linked with hydrogen or calcium. By blocking the entry of sodium into distal convoluted tubular cells, potassium loss through potassium channels is diminished (Scoble et al, 1986).

Amiloride has some antihypertensive effect of its own (Katzman et al, 1988) and may therefore potentiate the effect of thiazide diuretic while at the same time blunting the renal wastage of potassium. It is largely used in combination with HCTZ as Moduretic, containing 50 mg of HCTZ and 5 mg of amiloride.

Side effects have been infrequent; nausea, flatulence, and skin rash have been the most frequent and hyperkalemia the most serious. However, a disturbingly large number of cases of hyponatremia in elderly patients have been reported after its use (Millson et al, 1984).

## ADRENERGIC-INHIBITING DRUGS

This group of drugs includes some that act centrally, others peripherally, either on alpha- or beta-receptors. To understand the action of these drugs, let us briefly consider the workings of the sympathetic nervous system. The effects of the system are mediated by the actions of norepinephrine (noradrenaline) released locally from postganglionic nerve endings and epinephrine (adrenaline) released from the adrenal medulla; these actions begin with the binding of the catecholamines to receptors located on the external surface of the effector cell membrane. Receptor occupancy is transduced by specific guanine nucleotide binding (G) proteins into activation of second messengers within the cell, which in turn activate those responses characteristic of the particular tissue (Insel, 1989).

Ahlquist (1948) found that the responses to catecholamines in various tissues were mediated through two distinct types of receptors, termed alpha and beta, based upon different degrees of responsiveness to agonists (Fig. 7.14). Subsequently, two subtypes of beta-receptors, termed $beta_1$ and $beta_2$ (Lands et al, 1967), and two subtypes of alpha receptors, termed $alpha_1$ and $alpha_2$, have been characterized (Langer, 1974; Berthelsen and Pettinger, 1977).

Various sympathetic nervous system actions are mediated by different adrenergic receptor types. Some of the alpha and beta effects antagonize one another; others are complementary. A number of drugs act as either *agonists* (i.e., possess both affinity for and efficacy at receptors) or *antagonists* (i.e., possess affinity but no efficacy and, therefore, antagonize natural agonists). Weak agonists, termed *partial agonists*, cannot evoke the maximal response of which the cell is capable but have enough affinity for the receptor to antagonize the natural agonists.

Receptor numbers decrease after chronic exposure to agonists, i.e., desensitization, whereas receptor numbers increase after diminished ex-

Presynaptic          Postsynaptic

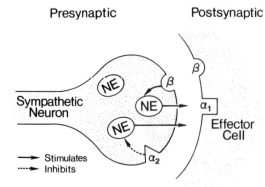

→ Stimulates
┄┄► Inhibits

**Figure 7.14.** Simplified schematic view of the adrenergic nerve ending showing that norepinephrine (*NE*) is released from the storage granules when the nerve is stimulated and enters the synaptic cleft to bind to alpha$_1$- and beta-receptors on the effector cell (postsynaptic). In addition, a short feedback loop exists, in which NE binds to alpha$_2$- and beta-receptors on the neuron (presynaptic), either to inhibit or to stimulate further release.

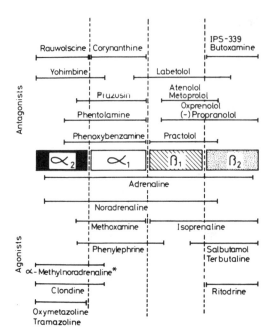

**Figure 7.15.** Schematic representation of range of actions of agonists and antagonists at adrenoceptors; some are used solely for purposes of defining subclass of receptor mediating an effect. *Length of bar* gives indication of occurrence of effect at subclass of receptor and indication of the chances of a clinically important effect being produced. (From Lees GM: *Br Med J* 283:175, 1981.)

posure to agonists, i.e., super sensitization (Sibley and Lefkowitz, 1988). The former likely explains the lesser response to exogenous catecholamines in patients with a pheochromocytoma; the latter, the tendency for patients treated with beta-blocking drugs to develop coronary ischemia when the drugs are withdrawn, at which time the increased number of receptors are suddenly exposed to agonist effects.

The range of actions of agonists and antagonists upon various adrenergic receptors is shown in Figure 7.15. Some of these agents are used only to identify the subgroups, but most are used for various effects upon the heart and vasculature. Those currently used to treat hypertension are shown in Table 7.4. Those that interfere with the normal release of norepinephrine at the nerve endings are referred to as peripheral neuronal blocking drugs. Another group act centrally by stimulating alpha-receptors. Others block the alpha- or beta-adrenergic receptor sites on the effector cells: Prazosin is one of the alpha-blockers and propranolol, the first widely used beta-blocker.

## PERIPHERAL ADRENERGIC INHIBITORS

### Reserpine

Although it also has central effects, the major hypotensive action of reserpine is peripheral (Boura and Green, 1984).

Reserpine is an effective, inexpensive, easy-to-take, and generally safe drug. When compared with methyldopa and propranolol, reser-

pine was found to be best (Finnerty et al, 1979). Reserpine was used in the original VA Cooperative Studies and in the more recent HDFP trial that proved the efficacy of drug therapy. In the United States, it is being used less and less. The reasons for this lesser use include these:

—Because it is an inexpensive generic drug, reserpine has no constituency pushing for its use.

—Reserpine has become old hat; the advent of every new "miracle" antihypertensive makes it look more and more outdated.

—The scare of cancer has tainted reserpine, although the claims have been refuted (Horwitz and Feinstein, 1985).

—The lurking specter of insidious depression also scares us away from its use although this seems to be a rare problem with current dosage.

### Chemistry

Reserpine, one of the many alkaloids of the Indian snakeroot *Rauwolfia serpentina*, has all of the desirable pharmacological actions of the various preparations prepared from the plant. Reserpine is absorbed readily from the gut, taken up rapidly by lipid-containing tissue, and bound to sites involved with storage of biogenic amines. Its effects start slowly and persist, so only one dose per day is needed.

### Mode of Action

Reserpine blocks the transport of norepinephrine into its storage granules so that less of the neurotransmitter is available when the adrenergic nerves are stimulated. The resultant decrease in sympathetic tone results in a decrease in peripheral vascular resistance. Catecholamines are also depleted in the brain, which may account for the sedative and depressant effects of the drug, and in the myocardium, which may decrease cardiac output and pose a problem to patients in terms of heart failure; ordinarily, though, its action is reflected only by a slight bradycardia (Cohen et al, 1968). At least in pituitary cells in vitro, reserpine acts as a calcium antagonist as well (Login et al, 1985).

### Clinical Use

By itself, reserpine, up to 0.5 mg/day, has limited antihypertensive potency, resulting in an average decrease of only 3/5 mm Hg. Combined with a thiazide, the reduction averaged 14/11 mm Hg (VA Cooperative Study, 1962). The potential of controlling mild hypertension with a single daily dose of reserpine plus a long-acting diuretic makes this combination very attractive—and it works. In a comparison of various regimens in patients with mild hypertension, a combination of *Rauwolfia* and thiazide worked even better than a beta-blocker plus a thiazide (VA Cooperative Study Group, 1977a).

### Dosage

With a diuretic, as little as 0.05 mg once daily will provide most of the antihypertensive effect of 0.25 mg and is associated with less lethargy and impotence (Participating VA Centers, 1982).

### Side Effects

Nasal stuffiness may be irritating, and increased gastric acid secretion may, rarely, activate an ulcer. The most serious problem is central nervous system (CNS) depression, which may simply tranquilize an apprehensive patient, or may be so severe as to lead to serious depression. The problem rarely occurs with doses of 0.25 mg per day or less (Goodwin and Bunney, 1971). Patients with past or present depression should not be given the drug, and all patients should be warned to stop the drug if they start feeling depressed or begin awakening early in the morning without being able to fall back to sleep.

## Guanethidine (Ismelin)

Guanethidine at one time was frequently used with many patients with moderate hypertension because it requires only one dose per day and has a steep dose-response relationship, thus producing an effect in almost every patient. As other drugs have become available, guanethidine has been relegated to use only if combinations of other drugs do not control the blood pressure (Joint National Committee, 1988).

### Chemistry

Guanethidine is one of a group of guanidine compounds that lowers blood pressure. Its absorption from the gut is limited and variable, ranging from 3 to 27% (McMartin and Simpson, 1971). The drug is taken into the adrenergic nerves by an active transport mechanism, the same pump that returns extracellular norepinephrine across the nerve membrane. This pump is inhibited by ephedrine, amphetamine, and tricyclic antidepressants (e.g., imipramine, amitriptyline), thereby accounting for the antagonism to the action of guanethidine seen in patients taking these drugs (Mitchell et al, 1970).

### Mode of Action

Once inside the adrenergic nerves, guanethidine initially blocks the exit of norepinephrine; it then causes an active release of norepinephrine from its storage granules, depleting the reserve pool of the neurotransmitter and decreasing the amount released when the nerve is stimulated. Myocardial catecholamine stores are partially depleted. The drug does not cross the blood-brain barrier, accounting for the absence of any sedative effect.

The interference with norepinephrine release causes a decrease in arteriolar constriction and a modest reduction in peripheral resistance. The depletion of myocardial catecholamine stores is responsible for a decrease in heart rate, stroke volume, and cardiac output. The blood pressure is reduced somewhat in the supine position, but much more so when the patient is upright since the normal vasoconstrictive response to posture is blunted.

### Clinical Use

Guanethidine is powerful and has a steep dose-response relationship so that the more drug given, the greater the effect. The appearance of minimal postural hypotension may be used as an indication that the therapeutic endpoint has been reached. Patients should protect themselves by sleeping with the head of the bed elevated, rising slowly from supine or sitting positions, and wearing effective elastic hose.

### Dosage

The amount required to lower standing blood pressure to an acceptable and tolerable level varies from 25 to 300 mg daily. The initial dose should be no more than 25 mg, and increments of 10 to 12.5 mg should be made no more often than every 3 to 5 days. The drug need be given only once daily, and the full hypotensive action of a given dose may not be manifest for some days.

### Side Effects

Most of the complications are expected, in keeping with the known effects of the drug: postural hypotension, fluid retention, diarrhea, failure of ejaculation.

### Guanadrel (Hylorel)

Guanadrel sulfate, a close relative to guanethidine, has almost all of the attributes of that drug with a shorter onset and offset of action that diminish the frequency of side effects and make it tolerable even among the elderly (Owens and Dunn, 1988). It is as effective as methyldopa and may be particularly useful in patients who cannot tolerate the CNS side effects of centrally acting drugs (Finnerty and Brogden, 1985).

### Bethanidine (Tenathan)

Bethanidine, another close relative to guanethidine, has comparable potency and side effects, except that it produces less diarrhea. The main difference is its shorter duration of action, 8 to 12 hours. In a controlled trial, bethanidine was less satisfactory than guanethidine (VA Cooperative Study, 1977b).

### Debrisoquin (Declinax)

Debrisoquin, another adrenergic neuronal blocker with a shorter duration of action than guanethidine, has not been approved for use in the United States. It has side effects and efficacy similar to those of guanethidine (Flammer et al, 1979), but about half of the patients require increases in dosage after achieving adequate control due to increased metabolic degradation of the drug.

## CENTRAL ALPHA-AGONISTS

The previous drugs inhibit release of catecholamines primarily from peripheral adrenergic neurons. We will now examine those that stimulate central alpha$_2$-adrenergic receptors that are involved in depressor sympathoinhibitory mechanisms (Bobik et al, 1986) (Fig. 7.16).

These drugs, including methyldopa, guanabenz, clonidine, and guanfacine, share certain characteristics (Henning, 1984):

—Their antihypertensive action involves a marked decline in sympathetic activity as is reflected in lower circulating levels of norepinephrine (Sullivan et al, 1986). However, the normal dynamic regulation of the circulation is little affected, so appropriate catechol responses can occur with stress, changes in posture, and other stimuli.

—They reduce the ability of the baroreceptor reflex to compensate for a decrease in blood pressure, accounting for the relative bradycardia and enhanced hypotensive action noted upon standing (Jarrott et al, 1987).

—Hemodynamically, they cause the blood pressure to fall by a modest decrease in both peripheral resistance and cardiac output, which may also involve venous dilation (Bentley, 1987).

—Plasma renin levels usually fall (Green et al, 1984), though this is not closely related to their antihypertensive effects (Weber et al, 1976).

—If given without a diuretic, fluid retention often accompanies the reduction in blood pressure. This may not occur with guana-

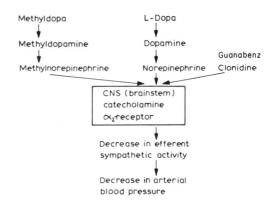

**Figure 7.16.** Schematic representation of the common mechanism probably underlying the hypotensive actions of methyldopa, L-dopa, clonidine, guanabenz, and guanfacine. (From Henning M: In: van Zwieten PA (ed). *Handbook of Hypertension, vol 3, Pharmacology of Antihypertensive Drugs*. Amsterdam: Elsevier, 1984, p 156.)

benz, which appears to be natriuretic (Gehr et al, 1986).

—These drugs appear to maintain renal blood flow despite a fall in blood pressure, presumably by reduction in renal vasoconstriction (Lowenstein et al, 1984).

—Their central site of action is responsible for some common side effects: sedation, decrease in alertness, and a dry mouth.

—When they are abruptly stopped, a rapid rebound and, rarely, an overshoot of the blood pressure may be experienced with or without accompanying features of excess sympathetic nervous activity. This discontinuation syndrome likely represents a sudden surge of catecholamine release, freed from the prior state of inhibition.

## Methyldopa (Aldomet)

From the early 1960s to the late 1970s when beta-blockers became available, methyldopa (Aldomet) was the most popular drug after diuretics used to treat hypertension.

### Chemistry

Methyldopa is the alpha-methylated derivative of dopa, the natural precursor of dopamine and norepinephrine. It was first used to treat hypertension because it inhibited the enzyme dopa decarboxylase, which is required to convert dopa to dopamine; it was thought that synthesis of norepinephrine should be inhibited and thereby sympathetic activity would be suppressed (Oates et al, 1960). When this mechanism was not substantiated, the false transmitter hypothesis was proposed: Methyldopa is metabolized to methylnorepinephrine, and this "false transmitter" should invoke less of a response than norepinephrine. The problem with this hypothesis was that the false transmitter was almost equipotent to the natural hormone.

The last and current hypothesis involves the formation of methylnorepinephrine and methylepinephrine (Goldberg et al, 1981), which act not as false transmitters but as potent agonists at alpha-adrenergic receptors within the central nervous system, similar to the action of clonidine (Henning, 1984)·(Fig. 7.16). The hypotensive action of both depends on the integrity of central adrenergic neurons in the lower brain stem (Jarrott et al, 1987).

### Clinical Use

Blood pressure is lowered maximally about 4 hours after an oral dose, and some effect per-

sists for up to 24 hours. Since it rarely produces serious postural hypertension and does not cause an increase in cardiac output, methyldopa has been recommended for use in patients with coronary and cerebral vascular complications and the elderly (Vandenburg et al, 1984). Left ventricular hypertrophy may regress, without apparent relation to changes in blood pressure (Fouad et al, 1982).

### Dosage

For most patients, therapy should be started with 250 mg 1 or 2 times per day, and the daily dosage can be increased to a maximum of 3.0 g on a twice-per-day schedule. In patients with renal insufficiency the dosage should be halved.

Absorption and metabolism of methyldopa may be slowed by concomitant intake of sulfate-containing drugs such as ferrous sulfate with a resultant decrease in its antihypertensive effect (Campbell et al, 1988).

### Side Effects (Table 7.7)

In addition to the anticipated postural hypotension and fluid retention, "autoimmune" side effects, including fever and liver dysfunction, are peculiar to methyldopa. These may reflect an inhibition of suppressor T cells with resultant unregulated autoantibody production by B cells

**Table 7.7. Side Effects of Methyldopa (Aldomet)**

Central nervous system
 Sleepiness (28%)[a]
 Loss of mental alertness (Adler, 1974)
 Decrease upper airway muscle tone (Lahive et al, 1988)
 Dry mouth (9%)
 Galactorrhea (Steiner et al, 1976)

Peripheral autonomic blockade
 Postural hypotension (15%)
 Impotence (2%) (Pillay, 1976)

Rebound (after 48 to 60 hr) (Houston, 1981)

"Autoimmune"
 Drug fever
 Positive Coombs' test (20%) (Carstairs et al, 1966)
 Hemolytic anemia (0.2%) (Shalev et al, 1983)
 Positive antinuclear antibodies (13%) (Wilson et al, 1978)
 Red cell aplasia (Itoh et al, 1988)
 Thrombocytopenia (Pai and Pai, 1988)
 Lupus-like syndrome (Dupont and Six, 1982)
 Liver dysfunction (Rodman et al, 1976)
  Abnormal tests (6.3%)
  Hepatitis and hepatic necrosis

Other inflammatory reactions
 Myocarditis (Seeverens et al, 1982)
 Pancreatitis (van der Heide et al, 1981)
 Colitis (Gloth and Busby, 1989)
 Retroperitoneal fibrosis (Ahmad, 1983)
 Skin rash (Wells et al, 1974)

[a]Incidence figures from Reid et al, 1984.

(Kirtland et al, 1980). Liver dysfunction usually disappears when the drug is stopped, but at least 83 cases of serious hepatotoxicity have been reported (Rodman et al, 1976), and the drug should probably not be given to patients with known liver disease.

Parkinsonian symptoms may appear, presumably by inhibiting the decarboxylase enzyme needed to convert dopa to dopamine. On the other hand, patients taking levodopa for therapy of parkinsonism may have a greater hypotensive effect from alpha-methyldopa and better control of the parkinsonism (Gibberd and Small, 1973).

Little data are available about lipid changes; in one study, total cholesterol was unchanged; HDL-cholesterol was lower by 10% (Leon et al, 1984).

Certain biochemical tests can be altered by methyldopa therapy:

—red color in both the aqueous and butanol layers of the modified Watson-Schwartz test for porphobilinogen (Pierach et al, 1977);
—higher urinary creatinine levels as determined by the autoanalyzer (Maddocks et al, 1973);
—lower urine vanillylmandelic acid (VMA) levels, whereas urine metanephrine and free catechols measured by fluorimetric assays are higher (Tyce et al, 1963).

Overall, in large surveys, the number and range of the adverse reactions to methyldopa are rather impressive (Lawson et al, 1978; Furhoff, 1978). In a comparison with a beta-blocker in which treatment was given for 2 years, four of 30 patients given an average dose of 308 mg of metoprolol had to have the drug withdrawn, but 17 of 26 patients given an average dose of 1120 mg of methyldopa had to have the drug stopped (Lorimer et al, 1980). In view of its unique and potentially serious side effects, I believe other central alpha-agonists should be used in place of methyldopa.

## Clonidine (Catapres)

The use of this drug has been limited by concern over a withdrawal syndrome (Neusy and Lowenstein, 1989), but its availability as a transdermal preparation has led to an increase in its use.

### Chemistry

Clonidine is an imidazoline derivative. It is readily absorbed and plasma levels peak within an hour (Davies et al, 1977). The plasma half-life is 6 to 13 hours. About 50% is excreted in the urine, mainly as unidentified metabolites. Intravenous clonidine is not available in the United States but is used elsewhere.

### Mode of Action

Clonidine binds to specific imidazole binding sites in the brain, sites that may be functional receptors that mediate its hypotensive action (Meeley et al, 1989). In experimental animals, clonidine activates opiate receptors in the brain, and this may play a role in its hypotensive action as well as explain its value for management of opiate withdrawal (van Giersbergen et al, 1989).

### Clinical Use

When taken orally, the blood pressure begins to fall within 30 minutes, with the greatest effect occurring between 2 and 4 hours. The duration of effect is from 12 to 24 hours.

A transdermal preparation designed to continuously deliver clonidine over a 7-day interval has been found to be effective and to cause milder side effects than oral therapy (Weber et al, 1984). Others, however, report considerable skin irritation and side effects similar to those seen with the oral drug (Langley and Heel, 1988) Rebound hypertension has been reported when the patch was discontinued (Metz et al, 1987).

The sympathetic nervous suppression induced by clonidine has been used to prevent the reflex sympathetic overactivity that follows vasodilator therapy with either hydralazine (Velasco et al, 1978) or minoxidil (Mitchell and Pettinger, 1978) and to serve as a screening test for pheochromocytoma (see Chapter 12). Clonidine has been effective in patients with renal insufficiency, and very little is eliminated during dialysis (Hulter et al, 1979).

Clonidine will smoothly lower markedly elevated blood pressure, referred to as "urgent hypertension" when an initial 0.1- to 0.2-mg dose is followed by hourly 0.05- to 0.1-mg doses (Jaker et al, 1989).

### Dosage

The starting dose should be 0.1 mg twice per day, with a maximum of 1.2 mg/day. Patients may be given most and perhaps all of the daily dose at bedtime to compensate for the sedative effect (Ram et al, 1979). The transdermal patch is available in 0.1-, 0.2-, and 0.3- mg/day doses.

### Side Effects

Clonidine and methyldopa share the two most common side effects, sedation and dry mouth, though they are more frequent with clonidine (Amery et al, 1970). These may dissipate over a few months, and some patients are less bothered by them 6 months after start of therapy. Rarely, hallucinations and other CNS effects are noted (Brown et al, 1980). Clonidine does not share the ''autoimmune'' hepatic and hematological derangements that frequently accompany methyldopa therapy.

*Rebound and Discontinuation Syndromes.* If antihypertensive therapy is inadvertently stopped abruptly, various ''discontinuation syndromes'' may occur: (1) a rapid asymptomatic return of the BP to pretreatment levels that occurs in the majority of patients; (2) a ''rebound'' of the blood pressure with rapid return of the BP plus symptoms and signs of sympathetic overactivity and possibly other cardiovascular events; and (3) an ''overshoot'' of the BP above pretreatment levels. In addition patients who suddenly stop use of beta-blockers may experience a different discontinuation syndrome manifested by the sudden appearance of coronary ischemia.

A discontinuation syndrome has been reported with most currently used drugs (Houston, 1981). The approximate total number of patients reported to have a discontinuation syndrome was highest with clonidine, followed by propranolol and methyldopa. In a carefully monitored study, rebound was not observed after withdrawal of propranolol, but some rise in systolic BP was seen in seven of 13 subjects after clonidine withdrawal (Neusy and Lowenstein, 1989). The discontinuation syndrome with central adrenergic inhibitors probably reflects a rapid return of catecholamine secretion that had been suppressed during therapy (Reid et al, 1977).

A number of factors may predispose certain hypertensive patients to a discontinuation syndrome. Those who take high doses of any antihypertensive drug are vulnerable, particularly if they have underlying severe hypertension and high levels of renin-angiotensin. Those who had been on a combination of a central adrenergic inhibitor (e.g., clonidine) and a beta-blocker may be particularly susceptible if the central inhibitor is withdrawn while the beta-blocker is continued (Lilja et al, 1982). This leads to a sudden surge in plasma catecholamines in a situation in which peripheral alpha-receptors are left unopposed to induce vasoconstriction because the beta-receptors are blocked and cannot mediate vasodilation. All antihypertensives should be stopped gradually, but if the above combination is being used, the beta-blocker should be discontinued in advance of the clonidine.

If a discontinuation syndrome appears, the previously administered drug should be restarted, and the symptoms will likely recede rapidly. If needed, labetalol will effectively lower a markedly elevated blood pressure (Mehta and Lopez, 1987).

*Other Problems.* Depression of sinus and atrioventricular (AV) nodal function may be common (Roden et al, 1988), and a few cases of severe bradycardia have been reported (Byrd et al, 1988). Large overdoses will lead to hypertension presumably by stimulation of peripheral alpha-receptors causing vasoconstriction (Hunyor et al, 1975). The antihypertensive effect of clonidine may be blunted by simultaneous intake of tricyclic antidepressants (Briant et al, 1973) and tranquilizers (van Zwieten, 1977).

Unlike methyldopa and reserpine, clonidine does not increase serum prolactin (Lal et al, 1975), but it will acutely raise growth hormone levels (Gil-Ad et al, 1979), a property taken advantage of to treat growth hormone deficient children (Pinton et al, 1985). The drug does not adversely affect lipoproteins or metabolic control in hypertensive diabetics (Nilsson-Ehle et al, 1988).

## Other Uses: Opiate Withdrawal

Clonidine has been found to be a safe and effective nonopiate treatment of opiate withdrawal, presumably by its activation of opiate receptors (Bond, 1986). Clonidine has also been given to people withdrawing from cigarette smoking, but, in a controlled study, it was found to have little benefit on withdrawal symptoms or smoking reduction (Franks et al, 1989).

Clonidine also suppresses menopausal hot flashes (Laufer et al, 1982) and diarrhea due to diabetic neuropathy (Fedorak et al, 1985) or ulcerative colitis (Lechin et al, 1985).

## Guanabenz (Wytensin)

This drug, structurally similar to clonidine, also acts as a central alpha$_2$-agonist, resulting in a decrease of sympathetic outflow from the brain (Bonham et al, 1984). However, it has some distinctive features that make it an attractive choice for a centrally acting agent.

## Chemistry

Guanabenz is an aminoguanidine whose absorption is complete, with peak blood levels reached 2 to 5 hours after oral intake (Holmes et al, 1983). It is extensively metabolized, and its mean plasma half-life is 14 hours.

### Mode of Action

The drug acts centrally in a manner similar to clonidine. Effective control of blood pressure is not associated with changes in renal blood flow, sodium balance, or plasma renin activity (Mosley et al, 1984). Patients on long-term therapy tend to lose a few pounds in body weight, attributed to a natriuresis that in turn may be explained by its effect on chloride reabsorption in the papillary collecting duct (Stein and Osgood, 1984) as well as by its lesser alpha$_1$-mediated vasoconstrictor effect in the kidneys, as compared with that of clonidine (Wolff et al, 1984).

### Clinical Use

In usual doses, guanabenz is effective as an antihypertensive, equal to methyldopa, clonidine, or propranolol (Bauer, 1983). In clinical use, it causes side effects similar to those of clonidine, but unlike these other agents it offers the advantages of not causing reactive fluid retention, so it has been approved for initial use as monotherapy. Moreover, its use is usually associated with slight lowering of serum cholesterol in contrast to the tendency of adverse lipid changes with diuretics and many beta-blockers (Kaplan and Grundy, 1988). The drug can be safely used in diabetics (Gutin and Tuck, 1988) and asthmatics (Deitch et al, 1984).

### Dosage

Therapy should begin with 4 mg twice per day, with increments up to a total of 64 mg/day.

### Side Effects

The side effects mimic those seen with other central alpha-agonists, with sedation and dry mouth the most prominent, being seen in 20 to 30% of patients. Weakness and dizziness each occur in about 6%, whereas GI complaints are rare. A withdrawal syndrome may occur if the drug is stopped abruptly (Ram et al, 1979).

### Guanfacine (Tenex)

Another clonidine-like drug, guanfacine appears to enter the brain more slowly and to maintain its antihypertensive effect longer (Dollery and Davies, 1980). These differences translate into a once-per-day dosage and, perhaps, fewer CNS side effects (Jerie and Lasance, 1984).

Withdrawal symptoms are less common than with clonidine (Wilson et al, 1986).

### Lofexidine

This is another imidazoline derivative, very similar to clonidine in hemodynamics (Fouad et al, 1981), clinical effectiveness (Garrett and Kaplan, 1981), and side effects (Schultz et al, 1981). It has been effective in managing withdrawal from both opiates (Washton et al, 1981) and alcohol (Cushman et al, 1985).

### Other Agents

A number of other centrally acting alpha$_2$-agonists are under investigation (van Zwieten, 1988). None appears to be free from the sedative liability of those now available (Sweet, 1984).

## ALPHA-ADRENERGIC RECEPTOR BLOCKERS

Selective alpha$_1$-blockers have had a relatively small share of the overall market for antihypertensive drugs in the United States. Until 1987, prazosin (Minipress) was the only alpha-blocker available but terazosin (Hytrin) and doxazosin (Cardura) have been approved and others likely soon will be, along with longer acting formulations of prazosin. The availability of more of these drugs and the increasing awareness of their special ability to improve lipid levels suggest that their use will expand considerably.

Nonselective alpha-blockers are used almost exclusively in the medical management of pheochromocytoma since they were only minimally effective in primary hypertension and caused considerable side effects. These drugs, phenoxybenzamine and phentolamine, are covered in Chapter 12 under medical management of pheochromocytoma.

When the two major subtypes of alpha receptors were identified, prazosin, which had been characterized as a nonspecific vasodilator, was recognized to act as a competitive antagonist of postsynaptic alpha$_1$-receptors (van Zwieten, 1984). It remains as the prototype of this class of drugs but a number of others share this action, some almost exclusively, others with other effects as well (Cubeddu, 1988) (Table 7.8).

The major action of prazosin and the other drugs that act primarily as alpha$_1$-receptor antagonists is to block the activation of postsynaptic alpha$_1$-receptors by circulating or neurally-released catecholamines, an activation that normally induces vasoconstriction. This blockade dilates both resistance and capacitance vessels.

**Table 7.8. Additional Properties of Various Alpha$_1$ Antagonists$^a$**

| | Alpha$_2$ | | CNS | Other |
| | Antagonist | Agonist | (SNS) | Effects |
|---|---|---|---|---|
| Prazosin | | | + | |
| Doxazosin | | | ? | |
| Terazosin | | | ? | |
| Trimazosin | | | ? | Vasodilator |
| Indoramin | | | + | H$_1$, 5HT |
| Urapidil | | + | + | DA |
| Ketanserin | | | − | 5HT$_2$ |
| Labetalol | | | ? | B$_1$, B$_2$ |
| Phentolamine | + | | − | |
| Phenoxybenzamine | + | | − | H$_1$, 5HT, DA |

$^a$From Cubeddu LX: *Am Heart J* 116:133, 1988.

H$_1$ = histamine 1 receptor antagonist; 5HT = serotonin receptor antagonist; DA = dopamine receptor antagonist; B$_1$- and B$_2$-adrenergic receptor antagonist; SNS = sympathetic nervous system; CNS = central nervous system; ? = unknown; + = demonstrated effect; − = no effect.

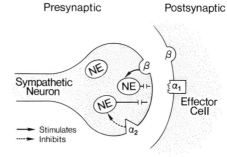

**Prazosin Inhibits Postsynaptic $\alpha_1$ Receptor But Not Presynaptic $\alpha_2$ Receptor**

**Figure 7.17.** Schematic view of the action of prazosin as a postsynaptic alpha-blocker. By blocking the alpha$_1$-adrenergic receptor on the vascular smooth muscle, catecholamine-induced vasoconstriction is inhibited. The alpha$_2$-receptor on the neuronal membrane is not blocked; therefore inhibition of additional norepinephrine release by the short feedback mechanism is maintained.

Peripheral resistance falls without major changes in cardiac output, in part because of a balance between a decrease in venous return (preload) and a slight degree of reflex sympathetic stimulation as a consequence of the vasodilation.

At a cellular level, alpha$_1$-receptor blockers act in a manner analogous to calcium entry blockers. The activation of alpha$_1$-adrenergic receptors by agonists leads to a mobilization of stored calcium within cells. There is evidence for two subtypes of alpha$_1$-receptors, one promoting influx of calcium into cells, the other acting to increase intracellular release of calcium via the inositol phospholipid pathway (Minneman, 1988). Blockade of these alpha$_1$-receptors, then, likely induces vasodilation by reducing levels of intracellular calcium.

The hemodynamic effects of these drugs occur by a relatively selective blockade of the postsynaptic alpha$_1$-receptor (Fig. 7.17). The presynaptic alpha$_2$-receptors remain open, capable of binding neurotransmitter and thereby inhibiting the release of additional norepinephrine (NE) through a direct negative feedback mechanism. This inhibition of NE release explains the lack of tachycardia, increased cardiac output, and rise in renin levels that characterize the response to drugs that block both the presynaptic alpha$_2$-receptor and postsynaptic alpha$_1$-receptor, e.g., phentolamine. Despite this selective blockade, neurally mediated responses to stress and exercise are unaffected, and the baroreceptor reflex remains active. However, the decrease in preload and the blockade of alpha$_1$-receptors largely prevent the reflex sympathetic activation seen with direct vasodilators, e.g., hydralazine.

Accompanying these desirable attributes, other pharmacological actions may lessen the usefulness of these drugs: They relax the venous bed as well and, at least initially, may affect the visceral vascular bed more than the peripheral vascular bed; the subsequent pooling of blood in the viscera may explain the propensity to first-dose hypotension (Jauernig et al, 1978). Since baroreceptors are active, plasma NE rises after the blood pressure falls, which may limit their antihypertensive potency (Eklund et al, 1983). Volume retention is common (Bauer, 1985), perhaps because renin and aldosterone levels are less suppressed than they are with other adrenergic-inhibiting drugs.

Prazosin and other members of this class may also exert some CNS effects that add to their antihypertensive efficacy (Cubeddu, 1988) and side effects. In particular, prazosin may aggravate cataplexy in dogs (Mignot et al, 1988) and people (Guilleminault et al, 1988).

The overall favorable hemodynamic and lipid effects and the relative lack of CNS and metabolic side effects make alpha$_1$-blockers particularly attractive as first line therapy.

### Prazosin (Minipress)

#### Chemistry

A quinazoline derivative, prazosin is rapidly absorbed, reaching maximal blood levels at 2 hours and having a plasma half-life of about 3 hours (Schäfers and Reid, 1989). The drug is highly bound to plasma proteins but, in dogs, is rapidly taken into vascular smooth muscle cells. It is metabolized in the liver and excreted largely via bile and feces.

## Clinical Use

Prazosin is effective in lowering the blood pressure, equivalent to beta-blockers (Alderman, 1989), ACE inhibitors (Cheung et al, 1989), or hydrochlorothiazide (Stamler et al, 1988). It works equally in black and nonblack patients (Batey et al, 1989) and in the elderly (Cheung et al, 1989). Prazosin can be effectively combined with a diuretic, beta-blockers, or calcium entry blockers (Schäfers and Reid, 1989). Prazosin is effective in more severe hypertensives (McAreavey et al, 1984) and in those with chronic renal failure (Lameire and Gordts, 1986). In the presence of renal failure, the hypotensive action is enhanced, so lower doses should be used.

Prazosin does not alter plasma renin levels and may be useful in controlling the hypertension of patients who are undergoing dynamic tests of their renin-angiotensin system (Webb et al, 1987).

Overall, the drug is quite well tolerated, with relatively little sedation, dry mouth, or impotence, as may be seen with central adrenergic agonists. Furthermore, prazosin does not block beta-receptors, so bronchospasm, poor peripheral circulation, and reduced cardiac output are not potential problems as they are with beta-blockers. During isotonic exercise, prazosin does not reduce performance as do beta-blockers but, on the other hand, it will not reduce the exercise-associated rise in systolic pressure as will beta-blockers (Thompson et al, 1989). During isometric exercise, prazosin will suppress the pressor response better than will a beta-blocker (Hamada et al, 1987).

## Ancillary Effects

*Cardiac.* In dogs, selective alpha$_1$-blockade with prazosin will increase coronary blood flow during induced hypoperfusion (Liang and Jones, 1985) and prevents fatal arrhythmias after acute ischemia (Wilber et al, 1987). In people with coronary disease, alpha$_1$-blockade may be either beneficial or harmful (Feigl, 1987). By limiting the vasoconstriction that is a normal part of the sympathetic activation that occurs during exercise or emotional stress, an alpha$_1$-blocker could improve coronary flow if the vasoconstriction is mainly at the stenotic segment but could worsen coronary flow if the vasoconstriction primarily involves small vessels beyond the stenosis.

Left ventricular hypertrophy has been shown to regress after prazosin therapy (Ram et al, 1989). This is not surprising since alpha$_1$-receptor stimulation is the molecular mediator of cardiac myocyte hypertrophy (Bishopric et al, 1987).

As a balanced arteriolar and venous dilator, prazosin seemed to be a useful drug for treating congestive heart failure (Miller et al, 1977) but tolerance usually develops (Awan et al, 1981).

*Genital.* The nonselective alpha$_1$- and alpha$_2$-blocker phentolamine is being widely used by injection directly into the penis to increase arterial inflow in patients with erectile impotence (Levine et al, 1989). In one small trial, oral phentolamine was also helpful in eight of 16 patients (Gwinup, 1988). No data are available as to whether oral prazosin will have any such effect. On the other hand, prazosin has been found to at least temporarily relieve most of the obstructive symptoms of benign prostatic hypertrophy (BPH) apparently by relaxing the tone of prostatic muscle (Lepor, 1989). A review of all medical therapies for BPH concluded that "Prazosin and similar alpha$_1$-adrenergic antagonists seem certain to fulfill a role in the short-term management of BPH, especially for relief of symptoms in patients awaiting surgery or in those who are otherwise unfit for operation" (Editorial, *Lancet*, 1988).

*Lipid Effects.* As first noted by Leren et al (1980), a generally favorable effect of prazosin and other alpha-1 blockers on blood lipid levels has been well established, with a decrease in total and LDL-cholesterol and triglycerides and a rise in HDL-cholesterol usually being observed (Grimm, 1989). In a 6-month study comparing prazosin with metoprolol, the mean difference in serum cholesterol at the end of the trial was about 15 mg/dl or about 9% of the pretreatment value (Lithell et al, 1988). This favorable effect of an alpha$_1$-blocker versus the equally widely recognized detrimental effect of beta-blockers and diuretics could have a significant impact on overall cardiovascular risk. Provocatively, in experimental animals, alpha$_1$-blockers have been found to reduce atherogenesis (Kowala and Nicolosi, 1989).

*Other Metabolic Effects.* Prazosin does not alter glucose tolerance in diabetics (Ferlito et al, 1983). In obese normoglycemic hypertensives, prazosin has been found to actually improve the disappearance rate of glucose during an intravenous glucose tolerance test and reduce both the peak and the total insulin response (Pollare et al, 1988). In view of the hyperinsulinemia noted in both obese and nonobese hypertensives described in Chapter 3, this could add to the antihypertensive effect of the drug.

## Dosage

The initial dose should be 1 mg, either at bedtime or on a morning when the patient may be relatively inactive, in case first-dose hypotension occurs. Dosage should be titrated upward, with a total daily dose of up to 20 mg sometimes required. The drug should be given 2 times a day although some patients may maintain control with once-a-day therapy (Soltero et al, 1986). A rate-controlled, osmotic pump delivery system will provide more certain 24-hour efficacy (Elliott et al, 1988). No real tolerance to the antihypertensive action of the drug has been seen after 4 to 7 years of continual use (New Zealand Hypertension Study Group, 1980; Walker et al, 1981). However, if reactive fluid retention occurs, the blood pressure may rise, only to fall again with the addition of a small dose of diuretic.

## Side Effects

Side effects include headache, drowsiness, fatigue, and weakness—likely nonspecific effects of a lowering of the blood pressure. For most patients, the side effects diminish with continued therapy. Impotence is likely infrequent (Scharf and Mayleben, 1989), but no large-scale comparative sudies have been published. Rarely, a first-dose response, with postural hypotension developing in 30 to 90 minutes, is seen (Bendall et al, 1975). However, even massive overdoses may not do much harm if the patient stays supine (McClean, 1976). The degree of first-dose hypotension has been found to correlate inversely with the baseline plasma renin activity (Nicholson et al, 1985). The problem can generally be avoided by initiating therapy with a small dose and making sure the patient is not already volume depleted as a result of diuretic therapy.

## Terazosin (Hytrin)

The second alpha$_1$-blocker to be approved for use in the United States, this drug is similar in every way to prazosin except that it has a longer duration of action that allows for once-a-day dosage (Frishman et al, 1988). It provides similar improvements in lipids as seen with prazosin (Luther et al, 1989).

The major characteristics of terazosin and the other not-yet- approved alpha$_1$-blockers are shown in Table 7.9.

## Doxazosin (Cardura)

As seen in Table 7.9, doxazosin has a slower onset of peak action, which probably will translate into a low incidence of first-dose hypotension and a long duration of action translating into a once-a-day dosage. The drug has antihypertensive efficacy equal to beta-blockers (Lijnen et al, 1989) or ACE inhibitors (Taylor et al, 1988). As with prazosin, serum lipids are often improved (Ames and Kiyasu, 1989) while insulin sensitivity is not impaired (Scheen et al, 1989).

## Other Agents

### Trimazosin and Alfuzosin

These drugs, also structurally related to prazosin, may lower the blood pressure by direct arteriolar dilation in addition to alpha$_1$-blockade (Van Kalken et al, 1986; di Priolo et al, 1988).

### Indoramin

Also similar in structure and effect to prazosin, indoramin has been introduced for clinical use in numerous places outside the United States. It differs from prazosin in having a direct effect upon the heart, reducing contractile force and rate, and it may cause more sedation and other central effects (Holmes and Sorkin, 1986).

### Urapidil

Chemically different, this phenylpiperazine derivative also appears to have a somewhat different mode of antihypertensive action beyond blocking alpha$_1$-receptors. Experiments in animals support an interaction with serotonin receptors in the brain (Kolassa et al, 1989).

### Ketanserin

Though included in a survey of alpha-blocking agents (Cubeddu, 1988), this quinazoline

**Table 7.9. Comparative Characteristics of Alpha$_1$ Antagonists**[a]

| Drugs | Duration of Action (hr) | Peak of Action (hr) | Therapeutic Dose (mg) | Frequency of Administration (times/day) |
|---|---|---|---|---|
| Prazosin | 4–6 | 0.5 | 2–20 | 2 or 3 |
| Terazosin | >18 | 1–1.7 | 1–40 | 1 or 2 |
| Doxazosin | 18–36 | 6 | 1–16 | 1 |
| Trimazosin | 3–6 | 3–6 | 100–900 | 2 or 3 |
| Indoramin | >6 | 2 | 50–150 | 2 or 3 |
| Urapidil | 6–8 | 3–5 | 15–120 | 1 or 2 |
| Ketanserin | >12 | 1–2 | 20–40 | 1 or 2 |

[a]From Cubeddu LX: *Am Heart J* 116:133, 1988.

derivative is also a selective blocker of 5-hydroxytryptamine$_2$(5-HT$_2$)-serotonergic receptors, likely at lower concentrations than needed for its alpha$_1$-adrenergic blocking effect (Vanhoutte et al, 1983). The drug may turn out to be a useful agent for peripheral vascular disease (DeCree et al, 1984).

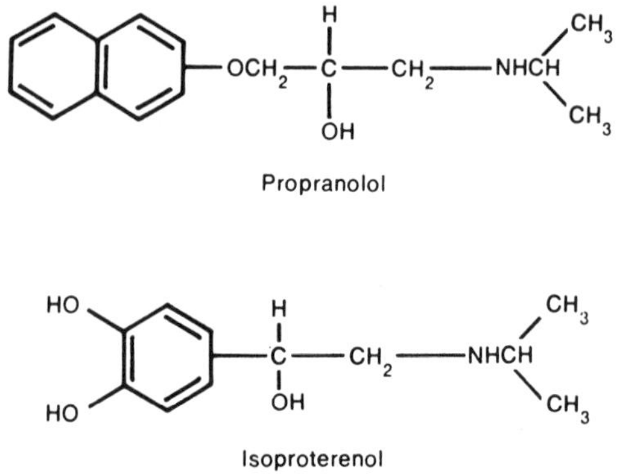

### Dihydroergotoxine

This ergot derivative has multiple cardiovascular effects, among which are postsynaptic alpha$_1$- and alpha$_2$-receptor antagonism (Woodcock et al, 1984). It has been used in Europe for treatment of hypertension.

## BETA-ADRENERGIC RECEPTOR BLOCKERS

Beta-adrenergic blocking agents have become the most popular antihypertensive drugs after diuretics (Fig. 7.3). Though they are no more effective than other antihypertensive agents and may on occasion induce serious side effects, they are generally well tolerated, and they offer the special advantage of relieving a number of concomitant diseases. The hope that they would provide special primary protection against initial coronary events remains unproved: When compared with a diuretic, no significant difference between the two drugs in protecting against coronary mortality was noted in two large trials (Medical Research Council Working Party, 1985; Wilhelmsen et al, 1987) but the half of the patients in the latter trial who received the beta-blocker metoprolol did have a lower coronary death rate than did those on a diuretic (Wikstrand et al, 1988). This important issue is covered in more detail in Chapter 5.

### Chemistry

These agents are chemically similar to beta-agonists and to each other (Fig. 7.18). Powell and Slater reported in 1958 that isoproterenol (isoprenaline) with chlorine substituted for hydroxyl groups on the ring (dichloroisoprenaline, or DCI) blocked the depressor and vasodilator effects of isoproterenol. Shortly thereafter, Moran and Perkins (1958) showed that DCI blocked adrenergic stimulation of the heart and coined the term "beta-adrenergic blocking drug." DCI also had sympathomimetic effects, so when James Black began his search for drugs that would block only the adrenergic receptors, a series of other compounds were synthesized (Black and Stephenson, 1962). Propranolol was synthesized in 1963, described first in 1964 (Black et

**Figure 7.18.** Structure of propranolol and the beta-agonist isoproterenol.

al, 1964), shown to be effective in treatment of hypertension that same year (Prichard and Gillam, 1964), and marketed in England in 1965. The time from first animal testing to clinical availability in England took a remarkably short 2 2/3 years.

Since then a large series of similar drugs have been synthesized and about 14 brought to market, 10 in the United States as of September 1990. They differ in a number of ways (Table 7.10), some having clinical significance, others such as the membrane-stabilizing effect probably irrelevant (Frishman, 1987; Reid, 1988a). The various beta-blockers can be conveniently classified by their relative selectivity for the beta$_1$-receptors (primarily on the heart) and presence of intrinsic sympathomimetic activity (ISA), also referred to as partial agonist activity (Fig. 7.19).

### Mode of Action

Their competitive inhibition of beta-adrenergic activity produces numerous effects on functions that regulate the blood pressure including a decrease in cardiac output, a decrease in renin release, perhaps a decrease in central sympathetic nervous activity and a probable decrease in peripheral vascular resistance.

The traditional view has been that the primary effect was a reduction in cardiac output by 15 to 20% resulting from the blockade of cardiac beta$_1$-receptors thereby reducing both heart rate and myocardial contractility (Tarazi and Dustan, 1972). However, this view has been challenged, in part because of studies with a pure beta$_2$-blocking agent (ICI 118551) without beta$_1$ (cardiac) blocking action that produces an antihypertensive effect comparable to propranolol (Vincent et al, 1987).

**Table 7.10. Pharmacological Properties of Some Beta-Blockers**

| Drug | Trade Name | Cardioselectivity | Intrinsic Sympathomimetic Activity | Membrane Stabilizing Activity | Lipid Solubility | Maximum Daily Dose (*mg*) |
|---|---|---|---|---|---|---|
| Acebutolol | Sectral | + | + | + | + | 1200 |
| Alprenolol | Aptin | − | + + | + | + + + | 400 |
| Atenolol | Tenormin | + | − | − | − | 20 |
| Betaxolol | Kerlone | + | 0 | 0 | + + | 400 |
| Bisoprolol | Concor | + | 0 | 0 | + + | 20 |
| Carteolol | Cartrol | − | + | 0 | − | 40 |
| Carvedilol | BM 14190 | − | 0 | + + | + + | 100 |
| Celiprolol | Selectol | + | +? | 0 | − | 600 |
| Dilevalol | Unicard | − | + | 0 | + + + | 800 |
| Esmolol | Brevibloc | + | 0 | 0 | − | 300μg/kg/min/I.V. |
| Labetalol | Normodyne, Trandate | − | +? | 0 | + + + | 2400 |
| Metoprolol | Lopressor | + | − | + | + + + | 300 |
| Nadolol | Corgard | − | − | − | − | 160 |
| Oxprenolol | Trasicor | − | + + | + | + + + | 480 |
| Penbutolol | Levatol | − | + | + | + + + | 80 |
| Pindolol | Visken | − | + + + | + | + | 45 |
| Propranolol | Inderal | − | − | + + | + + + | 320 |
| Sotalol | Sotacor | − | − | − | − | 600 |
| Timolol | Blocadren | − | − | − | + + | 60 |

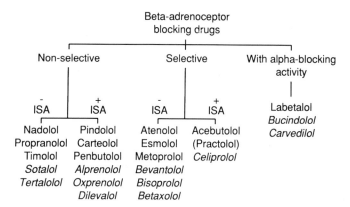

**Figure 7.19.** Classification of beta-adrenoceptor blockers based on cardioselectivity and intrinsic sympathomimetic activity (*ISA*). Those not approved for use in the United States are in *italics*.

## Acute

These investigators have examined the hemodynamic changes during the first 24 hours after administration of four beta-blockers with disparate characteristics: (1) acebutolol: beta$_1$-selective with moderate ISA; (2) atenolol: beta$_1$-selective, no ISA; (3) pindolol: non-selective with strong ISA, and 4) propranolol: nonselective, no ISA (van den Meiracker et al, 1988). The blood pressure fell quickest after pindolol, which induced no fall in cardiac output (CO) nor rise in systemic vascular resistance (SVR) (Fig. 7.20). With the other three drugs, the fall in blood pressure was a bit delayed during which time CO fell and SVR rose. This hemodynamic profile is the one generally provided as the mode of action for the antihypertensive action of beta-blockers. Note, however, what followed after 3 to 4 hours with the three agents without strong ISA: CO returned to normal and SVR fell to below normal.

The authors conclude ". . . that the most important hemodynamic change during the onset of the hypotensive action of beta-adrenoceptor antagonists is vasodilation. . . . It is the ability of these drugs to interfere with sympathetic vasoconstrictor nerve activity that is likely responsible for their blood pressure-lowering efficacy."

## Chronic

Man in't Veld et al (1988a) reviewed the literature on acute and chronic hemodynamic

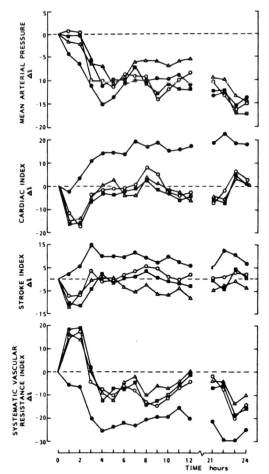

**Figure 7.20.** Plots of time course of percentage changes in systemic hemodynamics after the first oral doses of either acebutolol (■), atenolol (△), pindolol (●), or propranolol (○). First oral dose was given at time 0. (From van den Meiracker AH et al: *Circulation* 78:957, 1988.)

changes with beta-blockers, covering 85 studies on 10 drugs in a total of 912 patients, and observed a fairly uniform pattern: Cardiac output usually fell acutely (except with high-ISA pindolol) and remained lower chronically; peripheral resistance, on the other hand, usually rose acutely but universally fell toward if not to normal chronically (Fig. 7.21). They documented these effects in a study of the four agents shown in Figure 7.20 administered for 3 weeks (van den Meiracker et al, 1989.) The situation likely reflects a partial return or adaptation of the initially elevated SVR, either by readjustment of baroreceptor sensitivity (Scott, 1983) or by inhibition of norepinephrine release from sympathetic nerves by blockade of the presynaptic receptors (Thadani, 1983), or by a decrease in alpha-receptor-mediated vasoconstriction in some

unexplained manner (Bolli et al, 1982). Despite these adaptations, patients on beta-blockers have persistently impaired vasodilation in response to exercise or epinephrine (Lenders et al, 1988).

### Plasma Catechols

Despite the probable adaptation of peripheral resistance, plasma catecholamine levels are increased after beta-blockade (Lijnen et al, 1979) reflecting a sharp reduction in the clearance of both epinephrine and norepinephrine from the circulation during beta-blockade (Cryer et al, 1980) as well as some baroreflex-mediated activation of the sympathetic nervous system.

### Renin Release

Renin levels usually fall promptly after beta-blocker therapy, presumably reflecting the beta$_2$-receptor mediation of renin release. After 18 weeks of beta-blocker therapy, active renin fell but prorenin rose, and there was a highly significant correlation between the combination of the pretreatment values of active renin, prorenin, and aldosterone with the fall in blood pressure (McKenna and Davison, 1986).

### Pharmacological Differences

Three major differences have an impact upon the clinical use of beta-blockers: lipid solubility, cardioselectivity, and intrinsic sympathomimetic activity. The first of these largely determines the duration and constancy of action. The latter two help determine the pattern of side effects.

### Lipid Solubility

Beta-blockers have varying degrees of lipid solubility (Fig. 7.22). Those that are more lipid soluble (lipophilic) tend to be taken up and metabolized extensively by the liver. As an example, with oral propranolol and metoprolol, up to 70% is removed on the first pass of portal blood through the liver. The bioavailability of these beta-blockers is therefore less after oral than after intravenous administration.

Those such as atenolol and nadolol, which are much less lipid soluble (lipophobic), escape hepatic metabolism and are mainly excreted by the kidneys, unchanged. As a result, their plasma half-life and duration of action are much longer, and they achieve more stable plasma concentrations. In addition, they enter the brain less and may thereby cause fewer CNS side effects (Conant et al, 1989).

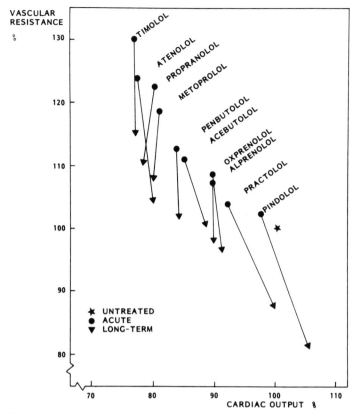

**Figure 7.21.** Hemodynamic interrelationships during acute (•) and long-term (▼) beta-blockade in hypertension. The *asterisk* indicates the situation before treatment. (From Man in't Veld AJ, Van den Meiracker AH, Schalekamp MA: *Am J Hypertens* 1:91, 1988a.)

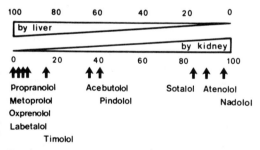

**Figure 7.22.** Relative degree of clearance by hepatic uptake and metabolism (liver) and renal excretion (kidney) of 10 beta-adrenoceptor-blocking agents. The differences largely reflect differences in lipid solubility, which progressively diminishes from left to right. [From Meier J: *Cardiology* 64(Suppl 1):1, 1979 and by permission of S Karger AG, Basel.]

## Cardioselectivity

All currently available beta-blockers antagonize cardiac $beta_1$-receptors competitively, so they all can be used to prevent angina or arrhythmias. However, there seems to be little difference in antihypertensive efficacy between those that are more or less cardioselective. The major issue revolves around protection from various side effects that might be anticipated from lesser degrees of blockade of $beta_2$-receptors in bronchi, peripheral vessels, and the pancreas.

The assumption that an agent with relative cardioselectivity is automatically preferable to one that is less so must be tempered by these considerations:

1. No beta-blocker is purely cardioselective, particularly in large doses.
2. No tissue contains exclusively only one subgroup of receptors: The heart has both, with $beta_1$ predominating; bronchioles have both, with $beta_2$ predominating.
3. When high endogenous catechol levels are needed, even minimal degrees of $beta_2$-blockade from a cardioselective drug may cause trouble. Under resting conditions, atenolol clearly causes no bronchospasm; however, during an attack of asthma, when the bronchial caliber is highly dependent on

sympathetic tone, bronchospasm may be worsened in its presence (Breckenridge, 1983).

4. Side effects may reflect not only a beta$_2$-blockade of peripheral vasodilation but also beta$_1$-mediated falls in cardiac output and limb blood flow.

Nonetheless, cardioselective agents have some advantages. For instance, they have been shown to disturb lipid and carbohydrate metabolism less than nonselective agents, and they will allow diabetics on insulin to raise the blood sugar more rapidly in the event of a hypoglycemic reaction (Lager et al, 1979). As concluded by Breckenridge (1983), "cardioselectivity is a property of limited clinical relevance with respect to efficacy but perhaps of slightly more importance with respect to toxicity."

On the other hand, in the presence of certain concomitant diseases, a nonselective beta$_2$-antagonist effect may be preferable. Examples include migraine and tremor, which seem to be helped because of blockade of beta$_2$-receptors. Also, beta$_2$-receptors are involved in stress-induced hypokalemia, so nonselective agents will block this fall in plasma $K^+$ more than selective ones will (Brown et al, 1983). This could have clinical relevance since stress-induced hypokalemia could be a mechanism for sudden death.

### Intrinsic Sympathomimetic Activity

Of those now available in the United States, pindolol and, to a lesser degree, acebutolol have intrinsic sympathomimetic activity that, on a molecular basis, appears to involve activation of cyclic adenosine monophosphate (AMP). As shown in Figure 7.23, rather than having two

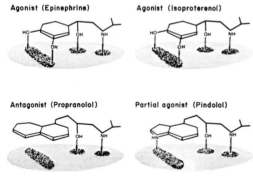

**Figure 7.23.** Major points of attachment for maximal stimulation (agonist, e.g., isoproterenol), less than optimal stimulation (partial agonist, e.g., pindolol), and no stimulation (antagonist, e.g., propranolol). (From Clark BJ: *Am Heart J* 104:334, 1982.)

sites of attachment for full stimulation of the beta-receptor (as does isoproterenol), these drugs have only one site of attachment, thereby producing partial stimulation but at the same time shielding the receptor from natural endogenous agonists. Those beta-blockers with neither site of attachment (such as propranolol) have only antagonist activity. As noted before, beta-blockers with ISA lower the blood pressure equally but cause less or no fall in cardiac output, heart rate, and renin levels (van den Meiracker et al, 1988) (Fig.7.20).

The presence of intrinsic sympathomimetic activity may be clinically reflected in various beneficial features: less bradycardia, less bronchospasm, less decrease in peripheral blood flow, and less derangement of blood lipids (Frishman, 1987). Moreover, cardiac output is well maintained during exercise with the high-ISA drug pindolol compared with propranolol (Ades et al, 1989). Whereas this could improve exercise performance and achievement of conditioning, it limits the reduction in systolic pressure obtained with non-ISA beta-blockers.

### Clinical Use

As noted in Figure 7.20, beta-blockers begin to lower the blood pressure within hours, although the maximal effect may take longer (Man in't Veld et al, 1988a). One of the attractions of beta-blockers is the consistency of their antihypertensive action, which is little altered by changes in activity, posture, or temperature (Prichard and Gillum, 1969). Since the sympathetic nervous system is blocked, the hemodynamic responses to stress are reduced, but most patients can perform ordinary physical activities without difficulty. With more intense stress, however, the response may be blunted, probably enough to interfere with athletic performance (Chick et al, 1988).

### Monotherapy

Beta-blockers have been proposed as initial monotherapy for most cases of hypertension (Laragh, 1976). However, propranolol by itself, in doses up to 480 mg per day, controlled only half of a group of patients with mild hypertension (VA Cooperative Study Group, 1977a). Moreover, a paradoxical rise in pressure was noted in 11% of low-renin patients given a beta-blocker (Drayer et al, 1976), probably reflecting the combination of fluid retention and alpha-adrenergic-mediated peripheral and renal vasoconstriction that occurs in the face of blockade of beta$_2$-receptors in the vascular bed. In patients with normal or high renin, the inhibition of renin by the beta-blocker probably counteracts both of these antagonistic actions.

Two groups of patients who tend to have lower renin levels have also been claimed to respond less to beta-blockers—blacks and the elderly. The evidence showing a lesser response for blacks is persuasive and uniform (Cruickshank et al, 1988; Obel, 1989). However, the claim made by Bühler et al (1984) that the elderly are less responsive seems not to be valid: The elderly respond about as well as do younger patients (Massie, 1987; Freis et al, 1988; Man in't Veld et al, 1988b), and they respond as well to beta-blockers as to diuretics (Wikstrand et al, 1986).

Whereas blacks respond less well, men of Chinese descent are considerably more responsive as compared with American whites (Zhou et al, 1989).

## Comparability of Effects

Though the various beta-blockers have not all been tested against one another, they appear to have fairly equal antihypertensive efficacy (Davidson et al, 1976; Wilcox, 1978) although in randomized crossover studies, atenolol seems to be more effective (Wilcox, 1978; Van Rooijen et al, 1979; Scott et al, 1982).

In various clinical situations, preference may be given to beta-blockers with certain characteristics (Table 7.11). For the majority of patients with uncomplicated hypertension, considering all of these pharmacological and clinical features, there seems to be some advantage in choosing a relatively cardioselective, lipid-insoluble agent with ISA to provide the certainty of prolonged action and the likelihood of fewer side effects. In the future, beta-blockers that also have a vasodilatory effect, e.g. carvedilol or celiprolol, may be especially favored (Opie, 1988a).

## Special Uses for Beta-Blockers in Hypertensives

*Coexisting Coronary Disease.* Even without firm proof that beta-blockers protect hypertensive patients from coronary events, the antiarrhythmic and antianginal effects of the drugs make them especially useful in hypertensive patients with coexisting coronary disease (Lee et al, 1989). On the other hand, patients with variant angina due to coronary spasm may have their problem made worse with these drugs, presumably from unopposed alpha-adrenergic vasoconstriction (Nielsen et al, 1987).

A beneficial effect of beta-blockers in patients with acute myocardial infarction, both intravenously for acute intervention and orally for chronic use, has been clearly documented (Yusuf et al, 1988). In this overview of the results of randomized clinical trials, intravenous beta-blockers are shown to reduce mortality in patients with acute myocardial infarction by 13% (95% confidence interval -2 to -25) and oral beta-blockers to reduce long-term mortality post-MI by 22% (95% confidence interval -16 to -30). The ultrashort acting intravenous agent esmolol

**Table 7.11.  Situations Affecting the Choice of Beta-Blocker**

| Condition | | Relative Contraindication | If used, Type of Beta-Blocker Preferred |
|---|---|---|---|
| Cardiac | Left ventricular failure | Almost always | High ISA[a] |
| | High-degree heart block | Almost always | High ISA |
| | Severe bradycardia | Often | High ISA |
| | Variant (Prinzmetal's) angina | Usual | High ISA |
| | Angina | None | Little ISA |
| Peripheral vascular | Severe claudication | Almost always | Cardioselective, high ISA (small dose) |
| Pulmonary | Bronchospasm, asthma | Always | |
| | Chronic airways disease | Often | Cardioselective (small dose) |
| Central nervous | Severe depression | Usual | Lipid-insoluble |
| | Difficult sleep, dreams | Rare | Lipid-insoluble |
| | Fatigue | Rare | Lipid-insoluble |
| | Migraine | None | Noncardioselective |
| Diabetes mellitus | Insulin-requiring | Often | Cardioselective |
| | Noninsulin-requiring | Rare | Cardioselective |
| Lipid disorders | High triglycerides Low HDL-cholesterol | Often | High ISA |
| Liver disease | | Rare | Lipid-insoluble |
| Renal Disease | | Rare | Lipid-soluble |

[a]ISA, intrinsic sympathomimetic activity.

may be useful in patients with acute MI even in the presence of moderate left ventricular dysfunction (Kirshenbaum et al, 1988).

*Patients Needing Antihypertensive Vasodilator Therapy.* If a diuretic and an adrenergic blocker are inadequate to control blood pressure, addition of a vasodilator is the logical third step. When used alone, direct vasodilators set off reflex sympathetic stimulation of the heart. The simultaneous use of beta-blockers prevents this undesired increase in cardiac output, which not only bothers the patient but also dampens the antihypertensive effect of the vasodilator.

*Patients with Hyperkinetic Hypertension.* Some hypertensive patients have increased cardiac output that may persist for many years. Beta-blockers should be particularly effective in such patients, but a reduction in exercise capacity may restrict their use in young athletes.

*Patients with Marked Anxiety.* The somatic manifestations of anxiety—tremor, sweating, and tachycardia—can be reduced with beta-blockers, which has been found useful for violin players, surgeons and race-car drivers (Tyrer, 1988). This may extend to patients with alcohol withdrawal (Kraus et al, 1985). Timolol was found to be useful as a nonsedative, antianxiety premedication for patients undergoing day surgery (Mackenzie and Bird, 1989). Atenolol protected patients with acute head injury from stress-induced cardiac damage (Cruickshank et al, 1987).

Other conditions for which beta-blockers may be useful include migraine, intention tremor, and glaucoma. Timolol eyedrops may cause systemic effects whereas a newer agent, metipranolol, causes less (Bacon et al, 1989).

## Dosage

Most of the drugs have a flat dose-response curve as has been demonstrated for propranolol: The response to 40 mg twice daily was equal to that found with 80, 160, or 240 mg twice daily (Serlin et al, 1980). With atenolol, 25 mg/day was as effective as 50, 75, or 100 mg (Marshall et al, 1979).

Lipid-insoluble agents are removed mainly by renal excretion and have relatively longer serum half-lives. In patients with renal insufficiency, higher blood levels are seen with usual doses (McAnish et al, 1980). Though there is little evidence of greater effects—either good or bad—from these higher blood levels, the doses should be progressively reduced in those with renal insufficiency.

All beta-blockers act longer on the blood pressure than the pharmacokinetics data would imply. In moderate doses, most beta-blockers will likely keep the blood pressure down when given once daily (Watson et al, 1979; Johansson et al, 1980). To ensure adequate control, early morning blood pressures should be measured before the daily dose is taken.

## Drug Interactions (Table 7.12)

Most of those listed in Table 7.12 relating to interference with metabolism are of little clinical significance. However, those related to beta-blockade may be serious, including potentiation of side effects of antiarrhythmic drugs and hypotension with calcium antagonists or alpha-blockers (Beeley, 1984). Other interactions lead to pressor reactions: In addition to that noted during hypoglycemia, serious hypertension may occur when exogenous sympathomimetics (diet pills, nose drops) are ingested, although in a careful study, propranolol antagonized the pressor effect of phenylpropanolamines (Pentel et al, 1985).

Some interactions interfere with beta-blockers, including the action of nonsteroidal antiinflammatory agents (Durao et al, 1977; Webster, 1985).

## Interactions with Food, Drink, and Cigarettes

Simultaneous ingestion of protein-rich food increases bioavailability of propranolol apparently by a decrease in hepatic clearance and not by an increase in hepatic blood flow (Modi et al, 1988). Alcohol ingestion reduced plasma propranolol (Sotaniemi et al, 1981) as did smoking (Feely et al, 1981), both presumably from increased hepatic oxidative metabolism. These effects point to a need to maintain a constant pattern of beta-blocker intake, at the same time each day and in the same relation to food intake.

## Side Effects

The side effects of beta-blockers reflect the blockade of both beta$_1$- and beta$_2$-receptors (Frishman, 1988). Those that are more cardioselective would be expected to induce fewer beta$_2$ effects, and this has been noted (Fodor et al, 1987) (Fig. 7.24). In this single-blind study of 52 hypertensive patients who had a past history of side effects with beta-blocker therapy, three 8-week courses of beta-blocker therapy

**Table 7.12. Drug Interactions with Beta-Adrenoceptor Antagonists[a]**

| Drugs Interfering | Mechanism | Effect |
| --- | --- | --- |
| *Due to beta-adrenoceptor blockade* | | |
| Sympathomimetic amines (including common cold remedies), adrenaline | Unopposed alpha-receptor stimulation | Hypertensive crisis |
| Ergotamine | Additive vasoconstrictor effect | Hypertensive crisis |
| Clonidine withdrawal | Unopposed alpha-receptor stimulation | Hypertensive crisis |
| Verapamil, diltiazem, antiarrhythmic agents | Additive depression of sinoatrial/atrioventricular conduction | Bradycardia, AV conduction asystole |
| Nifedipine, verapamil, diltiazem, antiarrhythmic agents | Additive negative inotropic effect | Cardiac failure |
| $Beta_2$-agonists | $Beta_2$-receptor blockade | Antagonism of $Beta_2$-receptor mediated bronchodilatation |
| *Interference with metabolism* | | |
| Cimetidine, chlorpromazine | Decreased hepatic metabolism | Increased plasma levels of certain beta-blockers |
| Hydralazine | Decreased hepatic clearance | Increased plasma levels of certain beta-blockers |
| Thyroxine, rifampicin | Increased metabolism | Decreased plasma levels of certain beta-blockers |
| *Others* | | |
| NSAIDs | Sodium retention | Antagonism of antihypertensive effect |
| Diuretics | Hypokalaemia | Risk of ventricular arrhythmias with sotalol |
| Insulin | Masking of adrenergic response to hypoglycaemia and inhibition of glycaemic response to hypoglycaemia | Masking of hypoglycaemia symptoms and delaying recovery from hypoglycaemia |

[a]From McMurray, JJV, Struthers AD: *Med Int* 60:2459, 1988.

were given in doses needed to control the blood pressure. The first course was with propranolol 40 to 160 mg twice daily, the second with atenolol, 50 to 100 mg once daily, the third with the previously used dose of propranolol. Most side effects were more common with the nonselective lipid-soluble propranolol and most recurred at a similar frequency on rechallenge with that drug.

## Central Nervous System

As noted in Figure 7.24, central nervous system side effects—insomnia, nightmares, depressed mood—occur in some patients but less with the lipid-insoluble agents (Kostis and Rosen, 1987). The very frequent side effects of centrally acting adrenergic inhibiting drugs—sedation and dry mouth—are very rare.

Moreover, two major problems—depression and cognitive side effects, e.g., memory, motor performance, abstraction—which are widely perceived to be commonly seen may not be. In a review of 55 published studies, beta-blocker use was found to worsen cognitive function in 17%, improve function in 16%, and have no significant effect in the rest (Dimsdale et al, 1989). As for depression, most short-term studies show little effect on mood (Blumenthal et al, 1988) and major depression was slightly less frequent in a group of patients on beta-blockers than in those on other medications for chest pain (Carney et al, 1987).

## Carbohydrate Metabolism

Diabetics may have additional problems with beta-blockers. The responses to hypoglycemia, both the symptoms and the counterregulatory hormonal changes that raise the blood sugar, are largely mediated by epinephrine, particularly in those who are insulin dependent since they are usually also deficient in glucagon (Popp et al, 1984). If they became hypoglycemic, the beta-blockade of epinephrine responses would delay the return of the blood sugar (Lager et al, 1979). The more cardioselective beta-blockers are preferable for those susceptible to hypoglycemia

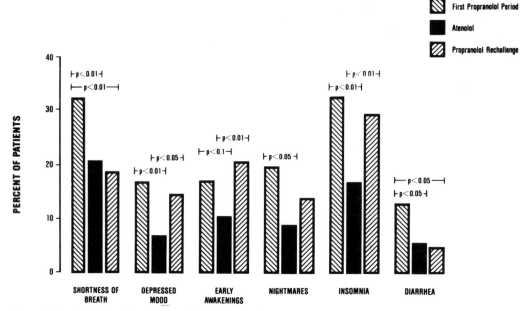

**Figure 7.24.** Overall incidence rates of side effects during 8 weeks of treatment with propranolol and atenolol (N = 52) (ANOVA). (From Fodor JG, et al: *J Clin Pharmacol* 27:892, 1987.)

(Clausen-Sjöbom et al, 1987), but all may delay recovery. Moreover, hypoglycemia reactions may precipitate a marked rise in blood pressure, even to the level of a hypertensive crisis (Mann and Krakoff, 1984). The only symptom of hypoglycemia may be sweating, which may be enhanced in the presence of a beta-blocker (Molnar et al, 1974) so that the patient should be advised to use sweating as a sign of hypoglycemia.

Those diabetics not on insulin may become more hyperglycemic when given a beta-blocker but much more so when they are also given a diuretic (Dornhorst et al, 1985).

The larger population of nondiabetic hypertensives may be at a higher risk for developing overt diabetes when treated with beta-blockers. Both metoprolol and atenolol given for 16 weeks significantly inhibited glucose uptake mediated by insulin; the insulin resistance was accompanied by higher plasma insulin levels (Pollare et al, 1989c). In a 12-year follow-up of 98 women on a beta-blocker, the relative risk for developing diabetes was 6.1 times greater for them than for women on no antihypertensive drugs (Bengtsson et al, 1984). In another 9-year prospective study, the incidence of diabetes was 6-fold higher among 67 men who took a beta-blocker (35 also took a diuretic) than seen in a matched group of nontreated normotensives (Skarfors et al, 1989).

**Lipid Metabolism**

Beta-blockers without ISA clearly raise serum triglycerides and lower HDL-cholesterol (Weidmann et al, 1985; Lardinois and Neuman, 1988) (Fig. 7.25). The effects may be less with cardioselective agents (Day et al, 1982) and even less or not seen with those having ISA (Weidmann et al, 1985; Terént et al, 1989). The inability of beta-blocker-based antihypertensive therapy to clearly reduce coronary mortality, as reviewed in Chapter 5, has only naturally led to speculation that the lipid changes are responsible for this lack of primary protection (Lithell et al, 1988).

The mechanism for this effect is unknown. One proposed mechanism: Day et al (1982) observed a delay in the clearance of intravenous soya oil given to 25 patients on a beta-blocker that they attributed to an inhibition of lipoprotein lipase activity by unopposed alpha-stimulation. Another has been suggested by the finding of increased peripheral production of HDL-cholesterol during exercise, interpreted as a reflection of an increased delivery of substrates for lipoprotein lipase through the increased muscle blood flow (Ruys et al, 1989). Peripheral vasoconstriction induced by non-ISA beta-blockers could then be reflected in lower peripheral HDL production.

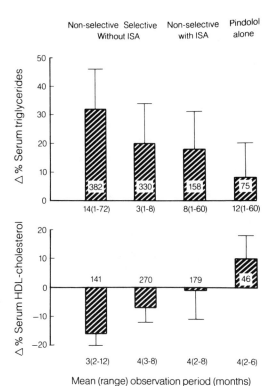

**Figure 7.25.** Mean percentage of responses of serum triglycerides and HDL-cholesterol to monotherapy with different types of beta-blockers (mean ± SD). *ISA*, intrinsic sympathomimetic activity. *Numbers in bar columns*, total numbers of reported cases used for analysis. (From Weidmann P, Uehlinger DE, Gerber A: *J Hypertens* 3:297, 1985.)

### Renal Function

A 20% fall in glomerular filtration rate and renal blood flow (RBF) has been observed in normotensive and hypertensive patients with normal kidney function who were given propranolol (Bauer and Brooks, 1979). The decrease in RBF was related to a fall in cardiac output accompanied by renal vasoconstriction from unopposed alpha-adrenergic tone. No such falls in renal function were noted in patients given the cardioselective agent atenolol (Wilkinson et al, 1980) or nadolol (Textor et al, 1982). Despite the potential problem, renal dysfunction is rarely seen, even in those who have underlying renal insufficiency (Epstein and Oster, 1985).

### Potassium

A slight rise in serum potassium may be seen with chronic use of beta-blockers (Traub et al, 1980). During exercise, the rise may be even greater (Carlsson et al, 1978). These effects likely reflect blockade of the beta$_2$-mediated epineph-

rine activation of the Na$^+$, K$^+$-ATPase pump that normally transports potassium from extracellular fluid into cells (Rosa et al, 1980). As noted earlier, during stress plasma K$^+$ may fall as much as 1.0 mmol/liter; the effect can be blocked by beta$_2$-receptor blockade.

In addition, the beta-blocker suppression of renin release could reduce the secondary aldosteronism seen with diuretic therapy. Despite this, beta-blocking therapy may not protect against diuretic-induced hypokalemia (Carriere et al, 1984; Steiness, 1984). This may reflect some K$^+$-wasting from the beta-blocker: A cumulative 150-mmol negative potassium balance was measured in seven patients given timolol for 8 days (Steiness, 1984).

### Calcium Metabolism

After 6 months on propranolol, plasma-ionized calcium and phosphate levels increased and parathyroid hormone levels decreased (Hvarfner et al, 1988). This pattern was attributed to reduced calcium binding to albumin, increasing ionized calcium, which suppresses PTH.

### Exercise Capacity

Beta-blockers will reduce the ability to perform exercise, in part because of the more rapid onset of the feeling of fatigue and the subjective perception that exercise is harder to perform, which may arise more from central than peripheral mechanisms (Cooper et al, 1988). However, in addition, beta$_2$-blockade interferes with circulatory and metabolic response to exercise (Cleroux et al, 1989) and impairs the attainment of conditioning (McLeod et al, 1984). Nonetheless, conditioning can be attained (Chick et al, 1988), likely with less difficulty with cardioselective agents (Ades et al, 1988). High ISA drugs, e.g., pindolol, allow maintenance of normal cardiac output (Ades et al, 1989) but do not appear to maintain exercise tolerance any better than non-ISA drugs, e.g., propranolol (Duncan et al, 1989).

Despite these problems with performance, beta-blockers are considered the drugs of choice for suppressing excessive rises in blood pressure during isotonic exercise (Klaus, 1989). They may not do so well in suppressing the rise during isometric exercise (Hamada et al, 1987).

### Pregnancy

Intrauterine growth retardation, respiratory distress, bradycardia, and hypoglycemia have been observed in some fetuses when beta-blockers are given during pregnancy, but as noted in Chapter 11, overall results seem as good or better than with other drugs. The drugs enter breast milk but only in very low concentrations (Liedholm et al, 1981).

### Impotence

Impotence has been noted with beta-blockers, as with all antihypertensive agents, as noted earlier in this chapter (Croog et al, 1986). In the MRC trial, the frequency of impotence elicited by a questionnaire increased from 10.1% among those on placebo to 13.2% for those on propranolol (Medical Research Council Working Party, 1981).

### Skin and Connective Tissue

Practolol, the only beta-blocker to possess an acetanilide structure, is the only one to cause a serious and progressive oculomucocutaneous syndrome (Editorial, *Br Med J*, 1977).

Despite isolated case reports, there does not appear to be a causal connection between beta-blockers and retroperitoneal fibrosis (Pryor et al, 1983). Psoriasis has been worsened by use of beta-blockers (Savola et al, 1987).

### Discontinuation Syndromes

In hypertensives taking beta-adrenergic blockers, abrupt cessation may lead to withdrawal symptoms suggestive of sympathetic overactivity (Houston, 1988). However, the more frequent and serious discontinuation syndrome is seen in patients with underlying coronary artery disease who may develop angina, infarction, or sudden death (Miller et al, 1975). These ischemic episodes likely reflect the phenomenon of supersensitivity: An increased number of beta-receptors appear in response to the functional blockade of receptors by the beta-blocker; when the beta-blocker is discontinued and no longer occupies the receptors, the increased number of receptors are suddenly exposed to endogenous catecholamines, resulting in a greater beta-agonist response for a given level of catechols. Hypertensives, with a high frequency of underlying coronary atherosclerosis, may be particularly susceptible to this type of withdrawal syndrome, so when the drugs are discontinued, their dosage should be cut by half every 2 or 3 days and the drugs stopped after the third reduction.

### Overdose

Massive intoxication of beta-blockers may cause profound hypotension, seizures, and coma, which are usually responsive to appropriate beta-agonist therapy (Warwick and Boulton-Jones, 1989). Membrane stabilizing activity (MSA), a pharmacological property usually given little attention, may be responsible for the higher rate of deaths from overdoses of drugs that have MSA (e.g., propranolol) than from those that do not (e.g., atenolol) (Henry and Cassidy, 1986).

## ALPHA- AND BETA-RECEPTOR BLOCKERS

Modification of the conventional beta-blocker structure has provided agents with combined alpha- and beta-blocking properties. Labetalol is now available, and a number of other blockers are being investigated, including dilevalol, an R,R isomer of labetalol, (Strom et al, 1989); carvedilol (Cubeddu et al, 1987); prizidilol (Lund-Johansen, 1988); and medroxalol (Williams et al, 1987b). Yet another, bufuralol, appears to vasodilate because of beta$_2$ stimulation along with its beta$_1$-blocking effect (Pfisterer et al, 1984). The following relates only to labetalol.

### Chemistry

Oral labetalol is rapidly absorbed, is lipid soluble, undergoes first-pass metabolism in the liver, and is about 33% bioavailable (Goa et al, 1989). Bioavailability increases with the patient's age because of decreased clearance of the drug (Abernethy et al, 1987). When administered with food, the bioavailability may be increased by a third, but at the same time absorption is slowed so that the time of maximal drug concentration increases from 1 hour after intake to 3 hours (Daneshmend and Roberts, 1982).

### Mode of Action

Labetalol is a nonselective beta$_1$- and beta$_2$-receptor blocker and is, like prazosin, highly selective for alpha$_1$-receptors. The ratio of alpha- to beta-blocking action has been estimated as between 1:3 and 1:7. The ratio may fall with increasing plasma concentrations because the upper plateau of the dose-response curve for beta-blockade may be reached at lower plasma concentration, whereas maximal alpha-blockade may not occur until plasma concentrations are much higher (Louis et al, 1984).

The hemodynamic consequences of the combined alpha- and beta-blockade are a fall in blood pressure mainly via a fall in systemic vascular resistance with little effect on cardiac output (Opie, 1988c) (Fig. 7.26). Note the distinct hemodynamic differences between classical beta-blockers and labetalol.

With chronic therapy, renal vascular resistance and forearm resistance are reduced. Coronary blood flow is slightly decreased but less than with conventional beta-blockers.

Acutely, plasma renin activity decreases and then rises, whereas norepinephrine levels increase (Vlachakis et al, 1984). Chronically, PRA is increased, and plasma aldosterone is unchanged (Weidmann et al, 1978). These authors reported increased urinary excretion of catecholamines, but this has subsequently been found to be a chemical interference and not a true increase in excretion (Hamilton et al, 1978). However, it remains a source of major diagnostic confusion if workup for pheochromocytoma is done while the patient is on labetalol (see Chapter 12).

## Clinical Use

Given orally, labetalol is effective in patients with mild to severe hypertension (Wallin and O'Neill, 1983). It maintains good 24-hour control and blunts early morning surges in pressure when given twice daily (DeQuattro et al, 1988). It has been reported to be more effective than propranolol in black hypertensives (El-Ackad et al, 1984) and the elderly (Buell et al, 1988). Its effect on supine blood pressure is comparable to that of a beta-blocking drug, but its effect on standing blood pressure is greater. The antihypertensive effect has been found to be similar to that of a beta-blocker and hydralazine (Barnett et al, 1978), and it is effective in patients with renal insufficiency (Williams et al, 1978). Fluid retention may develop when it is used alone, so a diuretic may be needed (Weidmann et al, 1978).

Labetalol has been used both orally and intravenously to treat hypertensive emergencies including postoperative hypertension (Leslie et al, 1987). The drug can be used to treat hypertensives with angina (Opie, 1988c) or with vasospastic side effects of beta-blockers (Eliasson et al, 1984). Despite its antihypertensive effect, it has been said not to reverse echocardiographic left ventricular hypertrophy (Weinberg et al, 1984). It has been successfully used to treat

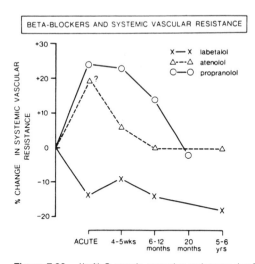
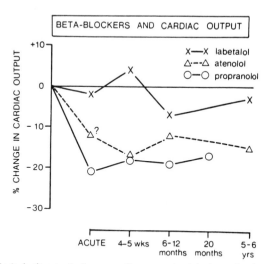

**Figure 7.26.** (*Left*) Systemic vascular resistance (or SVR index) after acute therapy, after approximately 1 month of therapy, after 6 to 12 months, and after 5 to 6 years of therapy with labetalol, atenolol, or propranolol. Data (from Jokes AM, Thompson FD: *Br J Clin Pharmacol* 3(Suppl):789, 1976) for acute labetalol; (from Tsukiyama H, Otsuka K, Higuma K: *Br J Clin Pharmacol* 13:269S, 1982) for 4 to 5 weeks; and (from Lund-Johansen P: *Am J Med* 75:24, 1983) for 1 to 6 years of labetalol. For atenolol, acute data estimated (from Holtzman JL, Finley D, Johnson B, et al: *Clin Pharmacol Ther* 40:268, 1986); 4- to 5-week data averaged (from Tsukiyama H, Otsuka K, Higuma K: *Br J Clin Pharmacol* 13:269S, 1982) and (Dreslinski GR, Messerli FH, Dunn FG, et al: *Circulation* 65:1365, 1982); 1- to 5-year data from (Lund-Johansen P: *J Cardiovasc Pharmacol* 1:487, 1979). For propranolol data, see (Tarazi RC, Dustan HP: *Am J Cardiol* 29:633, 1972) except for 5-week data (Tsukiyama H, Otsuka K, Higuma K: *Br J Clin Pharmacol* 13:269S, 1982). (*Right*) Cardiac output (or cardiac index) for same groups as in left, with same data sources. (From Opie LH: *Cardiovasc Drugs Ther* 2:369, 1988c.)

hypertension during pregnancy (Lunell et al, 1981).

## Side Effects

In a multicenter trial, 22% of 128 patients withdrew from therapy with labetalol because of side effects (New Zealand Hypertension Study Group, 1981). Symptomatic orthostatic hypotension, the most common side effect, is seen most often during initial therapy, when large doses are used, or during hot weather. Labetalol has occasionally caused a paradoxical increase in blood pressure in patients with pheochromocytoma and in those receiving other antihypertensive medication (Briggs et al, 1978). A variety of other side effects have been seen (Brogden et al, 1978), including intense scalp itching (New Zealand Hypertension Study Group, 1981) and ejaculatory failure (O'Meara and White, 1988). Bronchospasm is less likely to occur with labetalol than with a beta-blocking drug but has been reported occasionally (Light et al, 1983). An increased titer of antinuclear and antimitochondrial antibodies has developed in some patients (Wilson et al, 1980). Although a systemic lupus syndrome has not been reported, lichenoid skin eruptions have been (Prichard, 1984). Hepatic dysfunction occurs rarely but, in a few cases, has been fatal (Douglas et al, 1989).

In keeping with its alpha-blocking effect, labetalol apparently does not adversely alter blood lipids, as do conventional beta-blockers (Lardinois and Neuman, 1988).

## Dilevalol

The R,R-stereoisomer of labetalol differs in being a selective beta$_2$-agonist with nonselective beta-adrenergic blocking effects but is similar in that it also reduces blood pressure mainly by peripheral vasodilation (Strom et al, 1989). In doses of 400 to 1600 mg once daily, it does not adversely alter lipids and may raise HDL-cholesterol in patients with initially low levels (Materson et al, 1989).

## DIRECT VASODILATORS

Drugs that enter the vascular smooth muscle cell to cause vasodilation are termed *direct* vasodilators. This is in contrast to those that vasodilate in other ways, by inhibiting hormonal vasoconstrictor mechanisms (e.g., ACE inhibitors), or by preventing the calcium entry into the cells that initiate constriction (e.g., calcium entry blockers), or by blocking alpha-receptor mediated vasoconstriction (e.g., alpha$_1$-blockers).

The direct vasodilators set off baroreceptor reflex-mediated sympathetic stimulation that precludes their use as initial therapy and positions them largely as the third drug to be added to a diuretic and an adrenergic inhibitor. Since the other three types of vasodilators in some manner blunt sympathetic activation, they increasingly are being used as the initial or the second drug in therapy.

Vasodilators differ considerably in their power, mode of action, and relative activities on arteries and veins (Table 7.13).

## Hydralazine (Apresoline)

### Chemistry

One of several phthalazine derivatives with hypotensive action, hydralazine is the only one approved for use in the United States. Hydralazine is well absorbed from the gut; a maximal blood level is reached in an hour; the plasma half-life is 2 to 3 hours but some persists for up to 24 hours, and it remains even longer within the walls of muscular arteries (Talseth, 1976a).

The inactivation of hydralazine involves acetylation in the liver by the enzyme N-acetyltransferase. The level of this enzyme activity is genetically determined: Rapid acetylation is probably coded for by an autosomal dominant gene; slow acetylators are homozygotes for the allele coding for slow acetylation (Batchelor et al, 1980). As we shall see, Perry et al (1970) showed that those who develop a lupus-like toxicity tend to be slow acetylators and thus are exposed to the drug longer.

In patients with impaired renal function, the plasma half-life is greatly prolonged, perhaps because of a decrease in both renal clearance and metabolic conversion (Talseth, 1976b).

**Table 7.13. Vasodilator Drugs Used to Treat Hypertension**

| Drug | Relative Action on Arteries (A) or Veins (V) |
|---|---|
| Direct | |
|   Hydralazine | A >> V |
|   Minoxidil | A >> V |
|   Nitroprusside | A + V |
|   Diazoxide | A > V |
|   Nitroglycerin | V > A |
| Calcium entry blockers | A >> V |
| Angiotensin converting enzyme inhibitors | A > V |
| Alpha-blockers | A + V |

## Mode of Action

The drug acts directly to relax the smooth muscle in the walls of peripheral arterioles, the resistance vessels more so than the capacitance vessels, thereby decreasing peripheral resistance and blood pressure (Finkelstein et al, 1988).

*Compensatory Responses.* Coincidental to the peripheral vasodilation, the heart rate, stroke volume, cardiac output, and myocardial oxygen requirement rise. Most of this appears to reflect baroreceptor-mediated reflex increase in sympathetic discharge (Fig. 7.27) with a close correlation between tachycardia and plasma norepinephrine levels (Lin et al, 1983). Direct stimulation of the heart (Khatri et al, 1977) and central nervous system effects may also be involved (Gupta and Bhargava, 1965).

In addition, the sympathetic overactivity and the fall in blood pressure increase renin release (Ueda et al, 1968) that, with the catecholamines, counteracts the vasodilator's effect. Beyond these effects that can be prevented by sympathetic blockers, direct vasodilators cause sodium retention, and this is preventable by concomitant diuretic therapy (Fig. 7.27).

## Clinical Use

These compensatory responses sharply limited the use of hydralazine by itself. Furthermore, the average reduction in blood pressure with 200 mg of hydralazine per day plus a thiazide was only 11/12 mm Hg, but when reserpine, 0.25 mg twice daily, was added, the hypotensive effect of the three agents was superior to that of any two, producing an average blood pressure reduction of 23/21 mm Hg (VA Cooperative Study, 1962). Moreover, the bothersome cardiac side effects of hydralazine were neutralized by the adrenergic blocking action of the reserpine. More recently, a beta-blocker has usually been combined with hydralazine and a diuretic in the treatment of more severe hypertension (Eggertsen and Hansson, 1985).

In older patients, with less responsive baroreceptor reflexes, hydralazine may lower the blood pressure without causing sympathetic overactivity (VA Cooperative Study Group, 1981b).

Nonsteroidal antiinflammatory drugs (NSAIDs) such as indomethacin attenuate the hypotensive action of hydralazine (Cinquegrani and Liang, 1986).

## Dosage

Alone or in combination, hydralazine should usually be started at 25 mg 2 times per day. Though the drug has usually been prescribed in three and four doses daily, the good and bad effects are similar for two doses as for four doses daily (O'Malley et al, 1975).

The maximal dose, although often stated to be 400 mg, should probably be limited to 200 mg per day for two reasons: to lessen the likelihood of a lupus-like syndrome and because higher doses seldom provide additional benefit. In one study, when hydralazine was added to therapy with a diuretic and a beta-blocker, 50 mg twice daily gave as much antihypertensive effect as did 100 or 200 mg twice daily (Vandenburg et al, 1982).

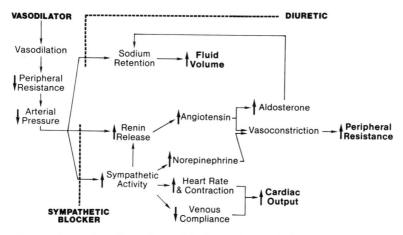

**Figure 7.27.** Primary and secondary effects of vasodilator therapy in essential hypertension and the manner by which diuretic and beta-adrenergic blocker therapy can overcome the undesirable secondary effects. (From Koch-Weser J: *Arch Intern Med* 133:1017, 1974, copyright 1974, American Medical Association.)

## Side Effects

Four kinds of side affects are seen: those due to reflex sympathetic activation, those due to fluid retention, those due to a lupus-like reaction, and nonspecific problems. As noted, the headaches, flushing, and tachycardia should be anticipated and prevented by concomitant use of adrenergic inhibitors. Unless an adrenergic inhibitor is also used, the drug should be given with caution to patients with coronary artery disease and should be avoided in patients with a dissecting aortic aneurysm or recent cerebral hemorrhage, in view of its propensity to increase cardiac output and cerebral blood flow (Schroeder and Sillesen, 1987).

The lupus-like reaction has been described by Perry (1973), reviewing his experience with 371 patients given the drug for as long as 20 years: An early, febrile reaction resembling serum sickness was seen in 11 patients; late toxicity developed in 44 (with serious symptoms in 14), resembling systemic lupus erythematosus or rheumatoid arthritis. These symptoms almost invariably went away when therapy was stopped or the dosage was lowered; this late toxicity occurred only among the one-half of the population who are slow acetylators of the drug. Though Perry noted that remissions of serious hypertension may occur more frequently and overall survival may be better among patients who develop toxicity (Perry et al, 1977), rapidly progressive renal damage has been reported (Sturman et al, 1988).

Susceptibility to hydralazine-induced lupus, as with idiopathic lupus, may depend partly upon genetically determined lower levels of the classical pathway complement protein, C4 (Speirs et al, 1989).

The syndrome is clearly dose dependent. In a prospective study of 281 patients, no cases of the lupus syndrome were seen in those taking 50 mg daily whereas it was seen in 5.4% taking 100 mg daily and in 10.4% with 200 mg daily (Cameron and Ramsay, 1984). The incidence was 4-fold higher in women than in men, and 19.4% of women taking 200 mg daily developed the syndrome. The incidence of a positive antinuclear antibody titer of 1:20 or higher is even greater: Whereas 50% of patients taking hydralazine did so, only 3% developed the lupus syndrome (Mansilla-Tinoco et al, 1982).

Other side effects include anorexia, nausea, vomiting, and diarrhea and, less commonly, paresthesias, tremor, and muscle cramps.

One seldom considered advantage of hydralazine is that it usually *lowers* serum cholesterol, as noted in 1955 (Perry and Schroeder, 1955) and reconfirmed more recently (Lopez et al 1983). These authors noted a fall in LDL and a rise in HDL cholesterol levels with hydralazine. The same good lipid effects have been noted with minoxidil (Johnson et al, 1986).

One additional potential disadvantage of hydralazine (and other direct vasodilators) is its failure when given alone to regress left ventricular hypertrophy, presumably because of its marked stimulation of sympathetic nervous activity (Leenen et al, 1987).

### Minoxidil (Loniten)

More potent than hydralazine, minoxidil has become a mainstay in the therapy of severe hypertension associated with renal insufficiency (see Chapter 9). Its propensity to grow hair precludes its use in many women, but this effect has led to its use as a topical ointment for male pattern baldness. Some of the drug is absorbed: Slight but significant increases in left ventricular (LV) end-diastolic volume, cardiac output, and LV mass were recorded after 6 months' use of topical minoxidil (Leenen et al, 1988). Orally, the drug is effective when used with diuretics and adrenergic inhibitors, controlling perhaps 75% of patients previously resistant to multiple drugs (Mitchell and Pettinger, 1978; Keusch et al, 1978; Taverner et al, 1983).

### Chemistry

A piperidinopyrimidine derivative, minoxidil is well absorbed, and peak plasma levels are reached within 1 hour (Pettinger, 1980). Though its plasma half-life is only 4 hours, antihypertensive effects persist for about 24 hours, and it can be used once daily (Johnson et al, 1986). It is metabolized in the liver, and the inactive glucuronide is excreted mainly in the urine. Daily doses vary from 2.5 to 60 mg.

### Mode of Action

Minoxidil induces smooth muscle relaxation by increasing potassium permeability, which in turn inhibits calcium influx, a mechanism apparently unique among currently available vasodilators (Meisheri et al, 1988).

*Compensatory Reactions.* Since it is both more potent and longer lasting than hydralazine, it is not surprising that minoxidil turns on the various reactions to direct arteriolar vasodilation to an even greater degree. Therefore, large doses of potent diuretics and adrenergic blockers will be needed in most patients.

## Clinical Use

When combined with these other drugs, minoxidil may provide excellent control of the blood pressure, even in patients with severe renal insufficiency. Thereby renal function may improve, particularly in those who present with malignant hypertension (Mitchell et al, 1980). However, the propensity to reactive fluid retention precludes the use of even small doses of minoxidil as a third drug in the treatment of more moderate hypertension (Westwood et al, 1986).

## Side Effects

Very rarely, profound hypotension may follow the initial dose (Allon et al, 1986). The most common side effect, seen in about 80%, is hirsutism, beginning with fairly fine hair on the face and then with coarse hair increasing everywhere, including the external ear canal to the extent of causing hearing loss (Toriumi et al, 1988). It is apparently related to the vasodilation and not to hormonal effects (Feldman and Puschett, 1980). The hair gradually disappears when the drug is stopped.

Beyond generalized volume expansion, pericardial effusions appear in about 3% of the patients who receive minoxidil (Martin et al, 1980). Since most of these patients had severe renal disease, many being on dialysis, it is difficult to ascribe the effusion specifically to minoxidil. However, in a few cases without renal or cardiac failure, effusions appear and may disappear, despite continuation of minoxidil (Houston et al, 1981).

Two other prior concerns about cardiopulmonary side effects have not been substantiated. Right atrial fibrotic lesions were noted in dogs given massive doses of minoxidil but have not been described in man (Sobota et al, 1980). Pulmonary hypertension has been reported, but this likely reflects the presence of high pulmonary vascular resistance before minoxidil was administered (Atkins et al, 1977).

## Investigational Drugs

A number of direct-acting vasodilators are under clinical study, including caldralazine (Persson et al, 1987); endralazine (Kindler et al, 1987); pinacidil (Goldberg et al, 1989); carprazidil (Gerber et al, 1984); and cyclosidimine (Shanks et al, 1984).

Nitrates, by their vasodilating properties akin to endothelium-derived relaxing factor, can also be used as antihypertensives, both transdermal nitroglycerin (Simon et al, 1986) and sublingual isosorbide (Fontanet et al, 1987).

Intravenous direct vasodilators, in particular diazoxide and nitroprusside, are considered in the next chapter.

## CALCIUM ENTRY BLOCKERS

These drugs, here referred to as calcium entry blockers (CEBs), are called calcium antagonists by their discoverer, the German physiologist Albrecht Fleckenstein (1967). Since their introduction as antianginal agents in the 1970s but even more since their approval as antihypertensives in the 1980s, they have been increasingly used to treat hypertension and they are included among the recommended choices for initial monotherapy in the 1988 Joint National Committee (JNC-4) report (Joint National Committee, 1988).

These drugs work by inhibiting the entry of calcium into cardiac and smooth muscle cells through calcium-permeable channels in the cell plasma membrane. The movement of calcium through these channels is much slower than that of sodium during depolarization, so they are referred to as "slow channels." As detailed in Chapter 3, a rise in intracellular calcium is intimately involved in smooth muscle contraction so these drugs act at a critical, basic level to lower the blood pressure. They may do even more: In vitro, they inhibit the action of platelet-derived growth factor on vascular smooth muscle cells (Block et al, 1989), so they may be capable of interrupting the hypertrophy induced by various growth factors that establishes the hypertensive process.

Until recently, only three CEBs were available in the United States and most of the rest of the world: nifedipine, verapamil, and diltiazem. Nicardipine is the first of a large number of "second generation" drugs, mostly dihydropyridines, which are being introduced, and the total number of CEBs to be marketed will likely rival the beta-blockers (Feely et al, 1988).

The currently available CEBs differ in their molecular structure, their sites and modes of action upon the slow channel, and their effects upon various other cardiovascular functions (Das, 1988). There are, therefore, differences in clinical actions and marked variations in side effects between the three types of CEBs now available. Although they are all effective antihypertensive agents, the dihydropyridines are the most potent peripheral vasodilators and, although all CEBs have a negative inotropic effect in vitro, only verapamil and diltiazem exhibit these effects in vivo whereas the dihydropyridines have little effect on atrioventricular conduction (Opie, 1988b) (Table 7.14).

## Chemistry

These agents include some that are related to papaverine (verapamil), others that are dihydropyridines (nifedipine, nicardipine, etc.), and others that are benzothiazepines (diltiazem) (Fig. 7.28). Their selective action on the slow channels distinguishes them from other vasodilators that appear to interfere with the availability of calcium ions within cells in other ways (Zsoter and Church, 1983).

## Mode of Action

The CEBs lower the blood pressure by interfering with calcium-dependent contractions of vascular smooth muscle, thereby producing a fall in peripheral vascular resistance (Lund-Johansen and Omvik, 1987). The dihydropyridines are the most powerful in relaxing peripheral vascular smooth muscles and thereby are more likely to activate baroreceptor reflexes that lead to an increase in plasma catecholamines and heart rate (Opie, 1988b). The negative chronotropic effects of verapamil and diltiazem may block this reflex sympathetic stimulation and result in a decreased heart rate (Table 7.14).

The possibility has been raised that CEBs not only lower the blood pressure but actually correct an underlying defect responsible for the increased pressure—the increased intracellular calcium concentration described in Chapter 3 that may, in turn, be the final pathway to vascular hypertrophy (Block et al, 1989). Moreover, the presumed defect in the transport of sodium across cell membranes that is in turn thought to be responsible for the increase in free intracellular calcium has been shown to be decreased after therapy with verapamil (Gray et al, 1984) or diltiazem (Khalil-Manesh et al, 1987), and the membrane fluidity of red blood cells is increased by both of these CEBs (Tsuda et al, 1988).

As attractive as this seems to be, caution has been advised in interpreting a greater effect of CEBs in hypertensives that may be simply proportional to the degree of hypertension, rather than a specific reversal of an underlying abnormality.

CEBs may reduce calcium entry in ways beyond their blockade of voltage-sensitive slow channels. van Zwieten et al (1987) have provided evidence that they may also block receptor-operated channels, involving both alpha-adrenoreceptors and angiotensin II receptors, which trigger the influx of calcium into cells. The dihydropyridine nicardipine, but not verapamil, provided functional alpha-antagonism (Pedrinelli et al, 1989). CEBs decrease vascular (and adrenal) responsiveness to angiotensin II (Millar et al, 1981) and induce a mild natriuresis (Reams et al, 1988) that could also contribute to their antihypertensive action.

## Clinical Use

The currently available calcium antagonists seem comparable in their antihypertensive potency (Frishman et al, 1988) although no direct comparisons have been made between them. They have been used alone, in combination with other agents, and in the treatment of refractory hypertension and hypertensive crisis (Kaplan, 1989c).

In the usual circumstances of mild to moderate hypertension, any of these drugs, when given alone, will control the hypertension of about two-thirds of patients. This has been seen with nifedipine (Hallin et al, 1983), nicardipine (Leonetti and Zanchetti, 1988), diltiazem (Pool et al, 1986), and verapamil (Zachariah et al, 1987).

In patients inadequately controlled on two drugs, i.e., a diuretic and an ACE inhibitor, the addition of a CEB (nifedipine) will usually provide satisfactory control (Mimran and Ribstein, 1985). Caution is advised against combining ei-

**Table 7.14. Pharmacological Effects of Calcium Entry Blockers[a]**

| | Diltiazem | Verapamil | Nifedipine | Nicardipine |
|---|---|---|---|---|
| Heart Rate | ↓ | ↓ | ↑ − | ↑ − |
| Myocardial Contractility | ↓ | ↓ ↓ | ↓ − | ↑ − |
| Nodal Conduction | ↓ | ↓ ↓ | − | − |
| Peripheral Vasodilation | ↑ | ↑ | ↑ ↑ | ↑ ↑ |

[a] ↓, decrease, ↑, increase, −, no change.

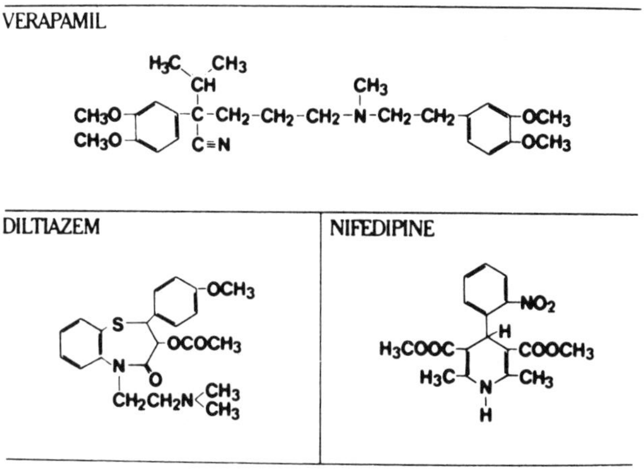

VERAPAMIL

DILTIAZEM

NIFEDIPINE

**Figure 7.28.** Structure of three calcium antagonists.

ther diltiazem or verapamil with a beta-blocker because of the potential for AV conduction problems.

## Duration of Action

Most of the studies of these agents have been performed with formulations requiring two or three doses per day. Longer-lasting formulations are available, along with other calcium entry blockers with inherently longer duration of action, such as nitrendipine (Ram et al, 1984).

The fall in blood pressure, measured by ambulatory monitoring, is maintained throughout the 24 hours with three doses a day of the regular preparations. With the sustained-release formulation of verapamil, some have noted 24-hour control with once-a-day dosage (Zachariah et al, 1987) but others have found the effect to wear out after about 20 hours (Cardillo et al, 1988). With the sustained-release form of diltiazem, equal efficacy was observed with once-daily and twice-daily dosages in one study (Mooser et al, 1988) but the drug is recommended for twice-a-day dosage . A twice-a-day "retard" tablet of nifedipine is now available (Cappuccio et al, 1986) as is a once-a-day formulation using an osmotic displacement gastrointestinal therapeutic system (GITS) (Phillips et al, 1989).

## Different Responses by Age

Bühler and coworkers (1984) found the response to calcium antagonists used alone is directly and strongly related to the age and pretreatment renin levels of the patient: The older the patient and the lower the PRA, the better

the response, which is opposite to that seen with beta-blockers (Fig 7.29). Other investigators have found that CEBs are particularly effective in the elderly (Stessman et al, 1985; Landmark, 1985), and some report an inverse correlation with age as do Bühler et al (Pedrinelli et al, 1986; Weinberger, 1987; Meredith et al, 1987; M'Buyamba-Kabangu et al, 1988). However, the

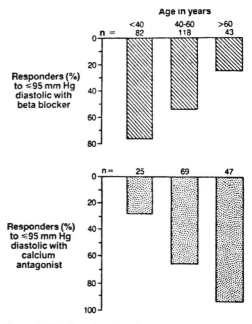

**Figure 7.29.** Fraction of patients who respond with a diastolic blood pressure of 95 mm Hg or less during antihypertensive therapy with beta-blockers (*top*) or calcium entry blockers (*bottom*) in three age groups with essential hypertension. (From Bühler FR, Bolli P, Kiowski W, et al: *Am J Med* 77:36, 1984.)

majority of published reports that compared younger with older patients and that provide actual data on the degree of reduction of blood pressure fail to document a significant difference (Ueda et al, 1986; Pool et al, 1986; Massie et al, 1987, Abernethy and Montamat, 1987; Mehta et al, 1987; Leonetti and Zanchetti, 1988; Ferrara et al, 1988). According to one analysis of the accumulated correlation data, only about 10% of the variance in the fall of blood pressure is attributable to age (Swales, 1987).

What some have noted as an apparently greater antihypertensive effectiveness of CEBs in the elderly may reflect the characteristically higher blood pressure levels of the elderly and the more pronounced efficacy of CEBs as the level of blood pressure increases.

There may be yet another reason why elderly patients appear to be more responsive than younger patients to CEBs: Pharmacokinetic changes have been noted in elderly patients that increase the bioavailability of verapamil (Abernethy et al, 1986), diltiazem (Abernethy and Montamat, 1987), nifedipine (Robertson et al, 1988), and nicardipine (Forette et al, 1985). Thus, they may be exposed to more active drug at any given dose level than would younger patients.

### Race

Although less information is available concerning differences between blacks and nonblacks in their response to CEBs, most comparisons have shown that blacks respond somewhat *less* to them in the same way that they respond less to both beta-blockers and angiotensin-converting enzyme inhibitors. In four studies involving sizeable numbers of blacks and nonblacks with comparable pretreatment blood pressure, similar results have been noted: With verapamil (Cubeddu et al, 1986), nitrendipine (Moser et al, 1984; Weinberger, 1987), or diltiazem (Massie et al, 1987), nonblack patients had slightly to significantly greater responses than did the black patients. Therefore, the hypothesis that the black population, with generally lower renin levels, should exhibit a greater responsiveness to CEBs is not supported by the published findings (Waeber et al, 1985).

### Additive Effect of Diuretic or Low Sodium Intake

As a corollary to the (unproven) thesis that CEBs are more effective in patients with lower renin levels, a decrease in the antihypertensive efficacy of these drugs has been claimed under two conditions wherein renin levels are raised: dietary sodium restriction (Valdes et al, 1982) and concomitant diuretic therapy (Rosenthal, 1982).

Numerous studies have examined these relationships. In general, the findings support the view that dietary sodium restriction does reduce (but not abolish) the antihypertensive effect of CEBs (Bellini et al, 1984; Morgan et al, 1986; Leonetti et al, 1987; Nicholson et al, 1987; MacGregor et al, 1987). The number of dihydropyridine receptors on cell membranes of hypertensive rats is increased with sodium loading (Garthoff and Bellemann, 1987) which could provide additional sites of action for the CEBs to explain the apparent potentiation of their antihypertensive action.

On the other hand, most studies have shown an additional antihypertensive effect when diuretics are combined with CEBs (Sever and Poulter, 1987). Subsequent to that review, additional and mostly larger scale studies have, by a count of eight to two, shown an additive effect from diuretics. Of those that showed an additive effect, three used nifedipine (Ferrara et al, 1987; Zezulka et al, 1987; Zusman et al, 1987), three diltiazem (Massie et al, 1987; Frishman et al, 1987; Weir et al, 1989), one nicardipine (Fagan et al, 1986), and one amlodipine (Glasser et al, 1989). Of the studies that did not show an additive effect from diuretics, one used diltiazem and involved only 22 patients (Schulte et al, 1987), the other used verapamil and involved only 13 patients (Nicholson et al, 1989).

### Natriuretic Effects

The overall published data, then, support an additive effect of diuretics when added to a CEB. Nonetheless, there is a rational explanation for at least a lesser potentiation by diuretics when added to CEBs than to other antihypertensive agents: The CEBs themselves are mildly natriuretic and, having shrunken the vascular volume, thereby would tend to leave less room for additional action from a diuretic.

This natriuretic effect has been amply demonstrated for nifedipine (Ene et al, 1985), nitrendipine (Ene et al, 1985), nicardipine (Baba et al, 1987), isradipine (Krusell et al, 1987), and verapamil (Hughes et al, 1988). In most, the effect has been studied for only brief periods, but a continued, long-term effect has been observed with isradipine (Krusell et al, 1987).

The increased excretion of sodium and water likely reflects the unique ability of CEBs, unlike other vasodilators, to maintain or increase the glomerular filtration rate (GFR), which, in turn, has been attributed to their selective vasodilatory action on the renal afferent arterioles (Loutzenhiser and Epstein, 1988). These effects likely persist, but, at least in one study with nicardipine (Smith et al, 1987), the acute increases in GFR and renal plasma flow were not maintained after 6 weeks, even though overall renal vascular resistance was still below baseline.

**Potential for Good or Bad Renal Effects**

On the surface, this preferential vasodilation of afferent arterioles with increases in GFR, renal blood flow, and natriuresis appears to favor the use of CEBs as a way of maintaining good renal function. However, a large body of experimental data has suggested that increased renal plasma flow and GFR may have a deleterious effect upon the progression of glomerulosclerosis. Increased glomerular perfusion, particularly in the face of systemic hypertension, is viewed as being responsible for the progressive loss of renal function once the process of nephron loss begins in the course of any type of renal disease (Brenner et al, 1988).

The effect of CEBs on renal function remains uncertain. Two experimental studies have been reported using the same strain of rats who had renal damage produced in the same manner, i.e., subtotal nephrectomy. The results are disparate: One (Harris et al, 1987) found that verapamil provided excellent protection against progression of renal failure over 15 weeks; the other (Jackson and Johnston, 1988) found that the CEB felodipine provided less protection than did the ACE inhibitor enalapril over 5 weeks. The only long-term study in humans with renal insufficiency found that nisoldipine given to 14 patients with moderate renal insufficiency slowed the rate of progression of their disease compared with that noted in 11 patients given "standard" antihypertensive therapy plus placebo (Eliahou et al, 1988). The blood pressures were similar in both groups but the pretreatment rate of loss of renal function was considerably faster in those given nisoldipine, so the results of this study must be considered only suggestive.

Obviously more information is needed about the long-term effects of CEBs in patients with renal insufficiency. Until that is available, CEBs can be used with assurance that they will likely preserve or even improve renal function in patients whose renal status is normal and likely will not cause rapid deterioration of renal function in those whose renal status is impaired.

**Issue of Cardioprotection**

CEBs were first made available as coronary vasodilators for the treatment of coronary artery disease (CAD) and are widely used for this purpose. Since many hypertensive patients also have CAD, the use of a CEB to treat both diseases is obviously rational and has been advocated (O'Rourke, 1985).

Beyond their unequivocal effects of improving myocardial blood flow while decreasing myocardial oxygen demand, CEBs have other features that suggest that they could protect patients from progression of CAD, i.e., cardioprotection. These include: (1) a variety of antiatherogenic effects in experimental animals (Weinstein and Heider, 1989); (2) an antithrombotic effect (for nifedipine but not verapamil) in rodent thrombosis models (Myers et al, 1986); (3) protection of jeopardized myocardium in a number of animal models of acute myocardial ischemia (Kingma and Yellon, 1988); (4) preliminary evidence that nicardipine, when given directly into the coronary artery after angioplasty, reduced signs of ischemia and release of thromboxane (Hanet, et al, 1987); and (5) the lack of adverse effects of these drugs on lipids, glucose, and potassium levels compared with what may be seen with diuretics or beta-blockers (Kaplan, 1989c).

Despite these favorable features, currently available CEBs have not been found to be cardioprotective either during or after myocardial infarction. As reviewed by Yusuf et al (1988), none of the four trials of nifedipine, three trials of verapamil, and one trial of diltiazem in acute myocardial infarction have shown a clear reduction in mortality, morbidity, or even enzyme release. Similarly, in four long-term trials after myocardial infarction, no benefit has been seen.

There are no data on the effect of CEBs on primary prevention of CAD in patients with hypertension. Their potential benefit in this regard cannot be excluded even though they do not appear to provide secondary prevention after an acute infarction. Witness the reverse situation with beta-blockers: They do provide secondary cardioprotection but in three of four trials they have not been shown to provide primary protection, as described in Chapter 5.

In concert with most antihypertensive drugs, the CEB diltiazem has been shown to reduce left ventricular mass and end-diastolic dimension without changing diastolic filling indices (Szlachcic et al, 1989).

CEBs do not impair the cardiac response to exercise and are clearly superior to beta-blockers in maintaining exercise capacity (Szlachcic et al, 1987).

### Use in Hypertensive Urgencies

Nifedipine capsules have been widely utilized to provide fast reduction in blood pressures deemed to be so high as to need immediate relief (Bertel et al, 1983) (Fig. 7.30). The nifedipine has often been administered by opening the capsule and squirting the drug under the tongue. Although this was thought to provide an even more rapid antihypertensive effect, absorption from the limited sublingual vascular bed is much slower and less complete than if the drug is swallowed (van Harten et al, 1987).

The slower sublingual route is probably preferable so as not to lower the blood pressure too much, too fast. Symptomatic hypotension with ischemic damage to the brain (Nobile-Orazio and Sterzi, 1981) and heart (O'Mailia et al, 1987)

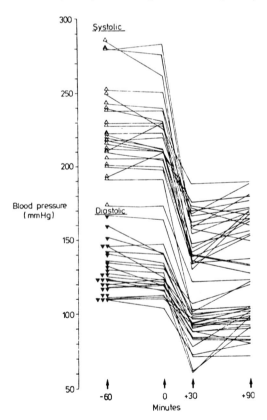

**Figure 7.30.** Effect of 10 to 20 mg nifedipine by mouth in hypertensive emergencies. N = 25. (From Bertel O, et al: *Br Med J* 286:19, 1983.)

have been noted after nifedipine. Most instances have involved inappropriate use of the drug, either to patients whose blood pressure was not in need of rapid reduction or in too high a dose, particularly superimposed on other drugs (Bertel, 1987).

If used appropriately, nifedipine is a generally safe and effective way to lower severe hypertension (Phillips et al, 1989. The best way is to give 5 mg, one-half of a capsule, by mouth or sublingually; if less than the desired effect is seen in 20 to 30 minutes, a second 5- or 10-mg dose can be given.

Nifedipine has been successfully used sublingually to manage perioperative hypertension (Adler et al, 1986) and by nasogastric tube in neurosurgical patients (Tateishi et al, 1988). If a slower and longer duration of action is desired, it can be given per rectum, inserting perforated capsules (Ishikawa et al, 1986).

### Other Calcium Antagonists

Most of the "second generation" now under clinical investigation are dihydropyridine derivatives, not too dissimilar from nifedipine (Freedman and Waters, 1987). These include nitrendipine (Byyny et al, 1989); felodipine (Elmfeldt et al, 1987); amlodipine (Frick et al, 1989); isradipine (Shepherd et al, 1989); nisoldipine (van Harten et al, 1989), and nimodipine. This latter agent appears to selectively dilate cerebral arteries (McCalden et al, 1984) and has been found to improve neurological outcome in men after an acute ischemic stroke (Gelmers et al, 1988) or subarachnoid hemorrhage (Pickard et al, 1989). Moreover, it facilitates associative learning in older rabbits (Deyo et al, 1989), so obviously it will be extensively studied for a possible protective effect against the neurological loss that often accompanies aging.

### Additional Effects

Even if CEBs do not prove beneficial in maintaining cerebral function with age, they have a number of other potential uses in keeping with the role of calcium in the contraction of smooth muscle (Table 7.15).

### Side Effects

Despite all of these real and potential advantages, side effects will likely preclude the use of these drugs in perhaps 15% of patients (Table 7.16). Most of these—the headaches, flushing, local ankle edema—are related to the vasodilation for which the drugs are given. With slow-

**Table 7.15. Prospective Uses for Calcium Entry Blockers**

Cardiovascular
  Migraine (Tietze et al, 1987)
  Raynaud's phenomenon (Nilsson et al, 1987)
  Nocturnal leg cramps (Baltodano et al, 1988)
  Subarachnoid hemorrhage (Flamm, 1989)
  Ischemic stroke (Gelmers et al, 1988)
  Hypertrophic cardiomyopathy (Opie, 1988)
  Pulmonary hypertension (Opie, 1988)
  Inhibit platelet activation (Addonizio, 1986)

Noncardiovascular
  Asthma (Massey et al, 1988)
  Esophageal motility disorders (Schwartz et al, 1984)
  Myometrial hyperactivity (Andersson, 1982)
  Biliary or renal colic (Bortolotti et al, 1987)

**Table 7.16. Relative Frequency of Side Effects of Calcium Entry Blockers**

| Effect | Verapamil | Diltiazem | Nifedipine | Nicardipine |
|---|---|---|---|---|
| Cardiovascular system | | | | |
| Hypotension | + | + | + | + |
| Flush | + | − | + + | + + |
| Headache | + | + | + + | + + |
| Ankle edema | + | + | + + | + |
| Palpitation/chest pain | − | − | + | + |
| Conduction disturbances | + + | + | − | − |
| Heart failure | + | − | (+) | − |
| Bradycardia | + + | + | − | − |
| Gastrointestinal tract | | | | |
| Nausea | + | + | + | + |
| Constipation | + + | (+) | − | − |

release formulations, in particular the nifedipine GITS preparation, vasodilatory side effects (with the exception of dependent edema) are markedly reduced (Frishman et al, 1989). Gastrointestinal problems may arise, with constipation a particular effect of verapamil. Nifedipine and nicardipine are particularly prone to cause edema in dependent areas that is caused not by generalized fluid retention but by vasodilation (Tordjman et al, 1985). It should be no surprise that, in a few patients, the antihypertensive effect may be so marked as to reduce the blood flow and induce ischemia of vital organs such as the brain (Nobile-Orazio and Sterzi, 1981), retina (Pitlik et al, 1983), or myocardium (O'Mailia et al, 1987). In patients with renal insufficiency, acute, reversible worsening of renal function may appear (Diamond et al, 1984) but renal function is usually well preserved (Saruta, 1989). The effect of verapamil on cardiac conduction has also given rise to concern about its concomitant use with beta-blockers. Though such an effect may rarely occur in patients given this

drug for coronary disease (Winniford et al, 1982), it seems not to be a common problem in the treatment of hypertension.

Concerns have been voiced over potential adverse effects of CEBs on calcium absorption and excretion. Verapamil use has not been found to alter either intestinal absorption or renal excretion in one study (Sjöden et al, 1987) but to increase renal excretion of calcium in another (Hvarfner et al, 1988). We have noted a decrease in the fractional absorption of $^{47}Ca$ and an increase in calcium excretion in 10 patients given nifedipine for 2 weeks (Breslau et al, 1988).

The secretion of various hormones involves movement of calcium into the endocrine cells. In the presence of CEBs, the steroidogenic response of the adrenal to either ACTH or angiotensin may be partially impaired (Favre et al, 1988), but this seems only to reduce the tendency for fluid retention. The secretion of other hormones seems not to be impaired (Millar and Struthers, 1984) despite some scattered reports of inhibition of pituitary hormone release (Veldhuis et al, 1985) and insulin secretion (Roth et al, 1989). After a review of 74 papers on the effects of CEBs in nondiabetic and 35 in diabetic patients, Trost and Weidmann (1987) concluded that these drugs do not have unfavorable effects on glucose homeostasis. Unlike beta-blockers, CEBs do not decrease insulin sensitivity (Pollare et al, 1989b).

Two other problems not infrequently observed with other antihypertensives are also less common with CEBs: Serum lipids are not adversely altered (Trost and Weidmann, 1987) and impotence seems to be rare (King et al, 1983) although a total of 31 patients have been reported to have developed gynecomastia (Tanner and Bosco, 1988).

Though nifedipine will lower the blood pressure of women with pregnancy-induced hypertension (Walters and Redman, 1984), it also will inhibit uterine contractions.

Rarely, nifedipine has been reported to cause nocturia (Williams and Donaldson, 1986) and nicardipine urinary retention (Eicher et al, 1987). Even more rarely, hepatic toxicity has been noted with diltiazem (Shallcross et al, 1987) and nifedipine (Abramson and Littlejohn, 1985). Eye pain, possibly due to ocular vasodilation, has been noted with nifedipine (Coulter et al, 1988). A wide spectrum of adverse cutaneous reactions, some quite serious, have been reported to occur rarely with various CEBs (Stern and Khalsa, 1989).

In patients given CEBs, increased blood levels and occasional toxicity have been reported with digoxin, theophylline, and phenytoin. Blood levels of quinidine and lithium may decrease (Halperin and Cubeddu, 1986). Hypotension may occur in patients receiving prazosin or beta-blockers, with the latter drugs perhaps because their hepatic degradation is slowed (Tateishi et al, 1989).

Overdoses usually are manifested by hypotension and conduction disturbances and can usually be overcome with parenteral calcium and dopamine (Herrington et al, 1986; Jakubowski and Mizgala, 1987).

### Overall Impression

The favorable balance between good and bad appears so large that it is no wonder that these agents have become major drugs for the treatment of various forms of hypertension. They are rarely contraindicated and often indicated for the treatment of hypertensive patients with a variety of concomitant conditions. With the availability of formulations that are effective on a once or, at most, twice per day schedule, and with the continued publication of such glowing reports of efficacy and relative safety of these drugs, their future looks even more promising.

### ANGIOTENSIN-CONVERTING ENZYME INHIBITORS

As detailed in Chapter 3, there are four ways to reduce the activity of the renin-angiotensin system in humans (Fig. 7.31). The first, the use of beta-blockers to reduce renin release from the juxtaglomerular (JG) cells, has been widely used. The second, the direct inhibition of the activity of renin, is being actively investigated (Verburg et al, 1989). The third way to block the system

is to use a competitive antagonist that attaches to angiotensin receptors but does not induce its cellular effects. Such an antagonist, saralasin, was available for a short time as a test for angiotensin-induced hypertension, and others are under investigation (Wong et al, 1989). The fourth, the use of agents that inhibit the enzyme responsible for conversion of inactive angiotensin I to active angiotensin II, has become feasible with the availability of angiotensin-converting enzyme inhibitors (ACEIs). The first of these, captopril, was introduced in 1981 for use in those resistant to other medications. After lower doses of captopril were found to be both effective and well tolerated in patients with mild hypertension, it was approved in July 1985 for the entire spectrum of hypertension. Enalapril was approved in December 1985 and lisinopril in 1987. A large number of other ACEIs are under active investigation (Waeber et al, 1989).

### Chemistry

After peptides from the venom of the Brazilian viper *Bothrops jararaca* were discovered to be ACEIs (Ondetti et al, 1971), one, a nonapeptide (teprotide), was found to effectively lower the blood pressure when used intravenously (Gavras et al, 1974). From study of the interaction of ACE and angiotensin, a model of the active site of the enzyme was developed and potent orally effective ACEIs were designed (Fig. 7.32) (Ondetti et al, 1977).

Three chemically different classes of ACEIs have been developed: sulfhydryl-containing, e.g., captopril; carboxy-alkyldipeptides, e.g., enalapril and lisinopril; and phosphorus-containing, e.g., fosinopril. Their different structures influence their tissue distribution and routes of elimination (Ondetti, 1988), differences that could

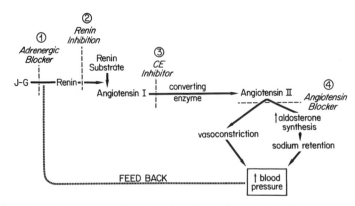

**Figure 7.31.** Renin-angiotensin system and four sites where its activity may be inhibited.

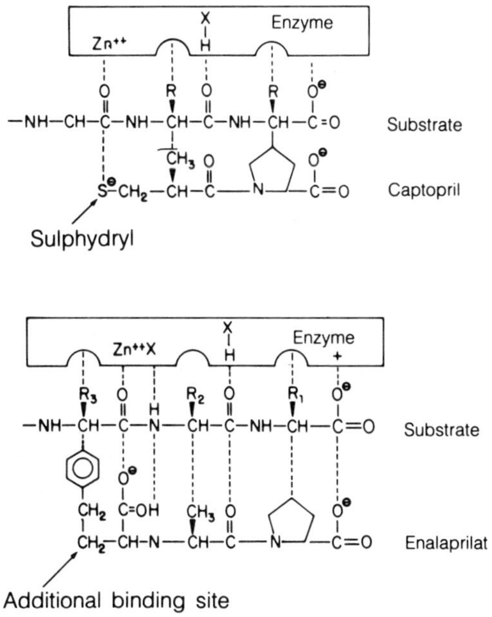

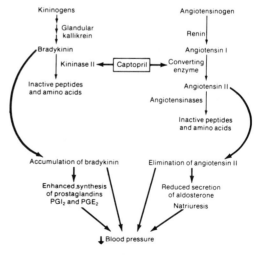

**Figure 7.32.** Hypothetical model of angiotensin-converting enzyme. [From Abrams WB, Davies RO, Gomez HJ: *J Hypertension* 2(Suppl 2):31, 1984.]

have an impact upon their effects on various organ functions beyond their shared ability to lower the blood pressure by blocking the circulating renin-angiotensin mechanism. In particular, the sulfhydryl-containing ACEIs undergo reversible modifications to form disulfides that can regenerate captopril and thereby constitute depot forms of the drug. Moreover, the conversion of captopril into disulfides can occur through interaction with free radicals, so the process may serve as a recyclable free radical scavenger, which could provide a cardioprotective effect (Chopra et al, 1989).

### Pharmacokinetics

*Captopril.* About 70% of a dose is rapidly absorbed and maximal concentrations are reached within 30 to 60 minutes. Most is excreted intact in the urine with a mean elimination half-life of 2 hours with normal renal function but a progressively longer one with renal insufficiency, requiring dose adjustments. This is also true for the other available ACEIs.

*Enalapril maleate* is a prodrug for the active compound, enalaprilat. The maleate ester increases oral absorption and the prodrug is rapidly deesterified in the liver. About 60% of an oral dose is bioavailable with peak levels of enalaprilat reached at about 4 hours.

*Lisinopril*, the lysine analogue of enalaprilic acid, is more slowly absorbed with an average bioavailability of 25% and peak serum levels reached about 6 to 10 hours after a dose.

All three of the ACEIs can be administered with food, although the absorption of captopril is delayed (Belz et al, 1988). Since renal function is usually reduced in the elderly, the half-life and efficacy of the drugs are prolonged in older patients.

### Pharmacodynamics

The pharmacodynamic behavior of ACEIs may be assessed in multiple ways including changes in the circulating levels of ACE, angiotensin I and II and renin, hemodynamics changes, and blockade of agonists. Findings with different assessments differ, and there are multiple interactions between blood and tissue effects that all add up to a complicated model to explain the dynamic effects of these drugs (Belz et al, 1988).

### Mode of Action (Fig. 7.33)

The most obvious manner by which ACEIs lower the blood pressure is to markedly reduce the circulating levels of angiotensin II, thereby removing the direct vasoconstriction induced by this peptide. At the same time, the activity of ACE within vessel walls and multiple tissues, including brain and heart, is inhibited, apparently to variable degrees by different ACEIs (Cushman et al, 1989).

The presence of the complete renin-angiotensin system within various tissues, including vessel walls (Dzau, 1987), heart (Linz et al, 1989),

**Figure 7.33.** Mechanisms by which captopril may lower the blood pressure.

and brain (Unger et al, 1988), is certain. What remains uncertain is the role of these tissue renin-angiotensin systems in pathophysiology and the contribution of the effect of ACEIs upon tissue ACE in their antihypertensive effects.

The reduction by ACEIs of circulating and tissue angiotensin II levels leads to multiple other effects beyond direct vasodilation that likely contribute to their antihypertensive effect. These include:

—a decrease in aldosterone secretion (Ramirez et al, 1988) that may cause natriuresis or, at least, a lack of reactive renal sodium retention as the blood pressure falls;

—a blunting of the expected increase in sympathetic nervous system activity typically seen after vasodilation, an effect that may involve both a decrease in sympathetic activity (Zimmerman et al, 1984) and an increase in parasympathetic activity (Ajayi et al, 1985). As a result, heart rate is not increased and cardiac output does not rise as seen with direct vasodilators such as hydralazine.

Although most if not all of ACEIs antihypertensive effects are mediated via reduction in angiotensin II levels, with the use of ultrasensitive assays that are capable of measuring low levels even in the face of the very high levels of angiotensin I, Nussberger et al (1989) have shown that some angiotensin II is present even at the peak of ACEIs action and that the levels rise considerably while the effects of the drugs are maintained. These rises in angiotensin II may reflect a ''break-through'' from the progressively higher levels of renin, ACE, and angiotensin I that build up in front of the site of ACE inhibition (Waeber et al, 1989).

### Effects Other Than on Angiotensin II

As shown in Figure 7.33, ACE is the same enzyme responsible for the breakdown of bradykinin, a vasodilatory peptide. The role of the presumably elevated levels of active bradykinin after ACEI administration remains uncertain (Brunner et al, 1988). However, high levels of bradykinin may be responsible for the frequent cough and rare angioneurotic edema seen with ACEI use.

Also shown in Figure 7.33 is an enhanced synthesis of vasodilatory prostaglandins, presumably via activation by bradykinin of phospholipases that release the precursor arachidonic acid from membrane phospholipids. A role of these prostaglandins in the action of ACEIs has

been suggested by a reduction in their antihypertensive efficacy when prostaglandin synthesis is blocked by NSAIDs such as indomethacin (Fujita et al, 1981). Although this may reflect the removal of an ACEI effect, it should be remembered that NSAIDs also blunt the effect of multiple other antihypertensive drugs, including diuretics and beta-blockers.

### Ancillary Effects

Regardless of how ACEIs lower the blood pressure, they do so in a manner that tends to protect the function of three vital organs—the heart, the brain, and the kidneys. As for the heart, cardiac output and heart rate are minimally altered and coronary perfusion may be increased by removal of the local vasoconstrictive effect of angiotensin II (Van Gilst et al, 1988). In experimental models of myocardial ischemia, captopril attenuates reperfusion-induced myocardial dysfunction, perhaps by scavenging free radicals (Westlin and Mullane, 1988). In patients who have had a myocardial infarction, captopril started a week later led to improved cardiac function (Sharpe et al, 1988) and attenuated progressive ventricular dilatation and dysfunction (Pfeffer et al, 1988). Beyond these protective effects, ACEIs, in common with most antihypertensive drugs, regress left ventricular hypertrophy and also reduce arterial compliance (Asmar et al, 1988). As will be noted later, ACEIs have become essential drugs in the treatment of congestive heart failure, presumably by their special balance of reducing afterload and inflow.

Cerebral blood flow is well maintained and there may be a downward shift in the limits of autoregulation, interpreted as the result of ACEI-induced decreases in sympathetic nervous activity (Waldemar et al, 1989). This effect may be responsible for the preservation or actual increase in cerebral blood flow seen in patients with congestive heart failure given an ACEI (Paulson et al, 1984).

The kidneys may also be specially protected by preferential vasodilatation of the efferent arterioles. Angiotensin II preferentially constricts these vessels, and its removal provides preferential dilatation. Thereby renal blood flow is increased but, more importantly, intraglomerular pressure is simultaneously reduced. As is further described in Chapter 9, this action of ACEIs may give them a unique protective effect in patients susceptible to progressive damage from glomerular hypertension, extending even to normotensive diabetics (Romanelli et al, 1989).

Beyond these potential benefits, captopril has also been shown to increase sensitivity to insulin and lower plasma insulin levels (Pollare et al, 1989a), which, in view of the adverse implications of hyperinsulinemia described in Chapter 3, could translate into another special advantage of this ACEI.

## Differences between ACEIs

Although some claim that distinct differences in tissue distribution and routes of elimination between various ACEIs may be reflected in different antihypertensive potencies and ancillary properties (Cushman et al, 1989), in most obvious ways all ACEIs seem quite alike. Nonetheless, much remains unknown about their modes of action (Brunner et al, 1988) and those that contain a sulfhydryl group, e.g., captopril, may provide a number of special properties such as free radical removal.

## Clinical Effects

A rather remarkable turnabout has occurred in the few years since captopril was approved "only for use in patients with severe hypertension unresponsive to other agents." ACEIs are now included among the drugs recommended for initial monotherapy of patients with mild and moderate hypertension (Joint National Committee, 1988). This turnabout reflects the use of smaller doses, the recognition of equal efficacy but apparently fewer side effects, and the potential for some special advantages not provided by other drugs now available (Williams, 1988).

## Monotherapy

An immediate fall in blood pressure occurs in about 70% of patients given captopril, and the fall is sometimes rather precipitous (Case et al, 1980). Such a dramatic fall is more likely in those with high renin levels, particularly if they are volume depleted by prior dietary sodium restriction or diuretic therapy. In patients collected from multiple clinical trials, the mean fall in blood pressure was 11% in those with low renin, 14% in those with normal renin, and 19% in those with high renin (Jenkins and McKinstry, 1979). The overall response rate to a moderate dose of any ACEI is equivalent to that seen with a diuretic (Johnston et al, 1984), a beta-blocker (Helgeland et al, 1986), or a calcium entry blocker (Morlin et al, 1987) with a

significant fall in blood pressure seen in 35 to 70% (Williams, 1988).

Black hypertensives, with lower renin levels as a group, have been found to respond less well to ACEIs than do white hypertensives (Weinberger, 1985; Pool et al, 1987). The addition of a diuretic will enhance their response (VA Cooperative Study, 1982b). On the other hand, elderly patients who also tend to have lower renin levels respond equally as well if not better than do younger patients (Reid et al, 1989).

As expected, patients with high renin forms of hypertension, i.e., renovascular hypertension, may respond particularly well to ACEIs (Jenkins and McKinstry, 1979) (Chapter 10). Excellent responses have been reported in patients with severe hypertension, renal failure, and hyperreninemia caused by connective tissue diseases (Strongwater et al, 1989). Patients with hypertension secondary to chronic renal parenchymal disease may also respond well (Abraham et al, 1988), presumably because they have inappropriately high renin levels and because they retain more of the drug.

## Combination Therapy

The addition of a diuretic, even in as low a dose as 6.25 mg of hydrochlorothiazide, will enhance the efficacy of an ACEI (Andrén et al, 1983) normalizing the blood pressure of another 20 to 25% of patients with mild to moderate hypertension more effectively than raising the dose of ACEI. In a group of 46 patients whose DBP remained above 90 mm Hg on 20 mg enalapril once daily, the half given 25 to 50 mg of hydrochlorothiazide had a subsequent greater fall in blood pressure by 11/6 mm Hg than did the half given 2 or 3 times more enalapril (Sassano et al, 1989). The marked additive effect of a diuretic likely reflects the ACEI blunting of the reactive rise of angiotensin II that usually occurs with diuretic use and that opposes the antihypertensive effect of the diuretic.

A calcium entry blocker will also add to the effect of an ACEI (Singer et al, 1987) whereas a beta-blocker may be less additive (Williams, 1988).

In patients with more severe hypertension, an ACEI may be more effective as the vasodilator in triple therapy than hydralazine (Laher et al, 1985). In a group of such patients with diastolic blood pressure above 95 mm Hg on a diuretic and beta-blocker combination; 85% normalized their blood pressure when captopril was added and 63% of these remained normotensive when the beta-blocker was then withdrawn (Muiesan et al, 1987).

Sublingual captopril is effective within 15 minutes in lowering the blood pressure in patients with severe hypertension, perhaps with fewer side effects and a longer duration of action than sublingual nifedipine (Hauger-Klevene, 1986).

## Use in Special Patients

*Renal Damage.* Patients who are predisposed to progressive renal damage may be particularly well treated with ACEIs. They include diabetics who frequently develop progressive nephropathy, intercapillary glomerulosclerosis or Kimmelstiel-Wilson's disease, and hypertensive patients with early renal insufficiency from nephrosclerosis. The rationale for the special attraction of ACEIs is their relatively greater vasodilation of renal efferent arterioles than of afferent arterioles, thereby reducing pressure within the glomeruli. As is described further in Chapter 9, intraglomerular hypertension is thought to be the major cause of the inexorably progressive loss of renal function that occurs once significant nephron loss has begun from any cause. Both experimental (Anderson et al, 1986) and clinical evidence (Bjorck et al, 1986; Parving et al, 1988) supports the effectiveness of ACEIs in reducing the rate of progression of renal damage.

Although the enthusiasm for the "renal protective" effect of ACEIs will likely continue to grow, the best long-term study showing protection of renal function in patients with diabetic nephropathy was done *without* the use of an ACEI (Parving et al, 1987). Thus much of what is being ascribed to ACEIs may reflect the value of any regimen that lowers systemic blood pressure without significantly reducing renal perfusion. Long-term studies with ACEIs are in process, and hopefully their place in the management of various nephropathies will soon be established.

In the meantime, careful monitoring of renal function is advised when using an ACEI in patients with hypertension and renal insufficiency. Some of these patients likely have bilateral renovascular disease and the use of ACEI may rapidly induce a usually reversible renal failure in this circumstance (see Side Effects). More of these patients may have unilateral renovascular disease where there are short-term benefits from ACEIs but likely long-term disadvantages, as is noted in Chapter 10.

*Congestive Heart Failure.* ACEIs are useful in the treatment of heart failure, whether caused by hypertension or not (Capewell et al, 1989). Both captopril and enalapril have been found to provide not only symptomatic relief but also prolonged survival for patients with severe CHF (CONSENSUS Trial Study Group, 1987; Newman et al, 1988). In one comparison, lisinopril was found to be more effective than captopril (Giles et al, 1989).

As effective as they are, ACEIs may produce declines in renal function, particularly when the systemic blood pressure falls in patients who start with low blood pressure and limited ability to improve cardiac output (Suki, 1989). The ACEI-induced decrease in angiotensin II levels obviously provides hemodynamic benefit but at the same time reduces GFR and, if the compensatory events are not adequate, may lead to progressive renal insufficiency.

*Coronary Disease.* ACEIs can reverse left ventricular hypertrophy (Asmar et al, 1988) and have been shown to attenuate the development of ventricular dilatation and dysfunction after an acute myocardial infarction (Pfeffer et al, 1988). They, therefore, are an attractive choice for hypertensive patients with coronary heart disease even though they do not provide the direct relief from ischemia as do beta-blockers or calcium entry blockers.

*Peripheral Vascular Disease.* ACEIs dilate both small and large arteries and improve walking distance in hypertensive patients with intermittent claudication (Roberts et al, 1987).

*Pulmonary Disease.* Even though they may induce a persistent cough, ACEIs are generally safe in patients with asthma (Boulet et al, 1989). However, patients with underlying bronchial hyperactivity seem to be more susceptible to the development of a cough (Kaufman et al, 1989).

*Nonmodulating Hypertensives.* According to the findings of Williams, Hollenberg, and coworkers described in Chapter 3, almost half of normal renin hypertensives are not capable of modulating their adrenal and renal responses to volume and angiotensin II in a normal manner. This "nonmodulation" is corrected by an ACEI (Dluhy et al, 1989), suggesting a defect in adrenal and renal receptor or postreceptor responses to angiotensin II. These patients may be the same as the "sodium-sensitive" population but there is now no certain way to identify them.

## Dosage

### Captopril

Initially, captopril was usually given in doses that are now known to be inordinately high, up to 300 mg 3 times per day. With more experience, doses have come down, particularly in the treatment of mild hypertensives. In the Veterans Administration (VA) Cooperative Study (1984) of 495 men with initial DBP between 92 and 109 mm Hg, the response was as good with 12.5 mg 3 times per day as with 25 mg or 50 mg 3 times per day. There is probably no need for using more than 150 mg per day.

The frequency of dosing may also be reduced. In the VA study (1984), 37.5 mg twice per day worked as well as the various doses given 3 times per day. In other studies, 50 to 100 mg given once per day provided good control of the blood pressure for 24 hours (Garanin, 1986; Conway et al, 1988; Frewin et al, 1989), but most have found twice-a-day dosing to be preferable (Pixley et al, 1989). A starting dose of 25 mg twice a day seems appropriate for most patients. Patients with CHF or on prior diuretic therapy should be started on 6.25 mg or less. Those with impaired renal function, e.g., creatinine clearance below 30 ml/min, should be given half of the usual doses.

### Enalapril

The effect of small doses may not last for the full 24 hours (Pixley et al, 1989) so that it should probably be given twice daily. In a controlled study, very little additional response was noted when doses were increased from 10 to 40 mg/day (Salvetti and Arzilli, 1989). Patients on a diuretic should be started with 2.5 mg.

### Lisinopril

Of all of the three currently available ACEIs, lisinopril is the only one with a certain 24-hour duration of action. The starting dose should be 2.5 mg for patients with renal insufficiency, 5 mg for those on a diuretic, 10 mg for most others (Heeg et al, 1989). The dose can be increased to 80 mg once a day.

## Drug Interactions

The addition of another antihypertensive to an ACEI will usually provide additional BP reduction. Greater effects are expected in situations where the other drug has stimulated renin-angiotensin activity, e.g., diuretics or direct vasodilators, or induced reactive renal fluid retention, e.g., alpha$_1$-blockers (Hodsman and Johnston, 1987).

### Nonsteroidal Antiinflammatory Drugs

NSAIDs will reduce the antihypertensive efficacy of ACEIs probably by blockade of ACEI-induced increased synthesis of vasodilatory prostaglandins (Witgall et al, 1982).

### Other Drugs

Probenecid decreases the excretion of organic acids such as ACEIs and thereby will increase their blood levels (Singhvi et al, 1982).

Lithium toxicity has been rarely reported in patients on lithium given an ACEI (Simon, 1988).

Antidiabetic agents may be potentiated, with induction of hypoglycemia (Rett et al, 1988).

## Side Effects

With the use of large doses of captopril in patients with severe hypertension and often renal insufficiency, a high incidence of side effects was reported after the drug was first introduced (Waeber et al, 1981). However, as smaller doses of drug have been used in patients with milder hypertension and normal renal function, the incidence of side effects has fallen significantly. For example, the incidence of neutropenia was 7.2% in patients with collagen vascular disease and impaired renal function and 0.4% with renal insufficiency from other causes but only 0.01% with normal renal function (Cooper, 1983).

The recognized side effects logically can be divided into three types: (1) those anticipated from their pharmacological efficacy; (2) those probably related to the chemical structure and perhaps more common with captopril with its sulfhydryl group; and (3) those that are nonspecific, as seen with any drug that lowers the blood pressure.

As to the relative incidence of side effects, postmarketing surveillance, practiced more assiduously in England than in the United States, provides data that are probably nonbiased (Table 7.17). Lisinopril likely shares most, if not all, of what is seen with the other two drugs (Andrivet et al, 1989).

### Anticipated from Pharmacological Efficacy

*First Dose Hypotension.* Hypotension may occur in those with high plasma renin levels (Hodsman and Johnston, 1987).

*Elevation of Plasma Potassium.* The inhibition of angiotensin II-mediated aldosterone secretion blunts potassium excretion, particularly

**Table 7.17. Comparison of Adverse Effects of Enalapril and Captopril in Patients with Hypertension**

| | Captopril (Blowers and Chalmers, 1988) | Enalapril (Inman et al, 1988) |
|---|---|---|
| No. of patients | 23,035 | 12,543 |
| Duration of treatment | one year | one year |
| | Adverse effects (%) | |
| Rash | 2.3 | 0.4 |
| Orthostatic symptoms | 2.7 | 5.1 |
| Cough | 0.9 | 2.9 |
| Taste disturbance | 0.7 | 0.2 |
| Blood dyscrasias | 0 | 0 |
| Renal impairment | 0.3 | 0.7 |
| Angioedema | 0.04 | 0.2 |

in patients with underlying renal insufficiency who are given potassium-sparing agents or potassium supplements (Burakis and Mioduch, 1984).

*Deterioration of Renal Function.* Intrarenal angiotensin II is an important contributor to the control of renal hemodynamics (Navar and Rosivall, 1984) and function (Siragy et al, 1988). Although a slight fall in renal blood flow, as reflected in a slight rise in serum creatinine, may occur in patients with primary hypertension or unilateral renovascular hypertension (Vetter et al, 1984), a severe deterioration of renal perfusion to the point of acute renal failure is seen almost only in those with marked stenoses in both renal arteries or in the artery supplying a solitary kidney wherein angiotensin II is critical for maintenance of renal blood flow beyond the stenoses (Hricik et al, 1983). Renal function usually returns when the drug is stopped.

*Pregnancy.* Clearly in animals (Broughton Pipkin et al, 1982) and likely in women (Boutroy et al, 1984), captopril will interfere with fetal growth, probably by decreasing uterine blood flow. Anuria may occur in the neonate (Schubiger et al, 1988).

*Blunting of Compensatory Responses to Volume Depletion.* An increase in angiotensin II is a major compensatory homeostatic response to volume depletion. Although only isolated cases have been reported (McMurray and Matthews, 1985), the potential for marked hypotension with prerenal azotemia in ACEI-treated patients who experience gastrointestinal fluid loss or other types of volume depletion should be remembered.

*Cough.* Almost never reported initially, cough may be the most frequent side effect of

ACEI therapy, reported in 5 to 20% of patients given one of these drugs (Goldszer et al, 1988). The mechanism for the dry, hacking, nonproductive but often intolerable cough may involve high levels of bradykinin that arise from the inhibition of the ACE that is also responsible for the inactivation of kinins. It is not accompanied by bronchospasm (Boulet et al, 1989) but may develop mainly in patients with underlying bronchial hyperreactivity (Kaufman et al, 1989). It seems to be more common in women (Morice et al, 1988). In one case, it was associated with a lymphocytic alveolitis (Kidney et al, 1989).

*Angioneurotic Edema.* This much less common but potentially much more serious side effect may also be induced by high levels of kinins (Williams, 1988).

**Related to the Chemical Structure**

These may be more common with captopril than with the nonsulfhydryl containing enalapril. Most but not all patients who experience one of these reactions while on high doses of captopril can be safely crossed over to enalapril (Rucinska et al, 1989).

*Taste Disturbance.* Although usually of little consequence and self-limited with continued drug intake, taste disturbance may be so bad as to interfere with nutrition. It appears to be related to the binding of zinc by the ACEI (Henkin, 1989).

*Rash.* The rash is usually a nonallergic, pruritic maculopapular eruption that usually appears during the first few weeks of therapy and may disappear despite continuation of the drug. A severe erythema and eczema may appear, possibly as an allergic reaction (Goodfield and Millard, 1985). Onycholysis has also been reported (Brueggemeyer and Ramirez, 1984).

*Proteinuria.* In patients with normal renal function, the development of proteinuria is rare. However, on rare occasions and usually only with high doses of an ACEI, what starts as only proteinuria may end up as a full-blown nephrotic syndrome. The problem may reflect an immune complex membranous glomerulopathy (Hoorntje et al, 1980) similar to that seen with other drugs which have a sulfhydryl group, but similar changes have been seen in renal biopsies from patients not receiving captopril.

*Leucopenia.* This reaction probably occurs exclusively in patients with underlying renal insufficiency (Cooper, 1983), particularly those with underlying immunosuppression either from a disease or from a drug. Though usually reversible, it may be fatal (Gavras et al, 1981b). There is no need to monitor white cell counts in patients with normal renal function. Even more rarely, thrombocytopenia alone may appear (Grosbois et al, 1989).

*Hypersensitivity Reactions.* Renal or skin manifestations may represent hypersensitivity reactions, particularly when they are associated with fever, arthralgias, and other such manifestations. In addition, the few cases of cholestatic jaundice (Rahmat et al, 1985) and pericarditis (Zatuchni, 1984) may represent hypersensitivity.

### Nonspecific Side Effects

As noted by Croog et al (1986), less interference in the quality of life was noted with captopril than with propranolol or methyldopa (Table 7.1). ACEIs seem to be "lipid neutral" (Koskinen et al, 1988), escaping another of the common biochemical side effects of both diuretics and beta-blockers. Headache, dizziness, fatigue, diarrhea, and nausea are all listed in reviews but seldom seem to be major problems. Sudden withdrawal does not frequently lead to a rebound (Vlasses et al, 1981). Overdose causes hypotension that should be easily managed with fluids and, if needed, dopamine (Augenstein et al, 1988).

### Perspective on the Use of ACEIs

Captopril when first introduced for use in severe hypertensives and in very high doses got a bad reputation that has quickly been overcome. On the basis of far fewer side effects with small doses given to patients with good renal function, ACEIs are being advocated for the larger population of milder hypertensives often for initial monotherapy.

If the apparent potential of ACEIs to provide special protection to the kidneys and heart is documented, these drugs will clearly be used progressively more for the treatment of all degrees of hypertension. In the near future, even more ACEIs will likely become available.

## DRUGS FOR THE FUTURE

A large number of new agents are in various phases of study (Taylor and Kaplan, 1989). Brief mention will be made of those that seem most likely to reach clinical use.

## Serotonin Antagonists

### Ketanserin

5-Hydroxytryptamine (5-HT) or serotonin is a central and peripheral neurotransmitter that is involved in the regulation of blood pressure. Ketanserin is a selective $5\text{-HT}_2$ receptor antagonist that lowers the blood pressure in humans (Staessen et al, 1988b). The mechanism is uncertain but likely also involves $alpha_1$-adrenergic receptor antagonism since pure $5\text{-HT}_2$ blockers are not antihypertensive (Scott et al, 1989). Ketanserin likely will not be introduced as an antihypertensive in the United States because it prolongs the QT interval that could predispose to serious ventricular arrhythmias (Cameron et al, 1988).

### Urapidil

This agent is thought to activate $5\text{-HT}_{1A}$ receptors in the CNS, thereby decreasing the firing of serotoninergic neurons and reducing sympathetic nervous activity (Kolassa et al, 1989).

## Dopamine Agonists

Dopamine, the precursor of norepinephrine, induces vasodilation and lowers the blood pressure (Goldberg, 1984). Exogenous dopamine also acts on $beta_1$-receptors to stimulate the heart and $alpha_1$- and $alpha_2$-receptors to cause vasoconstriction, so that it cannot be used to treat hypertension. However, selective dopamine agonists such as fenoldopam (SK-82526) may prove to be useful antihypertensive agents that also have a marked renal vasodilatory action (Ruilope et al, 1988).

Ergotoxine derivatives have a modest antihypertensive effect that may be induced by a dopaminergic mechanism (Uehlinger et al, 1989).

## Adenosine Receptor Agonists

Adenosine has a direct vasorelaxant effect and inhibits neurotransmitter release. Adenosine agonists are effective in experimental animals, lowering blood pressure while inhibiting renin release and causing a natriuresis (Taylor and Kaplan, 1989).

## Potassium Channel Openers

Pinacidil, nicorandil, and cromakalim are representatives of drugs that vasodilate by opening potassium channels and enhancing potassium efflux from vascular smooth muscle cells (Hamilton and Weston, 1989). Minoxidil and diazoxide may also work in the same manner (Cook, 1988).

### Renin Inhibitors

A number of direct inhibitors of renin (Verburg et al, 1989) and monoclonal antibodies and nonpeptide antagonists to angiotensin II (Zimmerman, 1989) are under investigation. They are attractive because their action would presumably inhibit the renin system without affecting bradykinin or other mechanisms.

### Atrial Natriuretic Peptide (ANP) Modulators

ANP is both natriuretic and vasodilatory and it lowers the blood pressure when given intravenously (Espiner and Richards, 1989). Since it is a relatively large peptide, it is not active orally, but work is being done to synthesize smaller sized peptides with comparable biological potency. In addition, inhibitors of the atriopeptidase enzyme that inactivates ANF are being investigated (Jardine et al, 1989).

### Phosphodiesterase Inhibitors

The vasorelaxation induced by ANP and other endogenous and exogenous agents is mediated by an increase in cyclic guanosine 3'5' monophosphate (cGMP). Inhibition of the phosphodiesterase enzyme will also raise cGMP levels and such inhibitors are under study as antihypertensives (Booth et al, 1987). This includes the agent flosequinan (BTS-49465) (Lewis et al, 1989).

### Conclusion

The number of drugs under investigation is obviously impressive. Time and the United States Food and Drug Administration will tell which of them have clinical usefulness. In the meantime, proper use of what is available will control virtually every hypertensive patient. We will have more and better drugs, perhaps available in easier to use, rate-controlled forms, so that a single capsule or a patch may provide smooth control over many days.

### CHOICE OF DRUGS: FIRST, SECOND, AND BEYOND

Let us now turn to the practical issue as to which of the many drugs now available (Table 7.18) should be the first, second, or subsequent choices in individual patients. Major changes in these choices are underway. In the United States, a diuretic was chosen as initial therapy up to

90% of the time for patients with mild hypertension in 1983 (Cloher and Whelton, 1986), but the use of diuretics has been falling since then and ACEIs and CEBs have been growing rapidly in popularity (Fig. 7.3). These changes in the use of drugs reflect multiple forces, not the least of which are the marketing campaigns fueled by the billions of dollars that await the winners.

In the next few pages, I will attempt to summarize the evidence and provide guidelines to the choices for therapy. At the onset, I reassert my opinion that considerable change is appropriate (Kaplan, 1983), but hopefully what follows will provide the hard data with which the individual reader can make his or her own conclusion. Despite my enthusiasm for change, I am well aware that I may be wrong and that the opinions of those who disagree should be respected. Perhaps the best course is to delete "right" and "wrong" because morality is not involved. Since no God-given directions for the treatment of hypertension were included on the tablets brought down by Moses, we should all recognize the frailties of human judgment.

Before proceeding into the specifics, we need to recall the overriding issue: to maximally reduce cardiovascular risk without decreasing (and hopefully improving) the enjoyment of life (Kaplan, 1988). The preferred qualities of the drugs are fairly obvious but none now available (or likely to become available) meets all of the criteria for perfection. Nonetheless, currently available choices come close and, used adroitly, they can provide almost all patients protection without much bother.

### Importance of the First Choice

More and more patients with milder and milder hypertension are being treated with drugs. As noted in Chapter 1, that number, in the United States alone, may include 40 million people. These people have two characteristics that must be kept in mind when their hypertension is treated: For the most part, they are asymptomatic; and for the majority, no overt cardiovascular harm would ensue if they were left untreated. The ethics of drug therapy for such patients were considered in Chapter 5.

When their first drug is chosen, that drug may be taken for 10, 20, 30, or 40 years. If it successfully lowers the blood pressure by 10 mm Hg, as it will in 50 to 60% of mild hypertensives, no more drugs may be needed. Recall, too, that the tendency of thiazide diuretics, the most commonly used antihypertensive, to raise serum cholesterol levels by 10 to 20 mg/dl was only recognized after they were taken for up to 20 years by millions of people. The need for certainty about long-term safety, in addition to efficacy, should be obvious.

Only since publication of the controlled clinical trials of drug treatment of mild hypertension—all but one of which used the same diuretic first, stepped care approach—have the risks of therapy become apparent, as noted in Chapter 5. Simply stated, the choices of therapy, particularly for the first drug, should be made with care. As summarized in Table 7.18, all drugs have adverse effects, and precautions are needed in the use of any and all.

## Joint National Committee Recommendations

The four reports—in 1977, 1980, 1984, and 1988—of the Joint National Committees provide recommendations of a group of knowledgeable experts as to what United States practitioners were and should be doing at the time of each report (Table 7.19). A diuretic was the sole recommendation for initial therapy in both the 1977 and 1980 reports. In the 1984 report, the option was changed to "begin with less than a full dose of either a thiazide-type diuretic or a beta-blocker." In the 1988 report, four choices were provided: diuretics, beta-blocker, ACEI, or CEB.

## Comparative Trials

The only trials that have compared the long-term ability of different drugs to protect patients from overall and cardiovascular morbidity and mortality—the only meaningful criterion—have examined only two classes: diuretics and beta-blockers. As described in Chapter 5, three of the four trials showed no difference between the two, whereas the MAPHY portion of the HAPPHY trial found the beta-blocker metoprolol to provide lower coronary mortality than did a diuretic. As noted in Chapter 5, the issue remains unsettled and, as for now, no one class of drug has been shown to be better in protecting against morbidity or mortality than any other. Unfortunately, no data are available with any agents other than diuretics and beta-blockers. Therefore, the decision to change to other drugs must be based on the possibility, or better the probability, but not the certainty that they will be better.

Numerous short-term randomized, blinded controlled trials have been done to answer the secondary questions as to whether one type of drug is more effective in reducing the blood pressure and less bothersome in causing adverse effects. In general, there is little to choose in regard to antihypertensive efficacy and what differences that are noted could be due to the use of nonequivalent doses of the two drugs. However, considerable differences have been observed as to side effects. Croog et al (1986) (Table 7.1) and Helgeland et al (1986) are well-controlled comparisons of three different drugs. In both of these, the ACEI came out best, with fewer adverse effects than the diuretic or beta-blocker in Helgeland and coworkers' and than the beta-blocker or the central alpha-agonist in Croog and coworkers. Recall, however, the loss of many of the advantages of captopril when a diuretic was added to achieve adequate antihypertensive efficacy. Clearly, comparisons to be fair need to be with equipotent amounts of drug since many side effects are almost certainly nonspecific as to drug but rather related to the degree of blood pressure fall.

Overall, as to the incidence of adverse effects, diuretics come out worse than beta-blockers (Wahl et al, 1986), alpha$_1$-blockers (Stamler et al, 1986), ACEIs (Zezulka et al, 1987), or CEBs (Leary and Van der Byl (1988). When beta-blockers are compared, they usually come out little different from either ACEIs (Herrick et al, 1989) or CEBs (Nifedipine-Atenolol Study Review Committee, 1988). Similarly ACEIs and CEBs are little different (Wolfson et al, 1988).

Unfortunately, there are almost no blinded crossover studies comparing two or more drugs in the same patients to explain what factors are responsible for individual variability. From the few that are available (Hornung et al, 1986; Bidiville et al, 1988; Menard et al, 1988), it is clear that some patients respond better to one type of drug than another, but there is no single factor that explains why those who respond do so. The individual patient comparative trial described earlier in this chapter (Guyatt et al, 1988) could be used to determine which is the best choice. Practically, however, there are some simpler guidelines that can be followed to ensure that each patient is given a *good* choice even if it is not the *best* choice. If the patient's pressure is well controlled and no bothersome or potentially hazardous adverse effects are present, there is no reason to keep searching for "the best." Likely more than one effective drug can be found for each patient. Rather than searching for per-

**Table 7.18.** **Oral Antihypertensive Drugs**

| Type of Drug | Daily Adult Dosage Minimum | Maximum mg/d | Number of doses daily | Frequent or Severe Adverse Effects[a] |
|---|---|---|---|---|
| **DIURETICS** | | | | |
| Thiazide-type | | | | |
|   Bendroflumethiazide (Naturetin) | 2.5 | 5 | 1 | Hypokalemia; hypomagnesemia; hy- |
|   Benzthiazide (Exna) | 12.5–25 | 50 | 1 | perglycemia; increased serum low |
|   Chlorothiazide (Diuril) | 125–250 | 500 | 1 | density lipoprotein cholesterol and |
|   Chlorthalidone (Hygroton) | 12.5–25 | 50 | 1 | triglyceride concentrations; hyper- |
|   Cyclothiazide (Anhydron) | 0.125–0.5 | 2 | 1 | uricemia; hyponatremia; hypercal- |
|   Hydrochlorothiazide (Esidrix) | 12.5–25 | 50 | 1 | cemia; pancreatitis; rashes and |
|   Hydroflumethiazide (Saluron) | 12.5–25 | 50 | 1 | other allergic reactions |
|   Indapamide (Lozol) | 2.5 | 5 | 1 | |
|   Methyclothiazide (Enduron) | 2.5 | 5 | 1 | |
|   Metolazone (Zaroxolyn, Diulo, Micronox) | 0.5–1.0 | 10 | 1 | |
|   Polythiazide (Renese) | 2 | 4 | 1 | |
|   Quinethazone (Hydromox) | 25 | 100 | 1 | |
|   Trichlormethiazide (Naqua) | 1–2 | 4 | 1 | |
| Loop diuretics | | | | |
|   Bumetanide (Bumex) | 0.5 | 5 | 2 | Dehydration; hypokalemia; hypo- |
|   Ethacrynic acid (Edecrin) | 25 | 100 | 2 | magnesemia; hyperglycemia; lipid |
|   Furosemide (Lasix) | 20–40 | 640 | 2–3 | changes as with thiazide-type di- |
| | | | | uretics; hyperuricemia; hypocal- |
| | | | | cemia; blood dyscrasias; rashes |
| Potassium-sparing agents | | | | |
|   Amiloride (Midamor) | 5 | 10 | 1 | Hyperkalemia; GI disturbances; rash; headache |
|   Spironolactone (Aldactone) | 25 | 100 | 1–2 | Hyperkalemia; GI disturbances; menstrual abnormalities; gyneco- mastia; rash; tumorigenic in rats |
|   Triamterene (Dyrenium) | 50 | 150 | 1 | Hyperkalemia; GI disturbances; in- creased blood urea nitrogen; met- abolic acidosis, nephrolithiasis |
| **ADRENERGIC INHIBITORS** | | | | |
| Peripheral-acting adrenergic inhibitors | | | | |
|   Guanadrel sulfate (Hylorel) | 10 | 100 | 2 | Similar to guanethidine, but less diarrhea |
|   Guanethidine (Ismelin) | 10 | 150 | 1 | Orthostatic hypotension; exercise hy- potension; diarrhea; bradycardia; sodium and water retention; retro- grade ejaculation |
| Rauwolfia alkaloids | | | | |
|   Rauwolfia (whole root) | 50 | 100 | 1 | Psychic depression; nightmares; na- |
|   Reserpine (Serpasil) | 0.05 | 0.25 | 1 | sal stuffiness; drowsiness; GI dis- turbances; bradycardia |
| Centrally acting alpha-blockers | | | | |
|   Clonidine (Catapres) | 0.1 | 1.2 | 2 | Sedation; dry mouth; rebound hyper- |
|   Clonidine TTS (Patch) | 0.1 | 0.3 | 1 q week | tension; headache; bradycardia; contact dermatitis from patches |
|   Guanabenz (Wytensin) | 4 | 64 | 2 | Similar to clonidine |
|   Guanfacine (Tenex) | 1 | 3 | 1 | Similar to clonidine, but milder |
|   Methyldopa (Aldomet) | 250 | 2000 | 2 | Sedation and other CNS symptoms; fever; orthostatic hypotension; bra- dycardia; GI disorders, including colitis; hepatitis; cirrhosis; hepatic necrosis; Coombs' positive hemo- lytic anemia; lupus-like syndrome; immune thrombocytopenia; red cell aplasia |
| Alpha₁-Adrenergic blockers | | | | |
|   Prazosin (Minipress) | 1–2 | 20 | 2 | Syncope with first dose; dizziness and vertigo; palpitations; fluid re- tention; headache; priapism |
|   Terazosin (Hytrin) | 1–2 | 20 | 1 | Similar to prazosin |

*continues*

**Table 7.18.** *Continued*

| Type of Drug | Daily Adult Dosage mg/d Minimum | Maximum | Number of doses daily | Frequent or Severe Adverse Effects[a] |
|---|---|---|---|---|
| **Beta-Adrenergic blockers** | | | | |
| Acebutolol (Sectral) | 200 | 1200 | 1 | Similar to propranolol, but less lipid changes and resting bradycardia; rare drug-induced lupus |
| Atenolol (Tenormin) | 25 | 150 | 1 | Similar to propranolol; relatively cardioselective at ≤ 100 mg/d |
| Metoprolol (Lopressor) | 50 | 200 | 1 | Similar to propranolol; relatively cardioselective at < 200 mg |
| Nadolol (Corgard) | 40 | 320 | 1 | Similar to propranolol |
| Pindolol (Visken) | 10 | 60 | 2 | Similar to propranolol, but less resting bradycardia and lipid changes |
| Propranolol hydrochloride (Inderal) | 40 | 320 | 2 | Fatigue; decreased exercise tolerance; increased serum triglycerides, decreased HDL cholesterol; bradycardia; vivid dreams or hallucinations; aggravation of peripheral vascular disease; increased airway resistance; mask symptoms of hypoglycemia; congestive heart failure; depression; rare blood dyscrasias and other allergic disorders; sudden withdrawal can lead to exacerbation of angina |
| Propranolol LA, long acting | 60 | 320 | 1 | |
| Timolol (Blocarden) | 20 | 80 | 2 | Similar to propranolol |
| **Combined alpha-beta-adrenergic blocker:** | | | | |
| Labetalol (Normodyne, Trandate) | 200 | 1800 | 2 | Similar to propranolol but more orthostatic hypotension; fever |
| **VASODILATORS** | | | | |
| **Direct** | | | | |
| Hydralazine (Apresoline) | 50 | 300 | 2 | Headache and dizziness; tachycardia; fluid retention; lupus-like syndrome; aggravation of angina; GI disturbances; rashes and other allergic reactions |
| Minoxidil (Loniten) | 2.5 | 80 | 1 | Marked fluid retention; hair growth on face and body; coarsening of facial features; tachycardia; aggravation of angina; thrombocytopenia; leukopenia |
| **Angiotensin-converting enzyme inhibitor** | | | | |
| Captopril (Capoten) | 25–50 | 300 | 1–3 | Cough; skin rash; loss of taste with anorexia; hypotension, particularly with a diuretic or volume depletion; angioedema; hyperkalemia if also on potassium supplements or potassium-retaining diuretics; acute renal failure with bilateral renal artery stenosis or stenosis of the artery to a solitary kidney; blood dyscrasias and renal damage are rare except in patients with renal dysfunction, and particularly in patients with collagen-vascular disease; may increase fetal mortality and should not be used during pregnancy. |
| Enalapril (Vasotec) | 2.5–5 | 40 | 1–2 | |
| Lisinopril (Prinivil, Zestril) | 5 | 40 | 1 | |
| **Calcium entry blocker** | | | | |
| Diltiazem SR (Cardizem SR) | 60 | 360 | 2 | Similar to verapamil |
| Nicardipine (Cardene) | | | 3 | Flushing; edema; tachycardia |
| Nifedipine (Procardia, Adalat) | 30 | 180 | 3 | Similar to nicardipine |
| Procardia XL | 30 | 180 | 1 | |
| Nitrendipine[b] | 5 | 40 | 1–2 | Similar to nicardipine |
| Verapamil SR (Calan SR, Isoptin SR) | 120 | 480 | 1–2 | Constipation; dizziness; edema; headache; bradycardia; AV block |

[a]All antihypertensive drugs can probably cause erectile impotence; spironolactone may cause loss of libido.
[b]Not yet approved for use in the United States (as of February 1990).

**Table 7.19. Drugs Recommended in the Four Joint National Committee Reports**

|  | JNC I (1977) | JNC II (1980) | JNC III (1984) | JNC IV (1988) |
|---|---|---|---|---|
| Step 1 | Thiazides | Thiazide | Thiazide or Beta-blocker | Thiazide, Beta-blocker, ACEI, or CEB |
| Step 2 | Propranolol Methyldopa Reserpine | Beta-blockers Clonidine Methyldopa Prazosin Rauwolfia | Adrenergic inhibitor or diuretic | Second drug of different class or Increase first drug or Substitute another drug |
| Step 3 | Hydralazine | Hydralazine | Hydralazine Minoxidil | Third drug of different class or Substitute second drug |

fection, we need simply to weed out the drugs that either produce little good effect or induce significant ill effects.

## Individualized Therapy (Fig. 7.34)

This approach is predicated on three major principles:

1. The first choice may be one of a variety of antihypertensives from each class of drugs—diuretics, centrally acting agents, alpha-blockers, beta-blockers, ACEIs, or CEBs.
2. The choice can be logically based on the type of patient and the presence of target organ damage or other cardiovascular risk factors.
3. Rather than proceeding with a second drug if the first does not work well or side effects ensue, a substitution approach is used—stop the first drug and try another from a different class.

Let us consider further these three principles.

## Characteristics of the Drugs (Table 7.20)

Each class of drugs has different features that make its members more or less attractive. In the past, diuretics were almost always chosen first, because they were considered free of significant side effects, easy to take, and inexpensive. Moreover, reactive fluid retention with other drugs used without a diuretic often blunted their effect, so the idea of using a diuretic first seemed

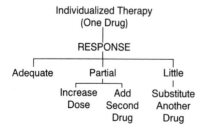

**Figure 7.34.** Individualized approach to the therapy of hypertension. The choice of initial therapy is based on multiple clinical features.

more logical. However, recognition of the "hidden" side effects and costs of diuretics, along with the lesser protection from coronary mortality in the trials wherein they were used, have caused many to doubt the wisdom of their routine use. At the least, these factors have led to the more widespread use of lower doses of diuretics and their combinations with potassium-sparing agents.

Beta-blockers have become increasingly popular. However, the need for caution and the contraindications to their use, along with recognition of their potential for altering lipids adversely, have put a damper on the enthusiasm for their use. The failure to find additional protection against coronary disease in trials with a beta-blocker, as described in Chapter 5, further weakened the argument for their use.

Drugs that act primarily as indirect vasodilators, alpha-blockers, ACEIs, and CEBs are being more widely advocated for initial therapy. There seems a certain logic for the use of drugs that induce vasodilation since an elevated peripheral resistance is the hemodynamic fault of established hypertension (Fig. 7.35).

Reserpine works as well as any of these with one dose a day. However, the concern about the subtle onset of depression and the recurrent (but unproved) claims of its carcinogenicity have caused many to stop using it.

## Characteristics of the Patients

Beyond the avoidance of certain drugs in certain patients, individual patient's characteristics may affect the likelihood of a good response to various classes of drugs. For example, an elderly, obese, black woman will likely respond better to a diuretic than to a beta-blocker or an ACEI. A younger, physically active, white man would likely respond particularly well to an alpha-blocker or an ACEI. In general, black patients tend to do better with a diuretic (VA Cooperative Study, 1982a), less well with a beta-

**Table 7.20. Choice of Initial Therapy**

| | Diuretics | Centrally Acting Agents | Alpha-Blockers | Beta-Blockers | Converting Enzyme Inhibitors | Calcium Antagonists |
|---|---|---|---|---|---|---|
| Hemodynamic effect | Initial volume shrinkage Peripheral vasodilation | Reduce cardiac output | Peripheral vasodilation | Reduce cardiac output | Peripheral vasodilation | Peripheral vasodilation |
| Side effects Overt | Weakness Palpitations | Sedation Dry mouth | Postural dizziness | Bronchospasm Fatigue Delay recovery hypoglycemia | Cough Taste disturbance Rash | Flushing Local edema Constipation (verapamil) |
| Hidden | Hypokalemia Hypercholes- terolemia Glucose intol- erance Hyperuricemia | Withdrawal syndrome Autoimmune syndromes (methyldopa) | | Glucose intol- erance Hypertrigly- ceridemia Decrease HDL- cholesterol | Leukopenia Proteinuria | AV conduction (verapamil, diltiazem) |
| Contraindica- tions | Preexisting volume contraction | Orthostatic hypotension Liver disease (methyldopa) | Orthostatic hypotension | Asthma Heartblock | Pregnancy | |
| Cautions | Diabetes mellitus Gout Digitalis toxicity | | | Peripheral vas- cular disease Insulin-requir- ing diabetes Allergy Coronary spasm Withdrawal angina | Renal insuffi- ciency Renovascular disease | Heart failure |
| Special advan- tages | Effective in blacks, elderly Enhance effectiveness of all other agents | No alteration in blood lipids No fluid reten- tion (guana- benz) | No decrease in cardiac out- put No alteration in blood lipids No sedation | Reduce recur- rences of coronary disease Reduce mani- festations of anxiety Coexisting angina, migrane, glaucoma | No CNS side effects Unload congestive heart failure No coronary vasoconstric- tion Possible renal protection | Effective in blacks, elderly No CNS side effects Coronary vaso- dilation |

blocker or an ACEI, and equally well with a CEB or alpha-blocker than do nonblack patients. The elderly tend to respond equally, if not better, to most classes than do the younger. However, for the individual patient, any drug may work well or poorly, and there is no set formula that can be used to predict success without side effects.

Even more than the demographic features, the presence of one or more concomitant disease features can provide a rational reason to choose or avoid one or another drug (Table 7.21). Patients with hypertension, usually being middle-aged or elderly, often have other medical problems, some related to their hypertension, others coincidental (Stewart et al, 1989).

As shown in Table 7.21, a hypertensive patient with angina would logically be given a beta-blocker or a CEB. Alpha-blockers, CEBs, and ACEIs are attractive choices for those in whom a diuretic or beta-blocker may pose particular problems, such as diabetics or hyperlipidemic patients.

*Making the Choice Based upon Renin Levels.* Laragh and coworkers, as far back as 1972 (Bühler et al, 1972) and persistently since (Laragh, 1989), have utilized the level of plasma renin activity (PRA) as a guide to the choice of initial therapy. As attractive as the concept is, in practice it often does not work (Weber and Drayer, 1984). To be sure, most studies do show that those with lower renin respond somewhat better to diuretics whereas those with higher renin respond better to beta-blockers and ACEIs. The elderly and blacks may respond particularly well to diuretics, perhaps because their renin

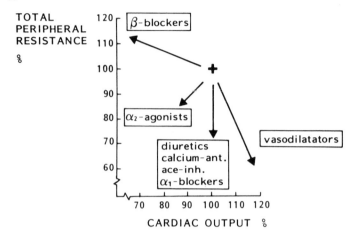

**Figure 7.35.** The major action of the seven classes of antihypertensive agents on peripheral resistance and cardiac output (From Man in't Veld et al: *Am J Hypertens* 1:91, 1988a.)

**Table 7.21. Concomitant Diseases and the Choice of Antihypertensive Drug Therapy**

| | Indications | Contraindications |
| --- | --- | --- |
| Diuretics | Congestive heart failure<br>Volume retention | Diabetes<br>Gout<br>Hypercholesterolemia |
| Central alpha-agonists | Withdrawal from addictive behaviors<br>(clonidine) (?) | Liver disease (methyldopa)<br>Autoimmune disease (methyldopa)<br>Depression |
| Alpha-blockers | Hypercholesterolemia<br>High level of physical activity | Postural hypotension |
| Beta-blockers | Coronary artery disease<br>Tachyarrhythmias<br>Migraine<br>Anxiety | Asthma<br>Diabetes requiring insulin<br>Bradyarrhythmias<br>Congestive heart failure<br>Peripheral vascular disease<br>Hypertriglyceridemia |
| ACE inhibitors | Congestive heart failure<br>Renal insufficiency (?)<br>Peripheral vascular disease | Renal failure<br>Renovascular hypertension<br>Volume depletion<br>Pregnancy |
| Calcium antagonists | Coronary artery disease<br>Tachyarrhythmias (verapamil)<br>Peripheral vascular disease | Bradyarrhythmias (verapamil) |

levels tend to be lower, whereas younger white patients may respond well to beta-blockers or ACEIs, perhaps because their renin levels are higher.

### Substitution Rather Than Addition

The traditional "stepped care" has usually meant that if the first drug does not work well, others would be added sequentially. This could mean that the patient is given one, two, or even three drugs, none of which works.

The wisdom of substitution rather than addition seems obvious. If the first choice, even if based on all reasonable criteria, does not lower the blood pressure much or is associated with persistent, bothersome side effects, that drug should be stopped and one from another class tried. Thereby, the least number of drugs should be needed to achieve the desired fall in blood pressure with the fewest side effects.

Patients with milder hypertension will often need only one drug. Therefore substitution should work for them. For those with more severe hypertension, the first drug may do all that is expected and still not be enough. Therefore, the addition of a second or, if needed, a third drug is logical.

## Cost as a Factor

For some patients, the cost of the medications used to treat hypertension may pose an obstacle to control of their disease (Shulman et al, 1986). The cost per tablet varies between a few cents for a generic hydrochlorothiazide or reserpine to almost 1 dollar for a brand-name ACEI or CEB. Practitioners concerned about the cost might then choose the least expensive agent.

However, there are additional factors that need to be considered. First the cost of the tablet may not be the major cost of the medication. If a diuretic causes hypokalemia that must be corrected, each dose of potassium supplement costs 25 to 40 cents and four to eight of these a day may be required. Diuretic-induced hyperlipidemia may be an even more serious albeit less obvious cost.

Secondly, most of the currently available tablets are designed to provide adequate and sustained antihypertensive efficacy for the majority of patients with mild hypertension with one or two doses a day, each dose of one tablet. This is in sharp contrast to the practices of the 1960s and 1970s when as many as 12 methyldopa and four hydralazine and multiple doses of other drugs were often prescribed. Thus the daily cost of the newer, trade-name medications will often be no more than the cost of one tablet per day. This compares with less than half of the cost of a pack of cigarettes or a six-pack of beer, two costs that certainly do not impede the consumption of either cigarettes or beer. Clearly, a half-dollar a day may pose a burden for many patients, but hopefully the cost of medication will not interfere with the provision of what is best for the individual patient. Nonetheless, lacking clear proof that one type of drug is clearly more protective against cardiovascular morbidity and mortality, the temptation to go with the least expensive cannot be discounted (Stason, 1989).

## Choice of Second Drug

Just as a thiazide diuretic has usually been chosen as first drug, a beta-blocker has most commonly been chosen as second, having taken over that position from methyldopa. Increasingly, other agents including ACEIs and CEBs are being chosen (Fig. 7.3). As noted in JNC-IV:

Combining antihypertensive drugs with different modes of action will often allow small doses of drugs to be used to achieve control, thereby minimizing the potential for dose-dependent side effects. If a diuretic is not chosen as the first drug, it will often be required as the second one since fluid retention (pseudotolerance) may be responsible in part for the suboptimal response to nondiuretic agents and since the addition of a diuretic will usually enhance the effects of other drugs. When additional drugs are added and the combination succeeds, a later attempt should be made to reduce the dose, if possible, to eliminate the initial drug.

The wisdom of adding a second drug rather than increasing the dose of the first has been widely accepted but inadequately tested. Nonetheless, there is no question that the addition of two drugs of dissimilar action will usually provide additional effect (Massie et al, 1987). In a group whose DBP remained above 95 mm Hg on 20 mg of enalapril who were randomly assigned to receive more enalapril or to have a diuretic added, those given the second agent did better than those given more of the first drug (Sassano et al, 1989). Clearly, the decision is easy if the dose of first drug is near the top of the dose-response curve: A second drug should be started. However, those on a submaximal dose of the first dose and tolerating it well could just as reasonably be given a larger dose rather than have a second drug started.

The choice of second drug depends largely on the nature of the first. If a diuretic is the first drug, the addition of an adrenergic inhibitor or an ACEI will usually provide significant additional antihypertensive effect. The addition of an alpha-blocker will minimize diuretic-induced hyperlipidemia (Stamler et al, 1988). Since they seldom cause sedation or dryness, as occurs frequently with central alpha-agonists, an alpha-blocker is a particularly attractive alternative to a beta-blocker as the second drug. If a nondiuretic agent is the first choice, a diuretic can be used as second. However, if a diuretic is to be avoided, combinations of a beta-blocker and a CEB (Nifedipine-Atenolol Study Review Committee, 1988) or of a CEB and an ACEI (Wolfson et al, 1988) will usually provide additive effects.

In the elderly, central alpha-agonists may be less attractive because of their tendency to cause sedation and prazosin may cause bothersome postural hypotension. However, all classes of drugs seem to work as well in the elderly as in the younger so that age per se is probably not an important determinant of the choice of therapy.

## Two Drugs as Initial Therapy

Since one-third to one-half of patients will end up on two drugs, some prefer to start with the combination of a diuretic and an adrenergic inhibitor. That practice is, in general, unwise for these reasons: (1) even with fairly high blood pressure, many will respond adequately to one drug, and there is no certain way to know who will need more than one; (2) if side effects appear, it is preferable to know which drug is responsible; (3) the dose-response curves differ with various drugs, so fixed-dose combinations may be inappropriate; and (4) except in those with dangerously high levels of blood pressure, a gradual, gentle reduction in pressure with one drug at a time is easier to tolerate than a sudden, drastic fall from two or more drugs.

## Combination Tablets

If the patient ends up on two drugs and the doses match the combinations available, such a combination tablet should be used. Of the combinations available, the addition of a potassium-sparing agent to a diuretic (Dyazide, Maxzide, Moduretic) is eminently sensible. Combinations of a diuretic plus almost every one of the other types of drugs are available. Caution is advised in not overdosing the diuretic if larger amounts of the other agent are needed.

## Choice of Third Drug

Hydralazine became the most popular third drug, added to a diuretic and an adrenergic inhibitor, in the late 1970s and early 1980s. This combination usually works, but others work as well. One controlled trial of five agents showed that minoxidil was most effective, labetalol and methyldopa were associated with a high prevalence of side effects, and hydralazine or prazosin were the most easily tolerated (McAreavey et al, 1984). Neither an ACEI nor a CEB was included in that trial and they are increasingly being added as the vasodilator in triple therapy.

## Choice of Fourth Drug

Few patients should need more than three drugs, particularly if the various reasons for resistance to therapy are considered. For those who do, the JNC-IV report recommends adding a fourth drug or having the patient evaluated for the reason behind resistance.

## Stepping Down or Off Therapy

Once a good response has occurred, patients may be able to reduce the amount or number of medications particularly if they have been on grossly excessive doses such as 100 mg a day of chlorthalidone (Grimm et al, 1985). Some may be able to discontinue all therapy, an idea advocated long ago (Page and Dustan, 1962) and frequently reiterated (Hudson, 1988; Alderman and Lamport, 1989). Patients able to stop therapy must be kept under surveillance since their hypertension may redevelop, although that may take some time. Overall, about 15% of those with moderate hypertension and from 30 to 50% of those with mild hypertension who have kept their DBP under 90 mm Hg on drugs will likely remain normotensive for at least 1 year off all drugs (Alderman and Lamport, 1989). That percentage can be increased by concomitant weight loss or sodium restriction (Stamler et al, 1987).

Whether it is worth the trouble to stop drug therapy completely is questionable. A more sensible approach would be to first decrease the dose of whatever is being used. That is feasible, without loss of control, in a significant number who are well controlled on a diuretic alone (Finnerty, 1984).

## Breaking Tablets in Half

One way to cut down on therapy may be to break tablets in half. Unfortunately some tablets, despite being scored, do not divide equally (Stimpel et al, 1985) in which case the better course would be to prescribe a smaller size.

## SPECIAL CONSIDERATIONS IN THERAPY

Despite apparently doing all of the right things, patients may be resistant to therapy and may have special problems that require special considerations.

## Resistant Hypertension

The reasons for a poor response are numerous (Table 7.22), with the most likely being volume overload due to either excessive sodium intake or inadequate diuretic (Ramsay et al, 1980; Graves and Buckalew, 1989). If the former is suspected, measurement of sodium in an overnight or 24-hour urine sample may be most revealing. If the latter is suspected, addition of furosemide, metolazone, or spironolactone may be useful, along with a lower sodium intake. If the response is still poor, it may be due to reactive hyperreninemia that may then respond to an ACEI or beta-blocker therapy (Gavras et al, 1981a).

Therapy of patients with very severe hyper-

**Table 7.22. Causes of Poor Response to Antihypertensive Drugs**[a]

Nonadherence to therapy
Drug related
  Doses too low
  Inappropriate combinations (e.g., two centrally acting
    adrenergic inhibitors)
  Rapid inactivation (e.g., hydralazine)
  Effects of other drugs
    Sympathomimetics
    Antidepressants
    Adrenal steroids
    Nonsteroidal antiinflammatory drugs
    Nasal decongestants
    Oral contraceptives
Associated conditions
  Increasing obesity
  Excess alcohol intake: ≥30 mL/d
  Renal insufficiency
  Renovascular hypertension
  Malignant or accelerated hypertension
  Other causes of hypertension
Volume overload
  Inadequate diuretic therapy
  Excess sodium intake
  Fluid retention from reduction of blood pressure
  Progressive renal damage

[a]From 1988 Joint National Committee: *Arch Intern Med* 148:1023, 1988.

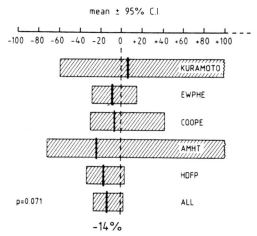

**Figure 7.36.** Differences in mortality from all causes between the actively treated group and the control group, in different trials of patients over age 60 with diastolic hypertension. For each trial, the difference and the 95% confidence limits are illustrated. A negative sign means a decrease in events in the actively treated group compared with the control group. In none of the trials was there a statistically significant reduction, nor was there one when the data from all trials were combined. (From Staessen et al: *J Cardiovasc Pharmacol* 12(Suppl 8):S33, 1988a.)

**Table 7.23. Factors That Might Contribute to Increased Risk of Pharmacological Treatment of Hypertension in the Elderly**

| Factors | Potential Complications |
|---|---|
| Diminished baroreceptor activity | Orthostatic hypotension |
| Decreased intravascular volume | Orthostatic hypotension dehydration |
| Sensitivity to hypokalemia | Arrhythmia, muscular weakness |
| Decreased renal and hepatic function | Drug accumulation |
| Polypharmacy | Drug interaction |
| CNS Changes | Depression, confusion |

tension in need of immediate reduction will be covered in the next chapter.

## Treatment of the Elderly Hypertensive

Many millions of people over age 65 have hypertension that in most is predominantly or purely systolic. As described in Chapter 4, the risks for such patients are significant, but there is no certainty either that the blood pressure can usually be reduced or that the risks of systolic hypertension can thereby be relieved. The initial results of the Systolic Hypertension in the Elderly Program (SHEP) showed that almost 80% of such patients do achieve a significant fall of systolic blood pressure at the end of 1 year on a small dose, 15 mg, of chlorthalidone (Hulley et al, 1985). The study is in progress but interim data reveal no striking reduction in morbidity or mortality (Perry et al, 1989). Multiple trials of treatment of diastolic hypertension in patients over age 60 performed in various counties have failed to document that people with significant diastolic hypertension above age 60 will benefit from therapy as determined by a decrease in overall or coronary mortality. (Staessen et al, 1988a) (Fig. 7.36). However, the mortality from stroke was reduced in these trials.

Since the elderly may have sluggish baroreceptor and sympathetic nervous responsiveness, as well as impaired cerebral autoregulation, therapy should be gentle and gradual, avoiding

drugs that are likely to cause postural hypotension or to exacerbate other common problems often seen among the elderly (Table 7.23). However, occasional reports of the serious consequences of inappropriate therapy with excessive doses of potent drugs (Ledingham and Rajagopalan, 1979; Jansen et al, 1986) should not deter appropriate therapy of those with diastolic hypertension (Applegate, 1989).

Until the results of the SHEP trial are in, sometime after 1992, a cautious but positive approach toward the treatment of systolic hypertension seems justified, using these guidelines:

—Treat all with a reasonable life expectancy who have systolic levels above 170 mm Hg, since that level is associated with significant risk from strokes and other cardiovascular diseases.

— Be sure that the elevated pressure is not "pseudohypertension" from calcified arteries too rigid to be compressed by the balloon cuff (Spence et al, 1978).

— Those who are obese or heavy salt users should be advised to reduce intake of calories and sodium. A low sodium diet has been shown to be as effective as a diuretic in such patients (Niarchos et al, 1984).

— The goal of therapy should probably be a systolic pressure of 160 mm Hg that can usually be reached without much of a fall in diastolic pressure.

— As shown in the 1-year feasibility trial for SHEP (Hulley et al, 1985), a low dose of a diuretic is a reasonable choice for initial monotherapy. CEBs, ACEIs, alpha-blockers, beta-blockers, and central alpha-agonists are also generally effective in the elderly.

— Use smaller doses, recognizing that the elderly may obtain greater effects that they can poorly tolerate (Tsujimoto et al, 1989).

— More careful attention to diuretic-induced potassium wastage may be warranted since elderly people may be more susceptible to cardiac complications from hypokalemia (Morgan et al, 1979) and more likely to become hypokalemic because of lesser potassium stores.

— The number of medications and the number of daily doses should be kept to a minimum, remembering that some of the elderly may have more trouble following complicated dosage schedules, reading the labels, and opening bottles with safety caps.

## Treatment of Patients with Cardiac Disease

Hypertensives often have coexisting coronary artery disease and may develop congestive heart failure. The presence of coronary artery disease favors the use of drugs such as CEBs or alpha-blockers that dilate the coronary vessels as well as peripheral ones. However, beta-blockers, which reduce cardiac work even though they may increase coronary and peripheral vascular resistance, have been successfully used. Since coronary spasm has been described with beta-blocker therapy (Kern et al, 1983) these agents should not be used in patients with known or suspected spasm. For hypertensives with heart failure, diuretics and ACEIs should be used. Low doses and careful monitoring are also needed in those elderly hypertensives thought to be in heart failure who have marked hypertrophic cardiomyopathy, since unloaders may make them hypotensive whereas beta-blockers or CEBs may make them better (Topol et al, 1985).

As noted in Chapter 4, left ventricular hypertrophy (LVH) is frequently present on echocardiography, even in patients with mild hypertension. A number of antihypertensive drugs have been shown to reverse LVH (Ram et al, 1989; White et al, 1989). At present, no clear guidelines can be given as to which type of drug is best to reverse LVH or even as to whether such reversal is a desirable goal of therapy, but a strong argument can be made for the use of drugs such as ACEIs, CEBs, and alpha-blockers that vasodilate without causing marked reflex sympathetic stimulation (Zusman, 1989).

## Treatment of Patients with Cerebrovascular Disease

Immediately after the onset of the manifestations of the stroke, blood pressure may become markedly elevated, only to fall precipitously if potent antihypertensive agents are given (Lavin, 1986). Brott and Reed (1989) provide these guidelines for antihypertensive therapy in acute stroke:

— If DBP is above 140 on two readings 5 minutes apart, use intravenous nitroprusside.

— If SBP is over 230 and/or DBP is 121-140 on 2 readings 20 minutes apart, use intravenous labetalol.

— If SBP is 180 to 230 and/or DBP is 105 to 120, defer emergency therapy in the absence of intracranial hemorrhage or left ventricular failure. If the elevation persists over an hour, use oral labetalol, nifedipine or captopril.

— If SBP is less than 180 and/or DBP is less than 105, antihypertensive therapy is usually not indicated

Concerns have been expressed over the potential for nitroprusside to induce further rises in intracranial pressure (Garner, 1986). In a study involving measurement of intracranial pressure in patients with hemorrhagic stroke and hypertension, barbiturates were found to be superior to nifedipine, reserpine, or furosemide in reducing both systemic and intracranial pressures (Hayashi et al, 1988). There is a great need for more such careful study of the treatment of acute stroke. In less well-controlled studies, beta-blockers were of no help (Barer et al, 1988) whereas the CEB nicardipine was helpful in relieving cerebral vasospasm (Flamm, 1989).

For chronic management in those who remain hypertensive, effective antihypertensive treatment has been shown to reduce recurrent strokes (Carter, 1970; HDFP, 1979; Tuomilehto et al, 1985). However, caution is advised: The blood pressure should be lowered gradually and without sudden drops so that cerebral blood flow will not fall. Elderly patients may have poor cerebral autoregulatory ability (Jansen et al, 1986), and that ability may be further impaired in the presence of cerebrovascular disease (Graham et al, 1984).

## Postural Hypotension

In addition to the elderly and those on adrenergic neuronal blockers, some patients may be susceptible to postural hypotension particularly with the first dose of medication. These include diabetics, patients with idiopathic autonomic failure, and patients with reduced central venous pressure or vagally mediated cardiac slowing (Semple et al, 1988).

Some of these patients have hypertension when supine and hypotension when upright (Frank et al, 1972). Presumably their loss of normal postural reflex vasoconstriction allows pooling of blood in the legs, depleting effective arterial blood volume and inducing fluid retention. When they are supine, the expanded overall body fluid volume causes the pressure to rise. Often these swings in pressure can be effectively modulated by sleeping with the head of the bed raised by 10 to 20° and effectively supporting the bottom half of the body with tightly fitting elastic supports such as the Jobst body stocking.

Beyond such physical support, various medications have been claimed but poorly documented to help. These include indomethacin (Kochar and Itskovitz, 1978) and pindolol (Man in't Veld and Schalekamp, 1981). The somatostatin analogue octreotide has been found to prevent postprandial hypotension in the elderly (Jansen et al, 1989) and orthostatic hypotension in patients with autonomic neuropathy (Hoeldtke and Israel, 1989), but it must be given subcutaneously. Avoidance of large meals and the ingestion of caffeine-containing beverages only in the early morning may be helpful.

## Paroxysmal Hypertension and Hypovolemia

Rarely, patients who are severely hypertensive when first seen rapidly go into peripheral vascular collapse when treated with antihypertensive agents (Cohn, 1966). These patients were

hypovolemic and hemoconcentrated, and their initial hypertension was at least partially a reflection of compensatory sympathetic nervous system overactivity and, very likely, an activated renin-angiotensin system. Their attempt to compensate for fluid volume depletion was reflected by tachycardia, sweating, and cool skin, as well as by hyperresponsiveness to various challenges of sympathetic function. When their compensatory support was removed, profound hypotension quickly followed.

Similar patients have been observed to have a fall in blood pressure as their shrunken fluid volume is replaced. In addition to quieting their disturbed sympathetic nervous system, fluid repletion may also lower their pressures by stopping the release of increased amounts of renin.

## Hypertension and Diabetes

Patients with diabetes and hypertension are susceptible to numerous problems in addition to their propensity to postural hypotension. If they develop nephropathy as evidenced by proteinuria, progressive deterioration of renal function is almost invariable. Aggressive management of their hypertension has been shown to slow the rate of fall in renal function (Parving et al, 1987). This is considered further in Chapter 9.

The choice of drugs should be carefully considered: Diuretics and beta-blockers may worsen glucose tolerance; beta-blockers may delay recognition and recovery from insulin-invoked hypoglycemia. Alpha-blockers, ACEIs, and CEBs may be appropriate choices (Trost, 1989), though many now choose a centrally acting alpha-agonist (Kaplan et al, 1987). Experimental (Anderson et al, 1986) and clinical (Romanelli et al, 1989) evidence is growing for a special effectiveness of ACEIs in limiting glomerular hypertension and proteinuria in diabetes.

## Hyperlipidemia

Hypertensives have a higher prevalence of hyperlipidemia even if they are on no therapy (MacMahon and MacDonald, 1986; Castelli and Anderson, 1986; Williams et al, 1988). Hypertension and hyperlipidemia are common to certain conditions including upper body obesity (Kaplan, 1989b), diabetes, and alcohol abuse, but even when these mechanisms are excluded, more hypercholesterolemia is found among hypertensives than age- and sex-matched normotensives.

Obviously, hypertensives should have assessment of their lipid status before institution of antihypertensive therapy and, if hyperlipidemia is present, appropriate diet and drug therapy provided to control the lipid problem. Unfortunately, the two most widely used antihypertensive agents, diuretics and beta-blockers, may induce hyperlipidemia, as described in the coverage of these drugs earlier in this chapter and summarized elsewhere (Lardinois and Neuman, 1988; Johnson and Danylchuk, 1989) (Table 7.24). The percentages given in Table 7.24 are based upon a thorough but not weighted analysis of published data. If either a diuretic or a non-ISA beta-blocker is used, the total and HDL-cholesterol levels should be rechecked after 2 to 3 months. If a significant alteration has occurred, another drug should be considered or an appropriate lipid-lowering regimen instituted. Fortunately, the other classes of drugs either are lipid neutral or may actually improve the lipid status (Table 7.24).

## Miscellaneous Diseases

### Peripheral Vascular Disease

Hypertension is a risk factor for the development of peripheral vascular disease. Lowering of the blood pressure, although it should slow the progression of atherosclerosis, may further impair already compromised peripheral circulation, particularly if the lowering is provided by non-ISA beta-blockers that induce peripheral vasoconstriction. Vasodilators are preferable, including ACEIs (Roberts et al, 1987) and CEBs (Rademaker et al, 1989).

### Asthma and Chronic Obstructive Pulmonary Disease

Patients with bronchospasm should not be given beta-blockers unless there is a powerful indication. ACEIs may cause a cough, perhaps most commonly in people who have underlying bronchial hyperreactivity (Kaufman et al, 1989). Some drugs used to treat pulmonary diseases may aggravate hypertension including sympathomimetic decongestants, e.g., phenylpropanolamine, or adrenal steroids.

### Gout

Thiazide-induced hyperuricemia is best neglected, but thiazides should not be given to patients who have gout unless their disease is well controlled with a uricosuric agent. Spironolactone can be used safely.

### Impotence and Other Sexual Dysfunction

Impotence, defined as the inability to obtain or maintain an erection, is seen in as many as 10 to 20% of middle-aged men and the prevalence is likely even greater among hypertensives even when they are on no treatment (Bansal, 1988). Numerous mechanisms may be involved including psychogenic factors (common), neurogenic causes (less common except among diabetics) (Tejada et al, 1989), hormonal deficiency (rare), and hemodynamic alterations (common particularly in those with other atherosclerotic risk factors such as smoking and hypercholesterolemia) (Virag et al, 1985).

Antihypertensive drugs are considered to be among the most common causes of impotence. In addition, they may cause retarded ejaculation, reduced desire for sex (libido) and, less frequently, gynecomastia. Most drug-induced problems of sexual dysfunction have been recognized in men. As many as 10% of women aged 35 to 59 have a significant sexual dysfunction (Osborn et al, 1988), but there are no data on the effects of antihypertensive drugs on sexual function among women.

Men may lose erectile potency whenever their blood pressure is lowered since much of the problem is due to vascular insufficiency of the penile artery from atherosclerosis that accompanies their hypertension. Beyond this nonspecific effect that applies to all antihypertensives,

**Table 7.24. Calculated Approximations of the Extent of Drug Effect on Plasma Lipids[a]**

| | Total Cholesterol | LDL Cholesterol | HDL Cholesterol | Triglycerides |
|---|---|---|---|---|
| Thiazides | +7% | +10% | + 2% | +14% |
| Beta-blockers | | | | |
|   Propranolol | 0 | − 3% | −11% | +16% |
|   Atenolol | 0 | − 2% | − 7% | +15% |
|   Pindolol | −1% | − 3% | − 2% | + 7% |
| Alpha$_1$-blockers | −4% | −13% | + 5% | − 8% |
| Central alpha$_2$-agonists | −7% | | | |
| Calcium entry blockers | 0 | 0 | 0 | 0 |
| ACE Inhibitors | 0 | 0 | 0 | 0 |

[a]Modified from Johnson and Danylchuk: Med Clin North Am 73:449, 1989.

impotence has been reported more frequently after the use of beta-blockers (Croog et al, 1988; Suzuki et al, 1988) or diuretics. In the MRC trial, impotence was noted in 10.1% of the men receiving placebo, 13.2% of those on propranolol, but 22.6% on the thiazide bendrofluazide (Medical Research Council Working Party, 1981). In another population of English men, hydralazine use was associated with more impotence than either beta-blockers or methyldopa (Bulpitt et al, 1989). In both Croog and associates' (1988) and Suzuki and associates'(1988) studies, captopril use was less likely to be associated with impotence than other drugs. Recall, however, that when a diuretic was added to captopril in order to achieve blood pressure control, the advantage of captopril was negated (Croog et al, 1988). There are really no good comparative studies to document the relative frequency of the problem with the various classes of drugs.

Before starting any antihypertensive drug therapy, the patient should be asked about sexual dysfunction and, if it is significant, evaluated as completely as feasible. The evaluation should include a careful history and examination for evidences of neurogenic, hormonal, or hemodynamic problems. Arterial inflow can be assessed by comparing penile blood pressure measured by Doppler ultrasound with brachial pressure (Bansal, 1988). Various therapies may then be provided, including oral yohimbine (Reid et al, 1987), nitroglycerin paste applied to the penile shaft (Owen et al, 1989), or intracorporeal injections of papaverine or prostaglandin $E_1$ (Sarosdy et al, 1989). Perhaps the most satisfactory is the penile pump, marketed in the United States as the ErecAid System by Osbon Medical Systems (P.O. Box 1478, Augusta, Georgia 30903). The cost is $300 but from what I have heard from patients, it is well worth the cost. If these do not work, a number of surgical procedures are available, including revascularization, but hopefully they will be needed much less as the penile pump is more widely used.

If the problem develops or is made significantly worse after starting any antihypertensive drug, that drug should be stopped. If the patient's hypertension is fairly mild, therapy should be withheld until return of pretreatment potency. When it returns, a very small dose of a drug from another class should be started, attempting to lower the blood pressure very slowly and gently. Some patients will become impotent whenever the systemic pressure is lowered very

much and, for them, medical or surgical management of the impotence may be required if the hypertension is to be controlled.

## Patients Who Are Pilots

Over the last few years the United States Federal Aviation Administration (FAA) has changed the regulations considerably as to the limits of blood pressure and the types of antihypertensive medications that can be taken by people who wish to be certified as a pilot. The maximum permitted blood pressure for 30 to 39 year old people is 145/92 or, if cardiac and renal function is normal, 155/98. The permissible levels increase with age. Most antihypertensive drugs can be used with the exceptions of those which may cause interference with alertness or performance including reserpine, guanethidine, guanadrel, and central alpha-agonists (methyldopa, clonidine, and guanabenz) (Federal Air Surgeon's Bulletin 86-1, April 1986).

## Anesthesia and Surgery

Hypertension, in the absence of significant coronary or myocardial dysfunction, does not add significantly to the cardiovascular risks of noncardiac surgery (Goldman, 1983). On the other hand, in the presence of preexisting disease, hypertension increases the risk of myocardial ischemia during anesthesia, and the prior administration of antihypertensive therapy reduces that risk (Stone et al, 1988). Therefore, patients on antihypertensive medications should continue on these drugs, as long as the anesthesiologist is aware of their use and takes reasonable precautions to prevent wide swings in pressure (Tinker et al, 1981).

Proof of the wisdom of this approach comes from studies such as those by Prys-Roberts et al (1971) who found that hypertensives on treatment had less trouble, particularly those whose hypertension was under good control. More recently, myocardial ischemia was detected in 11 of 39 untreated hypertensives but in none of 44 receiving atenolol, either chronically or a single dose 2 hours before induction (Stone et al, 1988).

### Specific Drugs

*Beta-Blockers.* As noted by Stone et al (1988), hypertensive patients being treated with beta-adrenergic blockers may have fewer problems with tachycardia, rises in pressure during intubation, dysrhythmias, or ECG evidence of myocardial ischemia, although they still may display an increase in blood pressure during surgery (Thulin et al, 1984). Patients on beta-blockers up until a few hours before anesthesia have been shown to have normal hemodynamic (Kopriva et al, 1978) and metabolic (Cooper et al, 1980) responses to surgery. Tinker et al (1981) point out that it is vital to continue beta-blocker therapy to prevent adrenergic-mediated imbalances of myocardial oxygen supply and demand, "more so during surgical stimulation." This is particularly essential in those with ischemic heart disease, who have been found to have recurrent angina and increased blood pressure when their beta-blocker therapy was stopped 4 days preoperatively (Ponten et al, 1982).

A special use for the short-acting intravenous beta-blocker, esmolol, has emerged: to attenuate the tachycardia and much of the pressor rise induced by intubation (Zsigmond et al, 1988). A single dose of a longer-acting oral agent 12 hours before will do much the same (Burns et al, 1988).

*Clonidine.* Oral therapy with this centrally acting alpha-agonist has been found to reduce the need for preoperative sedatives, intraoperative anesthetics, and postoperative narcotics (Flacke et al, 1987). Similar results were noted with oral therapy just 2 hours before both general (Ghignone et al, 1987) and ophthalmic (Ghignone et al, 1988) surgery.

*CEBs.* CEBs are the latest of the drugs whose primary action is vasodilation. As well reviewed by Fyman et al (1986), these drugs, including nitroprusside, nitroglycerin, hydralazine, and others, have been widely and successfully used in the perioperative period both to control hypertension and to improve cardiac performance. The CEBs, mainly verapamil, have been used increasingly during anesthesia for treatment of supraventricular tachycardia, hypertension, or coronary spasm. However, as reviewed by Merin (1987), "The administration of intravenous verapamil or diltiazem during open chest surgery in patients with depressed ventricular function anesthetized with potent inhalation anesthetics may be associated with further decreases in ventricular function."

The potential problems arise because of the similarity in pharmacological effects of the CEBs and inhalation anesthetics, both inducing negative inotropic and vasodilatory effects. In particular, isoflurane resembles the dihydropyridines (nifedipine and nicardipine) whereas halothane and enflurane are closer to verapamil and diltiazem (Lynch, 1988).

*ACEIs.* Less is known about the perioperative effects of ACEIs, but in one study of 22 patients given enalapril, 5 mg, 4 hours before anesthesia, the pressor response to intubation and surgery was reduced (Yates and Hunter, 1988).

**Preoperative Precautions**

The following precautions seem advisable in handling hypertensive patients before surgery:

1. If the blood pressure is uncontrolled and there is time available, therapy should be used to bring the pressure down.
2. If the patient is uncontrolled and must be operated on, special care should be taken to prevent a marked pressor response during intubation by preoperative reassurance and short-acting beta-blocker (esmolol). For those in whom beta-blockers are contraindicated, sublingual nifedipine (Puri and Batra, 1988), or oral clonidine (Flacke et al, 1987), or intravenous verapamil (Nishikawa and Namiki, 1989) has been shown to work well.
3. If the patient is potassium depleted, increased sensitivity to muscle relaxants and, as noted earlier in this chapter, cardiac arrhythmias may occur. A short infusion of 40 mmol of potassium, although it will raise plasma $K^+$ levels, may do little to correct longstanding intracellular potassium depletion, and more prolonged replacement therapy should be given.
4. In patients on adrenergic inhibitors, the pressor response to various sympathomimetic agents may be decreased, so larger doses may be needed to counteract hypotension.

**Postoperative Precautions**

A word of caution is necessary concerning control of hypertension postoperatively. When any antihypertensive drug is stopped before surgery, life-threatening hypertension may suddenly appear in the immediate postoperative period (Katz et al, 1976). This may be a particular problem with short-acting agents, especially clonidine.

For those in need of postoperative reduction in blood pressure, successful use of various parenteral forms of various agents has been reported including the short acting beta-blocker esmolol (Gibson et al, 1988), labetalol (Orlowski et al, 1989), and CEBs (Mullen et al, 1988). Epidural morphine given before surgery reduced the incidence of postoperative hypertension, presumably by attenuating the sympathetic response to surgery (Breslow et al, 1989).

On the other hand, significant lowering of pressure may occur as a nonspecific response to surgery and may persist for months (Volini and Flaxman, 1939). Do not be deceived by what appears to be an improvement in the patient's hypertension: Anticipate a gradual return to preoperative levels.

Special problems in postoperative patients after coronary bypass surgery, trauma, and burns are covered in Chapter 15. Anesthetic consid-

erations in patients with pheochromocytoma are covered in Chapter 12.

## CONCLUSION

The large numbers of drugs now available can be used to successfully treat virtually every hypertensive patient under most any circumstance. Even those at highest risk—the few who develop a hypertensive emergency—can be effectively treated, as is shown in the next chapter.

## References

Abernethy DR, Montamat SC: *Am J Cardiol* 60:116I, 1987.

Abernethy DR, Schwartz JB, Plachetka JR, et al: *Am J Cardiol* 60:697, 1987.

Abernethy DR, Schwartz JB, Todd EL, et al: *Ann Intern Med* 105:329, 1986.

Abdulla M, Norden A, Jagerstad M: *Lancet* 2:562, 1975.

Abraham PA, Opsahl JA, Halstenson CE, et al: *Arch Intern Med* 148:2358, 1988.

Abrams WB, Davies RO, Gomez HJ: *J Hypertension* 2(Suppl 2):31, 1984.

Abramson M, Littlejohn GO: *Med J Aust* 142:47, 1985.

Addonizio VP Jr, Fisher CA, Strauss JF III, et al: *Am J Physiol* 250:H366, 1986.

Ades PA, Gunther PGS, Meacham CP, et al: *Ann Intern Med* 109:629, 1988.

Ades PA, Wolfel EE, Hiatt WR, et al: *Eur J Clin Pharmacol* 36:5, 1989.

Adler AG, Leahy JJ, Cressman MD: *Arch Intern Med* 146:1927, 1986.

Adler S: *JAMA* 230:1428, 1974.

Ahlquist RP: *Am J Physiol* 153:586, 1948.

Ahmad S: *Am Heart J* 105:1037, 1983.

Ajayi AA, Campbell BC, Howie CA, et al: *J Hypertens* 3:47, 1985.

Alderman MH: *Am J Med* 86(Suppl 1B):1989.

Alderman MH, Lamport B: In: Kaplan NM, Brenner BM, Laragh JH (eds). *New Therapeutic Strategies in Hypertension.* New York: Raven Press, Ltd, 1989:171.

Allon M, Hall WD, Macon EJ: *Arch Intern Med* 146:2075, 1986.

Altura BM, Altura BT: *Drugs* 28(Suppl 1):120, 1984.

Amery A, Verstraete M, Bossaert H, et al: *Br Med J* 4:392, 1970.

Ames R: *Drugs* 36(Suppl 2):33, 1988.

Ames RP: *J Cardiovasc Pharmacol* 6:S466, 1984.

Ames RP: *Am J Hypertens* 2:98A, 1989 (abst).

Ames RP, Hill P: *Lancet* 1:721, 1976.

Ames RP, Kiyasu JY: *J Clin Pharmacol* 29:123, 1989.

Ames RP, Peacock PB: *Arch Intern Med* 144:710, 1984.

Andersen B, Snorrason SP, Ragnarsson J, et al: *Acta Med Scand* 218:449, 1985.

Anderson J, Godfrey BE, Hill DM: *Q J Med* 40:541, 1971.

Anderson S, Rennke HG, Brenner BM: *J Clin Invest* 77:1993, 1986.

Andersson KE: *Acta Obstet Gynecol Scand* 108 (Suppl):17, 1982.

Andersson PO, H-Anderson H, Hagman A, et al: *Clin Pharmacol Ther* 36:197, 1984.

Andren L, Weiner L, Svensson A, et al: *J Hypertension* 1(Suppl 2):384, 1983.

Andrivet P, Simonet T, Rieu P, et al: *Lancet* 1:434, 1989.

Applegate WB: *Ann Intern Med* 110:901, 1989.

Araoye MA, Chang MY, Khatri IM, et al: *JAMA* 240:1863, 1978.

Arndt K, Jick H: *JAMA* 235:918, 1976.

Asmar RG, Pannier B, Santoni JPh, et al: *Circulation* 78:941, 1988.

Atkins JM, Mitchell HC, Pettinger WA: *Am J Cardiol* 39:802, 1977.

Augenstein WL, Kulig KW, Rumack BH: *JAMA* 259:3302, 1988.

Awan NA, Lee G, De Maria AN, et al: *Am Heart J* 101:541, 1981.

Baba T, Ishizaki T, Murabayashi S, et al: *Clin Pharmacol Ther* 42:232, 1987.

Bacon PJ, Brazier DJ, Smith R, et al: *Br J Clin Pharmacol* 27:1, 1989.

Baltodano N, Gallo BV, Weidler DJ: *Arch Intern Med* 148:1969, 1988.

Bansal S: *Hypertension* 12:1, 1988.

Barer DH, Cruickshank JM, Ebrahim SB, et al: *Br Med J* 296:737, 1988.

Barnett AJ, Kalowski S, Guest C: *Med J Aust* 1:105, 1978.

Barry DI: *J Cardiovasc Pharmacol* 7:S94, 1985.

Batchelor JR, Welsh KI, Tinoco RM, et al: *Lancet* 1:1107, 1980.

Batey DM, Nicolich MJ, Lasser VI, et al: *Am J Med* 86(Suppl 1B):74, 1989.

Bauer GE, Hynyor SN, Stokes GS: In: Bulpitt CJ (ed). *Handbook of Hypertension, Epidemiology of Hypertension.* Amsterdam, Elsevier Science Publishers, 1985, vol 6.

Bauer JH: *Arch Intern Med* 143:1163, 1983.

Bauer JH: *J Clin Hypertens* 3:199, 1985.

Bauer JH, Brooks CS: *Am J Med* 66:405, 1979.

Baum C, Kannedy DL, Forbes MB, et al: *JAMA* 253:382, 1985.

Bause GS, Fleg JL, Lakatta EG: *Am J Cardiol* 59:874, 1987.

Beeley L: *Br Med J* 289:1330, 1984.

Beermann B, Grind M: *Clin Pharmacokinet* 13:254, 1987.

Beevers DG, Hamilton M, Harpur JE: *Postgrad Med J* 47:639, 1971.

Bellini G, Battilana G, Puppis E, et al: *Curr Ther Res* 35:974, 1984.

Belz GG, Kirch W, Kleinbloesem CH: *Clin Pharmacokinetics* 15:295, 1988.

Bendall MJ, Baloch KH, Wilson PR: *Br Med J* 2:727, 1975.

Bengtsson C, Blohme G, Lapidus L, et al: *Br Med J* 289:1495, 1984.

Bengtsson C, Lapidus L, Stendahl C, et al: *Acta Med Scand* 224:549, 1988.

Bentley GA: *Clin Exp Pharmacol Physiol* 14:465, 1987.

Berger L, Yu T: *Am J Med* 59:605, 1975.

Berglund G, Andersson O: *Lancet* 1:744, 1981.

Berglund G, Andersson O, Widgren B: *Acta Med Scand* 220:419, 1986.

Bertel O: *Arch Intern* 147:1683, 1987.

Bertel O, Conen D, Radü, et al: *Br Med J* 286:19, 1983.

Berthelsen S, Pettinger WA: *Life Sci* 21:595, 1977.

Bidiville J, Nussberger J, Waeber G, et al: *Hypertension* 11:166, 1988.

Bishopric NH, Simpson PC, Ordahl CP: *J Clin Invest* 80:1194, 1987.

Bjorck S, Nyberg G, Mulec H, et al: *Br Med J* 293:471, 1986.

Black DM, Brand RJ, Greenlick M, et al: *J Gerontol* 42:552, 1987.

Black JW, Crowther AF, Shanks RG, et al: *Lancet* 1:1080, 1964.

Black JW, Stephenson JS: *Lancet* 2:311, 1962.

Blackwell B: *N Engl J Med* 289:249, 1973.

Block LH, Emmons LR, Vogt E, et al: *Proc Natl Acad Sci USA* 86:2388, 1989.

Blowers D, Chalmers D: *Br Med J* 297:1269, 1988.

Blumenthal JA, Madden DJ, Krantz DS, et al: *Clin Pharmacol Ther* 43:429, 1988.

Bobik A, Jennings G, Jackman G, et al: *Hypertension* 8:16, 1986.

Bolli P, Amann FW, Burkart F, et al: *J Cardiovasc Pharamcol* 4:S162, 1982.

Bond WS: *J Clin Psychopharmacol* 6:81, 1986.

Bonham AC, Trapani AG, Portis LR, et al: *J Hypertens* 1(Suppl 2)543, 1984.

Booth RFG, Buckham SP, Lung DO, et al: *Biochem Pharmacol* 36:3517, 1987.

Boulet L-P, Milot J, Lampron N, et al: *JAMA* 261:413, 1989.

Boutroy MJ, Vert P, DeLigny BH, et al: *Lancet* 2:935, 1984.

Bortolotti M, Trisolino G, Barbara L: *JAMA* 258:3516, 1987.

Boura ALA, Green AF: In: Van Zwieten PA (ed). *Handbook of Hypertension,* Amsterdam: Elsevier Science Publishers, 1984, vol 3, p 220.

Bowden FJ: *Br Med J* 298:605, 1989.

Brater DC: *Drugs* 30:427, 1985.

Breckenridge A: *Br Med J* 286:1085, 1983.

Brenner BM, Garcia DL, Anderson S: *Am J Hypertens* 1:335, 1988.

Breslau NA, Ram CVS, Kaplan NM, et al: *J Bone Res* 3(Suppl 1):S12, 1988 (abstr.).

Breslow MJ, Jordan DA, Christopherson R, et al: *JAMA* 261:3577, 1989.

Briant RH, Reid JL, Dollery CT: *Br Med J* 1:522, 1973.

Briggs RSJ, Birtwell AJ, Pohl JEF: *Lancet* 1:1045, 1978.

Brogden RN, Heel RC, Speight TM, et al: *Drugs* 12:251, 1978.

Brooks BA, Lant AF, McNabb WR, et al: *Br J Clin Pharmacol* 17:497, 1984.

Brott T, Reed RL: *Stroke* 24:1, 1989.

Broughton Pipkin F, Symonds EM, Turner SR: *J Physiol* 323:415, 1982.

Brown MJ, Brown DC, Murphy MB: *N Engl J Med* 309:1414, 1983.

Brown MJ, Harland D, Murphy MB, et al: *Hypertension* 6(Suppl II):II–57, 1984.

Brown MJ, Salmon D,Rendell M: *Ann Intern Med* 93:456, 1980.

Brueggemeyer CD, Ramirez G: *Lancet* 1:1352, 1984.

Brunner HR, Waeber B, Nussberger J: *J Hypertension* 6(Suppl 3):S1, 1988.

Buell JC, Eliot RD, Plachetka JR, et al: *J Clin Pharmacol* 28:327, 1988.

Bühler FR, Bolli P, Kiowski W, et al: *Am J Med* 77:36, 1984.

Bühler FR, Laragh JH, Baer L, et al: *N Engl J Med* 287:1209, 1972.

Bulpitt CJ, Beevers DG, Butler A, et al: *J Hum Hypertens* 3:53, 1989.

Bulpitt CJ, Fletcher AE: *Am J Med* 84(Suppl 1B):40, 1988.

Burakis TG, Mioduch HJ: *Arch Intern Med* 144:2371, 1984.

Burns JMA, Hart DM, Hughes RL, et al: *Br J Anaesth* 61:345, 1988.

Bushinsky DA, Favus MJ, Coe FL: *Am J Physiol* 247:F746, 1984.

Byrd BF III, Collins HW, Primm RK: *Arch Intern Med* 148:729, 1988.

Byyny RL, LoVerde M, Mitchell W: *Am J Med* 86:49, 1989.

Cameron HA, Ramsay LW: *Br Med J* 289:410:1984.

Cameron HA, Waller PC, Ramsay LE: *Postgrad Med J* 64:112, 1988.

Campbell N, Paddock V, Sundaram R: *Clin Pharamcol Ther* 43:381, 1988.

Campese VM, Romoff M, Telfer N, et al: *Kidney Int* 18:351, 1980.

Campion EW, Glynn RJ, DeLabry LO: *Am J Med* 82:421, 1987.

Cannon PJ: Congestive Heart Failure: Diuretics. In: *Congestive Heart Failure: Clinician.* San Juan, Puerto Rico, Searle Laboratories, 1972.

Cannon PJ, Stason WB, Demartini FE, et al: *N Engl J Med* 275:457, 1966.

Capewell S, Taverner D, Hannan WJ, et al: *Br Med J* 299:942, 1989.

Cappuccio FP, Markandu ND, Tucker FA, et al: *Eur J Clin Pharmacol* 30:723, 1986.

Caralis PV, Materson BJ, Perez-Stable E: *Min Electrolyte Metab* 10:148, 1984.

Cardillo C, Musumeci V, Mores N, et al: *Cardiovasc Drug Ther* 2:533, 1988.

Carlson RV, Bailey RR, Begg EJ, et al: *Clin Pharmacol Ther* 40:561, 1986.

Carlsson E, Fellenius E, Lundborg P, et al: *Lancet* 2:424, 1978.

Carney RM, Rich MW, teVelde A, et al: *Am J Med* 83:223, 1987.

Carretta R, Fabris B, Bardelli M, et al: *J Hum Hypertens* 2:171, 1988.

Carriere S, Krip G, Randall R: *Curr Ther Res* 35:455, 1984.

Carstairs KC, Breckenridge A, Dollery CT, et al: *Lancet* 2:133, 1966.

Carter AB: *Lancet* 1:485, 1970.

Case DB, Atlas SA, Laragh JH, et al: *J Cardiovasc Pharmacol* 2:339, 1980.

Chaffman M, Heel RC, Brogden RN, et al: *Drugs* 28:189, 1984.

Chennavasin P, Seiwell R, Brater DC, et al: *Kidney Int* 16:187, 1979.

Cheung DG, Hoffman CA, Ricci ST, et al: *Am J Med* 86(Suppl 1B):87, 1989.

Chick TW, Halperin AK, Gacek EM: *Med Sci Sports Exerc* 20:447, 1988.

Chopra M, Scott N, McMurray J, et al: *Br J Clin Pharmac* 27:396, 1989.

Cinquegrani MP, Liang C-s: *Clin Pharmacol Ther* 39:564, 1986.

Clark BJ: *Am Heart J* 104:334, 1982.

Clausen TG, Brocks K, Ibsen H: *Acta Med Scand* 224:531, 1988.

Clausen-Sjöbom, Lins P-E, Adamson U, et al: *Acta Med Scand* 222:57, 1987.

Cleroux J, van Nguyen P, Taylor AW, et al: *J Appl Physiol* 66:548, 1989.

Cloher TP, Whelton PK: *Arch Intern Med* 146:529, 1986.

Cocco G, Iselin HU, Strozzi C, et al: *Eur J Clin Pharmacol* 32:335, 1987.

Cohen JD, Neaton JD, Prineas RJ, et al: *Am J Cardiol* 60:548, 1987.

Cohen SI, Young WM, Lau SH: *Circulation* 37:738, 1968.

Cohn JN: *N Engl J Med* 275:643, 1966.

Conant J, Engler R, Janowsky D, et al: *J Cardiovasc Pharmacol* 13:656, 1989.

CONSENSUS Trial Study Group: *N Engl J Med* 316:1429, 1987.

Conway J, Louwers P: *Circulation* 21:21, 1960.

Conway J, Way B, Boon N, et al: *J Hum Hypertens* 2:123, 1988.

Cook NS: *TIPS* 9:21, 1988.

Cooper GM, Paterson JL, Mashiter K, et al: *Br J Anaesth* 52:1291, 1980.

Cooper RA: *Arch Intern Med* 143;659, 1983.

Cooper RG, Stokes MJ, Edwards RHT, et al: *Br J Clin Pharmac* 25:405, 1988.

Cooper WD, Kuan P, Reuben SR, et al: *Eur Heart J* 5:464, 1984.

Cooperman LB, Rubin IL, *Am Heart J* 85:831, 1973.

Coulter DM: *Br Med J* 296:1086, 1988.

Cramer JA, Mattson RH, Prevey ML, et al: *JAMA* 261:3273, 1989.

Croog SH, Levine S, Sudilovsky A, et al: *Arch Intern Med* 148:788, 1988.

Croog SH, Levine S, Testa MA, et al: *N Engl J Med* 314:1657, 1986.

Cruickshank JK, Anderson NMcF, Wadsworth J, et al: *Br Med J* 297:1155, 1988.

Cruickshank JM: *Br Med J* 297:1227, 1988.

Cruickshank JM, DeGaute JP, Kuurne T, et al: *Lancet* 2:585, 1987.

Cryer PE, Rizza RA, Haymond MW, et al: *Metabolism* 29(Suppl 1):1114, 1980.

Cubeddu LX, Aranda J, Singh B, et al: *JAMA* 256:2214, 1986.

Cubeddu LX: *Am Heart J* 116:133, 1988.

Cubeddu LX, Fuenmayor N, Varin F, et al: *Clin Pharmacol Ther* 41:31, 1987.

Cumberbatch M, Morgan DB: *Clin Sci* 60:555, 1981.

Cull JD, Dorhani NO, Blaszkowski TP, et al: *JAMA* 253:3263, 1985.

Cushman DW, Wang FL, Fung WC, et al: *Am J Hypertens* 2:294, 1989.

Cushman P, Forbes R, Lerner W, et al: *Clin Exp Res* 9:103, 1985.

Dahlöf B, Hansson L, Acosta JH, et al: *Am J Hypertens* 1:38, 1988.

Daneshmend TK, Roberts CJC: *Br J Pharmacol* 14:73, 1982.

Das G: *Int J Clin Pharmacol Ther Toxicol* 26:575, 1988.

Davidson C, Thadani U, Singleton W, et al: *Br Med J* 2.7, 1976.

Davies DS, Wing LMH, Reid JL, et al: *Clin Pharmacol Ther* 21:593, 1977.

Day JL, Metcalfe J, Simpson CN: *Br Med J* 294:1145, 1982.

DeCree J, Leempoels J, Geukens H, et al: *Lancet* 2:775, 1984.

Degnbol B, Dorph S, Marner T: *Acta Med Scand* 193:407, 1973.

DeGoulet P, Menard J, Vu H-A, et al: *Br Med J* 287:88, 1983.

Deitch MR, Littman GS, Pascucci VL: *J Cardiovasc Pharmacol* 6:S818, 1984.

DeQuattro V, Lee DD-P, Allen J, et al: *Hypertension* 11(Suppl I):1–198, 1988.

Deyo RA, Straube KT, Disterhoft JF: *Science* (Wash DC) 243:809, 1989.

Diamond JR, Cheung JY, Fang LST: *Am J Med* 77:905, 1984.

Dimsdale JE, Newton RP, Joist T: *Arch Intern Med* 149:514, 1989.

di Priolo SL, Priore P, Cocco G, et al: *Eur J Clin Pharmacol* 35:25, 1988.

Dluhy RG, Smith K, Taylor T, et al: *Hypertension* 13:371, 1989.

Dollery CT, Davies DS: *Br J Clin Pharmacol* 10:5S, 1980.

Dornhorst A, Powell SH, Pensky J: *Lancet* 1:123, 1985.

Dørup I, Skajaa K, Clausen T, et al: *Br Med J* 296:455, 1988.

Douglas DD, Yang RD, Jensen P, et al: *Am J Med* 87:235, 1989.

Drayer JIM, Keim JH, Weber MA, et al: *Am J Med* 60:897, 1976.

Dreslinski GR, Messerli GH, Dunn FG, et al: *Circulation* 65:1365, 1982.

Duarte CG, Winnacker JL, Becker KL, et al: *N Engl J Med* 284:828, 1971.

Duke M: *JAMA* 239:43, 1978.

Duncan JJ, Vaandrager H, Farr JE, et al: *J Cardiopul Rehabil* 9:110, 1989.

Dupont A, Six R: *Br Med J* 285:693, 1982.

Durao V, Prata MM, Goncalves LMP: *Lancet* 2:1005, 1977.

Dustan HP, Tarazi RC, Bravo EL: *N Engl J Med* 286:861, 1972.

Dyckner T, Helmers C, Wester PO: *Acta Med Scand* 216:127, 1984.

Dykman D, Simon EE, Avioli LV: *Arch Intern Med* 147:1341, 1987.

Editorial: *Br Med J* 1:529, 1977.

Editorial: *Lancet* 1:1083, 1988.

Eggertsen R, Hansson L: *Int J Clin Pharmacol Ther Toxicol* 23:411, 1985.

Eicher JC, Chalopin JM, Tanter Y, et al: *JAMA* 258:3388, 1987.

Eklund B, Hjemdahl P, Seideman P, et al: *J Cardiovasc Pharmacol* 5:384, 1983.

El-Ackad TM, Curry CL, Hinds JE, et al: *Clin Res* 32:330A, 1984.

Eliahou HE, Cohen D, Ben-David A, et al: *Cardiovasc Drug Ther* 1:523, 1988.

Eliasson K, Danielson M, Hylander B, et al: *Acta Med Scand* 215:333, 1984.

Elliott HL, Vincent J, Meredith PA, et al: *Clin Pharmacol Ther* 43:582, 1988.

Elmfeldt D, Hedner T, Westerling S: *J Cardiovasc Pharmacol* 10 (Suppl 1):S154, 1987.

Ene MD, Williamson PJ, Roberts CJC, et al: *Br J Clin Pharmacol* 19:423, 1985.

Epstein M, Oster JR: *J Clin Hypertens* 1:85, 1985.

Eraker SA, Kirscht JP, Becker MH: *Ann Intern Med* 100:258, 1984.

Erne P, Bolli P, Bürgisser E, et al: *N Engl J Med* 310:1084, 1984.

Espiner EA, Richards AM: *Lancet* 1:707, 1989.

Fagan TC, Conrad KA, Mar JH, et al: *Clin Pharmacol Ther* 39:191, 1986 (abst #C40).

Favre L, Riondel A, Vallotton MB: *Am J Hypertens* 1:245, 1988.

Fedorak RN, Field M, Chang EB: *Ann Intern Med* 102:197, 1985.

Feely J, Crooks J, Stevenson IH: *Br J Clin Pharmacol* 12:73, 1981.

Feely J, Pringle T, Maclean D: *Br Med J* 296:705, 1988.

Feigl EO: *Circulation* 76:737, 1987.

Feldman HA, Puschett JB: *Curr Ther Res* 27:205, 1980.

Ferlito S, Puleo F, Carra G, et al: *J Endocrinol Invest* 6:199, 1983.

Ferrara LA, Pasanisi F, Marotta T, et al: *J Cardiovasc Pharmacol* 10(Suppl 10)S136, 1987.

Ferrara LA, Soro S, Marotta T, et al: *Am J Hypertens* 1:32A, 1988 (abst).

Finkelstein SM, Collins VR, Cohn JN: *Hypertension* 12:380, 1988.

Finnerty FA Jr: *Am J Cardiol* 53:1304, 1984.

Finnerty FA Jr, Brogden RN: *Drugs* 30:22, 1985.

Finnerty FA Jr, Davidov M, Mroczek WJ, et al: *Circ Res* 26 and 27 (Suppl I):1, 1970.

Finnerty FA Jr, Gyftopoulos A, Berry C, et al: *JAMA* 241:579, 1979.

Fitzgerald JD: *J Cardiovasc Pharamcol* 12(Suppl 8):S83, 1988.

Flacke JW, Bloor BC, Flacke WE, et al: *Anesthesiology* 67:11, 1987.

Flamm ES: *Am Heart J* 117:236, 1989.

Flammer J, Weidmann P, Gluck Z, et al: *Am J Med* 66:34, 1979.

Fodor JG, Chockalingam A, Drover A: *J Clin Pharmacol* 27:892, 1987.

Fonseca V, Phear DN: *Br Med J* 294:36, 1982.

Fontanet H, Garcia JC, del Rio J, et al: *Arch Intern Med* 147:426, 1987.

Forette F, Bellet M, Henry JF, et al: *Br J Clin Pharmac* 20:125S, 1985.

Fouad FM, Kanashima Y, Tarazi RC, et al: *Am J Cardiol* 49:795, 1982.

Fouad FM, Vidt DG, Williams H, et al: *Clin Pharmacol Ther* 29:498, 1981.

Frank JH, Frewin DB, Robinson SM, et al: *Aust NZ J Med* 1:1, 1972.

Franks P, Harp J, Bell B: *JAMA* 262:3011, 1989.

Freedman DD, Waters DD: *Drugs* 34:578, 1987.

Freis ED: *Clin Pharmacol Ther* 39:239, 1986.

Freis ED: *Arch Intern Med* 149:2640, 1989.

Freis ED, Reda DJ, Materson BJ: *Hypertension* 12:244, 1988.

Frewin DB, Buik C, Rennie G: *Eur J Clin Pharmacol* 36:11, 1989.

Frick MH, McGibney D, Tyler HM: *J Intern Med* 225:101, 1989.

Friedman E, Shadel M, Halkin H, et al: *Ann Intern Med* 110:24, 1989.

Frishman WH: *Am Heart J* 113:1190, 1987.

Frishman WH: *Hypertension* 11(Suppl II):II-21, 1988.

Frishman WH, Eisen G, Lapsker J: *Med Clin North Am* 72:441, 1988.

Frishman WH, Garofalo JL, Rothschild A, et al: *Am J Cardiol* 64:65F, 1989.

Frishman WH, Zawada ET, Smith LK, et al: *Am J Cardiol* 59:615, 1987.

Fujimura A, Ebihara A, Hino N, et al: *J Clin Pharmacol* 29:327, 1989.

Fujita T, Yamashita N, Yamashita K: *Clin Exp Hypertens* 3:939, 1981.

Fuller JH, Shipley MJ, Rose G, et al: *Br Med J* 287:867, 1983.

Furhoff A-K: *Acta Med Scand* 203:425, 1978.

Fyman PN, Cottrell JE, Kushins L, et al: *Can Anaesth Soc J* 33:629, 1986.

Garanin G: *Curr Ther Res* 40:567, 1986.

Garner L: *Arch Intern Med* 146:1454, 1986.

Garrett BN, Kaplan NM: *J Clin Pharmacol* 21:173, 1981.

Garthoff B, Bellemann P: *J Cardiovasc Pharmacol* 10(Suppl 10):S36, 1987.

Gavras H, Brunner HR, Laragh JH, et al: *N Engl J Med* 291:817, 1974.

Gavras H, Waeber B, Kershaw GR, et al: *Hypertension* 3:441, 1981a.

Gavras I, Graff LG, Rose BD, et al: *Ann Intern Med* 94:58, 1981b.

Gehr M, MacCarthy EP, Goldberg M: *Kidney Int* 29:1203, 1986.

Gelmers HJ, Gorter K, De Weerdt CJ, et al: *N Engl J Med* 318:203, 1988.

Gengo FM, Huntoon L, McHugh WB: *Arch Intern Med* 147:39, 1987.

Gerber A, Weidmann P, Bianchetti MG, et al: *Hypertension* 7(Suppl II):II-164, 1985.

Gerber A, Weidmann P, Saner R, et al: *Metabolism* 33:342, 1984.

Gerkens JF: *Clin Exp Pharmacol Physiol* 14:371, 1987.

Ghignone M, Calvillo O, Quintin L: *Anesthesiology* 67:3, 1987.

Ghignone M, Noe C, Calvillo O, et al: *Anesthesiology* 68:707, 1988.

Gibberd FB, Small E: *Med J* 2:90, 1973.

Gibson BE, Black S, Maass L, et al: *Clin Pharamcol Ther* 44:650, 1988.

Gifford RW Jr, Borazanian RA: *Hypertension* 12(Suppl I):I-119, 1989.

Gil-Ad I, Topper E, Laron Z: *Lancet* 2:278, 1979.

Giles TD, Katz R, Sullivan JM, et al: *JACC* 13:1240, 1989.

Gill JS, Beevers DG, Zezulka AV, Davies P: *Lancet* 1:567, 1985.

Gillum RF, Solomon HS, Kranz P, et al: *Arch Intern Med* 138:700, 1978.

Glasser ST, Chrysant SG, Graves J, et al: *Am J Hypertens* 2:154, 1989.

Gloth FM, Busby MJ: *Am J Med* 87:480, 1989.

Goa KL, Benfield P, Sorkin EM: *Drugs* 37:583, 1989.

Goldberg LI: *Am J Med* 77:37, 1984.

Goldberg MR, Gerkens JF, Oates JA, et al: *Eur J Pharmacol* 69:95, 1981.

Goldberg MR, Rockhold FW, Thompson WL, et al: *J Clin Pharmacol* 29:33, 1989.

Goldman L: *Ann Intern Med* 98:504, 1983.

Goldner MG, Zarowitz H, Akgum S: *N Engl J Med* 262:403, 1960.

Goldszer RC, Lilly LS, Solomon HS: *Am J Med* 85:887, 1988.

Gomez HJ, Cirillo (Rahway) VJ: *Prog Pharmacol* 6:1, 1986.

Good DW, Wright FS: *Am J Physiol* 236:F192, 1979.

Goodfield MJ, Millard IG: *Br Med J* 290:1111, 1985.

Goodwin FK, Bunney WE Jr: *Semin Psychiatry* 3:435, 1971.

Graham DI, McGeorge A, Fitch W, et al: *J Hypertens* 2:297, 1984.

Graves JW, Buckalew VM Jr: *Am J Hypertens* 2:50A, 1989 (abst).

Gray HH, Poston L, Hilton PJ, et al: *Br Med J* 288:673, 1984.

Green S, Zawada ET, Muakkassa W, et al: *Arch Intern Med* 144:1205, 1984.

Greenfield S, Kaplan S, Ware JE Jr: *Ann Intern Med* 102:520, 1985.

Grimm R, Neaton J, Elmer P, et al: *Circulation* 80:II–301, 1989 (abst).

Grimm RH Jr, Neaton JD, McDonald M, et al: *Am Heart J* 109:858, 1985.

Grosbois B, Milton D, Beneton C, et al: *Br Med J* 298:189, 1989.

Gross TP, Wise RP, Knapp DE: *Hypertension* 13(Suppl I):I–113, 1989.

Guilleminault C, Mignot E, Aldrich M, et al: *Lancet* 2:511, 1988.

Gupta KP, Bhargava KP: *Arch Int Pharmacodyn Ther* 155:84, 1965.

Gutin M, Tuck ML: *Curr Ther Res* 43:775, 1988.

Guyatt G, Sackett D, Adachi J, et al: *CMAJ* 139:497, 1988.

Gwinup G: *Ann Intern Med* 109:162, 1988.

Hallin L, Andren L, Hansson L: *J Cardiovasc Pharmacol* 5:1083, 1983.

Halperin AK, Cubeddu LX: *Am Heart J* 111:363, 1986.

Hamada M, Kazatani Y, Shigematsu Y, et al: *J Hypertension* 5:305, 1987.

Hamilton CA, Jones CH, Cargie HJ, et al: *Br Med J* 2:800, 1978.

Hamilton TC, Weston AH: *Gen Pharmacol* 20:1, 1989.

Hanet C, Rousseau MF, Vincent M-F: *Am J Cardiol* 59:1035, 1987.

Harris DCH, Hammond WS, Burke TJ, et al: *Kidney Int* 31:41, 1987.

Hauger-Klevene JH: *Lancet* 1:219, 1986.

Hayashi M, Kobayashi H, Kawano H, et al: *Stroke* 19:314, 1988.

Haynes RB: In: Robertson JIS (ed). *Handbook of Hypertension, Clinical Aspects of Essential Hypertension*. Amsterdam: Elsevier, 1983, vol 1, p 437.

Healy JJ, McKenna TJ, Canning BSTJ, et al: *Br Med J* 1:716, 1970.

Heer JF, De Jong PE, De Zeeuw D: *Lancet* 1:846, 1989.

Helgeland A, Hadelund CH, Strommen R, et al: *Lancet* 1:872, 1986.

Hendry BM, Ellory JC: *TIPS* 9:416, 1988.

Henkin RI: *N Engl J Med* 320:1751, 1989.

Henning M: In: van Zwieten PA (ed). *Handbook of Hypertension, Pharmacology of Antihypertensive Drugs*, vol 3, Amsterdam, Elsevier, 1984, p 156.

Henning R, Karlberg BE, Odar-Cederlöf I, et al: *Clin Pharmacol Ther* 28:707, 1980.

Henningsen NC, Bergengren B, Malmborg O, et al: *Acta Med Scand* 208:273, 1980.

Henry JA, Cassidy SL: *Lancet* 1:1414, 1986.

Herrick AL, Waller PC, Berkin KE, et al: *Am J Med* 86:421, 1989.

Herrington DM, Insley BM, Weinmann GG: *Am J Med* 81:344, 1986.

Hilton PJ: *Klin Wochenschr* 63 (Suppl III):49, 1985.

Hodsman GP, Johnston CI: *J Hypertension* 5:1, 1987.

Hoeldtke RD, Israel BC: *J Clin Endocrinol Metab* 68:1051, 1989.

Hohnloser SH, Verrier RL, Lown B, et al: *Am Heart J* 112:32, 1986.

Holland OB, Gomez-Sanchez CE, Kuhnert L, et al: *Arch Intern Med* 139:1015, 1979.

Holland OB, Kuhnert LV, Pollard J, et al: *Am J Hypertens* 1:380, 1988.

Holland OB, Nixon JV, Kuhnert L: *Am J Med* 70:762, 1981.

Hollenberg NK: *J Hypertension* 5(Suppl 1):S3, 1987.

Hollifield JW: *Am J Med* 77:28, 1984.

Holmes B, Brogden RN, Heel RC, et al: *Drugs* 26:212, 1983.

Holmes B, Sorkin EM: *Drugs* 31:467, 1986.

Holtzman JL, Finley D, Johnson B, et al: *Clin Pharmacol Ther* 40:268, 1986.

Hoorntje SJ, Kallenberg CGM, Weening JJ, et al: *Lancet* 2:1212, 1980.

Horan MJ, Page LB: *Hypertension* 11:1, 1988.

Hornung RS, Jones RI, Gould BA, et al: *Am J Cardiol* 57:93D, 1986.

Horwitz RI, Feinstein AR: *Arch Intern Med* 145:1873, 1985.

Hoss DM, Nierenberg DW: *Am J Med* 85:747, 1988.

Houston MC: *Am Heart J* 102:415, 1981.

Houston MC, Hodge R: *Am Heart J* 116:515, 1988.

Houston MC, McChesney JA, Chatterjee K: *Arch Intern Med* 141:69, 1981.

Hricik DE, Browning PJ, Kopelman R, et al: *N Engl J Med* 308:373, 1983.

Hudson MF: *J Hum Hypertens* 2:65, 1988.

Hughes GS Jr, Cowart TD, Oexmann MJ, et al: *Clin Pharmacol Ther* 44:400, 1988.

Hulley SB, Furberg CD, Gurland B, et al: *Am J Cardiol* 56:913, 1985.

Hulter HN, Licht JH, Ilnicki LP, et al: *J Lab Clin Med* 94:223, 1979.

Hunyor SN, Bradstock K, Somerville PJ, et al: *Br Med J* 4:23, 1975.

Hutcheon DF, Skinhøj, Andersen FJ: *Curr Ther Res* 43:55, 1988.

Hvarfner A, Bergström, Lithell H, et al: *Clin Sci* 75:543, 1988.

Hyman D, Kaplan NM: *N Engl J Med* 313:642, 1985.

Hypertension Detection and Follow-up Program Cooperative Group: *JAMA* 242:2562, 1979.

Inman WHW, Rawson NSB, Wilton LV, et al: *Br Med J* 297:826, 1988.

Insel PA: *Am J Hypertens* 2:112S, 1989.

Iseri LT, French JH: *Am Heart J* 108:188, 1984.

Ishikawa M, Yokota N, Sawazaki A, et al: *Am Heart J* 112:1116, 1986.

Itoh K, Wong P, Asai T, et al: *Am J Med* 84:1088, 1988.

Jackson B, Johnston CI: *J Hypertension* 6:495, 1988.

Jaker M, Atkin S, Soto M, et al: *Arch Intern Med* 149:260, 1989.

Jakubowski AT, Mizgala HF: *Am J Cardiol* 60:932, 1987.

Jansen PAF, Gribnau FWJ, Schulte BPM, et al: *Br Med J* 293:914, 1986.

Jardine AG, Connell JMC, Northridge DB, et al: *Am J Hypertens* 2:77A, 1989 (abst).

Jarrott B, Conway EL, Maccarrone C, et al: *Clin Exp Pharmacol Physiol* 14:471, 1987.

Jauernig RA, Moulds RFW, Shaw J: *Arch Int Pharmacodyn* 231:81, 1978.

Jeffcoate WJ: *Br Med J* 292:783, 1986.

Jefferson JW, Kalin NH: *JAMA* 241:1134, 1979.

Jenkins AC, McKinstry DN: *Med J Aust* 2(Suppl):32, 1979.

Jerie P, Lasance A: *Int J Clin Pharmacol Ther Toxicol* 22:170, 1984.

Jeunemaitre X, Charru A, Chatellier G, et al: *Am J Cardiol* 62:1072, 1988.

Jeunemaitre X, Chatellier G, Kreft-Jais C, et al: *Am J Cardiol* 60:820, 1987.

Jick H, Armstrong B: *Lancet* 2:368, 1975.

Jick H, Dinan BJ, Hunter JR: *J Urol* 127:224, 1982.

Jie K, van Brummelen P, Vermey P, et al: *Circ Res* 54:447, 1984.

Johansson BW: *Am J Cardiol* 57:34F, 1986.

Johansson BW, Dziamski R: *Drugs* 28 (Suppl 1):77, 1984.

Johansson SR, McCall M, Wilhelmsson C, et al: *Clin Pharmacol Ther* 27:593, 1980.

Johnson BF, Danylchuk MA: *Med Clin North Am* 73:449, 1989.

Johnson BF, Errichetti A, Urbach D, et al: *J Clin Pharmacol* 26:534, 1986.

Johnston CI, Arnolda L, Hiwatari M: *Drugs* 27:271, 1984.

1984 Joint National Committee: *Arch Intern Med* 144:1045, 1984.

1988 Joint National Committee: *Arch Intern Med* 148:1023, 1988.

Jokes AM, Thompson FD: *Br J Clin Pharmacol* 3(Suppl):789, 1976.

Jones B, Nanra RS: *Lancet* 2:1258, 1979.

Kaplan NM: *Ann Intern Med* 61:1079, 1967.

Kaplan NM: *Am J Cardiol* 51:1786, 1983.

Kaplan NM: *Am J Med* 77:1, 1984.

Kaplan NM: *Ann Intern Med* 109:36, 1988.

Kaplan NM: *Am J Hypertens* 2:213, 1989a.

Kaplan NM: *Arch Int Med* 149:1514, 1989b.

Kaplan NM: *JAMA* 262:817, 1989c.

Kaplan NM, Carnegie A, Raskin P, et al: *N Engl J Med* 312:746, 1985.

Kaplan NM, Grundy S: *Clin Pharmacol Ther* 44:297, 1988.

Kaplan NM, Rosenstock J, Raskin P: *Arch Intern Med* 147:1160, 1987.

Kassirer JP, Harrington JT: *N Engl J Med* 312:785, 1985.

Katz JD, Croneau LH, Barash PF: *Am Heart J* 92:79, 1976.

Katzman PL, Henningsen NC, Hulthen UL: *J Hum Hypertens* 2:147, 1988.

Kaufman J, Casanova JE, Riendl P, et al: *Chest* 95:544, 1989.

Kern MJ, Ganz P, Horowitz JD, et al: *Circulation* 67:1178, 1983.

Keusch GR, Weidmann P, Campese V, et al: *Nephron* 21:1, 1978.

Khalil-Manesh F, Venkataraman K, Samant DR, et al: *Hypertension* 9:18, 1987.

Khan MM, Logan KR, McComb JM, et al: *Am J Cardiol* 47:1301, 1981.

Khatri I, Uemura N, Notargiacomo A, et al: *Am J Cardiol* 40:38, 1977.

Kidney JC, O'Halloran DJ, Fitzgerald MX: *Br Med J* 299:981, 1989.

Kindler J, Rüegg PC, Neuray M, et al: *Eur J Clin Pharmacol* 32:367, 1987.

King BD, Pitchon R, Stern EH, et al: *Arch Intern Med* 143:1248, 1983.

Kingma JG Jr, Yellon DM: *Cardiovasc Drugs Ther* 2:313, 1988.

Kirtland HH, Mohler DN, Horwitz DA: *N Engl J Med* 302:825, 1980.

Klaus D: *Drugs* 37:212, 1989.

Knochel JP: *Am J Med* 77:18, 1984.

Kochar MS, Itskovitz HD: *Lancet* 1:1011, 1978.

Koch-Weser J: *Arch Intern Med* 133:1017, 1974.

Kohner EM, Dollery CT, Lowy C, et al: *Lancet* 1:986, 1971.

Kolassa N, Beller K-D, Sanders KH: *Am J Cardiol* 63:36C, 1989.

Kondowe GB, Deering AH, Riddell JG, et al: *Br J Clin Pharmacol* 25:315, 1988.

Kopriva CJ, Brown ACD, Pappas G: *Anesthesiology* 48:28, 1978.

Koskinen P, Manninen V, Eisalo A: *Br J Clin Pharmacol* 26:478, 1988.

Kostis JB, Breckenridge MB: *JACC* 13:13A, 1989.

Kostis JB, Rosen RC: *Circulation* 75:204, 1987.

Kowala MC, Nicolosi RJ: *J Cardiovasc Pharmacol* 13(Suppl 2):S45, 1989.

Kraus ML, Gottlieb LD, Horwitz RI, et al: *N Engl J Med* 313:905, 1985.

Krishna GG, Miller E, Kapoor S: *N Engl J Med* 320:1177, 1989.

Krishna GG, Shulman MD, Narins RG: *Semin Nephrol* 8:354, 1988.

Kroenke K, Wood DR, Hanley JF: *Arch Intern Med* 147:1553, 1987.

Krusell LR, Jespersen LT, Schmitz A, et al: *Hypertension* 10:577, 1987.

Kuller L, Farrier N, Caggiula A, et al: *Am J Epidemiol* 122:1045, 1985.

La Croix AZ, Wienphal J, White LR, et al: *N Engl J Med* 322:286, 1990.

Lager I, Blohme G, Smith U: *Lancet* 1:458, 1979.

Laher MS, O'Donohoe JF, O'Regan P, et al: *J R Soc Med* 78:367, 1985.

Lahive KC, Weiss JW, Weinberger SE: *Clin Sci* 74:547, 1988.

Lake CR, Ziegler MG, Coleman MD, et al: *Clin Pharmacol Ther* 26:428, 1979.

Lal S, Tolis G, Martin JB, et al: *J Clin Endocrinol Metab* 41:827, 1975.

Lameire N, Gordts J: *Eur J Clin Pharamcol* 31:333, 1986.

Landmark K: *J Cardiovasc Pharmacol* 7:12, 1985.

Lands AM, Arnold A, McAuliff JP, et al: *Nature* (Lond) 214:597, 1967.

Langer SZ: *Biochem Pharmacol* 23:1793, 1974.

Langley MS, Heel RC: *Drugs* 35:123, 1988.

Lant A: *Drugs* 31(Suppl 4):40, 1986.

Laragh JH: *Am J Med* 61:797, 1976.

Laragh JH: *Hypertension* 13(Suppl I):I-103, 1989.

Lardinois CK, Neuman SL: *Arch Intern Med* 148:1280, 1988.

Lasser NL, Grandits G, Caggiula AW: *Am J Med* 76:52, 1984.

Laufer LR, Erlik Y, Meldrum DR, et al: *Obstet Gynecol* 60:583, 1982.

Lavin P: *Arch Intern Med* 146:66, 1986.

Lawson DH: *Q J Med* 43:433, 1974.

Lawson DH, Glass D, Jick H: *Am Heart J* 96:572, 1978.

Leary WP, Reyes AJ: *Drugs* 28(Suppl 1):182, 1984.

Leary WP, Van der Byl: *S Afr Med J* 74:13, 1988.

Lechin F, van der Dijs B, Insausti CL, et al: *J Clin Pharmacol* 25:219, 1985.

Ledingham JGG, Rajagopalan B: *Q J Med* 48:25, 1979.

Lee DD-P, Kimura S, DeQuattro V: *Lancet* 1:403, 1989.

Leemhuis MP, van Damme KJ, Struyvenberg A: *Acta Med Scand* 200:37, 1976.

Leenen FHH, Smith DL, Farkas RM, et al: *Am J Med* 82:969, 1987.

Leenen FHH, Smith DL, Unger WP: *Br J Clin Pharmac* 26:481, 1988.

Lees GM: *Br Med J* 283:173, 1981.

Lemann J Jr, Gray RW, Maierhofer WJ, et al: *Kidney Int* 28:951, 1985.

Lemieux G, Beachemin M, Vinay P, et al: *Can Med Assoc J* 122:905, 1980.

Lenders JWM, de Boo Th, Lemmens WAJ, et al: *Clin Pharmacol Ther* 44:195, 1988.

Leon AS, Agre J, McNally C, et al: *J Clin Pharmacol* 24:209, 1984.

Leonetti G, Rupoli L, Gradnik R, et al: *J Hypertension* 5(Suppl 4):S57, 1987.

Leonetti G, Zanchetti A: *J Hypertension* 6 (Suppl 4):S655, 1988.

Leren P, Foss PO, Helgeland A, et al: *Lancet* 2:4, 1980.

Leslie JB, Kalayjian RW, Sirgo MA, et al: *Anesthesiology* 67:413, 1987.

Levine SB, Althof SE, Turner LA, et al: *J Urol* 141:54, 1989.

Levy D, Anderson KM, Plehn J, et al: *Am J Cardiol* 59:836, 1987.

Lewis EJ: *Am J Kid Dis* 10(Suppl 1):30, 1987.

Lewis HM, Kendall MJ, Smith SR, et al: *Br J Clin Pharmac* 27:547, 1989.

Lewis PF, Kohner EM, Petrie A, et al: *Lancet* 1:564, 1976.

Liang IYS, Jones CE: *Am J Physiol* 249:H1070, 1985.

Liedholm H, Melander A, Bitzen PO, et al: *Curr J Clin Pharmacol* 20:229, 1981.

Lief PD, Belizon I, Matos J, et al: *Program Am Soc Nephrol* 25A:66A, 1984.

Light RW, Chetty KG, Stansbury DW: *Am J Med* 75:109, 1983.

Lijnen PJ, Amery AK, Fagard RH, et al: *Br J Clin Pharmacol* 7:175, 1979.

Lijnen P, Staessen FJ, Lissens W, et al: *J Cardiovasc Pharmacol* 14:319, 1989.

Lilja M, Jounela AJ, Juustila HJ, et al: *Acta Med Scand* 211:375, 1982.

Lin M-S, McNay JL, Shepherd AMM, et al: *Hypertension* 5:257, 1983.

Linz W, Schölkens, Lindpaintner K, et al: *Am J Hypertens* 2:307, 1989.

Lithell H, Haglund K, Granath F, et al: *Acta Med Scand* 223:531, 1988.

Login IS, Judd AM, Cronin MJ, et al: *Am J Physiol* 248:E15, 1985.

Lopez LM, Aguila E, Baz R, et al: *Clin Res* 31:844A, 1983 [Abst].

Loube SD, Quirk RA: *Lancet* 1:1428, 1975.

Louis WJ, McNeil JJ, Drummer OH: *Drugs* 28(Suppl 2):16, 1984.

Loutzenhiser RD, Epstein M: *J Cardiovasc Pharmacol* 12(Suppl 6):S48, 1988.

Lowenstein I, Alterman L, Zelen R, et al: *J Clin Pharmacol* 24:436, 1984.

Lund-Johansen P: *J Cardiovasc Pharmacol* 1:487, 1979.

Lund-Johansen P: *Am J Med* 75:24, 1983.

Lund-Johansen P: *J Cardiovasc Pharamcol* 11(Suppl 1):S12, 1988.

Lund-Johansen P, Omvik P: *J Cardiovasc Pharmacol* 10 (Suppl 1):S139, 1987.

Lunell N-O, Hjemdahl P, Fredholm BB, et al: *Br J Clin Pharmacol* 12:345, 1981.

Luther RR, Glassman HN, Estep CB, et al: *Am Heart J* 117:842, 1989.

Lynch C: *Anesth Analg* 67:1036, 1988.

MacGregor GA, Banks RA, Markandu ND, et al: *Br Med J* 286:1535, 1983.

MacGregor GA, Pevahouse JB, Cappuccio FP: *J Hypertension* 5(Suppl 4):S127, 1987.

Mackenzie JW, Bird J: *Br Med J* 298:363, 1989.

MacMahon SW, Macdonald GJ: *Am J Med* 80(Suppl 2A):40, 1986.

Maddocks J, Hann S, Hopkins M, et al: *Lancet* 1:157, 1973.

Madias JE, Madias NE, Gavras HP: *Arch Intern Med* 144:2171, 1984.

MaGee PFA, Freis ED: *Hypertension* 8(Suppl II):II-135, 1986.

Magil AB, Balloon HS, Cameron EC, et al: *Am J Med* 69:939, 1980.

Man in't Veld AJ, Schalekamp MADH: *Br J Clin Pharmacol* 13:245S, 1982.

Man in't Veld AJ, Schalekamp MADH: *Br Med J* 282:929, 1981.

Man in't Veld AJ, Van den Meiracker AH, Schalekamp MA: *Am J Hypertens* 1:91, 1988a.

Man in't Veld AJ, Van den Meiracker AH, Schalekamp MA: *J Cardiovasc Pharmacol* 12(Suppl 8):S93, 1988b.

Mann SJ, Krakoff LR: *Arch Intern Med* 144:2427, 1984.

Mansilla-Tinoco R, Harland SJ, Ryan PJ, et al: *Br Med J* 284:936, 1982.

Marshall AJ, Heaton S, Barritt DW, et al: *Postgrad Med J* 55:537, 1979.

Martin BJ, Milligan K: *Arch Intern Med* 147:1768, 1987.

Martin WB, Spodick DH, Zins GR: *J Cardiovasc Pharmacol* 2(Suppl 2):S217, 1980.

Massey KL, Harman E, Hendeles L: *Eur J Clin Pharmacol* 34:555, 1988.

Massie B, MacCarthy EP, Ramanathan KB, et al: *Ann Intern Med* 107:150, 1987.

Massie BM: *Am J Cardiol* 60:1211, 1987.

Materson BJ, Vlachakis ND, Glasser SP, et al: *Am J Cardiol* 63:581, 1989.

McAnish J, Holmes BF, Smith S, et al: *Clin Pharmacol Ther* 28:302, 1980.

McAreavey D, Ramsey LE, Latham L, et al: *Br Med J* 288:106, 1984.

M'Buyamba-Kabangu J-R, Lepira B, Lijnen P, et al: *Hypertension* 11:100, 1988.

McCalden TA, Nath RG, Thiele K: *Stroke* 15:527, 1984.

McClean WJ: *Med J Aust* 1:592, 1976.

McClellan WM, Hall WD, Brogen D, et al: *Arch Intern Med* 148:525, 1988.

McInnes GT, Brodie MJ: *Eur J Clin Pharmacol* 34:605, 1988.

McInnes GT, Shelton JR, Harrison IR, et al: *Br J Clin Pharmacol* 14:449, 1982.

McKenna F, Davison AM: *Clin Nephrol* 25:149, 1986.

McKenna TJ, Donohoe JF, Brien TG, et al: *Br Med J* 2:739, 1971.

McKenney JM, Goodman RP, Wright JT Jr, et al: *Pharmacotherapy* 6:179, 1986.

McKibbin JK, Pocock WA, Barlow JB, et al: *Br Heart J* 51:157, 1984.

McLenachan JM, Henderson E, Morris KI, et al: *N Engl J Med* 317:787, 1987.

McLeod AA, Kraus WE, Williams RS: *Am J Cardiol* 53:1656, 1984.

McMartin C, Simpson P: *Clin Pharmacol Ther* 12:73, 1971.

McMurray J, Matthews DM: *Lancet* 1:581, 1985.

McMurray JJV, Struthers AD. *MEDICINE* 60:2459, 1988.

McVeigh G, Galloway D, Johnston D: *Br Med J* 297:95, 1988.

Medical Research Council Working Party: *Lancet* 2:539, 1981.

Medical Research Council Working Party: *Br Med J* 291:97, 1985.

Medical Research Council Working Party: *J Clin Pharmacol* 27:271, 1987.

Meeley MP, Towle AC, Ernsberger P, et al: *Hypertension* 13:341, 1989.

Mehta JL, Lopez LM: *Arch Intern Med* 147:389, 1987.

Mehta JL, Lopez LM, Deedwania PC, et al: *Am J Cardiol* 60:1096, 1987.

Meier J: *Cardiology* 64(Suppl 1):1, 1979.

Meisheri KD, Cipkus LA, Taylor CJ: *J Pharmacol Exp Ther* 245:751, 1988.

Menard J, Serrurier D, Bautier P, et al: *Hypertension* 11:153, 1988.

Meredith PA, Elliott HL, Ahmed JH, et al: *J Hypertension* 5(Suppl 5):S219, 1987.

Merin RG: *Anesthesiology* 66:111, 1987.

Messerli FH, Frohlich ED, Dreslinski GR, et al: *Ann Intern Med* 93:817, 1980.

Messerli FH, Ventura HO, Elizardi DJ, et al: *Am J Med* 77:18, 1984.

Metz S, Klein C, Morton N: *Am J Med* 82:17, 1987.

Middeke M, Weisweiler P, Schwandt P, et al: *Clin Cardiol* 10:94, 1987.

Mignot E, Guilleminault C, Bowersox S, et al: *J Clin Invest* 82:885, 1988.

Millar JA, McLean K, Reid JL. *Clin Sci* 61:65s, 1981.

Millar JA, Struthers AD: *Clin Sci* 66:249, 1984.

Miller RP, Woodworth JR, Graves DA, et al: *Curr Ther Res* 48:1133, 1988.

Miller RR, Awan NA, Maxwell KS, et al: *N Engl J Med* 297:303, 1977.

Miller RR, Olson HG, Amsterdam EA, et al: *N Engl J Med* 293:416, 1975.

Millson D, Borland C, Murphy P, et al: *Br Med J* 289:1308, 1984.

Mimran A, Ribstein J: *J Cardiovasc Pharmacol* 7:S92, 1985.

Minneman KP: *Pharmacol Rev* 40:87, 1988.

Mironneau J: *Am J Med* 84(Suppl 1B):10, 1988.

Mitchell HC, Graham RM, Pettinger WA: *Ann Intern Med* 93:676, 1980.

Mitchell HC, Pettinger WA: *JAMA* 239:2131, 1978.

Mitchell JR, Cavanaugh JH, Arias L, et al: *J Clin Invest* 49:1596, 1970.

Modi MW, Hassett JM, Lalka D: *Clin Pharmacol Ther* 44:268, 1988.

Molnar GW, Read RC, Wright FE: *Clin Pharmacol Ther* 15:490, 1974.

Mooser V, Waeber B, Nussberger J, et al: *J Hum Hypertens* 2:257, 1988.

Moran NC, Perkins ME: *J Pharmacol Exp Ther* 124:223, 1958.

Morgan DB, Davidson C: *Br Med J* 280:905, 1980.

Morgan T, Adam W, Carney S, et al: *Clin Sci* 57:335s, 1979.

Morgan T, Anderson A, Wilson D, et al: *Lancet* 1:793, 1986.

Morice A, Higenbottam TW, Brown MJ: *Br Med J* 297:1270, 1988.

Morlin C, Baglivo H, Boeijinga JK: *J Cardiovasc Pharmacol* 9(Suppl 3):S49, 1987.

Moser M, Lunn J, Nash DT, et al: *J Cardiovasc Pharmacol* 6:S1085, 1984.

Mosley C, O'Connor DT, Taylor A, et al: *J Cardiovasc Pharmacol* 6:S757, 1984.

Mroczek WJ, Davidov M, Finnerty FA Jr: *Am J Cardiol* 33:546, 1974.

Mroczek WJ, Leibel BA, Finnerty FA Jr: *Am J Cardiol* 29:712, 1972.

Mroczek WJ, Martin CH, Hattwick MAW, et al: *Curr Ther Res* 24:824, 1978.

Muiesan G, Alicandri C, Agabiti-Rosei E, et al: *J Clin Hypertens* 3:144, 1987.

Mullen JC, Miller DR, Weisel RD, et al: *J Thorac Cardiovasc Surg* 96:122, 1988.

Multicenter Study Group: *Acta Pharmacol Toxicol* 54(Suppl 1):47, 1984.

Murphy MB, Kohner E, Lewis PJ, et al: *Lancet* 2:1293, 1982.

Murray GD, Lesaffre E: *J Cardiovasc Pharmacol* 12(Suppl 8):S167, 1988.

Myers AK, Forman G, Duarte APT, et al: *Proc Soc Exp Biol Med* 183:86, 1986.

Nader PC, Thompson RJ, Alpern RJ: *Semin Nephrol* 8:365, 1988.

Navar LG, Rosivall L: *Kidney Int* 25:857, 1984.

Neusy A-J, Lowenstein J: *J Clin Pharmacol* 29:18, 1989.

Neuvonen PJ, Kivistö KT: *Med J Aust* 150:36, 1989.

Newman TJ, Maskin CS, Dennick LG, et al: *Am J Med* 84(Suppl 3A):140, 1988.

New Zealand Hypertension Study Group: *NZ Med J* 92:341, 1980.

New Zealand Hypertension Study Group: *NZ Med J* 93:215, 1981.

Niarchos AP, Laragh JH: *Am J Cardiol* 53:797, 1984.

Niarchos AP, Weinstein DL, Laragh JH: *Am J Med* 77:1061, 1984.

Nicar MJ, Peterson R, Pak CYC: *J Urol* 131:430, 1984.

Nicholson JP, Resnick LM, Pickering TG, et al: *Am J Med* 78:241, 1985.

Nicholson JP, Resnick LM, Laragh JH: *Ann Intern Med* 107:329, 1987.

Nicholson JP, Resnick LM, Laragh JH: *Arch Intern Med* 149:125, 1989.

Nielsen H, Mortensen SA, Sandøe: *Am Heart J* 114:192, 1987.

Nies AS, Gal J, Fadul S, et al: *J Pharmacol Exp Ther* 226:27, 1983.

Nifedipine-Atenolol Study Review Committee. *Br Med J* 296:468, 1988.

Nightingale SL, Morrison JC: *JAMA* 258:1200, 1987.

Nilsson-Ehle P, Ekberg M, Fridstrom P, et al: *Acta Med Scand* 224:131, 1988.

Nilsson H, Jonason T, Leppert J, et al: *Acta Med Scand* 221:53, 1987.

Nishikawa T, Namiki A: *Acta Anaesthesiol Scand* 33:232, 1989.

Nobile-Orazio E, Sterzi R: *Br Med J* 283:948, 1981.

Nordrehaug JE: *Acta Med Scand* 217:299, 1985.

Nordrehaug JE, von der Lippe G: *Br Heart J* 50:525, 1983.

Nussberger J, Waeber B, Brunner HR: *Am J Hypertens* 2:286, 1989.

Oates JA, Gillespie L, Udenfriend S, et al: *Science* (Wash DC) 131:1890, 1960.

Obel AO: *J Cardiovasc Pharmacol* 13:465, 1989.

O'Connor DT, Preston RA, Mitas JA II, et al: *Hypertension* 3:139, 1981.

O'Mailia JJ, Sander GE, Giles TD: *Ann Intern Med* 107:185, 1987.

O'Malley K, Segal JL, Israili ZH, et al: *Clin Pharmacol Ther* 18:581, 1975.

O'Meara J, White WB: *J Urol* 139:371, 1988.

Ondetti MA: *Circulation* 77(Suppl I):I–74, 1988.

Ondetti MA, Rubin B, Cushman DW: *Science* (Wash DC) 196:441, 1977.

Ondetti MA, Williams NJ, Sabo EF, et al: *Biochemistry* 10:4033, 1971.

Opie LH: *Am J Cardiol* 61:8C, 1988a.

Opie LH: *Cardiovasc Drugs Ther* 1:625, 1988b.

Opie LH: *Cardiovasc Drugs Ther* 2:369, 1988c.

Orlowski JP, Vidt DG, Walker S, et al: *Cleve Clin J Med* 56:29, 1989.

O'Rourke RA: *Am J Cardiol* 56:34H, 1985.

Osborn M, Hawton K, Gath D: *Br Med J* 296:959, 1988.

Osei K, Holland G, Falko JM: *Arch Intern Med* 146:1973, 1986.

Owen JA, Saunders F, Harris C, et al: *J Urol* 141:546, 1989.

Owens SD, Dunn MI: *Arch Intern Med* 148:1515, 1988.

Packer M, Gottlieb SS, Kessler PD: *Am J Med* 80(Suppl 4A):23, 1986.

Page IH, Dustan HP: *Circulation* 25:433, 1962.

Pai RG, Pai SM: *Am J Med* 85:123, 1988.

Papademetriou V, Burris JF, Notargiacomo

AV, et al: *Arch Intern Med* 148:1272, 1988.

Participating Veterans Administration Medical Centers: *JAMA* 248:2471, 1982.

Parving H-H, Andersen AR, Smidt UM, et al: *Br Med J* 294:1443, 1987.

Parving H-H, Hommel E, Smidt UM: *Br Med J* 297.1086, 1988.

Paton RR, Kane RE: *J Clin Pharmacol* 17:243, 1977.

Paulson OB, Jarden JO, Godtfredsen J, et al: *Am J Med* 76:91, 1984.

Pedrinelli R, Fouad FM, Tarazi RC, et al; *Arch Intern Med* 146:62, 1986.

Pedrinelli R, Taddei S, Salvetti A: *Clin Pharmacol Ther* 45:285, 1989.

Pentel PR, Asinger RW, Benowitz NL: *Clin Pharmacol Ther* 37:488, 1985.

Peroutka SJ, Snyder SH: *Mol Pharmacol* 16:687, 1979.

Perry HM Jr: Am J Med 54:58, 1973.

Perry HM Jr, Camel GH, Carmody SE, et al: *J Chron Dis* 30:519, 1977.

Perry HM Jr, Schroeder HA: *J Chron Dis* 2:520, 1955.

Perry HM Jr, Smith WM, McDonald RH, et al: *Stroke* 20:4, 1989.

Perry HM Jr, Tan EM, Carmody S, et al: *J Lab Clin Med* 76:114, 1970.

Persson B, Granerus G, Wysocki M, et al: *Eur J Clin Pharmacol* 31:513, 1987.

Pettinger WA: *N Engl J Med* 303:922, 1980.

Pfeffer MA, Lamas GA, Vaughan DE, et al: *N Engl J Med* 319:80, 1988.

Pfisterer M, Burckhardt D, Bühler FR, et al: *J Cardiovasc Pharmacol* 6:417, 1984.

Phillips RA, Ardeljan M, Goldman ME, et al: *Am J Hypertens* 2:196S, 1989.

Pickard JD, Murry GD, Illingworth R, et al: *Br Med J* 298:636, 1989.

Pierach CA, Cardinal RA, Petryka ZJ, et al: *N Engl J Med* 296:577, 1977.

Pillay VKG: *S Afr Med J* 50:625, 1976.

Pinton C, Corda R, Puggioni R, et al: *Lancet* 1:1482, 1985.

Pitlik S, Manor RS, Lipshitz I, et al: *Br Med J* 287;1845, 1983.

Pixley JS, Marshall MK, Stanley H, et al: *J Clin Pharmacol* 29:118, 1989.

Pollare T, Lithell H, Berne C: *N Engl J Med* 321:868, 1989a.

Pollare T, Lithell H, MBNrlin, et al: *J Hypertension* 7:551, 1989b.

Pollare T, Lithell H, Selinus I, et al: *Diabetologia* 31:415, 1988.

Pollare T, Lithell H, Selinus I, et al: *Br Med J* 298:1152, 1989c.

Ponten J, Biber G, Bjuro T, et al: *Acta Anaesthesiol Scand* 76:32, 1982.

Pool JL, Gennari J, Goldstein R, et al: *J Cardiovasc Pharmacol* 9(Suppl 3):S36, 1987.

Pool PE, Massie BM, Venkataraman K, et al: *Am J Cardiol* 57:212, 1986.

Popp DA, Tse TF, Shah SD, et al: *Diabetes Care* 7:243, 1984.

Porter JB, Jick H, Dinan BJ: *N Engl J Med* 304:954, 1981.

Powell CE, Slater IH: *J Pharmacol Exp Ther* 122:480, 1958.

Prichard BNC: *Drugs* 28(Suppl 1):51, 1984.

Prichard BNC, Gillam PMS: *Br Med J* 1:7, 1969.

Prichard BNC, Gillam PMS: *Br Med J* 2:725, 1964.

Prinoth M, Spahn H, Mutschler E: *Eur J Clin Pharmacol* 29:535, 1986.

Prisant LM, Beall SP, Jones KS, et al: *Clin Res* 37:17A, 1989 (abst).

Pryor PJ, Castle WM, Dukes DC, et al: *Br Med J* 287:639, 1983.

Prys-Roberts C, Meloche R, Foex P: *Br J Anaesth* 43:122, 1971.

Pullar T, Birtwell AJ, Wiles PG, et al: *Clin Pharmacol Ther* 44:540, 1988.

Puri GD, Batra YK: *Br J Anaesth* 60:579, 1988.

Rademaker M, Cooke ED, Almond NE, et al: *Br Med J* 298:561, 1989.

Ragnarsson J, Hardarson T, Snorrason SP: *Acta Med Scand* 221:143, 1987.

Rahmat J, Gelfand RI, Gelfand MC, et al: *Ann Intern Med* 102:56, 1985.

Ram CVS, Carnegie AL, Kaplan NM: In: Scriabine A, Vanov S, Deck K (eds). *Nitrendipine*. Baltimore: Urban & Schwarzenberg, 1984, p 501.

Ram CVS, Garrett BN, Kaplan NM: *Arch Intern Med* 141:1015, 1981.

Ram CVS, Gonzalez D, Kulkarni P, et al: *Am J Med* 86(Suppl 1B):66, 1989.

Ram CVS, Holland OB, Fairchild C, et al: *J Clin Pharmacol* 19:148, 1979.

Ramirez G, Ganguly A, Brueggemeyer CD: *J Clin Endocrinol Metab* 66:46, 1988.

Ramsay LE, McInnes GT, Hettiarachchi J, et al: *Br J Clin Pharmacol* 5:243, 1978.

Ramsay LE, Silas JH, Freestone S: *Br Med J* 281:1101, 1980.

Ramsey LE, Freestone S: *Br J Clin Pharmacol* 18:616, 1984.

Ray WA, Griffin MR, Downey W, et al: *Lancet* 1:687, 1989.

Reams GP, Hamory A, Lau A, et al: *Hypertension* 11:452, 1988.

Reed BR, Huff JC, Jones SK, et al: *Ann Intern Med* 103:49, 1985.

Reid JL: *Am Heart J* 116:1400, 1988.

Reid JL, Dargie HJ, Davies DS, et al: *Lancet* 1:1171, 1977.

Reid JL, Macdonald NJ, Lees KR, et al: *Am Heart J* 117:751, 1989.

Reid K, Morales A, Harris C, et al: *Lancet* 2:421, 1987.

Reinhart RA: *Arch Intern Med* 148:2415, 1988.

Rett K, Wicklmayr M, Dietze GJ: *N Engl J Med* 319:1609, 1988.

Roberts DH, Tsao Y, McLoughlin GA, et al: *Lancet* 2:650, 1987.

Robertson DRC, Waller DG, Renwick AG, et al: *Br J Clin Pharmac* 25:297, 1988.

Robertson JWK, Isles CG, Brown I, et al: *J Hypertension* 4:603, 1986.

Roden DM, Nadeau JHJ, Primm RK: *Clin Pharamcol Ther* 43:648, 1988.

Rodman JS, Deutsch DJ, Gutman SI: *Am J Med* 60:941, 1976.

Rosa RM, Silva P, Young J, et al: *N Engl J Med* 302:431, 1980.

Rosenberg L, Shapiro S, Slone D, et al: *N Engl J Med* 303:546, 1980.

Rosenthal J: In: Kaltenbach M, Neufeld HN (eds). Proceedings, 5th International Adalat Symposium. Oxfore-Princeton-Amsterdam: Excerpta Medica, 1982, p175.

Roth A, Miller HI, Belhassen B, et al: *Ann Intern Med* 110:171, 1989.

Rucinska EJ, Small R, Irvin J: *Int J Cardiol* 22:249, 1989.

Ruffolo RR Jr: *Fed Proc* 43:2910, 1984.

Ruilope LM, Robles RG, Miranda B, et al: *J Hypertension* 6:665, 1988.

Ruys T, Shaikh M, Nordestgaard BG, et al: *Lancet* 2:1119, 1989.

Sackett DL: *Can Med Assoc J* 121:259, 1979.

Sakhaee K, Nicar MJ, Glass K, et al: *J Clin Endocrinol Metab* 59:1037, 1984.

Salvetti A, Arzilli F: *Am J Hypertens* 2:352, 1989.

Salvetti A, Pedrinelli R, Bartolomei G, et al: *Eur J Clin Pharmacol* 33:221, 1987.

Sandström P-E, Sehlin J: *Am J Physiol* 255:E591, 1988.

Sarosdy MF, Hudnall CH, Erickson DR, et al: *J Urol* 141:551, 1989.

Saruta T: *Am Heart J* 117:243, 1989.

Sassano P, Chatellier G, Billaud E, et al: *J Cardiovasc Pharmacol* 13:314, 1989.

Savola J, Vehviläinen O, Väätäinen NJ: *Br Med J* 295:637, 1987.

Sawyer N, Gabriel R: *Postgrad Med J* 64:434, 1988.

Schäfers RF, Reid JL: Alpha Blockers. In: Kaplan NM, Brenner BM, Laragh JH (eds). *New Therapeutic Strategies in Hypertension*. New York: Raven Press Ltd, 1989, p 51.

Scharf MB, Mayleben DW: *Am J Med* 86(Suppl 1B):110, 1989.

Scheen AJ, Castillo M, Salvatore T, et al: *Curr Ther Res* 46:200, 1989.

Schoenfeld MR, Goldberger E: *Curr Ther Res* 6:180, 1964.

Schroeder T, Sillesen H: *Eur J Clin Invest* 17:214, 1987.

Schubiger G, Flury G, Nussberger J: *Ann Intern Med* 108:215, 1988.

Schulte K-L, Meyer-Sabellek W, Röcker, et al: *Am J Cardiol* 60:826, 1987.

Schultz HS, Chretien SD, Brewer DD, et al: *J Clin Pharmacol* 21:65, 1981.

Schwartz AB, Swartz CD: *JAMA* 230:702, 1974.

Schwartz ML, Rotmensch HH, Vlasses PH, et al: *Arch Intern Med* 144:1425, 1984.

Schwartz WB, de Strihou CVY, Kassirer JP: *N Engl J Med* 2:630, 1968.

Scoble JE, Sweny P, Varghese Z, et al: *Lancet* 2:326, 1986.

Scott AK, Rigby JW, Webster J, et al: *Br Med J* 284:1514, 1982.

Scott AK, Roy-Chaudhury P, Webster J, et al: *Br J Clin Pharmac* 27:417, 1989.

Scott EM: *J Autonom Pharmacol* 3:113, 1983.

Seeverens H, de Bruin CD, Jordans JGM: *Acta Med Scand* 211:233, 1982.

Semple PF, Thoren P, Lever AF: *J Hypertension* 6:601, 1988.

Serlin MJ, Orme ML'E, Baber NS, et al: *Clin Pharmacol Ther* 37:586, 1980.

Sever PS, Poulter NR: *J Hypertension* 5(Suppl 4):S123, 1987.

Shalev O, Mosseri M, Ariel I, et al: *Arch Intern Med* 143:592, 1983.

Shallcross H, Padley SPG, Glynn MJ, et al: *Br Med J* 295:1236, 1987.

Shanks RG, Balnave K, Russell C: *Br J Clin Pharmacol* 18:232, 1984.

Sharpe N, Smith H, Murphy J, et al: *Lancet* 1:255, 1984.

Shepherd AMM, Carr AA, Davidov M, et al: *J Cardiovasc Pharmacol* 13:580, 1989.

Shimizu T, Yoshitomi K, Nakamura M, et al: *J Clin Invest* 82:721, 1988.

Shulman NB, Martinez B, Brogan D, et al: *Am J Public Health* 76:1105, 1986.

Sibley DR, Lefkowitz RJ: *ISI Atlas of Sci: Pharmacol* 70, 1988.

Sica DA, Gehr TWB: *Nephrol* 51:454, 1989.

Simon G: *Am J Med* 85:893, 1988.

Simon G, Wittig VJ, Cohn JN: *Clin Pharmacol Ther* 40:42, 1986.

Singer DR, Markandu ND, Shore AC, et al: *Hypertension* 9:629, 1987.

Singhvi SM, Duchin KL, Willard DA, et al: *Clin Pharmacol Ther* 32:182, 1982.

Siragy HM, Lamb NE, Rose CE Jr, et al: *Am J Physiol* 255:F749, 1988. 1988.

Sjöden G, Rosenqvist M, Kriegholm E, et al: *Br J Clin Pharmac* 24:367, 1987.

Skarfors ET, Lithell HO, Selinus I, et al: *Br Med J* 298:1147, 1989.

Smith WM, Damato AN, Galluzzi NJ, et al: *Ann Intern Med* 61:829, 1964.

Smith SA, Rafiqi EI, Gardener EG, et al: *J Hypertension* 5:693, 1987.

Sobota JT, Martin WB, Carlson RG, et al: *Circulation* 62:376, 1980.

Solomon RJ: *Drugs* 28 (Suppl 1):66, 1984.

Soltero I, Colmenares A, Silva H: *Curr Ther Res* 40:739, 1986.

Sopko JA, Freeman RM: *JAMA* 238:608, 1977.

Sörgel F, Ettinger B, Benet LZ: *J Urol* 134:871, 1985.

Sotaniemi EA, Antilla M, Rautio A, et al: *Clin Pharmacol Ther* 29:705, 1981.

Speirs C, Fielder AHL, Chapel H, et al: *Lancet* 1:922, 1989.

Spence JD, Sibbald WJ, Cape RD: *Clin Sci Mol Med* 55:399s, 1978.

Staessen J, Fagard R, Lijnen P, et al: *J Cardiovasc Pharmacol* 12:718, 1988b.

Staessen J, Fagard R, Van Hoof R, et al: *J Cardiovasc Pharamcol* 12(Suppl 8):S33, 1988a.

Stamler R, Stamler J, Gosch FC, et al: *Am J Med* 80(Suppl 2A):1986.

Stamler R, Stamler J, Gosch FC, et al: *Hypertension* 12:574, 1988.

Stamler R, Stamler J, Grimm R, et al: *JAMA* 257:1484, 1987.

Stason WB: *Hypertension* 13(Suppl I):I-145, 1989.

Stein J, Osgood R: *J Cardiovasc Pharmacol* 6:S787, 1984.

Steiner J, Cassar J, Mashiter K, et al: *Br Med J* 1:1186, 1976.

Steiness E: *Clin Pharmacol Ther* 35:788, 1984.

Stenvinkel P, Alvestrand A: *Acta Med Scand* 224:89, 1988.

Stern R, Khalsa JH: *Arch Intern Med* 149:829, 1989.

Stessman J, Leibel B, Yagil Y, et al: *J Clin Pharmacol* 25:193, 1985.

Stewart AL, Greenfield S, Hays RD, et al: *JAMA* 262:907, 1989.

Stewart DE, Ikram H, Espiner EA, et al: *Br Heart J* 54:290, 1985.

Stimpel M, Vetter H, Kuffer B, et al: *J Hypertension* 3(Suppl 1):97, 1985.

Stone JG, Foex P, Sear JW, et al: *Anesthesiology* 68:495, 1988.

Strandgaard S, Haunsø S: *Lancet* 2:658, 1987.

Strandgaard S, Paulson OB: *Am J Hypertens* 2:486, 1989.

Strom BL: *N Engl J Med* 316:1456, 1987.

Strom BL, Carson JL, Schinnar R, et al: *Arch Intern Med* 147:954, 1987.

Strom JA, Vidt DG, Bugni W, et al: *Am J Cardiol* 63:251, 1989.

Strongwater SL, Galvanek EG, Stoff JS: *Arch Intern Med* 149:582, 1989.

Struthers AD, Whitesmith R, Reid JL: *Lancet* 1:1358, 1983.

Sturman SG, Kumararatne D, Beevers DG: *Lancet* 2:1304, 1988.

Suki WN: *Arch Intern Med* 149:669, 1989.

Sullivan PA, De Quattro V, Foti A, et al: *Hypertension* 8:611, 1986.

Sumner DJ, Meredith PA, Howie CA, et al: *Br J Clin Pharmacol* 26:715, 1988.

Suzuki H, Tominaga T, Kumagai H, et al: *J Hypertension* 6(Suppl 4):S649, 1988.

Swales JD: *J Hypertension* 5(Suppl 4):1987.

Sweet CS: *Hypertension* 6(Suppl II):II–51, 1984.

Swislocki ALM, Hoffman BB, Reaven GM: *Am J Hypertens* 2:419, 1989.

Szlachcic J, Hirsch AT, Tubau JF, et al: *Am J Cardiol* 59:393, 1987.

Szlachcic J, Tubau JF, Vollmer C, et al: *Am J Cardiol* 63:198, 1989.

Talseth T: *Eur J Clin Pharmacol* 10:183, 1976a.

Talseth T: *Eur J Clin Pharmacol* 10:311, 1976b.

Tannen RL: *Ann Intern Med* 98:773, 1983.

Tannenbaum PJ, Rosen E, Flanagan T, et al: *Clin Pharmacol Ther* 9:598, 1968.

Tanner LA, Bosco LA: *Arch Intern Med* 148:379, 1988.

Tarazi RC, Dustan HP: *Am J Cardiol* 29:633, 1972.

Tarazi RC, Dustan HP, Frohlich ED: *Circulation* 41:709, 1970.

Tateishi A, Sano T, Takeshita H, et al: *J Neurosurg* 69:213, 1988.

Tateishi T, Nakashima H, Shitou T, et al: *Eur J Clin Pharmacol* 36:67, 1989.

Taverner D, Bing RF, Heagerty A, et al: *Q J Med* 52:280, 1983.

Taylor DG, Kaplan HR: In: Kaplan NM, Brenner BM, Laragh JH (eds). *New Therapeutic Strategies in Hypertension*. New York: Raven Press, Ltd., 1989, p125.

Taylor SH, Lee PS, Sharma SK: *Am Heart J* 116:1820, 1988.

Tejada ISD, Goldstein I, Azadzoi K, et al: *N Engl J Med* 320:1025, 1989.

Temple R: *Med Cl N Amer* 73:495, 1989.

Terént A, Ribacke M, Carlson LA: *Eur J Clin Pharmacol* 36:347, 1989.

Textor SC, Fouad FM, Bravo EL, et al: *N Engl J Med* 307:601, 1982.

Thadani U: *Am J Cardiol* 52:10D, 1983.

Thompson PD, Cullinane EM, Nugent AM, et al: *Am J Med* 86(Suppl 1B):104, 1989.

Thulin T, Magnusson J, Werner O, et al: Program. *10th International Society of Hypertension*. Interkalen, Switzerland. June 1984, abstr 862.

Tietze KJ, Schwartz ML, Vlasses PH: *Drugs* 32:531, 1987.

Timmermans PBMWM: In: van Zwieten PA (ed). *Handbook of Hypertension, vol 3, Pharmacology of Antihypertensive Drugs*. Amsterdam: Elsevier, 1984.

Tinker JH, Noback CR, Vlietstra RE, et al: *JAMA* 246:1348, 1981.

Tohmeh JF, Shah SD, Cryer PE: *Am J Med* 67:772, 1979.

Topol EJ, Traill TA, Fortuin NJ: *N Engl J Med* 312:277, 1985.

Tordjman K. Rosenthal T, Bursztyn M: *Am J Cardiol* 55:1445, 1985.

Toriumi DM, Konior RJ, Berktold RE: *Arch Otolaryngol Head Neck Surg* 114:918, 1988

Traub YM, Rabinov M, Rosenfeld JB, et al: *Clin Pharmacol Ther* 28:765, 1980.

Trost BN: *Drugs* 38:621, 1989.

Trost BN, Weidmann P: *J Hypertension* 5 (Suppl 4):S81, 1987.

Tsuda K, Tsuda S, Minatogawa Y, et al: *Am J Hypertens* 1:283, 1988.

Tsujimoto G, Hashimoto K, Hoffmann BB: *Int J Clin Pharmacol Ther Toxicol* 27:102, 1989.

Tsukiyama H, Otsuka K, Higuma K: *Br J Clin Pharmacol* 13:269S, 1982.

Tuomilehto J, Nissinen A, Wolf E: *Br Med J* 291:857, 1985.

Tweeddale MG, Ogilvie RI: *N Engl J Med* 289:198, 1973.

Tyce GM, Sheps SG, Flock EV: *Mayo Clin Proc* 38:571, 1963.

Tyrer P: *Drugs* 36:773, 1988.

Ueda K, Kuwajima I, Murakami M, et al: Jpn Heart J 27:55, 1986.

Ueda H, Yagi S, Keneko Y: *Arch Intern Med* 122:387, 1968.

Uehlinger DE, Weidmann P, Gnaedinger MP: *Eur J Clin Pharmacol* 36:119, 1989.

Ullian ME, Linas SLi: *Semin Nephrol* 7:239, 1987.

Unger T, Badoer E, Ganten D, et al: *Circulation* 77(Suppl I):I–40, 1988.

Valdes G, Soto ME, Croxatto HR, et al: *Clin Sci* 63:447S, 1982.

van Brummelen P, Man in't Veld AJ, Schalekamp MADH: *Clin Pharmacol Ther* 27:328, 1980.

Vandenburg MJ, Cooper WD, Woollard ML, et al: *Eur J Clin Pharmacol* 26:325, 1984.

Vandenburg MJ, Wright P, Holmes J, et al: *Br J Clin Pharmacol* 13:747, 1982.

van den Meiracker AH, Man in't Verld AJ, Boomsma F, et al: *Circulation* 80:903, 1989.

van den Meiracker AH, Man in't Veld AJ, van Eck HJR, et al: *Circulation* 78:957, 1988.

Van der Linden W, Ritter B, Edlund G: *Br Med J* 289:654, 1984.

van Giersbergen PLM, Tierney SAV, Wiegant VM, et al: *Hypertension* 13:83, 1989.

Van Gilst WH, Scholtens E, De Graeff PA, et al: *Circulation* 77(Suppl I):I-24, 1988.

van Harten J, Burggraaf K, Danhof M, et al: *Lancet* 2:1363, 1987.

van Harten J, van Brummelen P, Danhof M, et al: *J Cardiovasc Pharmacol* 13:624, 1989.

Vanhoutte PM, Van Neuten JM, Symoens J, et al: *Fed Proc* 42:182, 1983.

van Kalken CK, van der Meulen J, Oe PL, , et al: *Eur J Clin Pharmacol* 31:63, 1986.

Van Rooijen GJM, Boer P, Dorhout-Mees EJ, et al: *Clin Pharmacol Ther* 26:420, 1979.

van Schaik BAM, Geyskes GG, Dorhout Mees EJ: *Nephron* 47:167, 1987.

van Zwieten PA: *J Pharm Pharmacol* 29:229, 1977.

van Zwieten PA: *Am J Cardiol* 61:6D, 1988.

van Zwieten PA: *J Hypertension* 6(Suppl 2):S3, 1988.

van Zwieten PA, Timmermans PBMWM, Van Brummelen P: *Am J Med* 77:17, 1984.

van Zwieten PA, Timmermans PBMWM, van Heiningen PNM: *J Hypertension* 5 (Suppl 4):S21, 1987.

Vardan S, Mehrotra KG, Mookherjee S, et al: *JAMA* 258:484, 1987.

Velasco M, Bertoncini H, Romero E, et al: *Eur J Clin Pharmacol* 13:317, 1978.

Veldhuis JD, Borges JLC, Drake CR, et al: *J Clin Endocrinol Metab* 60:144, 1985.

Verburg KM, Kleinert HD, Kadam JRC, et al: *Hypertension* 13:262, 1989.

Veterans Administration Cooperative Study Group on Antihypertensive Agents: *Arch Intern Med* 110:230, 1962.

Veterans Administration Cooperative Study Group on Antihypertensive Agents: *JAMA* 237:2303, 1977a.

Veterans Administration Cooperative Study Group on Antihypertensive Agents: *Circulation* 55:519, 1977b.

Veterans Administration Cooperative Study Group on Antihypertensive Agents: *Circulation* 64:772, 1981b.

Veterans Administration Cooperative Study Group on Antihypertensive Agents: *JAMA* 248:1996, 1982a.

Veterans Administration Cooperative Study Group on Antihypertensive Agents: *Br J Clin Pharmacol* 14:97S, 1982b.

Vetter H, Ramsey LE, Luscher TF, et al: *J Hypertension* 3(Suppl 1):1, 1985.

Vetter W, Wehling M, Foerster E-Ch, et al: *Klin Wochenschr* 62:731, 1984.

Vincent HH, Man in't Veld AJ, Boomsma F, et al: *Hypertension* 9:198, 1987.

Virag R, Bouilly P, Frydman D: *Lancet* 1:181, 1985.

Vlachakis ND, Barr J, Velasquez M, et al: *Clin Pharmacol Ther* 35:782, 1984.

Vlasses PH, Koffer H, Ferguson RK, et al: *Clin Exp Hypertens* 3:929, 1981.

Volini IF, Flaxman N: *JAMA* 112:2126, 1939.

Waeber B, Gavras I, Brunner HR, et al: *J Clin Pharmacol* 21:508, 1981.

Waeber B, Nussberger J, Brunner HR: *Hypertension* 7:223, 1985.

Waeber B, Nussberber J, Brunner HR: In: Kaplan NM, Brenner BM, Laragh JH (eds). *New Therapeutic Strategies in Hypertension*. New York: Raven Press, Ltd., 1989, p 97.

Wahl J, Singh BN, Thoden WR: *Am Heart J* 111:353, 1986.

Waldemar G, Schmidt JF, Andersen AR, et al: *J Hypertension* 7:229, 1989.

Walker RG, Whitworth JA, Saines D, et al: *Med J Aust* 2:146, 1981.

Wallin JD, O'Neill WM: *Arch Intern Med* 143:485, 1983.

Walters BNJ, Redman WG: *Br J Obstet Gynaecol* 91:330, 1984.

Washton AM, Resnick RB, Perzel JF Jr, et al: *Lancet* 1:991, 1981.

Watson RDS, Stallard TJ, Littler WA: *Lancet* 1:1210, 1979.

Webb DJ, Fulton JD, Leckie BJ, et al: *J Hum Hypertens* 1:195, 1987.

Weber MA, Case DB, Baer L, et al: *Am J Cardiol* 38:825, 1976.

Weber MA, Drayer JIM: *Am Heart J* 108:311, 1984.

Weber MA, Drayer JIM, Rev A, et al: *Ann Intern Med* 87:558, 1977.

Weber MA, Drayer JIM, McMahon FG, et al: *Arch Intern Med* 144:1211, 1984.

Webster J: *Drugs* 30:32, 1985.

Weidmann P, Uehlinger DE, Gerber A: *J Hypertension* 3:297, 1985.

Weidmann P, De Chatel R, Ziegler WH, et al: *Am J Cardiol* 41:570, 1978.

Weinberg P, Berezow J, Charlap S, et al: *Clin Res* 32:341A, 1984.

Weinberger MH: *J Cardiovasc Pharamcol* 7:S52, 1985.

Weinberger MH: *J Cardiovasc Pharmacol* 9(Suppl 4):S272, 1987.

Weinman EJ, Eknoyan G, Suki WN: *J Clin Invest* 55:283, 1975.

Weinstein DB, Heider JG: *Am J Med* 86(Suppl 4A):27, 1989.

Weir MR, Burris JF, Oparil S, et al: *Am J Hypertens* 2:21A, 1989 (abst).

Westlin W, Mullane K: *Circulation* 77(Suppl I):I–30, 1988.

Westwood BE, Wilson M, Heath WC, et al: *Med J Aust* 145:151, 1986.

Whang R: *Drugs* 28 (Suppl 1):143, 1984.

Whang R, Flink EB, Dyckner T, et al: *Arch Intern Med* 145:1686, 1985a

Whang R, Oei TO, Aikawa JK: *Arch Intern Med* 144:1794, 1984.

Whang R, Oei TO, Watanabe A: *Arch Intern Med* 145:655, 1985b.

Whelton PK: *Drugs* 28 (Suppl 1):54, 1984.

White WB, Schulman P, Karimeddini MK, et al: *Am Heart J* 117:145, 1989.

Widmann L, Dyckner T, Wester PO: *Eur J Clin Pharmacol* 33:577, 1988.

Wikstrand J, Warnold I, Olsson G, et al: *JAMA* 259:1976, 1988.

Wikstrand J, Westergren G, Berglund G, et al: *JAMA* 255:1304, 1986.

Wilber DJ, Lynch JJ, Montgomery DG, et al: *J Cardiovasc Pharmacol* 10:96, 1987.

Wilcox CS, Mitch WE, Kelly RA, et al: *J Lab Clin Med* 102:450, 1983.

Wilcox RG: *Br Med J* 2:383, 1978.

Wilhelmsen L, Berglund G, Elmfeldt D, et al: *J Hypertension* 5:561, 1987.

Wilkins RW: *Ann Intern Med* 50:1, 1959.

Wilkinson PR, Raftery EB: *Br J Clin Pharmacol* 4:289, 1977.

Wilkinson R, Stevens IM, Pickering M, et al: *Br J Clin Pharmcol* 10:51, 1980.

Williams G, Donaldson RM: *Lancet* 2:738, 1986.

Williams GH: *N Engl M Med* 319:1517, 1988.

Williams JG, DeVoss K, Craswell PW: *Med J Aust* 1:225, 1978.

Williams RL, Mordenti J, Upton RA, et al: *Pharmaceutical Res* 4:348, 1987a.

Williams RR, Hunt SC, Hopkins PN, et al: *JAMA* 259:3579, 1988.

Williams TC, Mac Carthy EP, Downs TR, et al: *Clin Pharmacol Ther* 42:76, 1987b.

Williams WR, Schneider KA, Borhani NO, et al: *Am J Prev Med* 2:248, 1986.

Wilson JD, Booth RJ, Bullock JY, et al: *Lancet* 2:312, 1980.

Wilson JD, Bullock JY, Sutherland DC, et al: *Br Med J* 1:14, 1978.

Wilson MF, Haring O, Lewin A, et al: *Am J Cardiol* 57:43E, 1986.

Wilson TW: *Clin Pharmacol Ther* 39:94, 1986.

Winer BM: *Circulation* 24:788, 1961.

Winniford MD, Markham RV Jr, Firth BG, et al: *Am J Cardiol* 50:704, 1982.

Witgall H, Hirsch F, Scherer B, et al: *Clin Sci* 62:611, 1982.

Wolff DE, Buckalew VM Jr, Strandhoy JW: *J Cardiovasc Pharmacol* 6:S793, 1984.

Wolfson P, Abernethy D, DiPette DJ, et al: *Am J Cardiol* 62:103G, 1988.

Wollam GL, Tarazi RC, Bravo EL, et al: *Am J Med* 72:929, 1982.

Wong PC, Price WA Jr, Chiu AT, et al: *Hypertension* 13:489, 1989.

Woo J, Woo KS, Kin T, et al: *Arch Intern Med* 147:1386, 1987.

Woodcock BG, Haberdank WD, Loh W, et al: *J Cardiovasc Pharmacol* 6:543, 1984.

Wyndham RN, Gimenez L, Walker WG, et al: *Arch Intern Med* 147:1021, 1987.

Yates AP, Hunter DN: *Anaesthesia* 43:935, 1988.

Yoshino G, Iwai M, Kazumi T, et al: *Curr Ther Res* 42:607, 1987.

Yu T, Berger L, Sarkozi L, et al: *Arch Intern Med* 141:915, 1981.

Yusuf S, Wittes J, Friedman L: *JAMA* 260:2088, 1988.

Zachariah PK, Sheps SG, Oshrain C, et al: *J Clin Hypertens* 3:536, 1987.

Zatuchni J: *JAMA* 251:343, 1984.

Zezulka AV, Gill JS, Dews I, et al: *Am J Cardiol* 59:630, 1987.

Zhou H-H, Koshakji RP, Silberstein DJ, et al: *N Engl J Med* 320:565, 1989.

Zidek W, Baumgart P, Karoff C, et al: *J Hypertens* 2 (Suppl 3):495, 1984.

Zimmerman BG: *Hypertension* 14:498, 1989.

Zimmerman BG, Sybert EG, Wong PC: *J Hypertension* 2:581, 1984.

Zsigmond EK, Barabas E, Korenaga GM: *Int J Clin Pharmacol Ther Toxicol* 26:225, 1988.

Zsoter TT, Church JG: *Drugs* 25:93, 1983.

Zusman RM: *Hypertension* 12:327, 1988.

Zusman RM: *Am J Hypertens* 2:200S, 1989.

Zusman R, Christensen D, Federman E, et al: *Am J Med* 82(Suppl 3B):37, 1987.

# 8 Hypertensive Emergencies and Urgencies

Life-threatening hypertension may occur in the course of any hypertensive disease but most commonly in the circumstances listed in Table 8.1. Of these, accelerated-malignant hypertension is most common. Although the incidence of accelerated-malignant hypertension may be diminishing and mortality from it is definitely falling (Bing et al, 1986; Kawazoe et al, 1988), the syndrome remains all too common, particularly among young and poor black and Hispanic men (Bennett and Shea, 1988). Therefore, clinicians must remain alert to the appearance of hypertensive emergencies and urgencies and must be aggressive in their management, since most who enter into these phases die if they are not treated.

## DEFINITIONS

The following definitions are generally accepted:

*Hypertensive Emergencies.* Situations wherein immediate reduction of blood pressure within minutes is needed, usually with parenteral therapy.

*Hypertensive Urgencies.* Situations wherein reduction of blood pressure is needed within a period of hours, usually with oral agents.

*Accelerated-Malignant Hypertension.* Until recently, the term "malignant" hypertension was used for the presence of papilledema (Grade 4 Keith-Wagener (K-W) retinopathy) whereas "accelerated" was used for the presence of hemorrhages and exudates (Grade 3 K-W retinopathy), both with markedly high blood pressure, the diastolic usually above 140 mm Hg. The funduscopic differences do not connote different clinical features or prognosis, so the term "accelerated-malignant" hypertension is recommended and will be used (Ahmed et al, 1986).

*Hypertensive Encephalopathy.* Sudden and usually marked elevation of blood pressure with severe headache and various alterations in consciousness, reversible by reduction of blood pressure.

## PATHOPHYSIOLOGY

### Accelerated-Malignant Hypertension

When blood pressure reaches some critical level, in experimental animals at a mean arterial pressure of 150 mm Hg, lesions appear in arterial walls, and the syndrome of accelerated-malignant hypertension begins (Fig. 8.1).

Though one or more humoral factors shown in Figure 8.1 may be involved in setting off the process (Möhring, 1977), including vasopressin (Hiwatari et al, 1986), the accelerated-malignant phase is likely to be a nonspecific consequence of very high blood pressure (Beilin and Goldby, 1977). Any form of hypertension may progress to the accelerated-malignant phase, some without activation of the renin-angiotensin or other humoral mechanisms (Gavras et al, 1975a).

In animal models, the level of the arterial pressure correlates closely with the development of fibrinoid necrosis, the experimental hallmark of accelerated-malignant hypertension (Giese, 1964; Byrom, 1974). In humans, fibrinoid necrosis is rare, perhaps because those who die acutely have not had time to develop the lesion and those who live with therapy are able to repair it. The typical lesions, best seen in the kidney, are hyperplastic arteriosclerosis and accelerated glomerular obsolescence (Jones, 1974).

**Table 8.1. Circumstances Requiring Rapid Treatment of Hypertension**

Hypertensive emergencies
  Cerebrovascular
    Hypertensive encephalopathy (any cause)
    Intracerebral hemorrhage
    Subarachnoid hemorrhage
  Cardiac
    Acute aortic dissection
    Acute left ventricular failure
    Acute or impending myocardial infarction
    After coronary bypass surgery
  Excessive circulating catecholamines
    Pheochromocytoma crisis
    Food or drug interactions with MAO inhibitors
  Eclampsia
  Head injury
  Postoperative bleeding from vascular suture lines
  Severe epistaxis
Hypertensive urgencies
  Accelerated-malignant hypertension
  Atherothrombotic brain infarction with severe
    hypertension
  Rebound hypertension after sudden cessation of
    antihypertensive drugs
  Surgical
    Severe hypertension in patients requiring immediate
      surgery
    Postoperative hypertension
    Severe hypertension after kidney transplantation
  Severe body burns

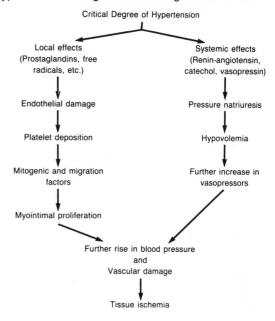

**Figure 8.1.** Scheme for initiation and progression of accelerated-malignant hypertension.

## Humoral Factors

There is support, however, for the involvement of factors other than the level of the blood pressure in setting off the accelerated-malignant phase, particularly since the range of pressures in patients with severe ''benign'' hypertension and accelerated-malignant hypertension may overlap (Kincaid-Smith, 1980). As shown on the *right side* of Figure 8.1, in both rats (Gross et al, 1975) and dogs (Dzau et al, 1981) with unilateral renal artery stenosis, the accelerated-malignant phase was preceded by natriuresis that markedly activated the renin-angiotensin system. The progression was delayed by giving saline loads after the natriuresis.

Whether these animal models involving a major insult to renal blood flow are applicable to human accelerated-malignant hypertension is uncertain. However, renal artery stenosis is a common cause of accelerated-malignant hypertension in humans, having been found in 35% of 123 patients seen at Vanderbilt with accelerated-malignant hypertension (Davis et al, 1979).

Evidence for the pathway shown in Figure 8.1 (*left*) comes from studies on cats made acutely and severely hypertensive, wherein the vascular damage could be inhibited by prior treatment with inhibitors of the cyclooxygenase enzyme involved in prostaglandin synthesis or by topical application of scavengers of free oxygen radicals (Kontos et al, 1981). These authors propose that the cascade starts with an increase in prostaglandin synthesis.

In humans, in addition to the presence of renal artery stenosis, the development of accelerated-malignant hypertension has been observed to be more common in association with cigarette smoking (Isles et al, 1979). High levels of serum immunologloglobulins are commonly found, likely as a consequence to vascular damage but possibly as a primary immunological disturbance (Hilme et al, 1989).

## Hypertensive Encephalopathy

Either with or without the structural defects of accelerated-malignant hypertension, progressively higher blood pressure can lead into the clinical picture of hypertensive encephalopathy. The brain dysfunction was once thought to reflect progressive vascular spasm and ischemia but is now considered to arise from a ''breakthrough'' hyperperfusion and leakage of fluid through the blood-brain barrier (Strandgaard and Paulson, 1989).

## Breakthrough Vasodilation

With changes in blood pressure, cerebral vessels dilate or constrict to maintain a relatively constant level of cerebral blood flow (CBF), the process of autoregulation (Fig. 8.2). These di-

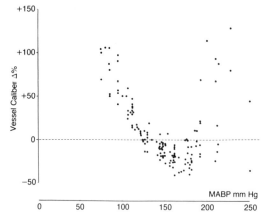

**Figure 8.2.** Observed change in the caliber of pial arterioles with a caliber less than 50 μm in eight cats, calculated as a percentage of change from the caliber at a mean arterial blood pressure (*MABP*) of 135 mm Hg. The blood pressure was raised by intravenous infusion of angiotensin II. (From MacKenzie ET, Strandgaard S, Graham DI, et al: Effects of acutely induced hypertension in cats on pial arteriolar caliber, local cerebral blood flow, and the blood-brain barrier. *Circ Res* 39:33, 1976 and by permission of the American Heart Association, Inc.)

rect measurements, taken in cats, show progressive dilation as pressures are lowered and progressive constriction as pressures rise (MacKenzie et al, 1976). Note, however, that when mean arterial pressures reach a critical level, around 180 mm Hg, the vessels suddenly dilate. The previously constricted vessels, unable to withstand such high pressures, are stretched and dilated, first in areas with less muscular tone, producing irregular sausage-string patterns, later diffusely, producing generalized vasodilation. This vasodilation allows a breakthrough of CBF, hyperperfusing the brain under high pressure, with leakage of fluid into the perivascular tissue leading to cerebral edema and the clinical syndrome of hypertensive encephalopathy (Strandgaard and Paulson, 1989).

In addition to hyperperfusion, a disruption of the blood-brain barrier related to alteration of endothelial surface charge likely contributes to the perivascular edema (Mayhan et al, 1989).

The ''breakthrough'' vasodilation mechanism for hypertensive encephalopathy shown experimentally in cats and baboons (Strandgaard et al, 1976) has also been demonstrated in humans (Strandgaard et al, 1973). By measuring CBF repetitively while arterial blood pressure is lowered by vasodilators or raised by vasoconstrictors, curves of autoregulation have been constructed. In normal humans, as in an-

imals, CBF is constant between mean arterial pressures of 60 and 120 mm Hg (Fig. 8.3). However, as shown in the curves for the upper two normotensive subjects whose pressure was raised beyond the limit of autoregulation, breakthrough hyperperfusion occurs.

Pressures such as these are handled without obvious trouble in chronic hypertensives, whose blood vessels adapt to the chronically elevated blood pressure with structural thickening (Folkow, 1987), presumably mediated by sympa-

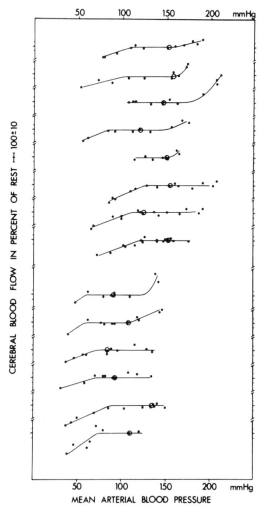

**Figure 8.3.** Curves of cerebral blood flow with varying levels of blood pressure in 14 people, the top 8 hypertensive, the bottom 6 normotensive. Each patient's habitual pressure is indicated by an open circle. The curves reflect autoregulation, with a shift to the right in the hypertensives. Both the lower and the upper limits of autoregulation are shown. Note the breakthrough of CBF when the upper limit is exceeded. (From Johansson B, Strandgaard S, Lassen NA: *Circ Res* (Suppl I)34 and 35:I-167; 1974.)

thetic nerves (Heistad, 1984). Thereby the entire curve of autoregulation is shifted to the right, shown in the *upper eight cases* in Figure 8.3. Even with this shift, breakthrough will occur if pressures are raised very high, to levels of 170 to 180 mm Hg, shown in the *upper five cases.*

These findings explain a number of clinical observations:

—Previously normotensive people who suddenly become hypertensive may develop encephalopathy at relatively low levels of hypertension. These include children with acute glomerulonephritis and young women with toxemia of pregnancy.

—Chronically hypertensive patients less commonly develop encephalopathy, and only at much higher pressures.

—When the blood pressure is lowered by antihypertensive drugs, chronic hypertensives often are not able to tolerate either sudden or drastic reductions without experiencing cerebral hypoperfusion—becoming weak and dizzy with postural hypotension. These symptoms may appear at levels of blood pressure that are still above the upper limit of normal and that are well tolerated by normotensives. The reason is that the entire curve of autoregulation shifts, so that the lower end is also moved with a fall-off of blood flow at levels of 100 to 120 mm Hg mean arterial pressure (Fig. 8.3). Fortunately, as detailed in Chapter 7, with time the curve can shift back toward the normal so that greater reductions in pressure can be tolerated. Unfortunately, the elderly may lose their ability to autoregulate, increasing their risk of brain damage from minor falls in blood pressure (Wollner et al, 1979).

—Maneuvers that increase CBF further and thereby increase intracranial pressure, such as $CO_2$ inhalation or cerebral vasodilators, e.g., hydralazine and nitroprusside, may be harmful in patients with encephalopathy.

—In experimentally infarcted brain tissue, autoregulation is lost; therefore, with high blood pressure, perfusion would be accentuated through the damaged tissue, leading to edema and compression of normal brain (Meyer et al, 1972). This provides experimental evidence for the clinical importance of carefully reducing the blood pressure in hypertensive stroke patients.

Thus, hypertensive encephalopathy is the consequence of progressively high arterial pressures that break through the protection of the blood-brain barrier and the autoregulation of CBF (Fig. 8.4).

## CLINICAL COURSE

### Predisposing Factors

Hypertensive encephalopathy and accelerated-malignant hypertension may appear with any form of hypertension. They develop in probably fewer than 1% of patients with primary hypertension. However, since 90% or more of hypertension is of unknown cause, i.e., primary, this is the most usual setting in which these syndromes appear. As noted above, encephalopathy is more common in those previously normotensive individuals whose pressures rise suddenly, as during toxemia of pregnancy. Accelerated-malignant hypertension often appears without encephalopathy, perhaps in those whose pressure rise more gradually.

Hypertensive emergencies may occur in patients taking monoamine oxidase inhibitors (MAO) who ingest tyramine-containing foods such as ripened cheese and red wine (Liu and Rustgi, 1987). They have also developed after intake of sympathomimetic drugs such as phenylpropanolamine (Pentel, 1984) or other pressors such as cocaine (Virmani et al, 1988).

### Signs and Symptoms

The common symptoms and signs are listed in Table 8.2. However, it is not uncommon to see patients, particularly young black men, who deny any prior symptoms when seen in the end stages of the hypertensive process with their

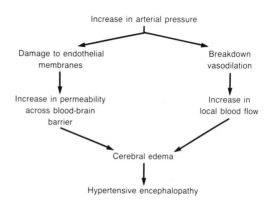

**Figure 8.4.** A scheme for the pathogenesis of hypertensive encephalopathy.

**Table 8.2. Clinical Characteristics of Hypertensive Emergencies**

Blood pressure: usually > 140 mm Hg diastolic
Funduscopic findings: hemorrhages, exudates, papilledema
Neurological status: headache, confusion, somnolence, stupor, visual loss, focal deficits, seizures, coma
Cardiac findings: prominent apical impulse, cardiac enlargement, congestive failure
Renal: oliguria, azotemia
Gastrointestinal: nausea, vomiting

kidneys destroyed, heart failing, and brain function markedly impaired.

The effects of the markedly elevated blood pressure are displayed in the optic fundi as demonstrated in monkeys with induced accelerated-malignant hypertension (Hayreh et al, 1985a,b, 1986). Beyond the chronic arteriolar sclerosis and hypertrophy, acute changes may include: arteriolar spasm, either segmental or diffuse; retinal edema, with a sheen or ripples; retinal hemorrhages, either superficial and flame shaped, or deep and dot shaped; retinal exudates, either hard and waxy from resorption of edema or cotton-wool, soft from ischemia; and papilledema and engorged retinal veins. In the monkeys, pinpoint, round periarteriolar transudates were particularly common, representing leakage from dilated arterioles (Hayreh et al, 1985b). These animals had optic neuropathy that was caused by ischemia of the nerve, leading Hayreh et al (1986) to caution against a precipitous reduction in pressure that could (and has) caused permanent blindness (Cove et al, 1979).

Rarely, enough fibrinoid necrosis occurs within abdominal arteries to produce major gut infarction with an acute abdomen as the presenting feature of malignant hypertension (Padfield, 1975). Rapidly progressive necrotizing vasculitis may present as a hypertensive emergency (O'Connell et al, 1985). An increased association between acute pancreatitis and malignant hypertension with renal failure has also been noted (Barcenas et al, 1978).

## Prognosis

Untreated patients with encephalopathy often become comatose and die. If treated by lowering the blood pressure, the encephalopathy usually dramatically clears. The danger from accelerated-malignant hypertension is not so acute, but if untreated, most patients will die within 6 months. One-year survival was only 10 to 20% without therapy (Keith et al, 1939; Harrington et al, 1959). With current therapy, *5-year* survivals of 60% (Kawazoe et al, 1988), 75% (Yu et al, 1986), and 82% (Bing et al, 1986) are seen, clearly indicative of the major protection provided by antihypertensive therapy.

### Importance of Renal Damage

Many patients when first seen with accelerated-malignant hypertension have significant renal damage, which markedly worsens their prognosis. In one series of 100 consecutive patients with malignant hypertension (Bing et al, 1986), the 5-year survival of those without renal impairment (serum creatinine less than 1.5 mg/dl) was 96%, no different from that of the general population. However, among those with renal impairment, 5-year survival fell to 65%. When vigorous antihypertensive therapy is begun, renal function often worsens transiently, but those who will eventually improve usually begin to do so within 2 weeks (Lawton, 1982). Marked and sustained improvement of renal function may occur after aggressive therapy of patients who present with acute renal failure (Isles et al, 1984), therapy that may need to include dialysis (Bakir et al, 1986).

### Causes of Death

Therapy utilized over the past 35 years has dramatically reduced immediate deaths from acute renal failure, hemorrhagic strokes, and congestive heart failure. With longer survival, death from an acute myocardial infarction is more likely (Barnett and Silberberg, 1973).

## EVALUATION

In addition to an adequate history and physical examination, a few laboratory tests should be done immediately to assess the patient's status (Table 8.3).

## Laboratory Findings

### Hematology and Urine Analysis

*Microangiopathic hemolytic anemia* with red cell fragmentation and intravascular coagulation may occur in accelerated-malignant hypertension, possibly originating from the fibrinoid necrotic arterial lesions (Gavras et al, 1975b).

The urine contains protein and red cells. In a few patients, acute oliguric renal failure may be the presenting manifestation of accelerated-malignant hypertension (Meyrier et al, 1984).

**Table 8.3. Initial Evaluation of Patients with Hypertensive Emergency/Urgency**

History
  Prior diagnosis and treatment of hypertension
  Intake of pressor agents: street drugs, sympathomimetics
  Symptoms of cerebral, cardiac, and visual dysfunction

Physical examination
  Blood pressure
  Funduscopic examination
  Neurological examination
  Cardiopulmonary status
  Body fluid volume assessment

Laboratory evaluation
  Hematocrit and blood smear
  Urine analysis
  Automated chemistry: creatinine, glucose, electrolytes
  Plasma renin and aldosterone (some cases)
  (Repeat plasma renin 1 hour after 25 mg captopril if renovascular hypertension is being considered)
  Spot urine for metanephrine if pheo is being considered
  Chest x-ray
  Electrocardiogram

## Blood Chemistry

Various features of *renal insufficiency* may be present, including metabolic acidosis, marked azotemia, and hypocalcemia.

*Hypokalemia* is present in about half of patients with accelerated-malignant hypertension, reflecting the secondary aldosteronism. Unlike the higher serum sodium level found in primary aldosteronism, this level is usually lower than normal in malignant hypertension.

## Renin-Aldosterone

*Plasma renin activity* (PRA) is usually increased, often to very high levels, in response to the intrarenal ischemia produced by the necrotic vascular lesions (Kawazoe et al, 1987).

*Aldosterone* secretion and excretion are usually increased and return to normal with control of the hypertension (Laragh et al, 1960). A few cases of primary aldosteronism (with solitary adrenal adenomas) have been associated with accelerated-malignant hypertension (Kaplan, 1963).

## Cardiography

The *electrocardiogram* (ECG) usually displays evidence of left ventricular hypertrophy, strain, and lateral ischemia. *Echocardiography* may show incoordinate contractions with impaired diastolic function and delayed mitral valve opening (Shapiro and Beevers, 1983).

## Central Nervous System

The *cerebrospinal fluid* is clear but usually under increased pressure. The *electroencephalogram* (EEG) may show varied, transient, focal, or bilateral disturbances. *Computed tomography* (CT) *scans* have revealed widespread areas of diminished density in the white matter that resolve after therapy and presumably represent focal collections of edema fluid (Rail and Perkin, 1980). *Magnetic resonance imaging* (MRI) shows more extensive, multifocal areas of extravasation (Hauser et al, 1988).

## DIFFERENTIAL DIAGNOSIS

Management of the patient with a hypertensive emergency or urgency usually does not require knowledge of the specific etiology since the first concern is to lower the blood pressure. However, the choice of therapy may differ with the diagnosis. A less aggressive approach may be indicated in patients with suggestive neurological features that represent another problem (Table 8.4).

Similar retinopathy with hemorrhages and even papilledema may, rarely, appear in severe anemia, collagen diseases, and subacute bacterial endocarditis. Some patients have pseudopapilledema associated with congenital anomalies, hyaline bodies (Drusen) in the disc, or severe farsightedness. The use of fluorescein fundus photography has greatly aided the distinction between the true and the pseudo states. In addition, benign intracranial hypertension may produce real papilledema but is usually a minimally symptomatic and self-limited process.

The differential of most of these conditions from a hypertensive crisis is usually rather easy clinically. However, aggressive lowering of the blood pressure should obviously be avoided in

**Table 8.4. Diseases That May Mimic a Hypertensive Emergency**

Acute left ventricular failure
Uremia from any cause, particularly with volume overload
Cerebral vascular accident
Subarachnoid hemorrhage
Brain tumor
Head injury
Epilepsy (postictal)
Collagen diseases, particularly lupus, with cerebral vasculitis
Encephalitis
Acute anxiety with hyperventilation syndrome
Drug ingestion: sympathomimetics (cocaine), phencyclidine
Acute intermittent porphyria
Hypercalcemia

some of the conditions, particularly after a cerebrovascular accident (CVA), when rapid decrease of cerebral blood flow may extend the lesion (Britton et al, 1980).

### Evaluation for Secondary Causes

Once other causes for the presenting picture than severe hypertension are excluded and necessary immediate therapy is provided, an appropriate evaluation for secondary causes for the hypertension should be performed as quickly as possible. It is far easier to obtain necessary blood and urine samples for required laboratory studies *before* institution of therapies that may markedly complicate subsequent evaluation. None of these procedures needs delay effective therapy.

### Renovascular Hypertension

Renovascular hypertension is by far the most likely secondary cause and unfortunately the one that may be least obvious by history, physical examination, and routine laboratory tests. Since the prevalence of renovascular hypertension is so high, there is an even greater need to rule it out before instituting therapy, if that therapy is to include an angiotensin-converting enzyme (ACE) inhibitor. As noted in Chapter 7, the use of ACE inhibitors in patients with bilateral renovascular disease may throw them into acute renal failure whereas those with unilateral renovascular disease may have loss of function of the involved kidney.

As described in Chapter 10, a single-dose captopril challenge test, measuring plasma renin activity before and 1 hour after 25 mg of captopril, appears to be a good screening study. It could be performed at the time the patient presents, since the captopril will almost certainly lower the blood pressure during the subsequent hour, protecting the patient while ruling out (or in) renovascular hypertension.

### Pheochromocytoma

A spot urine should be collected for metanephrine assay since pheochromocytoma is another possible cause and catechol measurements may be completely invalidated by labetalol and other antihypertensives drugs (see Chapter 12).

### Primary Aldosteronism

If significant hypokalemia is noted on the initial blood test, a plasma renin and aldosterone measurement should be obtained to rule out primary aldosteronism (see Chapter 13).

## TREATMENT FOR HYPERTENSIVE EMERGENCIES

When the blood pressure is so high as to threaten life, it should be lowered quickly. The majority of patients with the conditions shown in Table 8.1, e.g., intracerebral hemorrhage or acute myocardial infarction, will not be so hypertensive as to require immediate reduction in blood pressure. However, those with hypertensive encephalopathy must be treated. If the pressure is not reduced, cerebral edema will worsen, and the lack of autoregulation in ischemic brain tissue may result in further increases in the volume of the ischemic tissue, which may cause either acute herniation or more gradual compression of normal brain (Meyer et al, 1972). Moreover, with increased intracranial pressure, the Cushing reflex may cause the systemic pressure to rise further in an attempt to maintain cerebral blood flow (Jones, 1989).

On the other hand, as a result of too rapid lowering of pressure, hypoperfusion of the brain may occur, because of the shift of autoregulation previously described (Strandgaard and Paulson, 1989).

### Initiating Therapy

If the patient is encephalopathic or has evidence of a progressive stroke or myocardial ischemia, no more than a very few minutes should be taken to admit to an intensive care unit, place an intravenous access and, if possible, an intra-arterial line for continuous monitoring of the blood pressure. The initial blood and urine samples should be obtained and antihypertensive therapy should begin immediately thereafter.

### Monitoring Therapy

A number of parenteral (Table 8.5) and oral drugs are available to reduce the blood pressure in minutes. Abrupt falls should be avoided, and the goal of immediate therapy should be to lower the diastolic pressure only to about 110 mm Hg. The reductions may need to be even less if signs of tissue ischemia develop after therapy is begun. Most of the catastrophes seen with treatment of hypertensive emergencies were related to overly aggressive reduction of the blood pressure. In one report of 10 cases of cerebral complications in the treatment of accelerated hypertension, treatment acutely decreased blood pressure an average of 50%, with the diastolic falling below 90 mm Hg in eight of the 10 cases (Ledingham and Rajagopalan, 1979).

The dilemma is portrayed in two studies ap-

**Table 8.5. Parenteral Drugs for Treatment of Hypertensive Emergency (in Order of Rapidity of Action)**

| Drug | Dosage | Onset of Action | Adverse Effects |
|---|---|---|---|
| **Vasodilators** | | | |
| Nitroprusside (Nipride, Nitropress) | 0.25–10 μg/kg/min as IV infusion | Instantaneous | Nausea, vomiting, muscle twitching, sweating, thiocyanate, intoxication |
| Nitroglycerin | 5–100 μg/min as IV infusion | 2–5 min | Tachycardia, flushing, headache, vomiting, methemoglobinemia |
| Diazoxide (Hyperstat) | 50–100 mg/IV bolus repeated, or 15–30 mg/min by IV infusion | 2–4 min | Nausea, hypotension, flushing, tachycardia, chest pain |
| Hydralazine (Apresoline) | 10–20 mg IV / 10–50 mg IM | 10–20 min / 20–30 min | Tachycardia, flushing, headache, vomiting, aggravation of angina |
| Enalaprilat (Vasotec IV) | 1.25–5 mg q 6 hr | 15 min | Precipitous fall in BP in high renin states; response variable |
| Nicardipine | 5–10 mg/hr IV | 10 min | Tachycardia, headache, flushing, local phlebitis |
| **Adrenergic inhibitors** | | | |
| Phentolamine (Regitine) | 5–15 mg IV | 1–2 min | Tachycardia, flushing |
| Trimethaphan (Arfonad) | 0.5–5 mg/min as IV infusion | 1–5 min | Paresis of bowel and bladder, orthostatic hypotension, blurred vision, dry mouth |
| Esmolol (Brevibloc) | 500 μg/kg/min for 4 min, then 150–300 μg/kg/min IV | 1–2 min | Hypotension |
| Propranolol (Inderal) | 1–10 mg load; 3 ng/hr | 1–2 min | Beta-blocker side effect, e.g., bronchospasm, decrease cardiac output |
| Labetalol (Normodyne, Trandate) | 20–80 mg IV bolus every 10 min / 2 mg/min IV infusion | 5–10 min | Vomiting, scalp tingling, burning in throat, postural hypotension, dizziness, nausea |

pearing within 6 weeks of each other: in one, three children with severe *untreated* hypertension suffered permanent neurological damage; there was blindness in all three and paraplegia in one (Hulse et al, 1979); in the other study, blindness occurred in two young women soon after successful (and, in one case, quite gradual) treatment of malignant hypertension (Cove et al, 1979).

Particular care should be taken in elderly patients and in patients with cerebrovascular disease, either stroke or transient ischemic attacks (TIA), who are even more vulnerable to sudden falls in systemic blood pressure (Graham, 1989). As described in the preceding chapter, patients with acute stroke should have their blood pressure brought down only if it is extremely high and contributing to the neurological damage, as in the presence of intracranial hemorrhage (Brott and Reed, 1989).

If the neurological status worsens as treatment proceeds, intracranial pressure may be markedly elevated, most likely from the cerebral edema associated with the hypertensive emergency but also possibly by the further increase in cerebral blood flow invoked by antihypertensive drugs such as hydralazine (Schroeder and Sillesen, 1987) or nitroprusside (Cottrell et al, 1978a), which dilate cerebral vessels. In this situation, intracranial pressure should be measured and, if markedly elevated, reduced by appropriate therapies such as barbiturates, steroids, or osmotic agents (Brott and Reed, 1989).

## Cerebral Adaptation

The brain is relatively protected by a large degree of adaptability, likely developed to maintain the cerebral circulation during times of marked swings in systemic pressure for at least three reasons (Strandgaard and Paulson, 1989):

—Although the autoregulatory curve is shifted to the right in chronic hypertension, pressures can be lowered about 25% before reaching the lower limit, and symptoms may not occur until pressures are lowered another 25%.

—The brain, unlike the heart, can maintain metabolic functions despite a lower perfusion pressure by extracting more oxygen from the blood. Whereas coronary venous blood is usually only about 30% saturated (near the lower limit of oxygen removal), cerebral venous blood is usually about 60 to 70% saturated, so that considerably more oxygen can be extracted.

—As pressures are lowered over time, the structural changes responsible for the rightward shift in autoregulation recede and the curve returns towards normal, thereby improving the tolerance to a lower pressure.

Another factor likely responsible for the relative rarity of cerebral ischemia during therapy is the leftward shift of the lower limit of autoregulation induced by the action of certain antihypertensive drugs on the cerebral vessels. These include alpha-blockers and ACE inhibitors that, in different ways, both dilate large cerebral arteries and increase downstream pressure, causing smaller resistance vessels to constrict so that during a fall in pressure they provide a greater autoregulatory dilatory capacity than normal (Barry, 1989).

### Criteria for Drug Selection

The choice of therapy is based upon rapidity of action, ease of administration, and propensity for side effects. More studies are needed in humans of the effects of these various agents on CBF and autoregulation, intracranial pressure, and most importantly both immediate and eventual outcome.

The data that are available, mostly from animal studies, show that different drugs have different effects on the cerebral circulation (Barry, 1989; Strandgaard and Paulson, 1989) (Table 8.6). For example, diazoxide does not alter CBF until the systemic pressure reaches the lower limit of autoregulation; then CBF falls. Hydralazine raises CBF by directly dilating small resistance vessels, and it causes uneven perfusion and a loss of autoregulation. Captopril resets both the lower and upper limits of autoregulation to lower mean arterial pressures and shortens the autoregulatory plateau. In the words of Strandgaard and Paulson (1989): "From the point of view of the cerebral circulation, $\alpha$-blockers would appear to have the most ideal hemodynamic profile. Good studies of how clin-

ically commonly used $\alpha$-blockers affect CBF are however scant.'' With the use of available techniques to measure global and segmental CBF in man, such data should soon be available to provide more solid guidelines for the choice of an antihypertensive agent in the treatment of different types of hypertensive emergencies.

### Specific Indications (Table 8.7)

Although nitroprusside has been most widely used, the recognition of its propensity to increase intracranial pressure and the availability of additional effective parenteral agents have led me to downplay its use. Similarly, diazoxide seems to have outlived its usefulness and should be discarded along with intramuscular reserpine and intravenous methyldopa (because of their sedative effects). Both nitroprusside and diazoxide obviously work and, in thousands of patients, they have overcome hypertensive emergencies. Nonetheless, equally effective and likely safer agents are now available for the relatively few patients who need parenteral therapy.

Unfortunately there are no comparative studies to document the relative order of the choices listed in Table 8.7. Additional agents, e.g., the postsynaptic dopamine-1 receptor agonist fenoldopan (Bednarczyk et al, 1989), will likely soon be available along with more intravenous alpha-blockers, calcium entry blockers, and ACE inhibitors.

### Acute Aortic Dissection

Hypertension is frequently present in patients who suffer an acute aortic dissection. The usual patient is an elderly man with a long history of hypertension who presents with severe and persistent chest pain. If the event is suspected on clinical grounds, echocardiography or angiography will usually confirm the diagnosis (Erbel et al, 1989).

If the patient is hypertensive, the blood pressure should be reduced to nearly normal in a smooth and gentle manner, avoiding drugs such as direct vasodilators that reflexly stimulate cardiac output and may, thereby, increase the shearing forces that are dissecting the aorta. As described in Chapter 4, the stresses that damage the vessel wall are related not only to the mean pressure but also to the width of the pulse pressure and the maximal rate of rise of the pressure (dp/dt). Drugs that diminish dp/dt, such as trimethaphan or nitroprusside, particularly in com-

**Table 8.6. Effects of Antihypertensive Drugs on Cerebral Circulation in Hypertensive Rats[a]**

| Drug | Effect on Vessels | Effect on Cerebral Blood Flow | Effect on Autoregulation |
|------|-------------------|-------------------------------|--------------------------|
| Diazoxide | No effect[b] | No change[c] | Unchanged |
| Hydralazine Nitroprusside Calcium entry blockers | Dilate small resistance vessels | Increase | May be lost |
| Alpha-adrenergic blockers Ganglion-blockers (trimethaphan) | Dilate larger inflow tract arteries | No change[d] | Shift lower limit to a lower pressure level |
| Angiotensin converting enzyme inhibitors | Dilate large arteries with autoregulatory constriction of small resistance vessels | No change[d] | Shift lower and upper limits to a lower pressure level |

[a]Data from Barry DI: *Am J Cardiol* 63:14C, 1989; Strandgaard S, Paulson OB: *Am J Hypertens* 2:486, 1989.
[b]Diazoxide does not cross the blood-brain barrier.
[c]If systemic pressure is reduced below the lower limit of the cerebral autoregulatory curve, cerebral blood flow will fall proportionally.
[d]The shift of the lower limit of autoregulation enables CBF to be maintained at lower systemic pressures than usual.

bination with a beta-blocker, are the best to treat a dissection (De Sanctis et al, 1987).

The choice of definitive therapy of aortic dissection is usually surgical for those with proximal lesions, but chronic medical therapy seems better for those with distal lesions.

### Need for a Diuretic

An initial assessment of the patient's volume status is crucial. If, on the one hand, the patient is in heart failure or is otherwise obviously overloaded with fluid, a diuretic, usually intravenous furosemide or bumetanide, should be given. On the other hand, if the patient is volume depleted from pressure-induced natriuresis and prior nausea and vomiting, additional diuresis could be dangerous (Kincaid-Smith, 1980). In a few documented instances, volume expansion with intravenous saline has been shown to lower the blood pressure (Kincaid-Smith, 1973; Baer et al, 1977). Most of the patients whose blood pressure improved with salt repletion have had chronic renal disease, and it is likely that they start off with salt-wasting interstitial nephritis, as seen with analgesic nephropathy. However, once the pressure begins to fall, renal sodium retention usually begins, so a potent diuretic will likely then be needed to prevent progressive body fluid expansion.

### Specific Parenteral Drugs (Table 8.5)

#### Nitroprusside

*Clinical Use.* The blood pressure always falls when this drug is given, though it occasionally takes much more than the usual starting dose of 0.25 $\mu$g/kg/min for a response (Palmer and Lasseter, 1975; Cohn and Burke, 1979). The anti-

hypertensive effect disappears within minutes after the drug is stopped. Obviously, the drug should only be used in an intensive care unit, with constant monitoring of the blood pressure. A computer-controlled regulator of the rate of infusion has been described (Meline et al, 1985) but is not generally available.

*Mechanism of Action.* This exogenous nitrate apparently acts in the same manner as the endogenous vasodilator nitric oxide, now thought to be the endothelium-derived relaxing factor (Garg and Hassid, 1989). The drug is a direct arteriolar and venous dilator and has no specific effects—good or bad—on the autonomic or central nervous system (Shepherd and Irvine, 1986). The venous dilation reduces return to the heart causing a fall in cardiac output and stroke volume despite an increase in heart rate, while the arteriolar dilation prevents any rise in peripheral resistance as expected when cardiac output falls. Nitroprusside may cause redistribution of blood flow away from ischemic areas and potentially could increase the extent of myocardial damage in patients with coronary disease (Mann et al, 1978).

*Metabolism and Toxicity.* Nitroprusside is metabolized to cyanide and then to thiocyanate (Schulz, 1984). If high levels of thiocyanate (above 10 mg/100 ml) remain for days, toxicity may be manifested with fatigue, nausea, disorientation, and psychosis. Cyanide toxicity, usually heralded by a metabolic acidosis, may develop with high doses of nitroprusside given for prolonged periods. The high blood cyanide levels may be reduced by infusion of sodium thiosulfate or hydroxocobalamin (Cottrell and Tundorf, 1978).

Table 8.7. **Preferred Parenteral Drugs for Specific Hypertensive Emergencies (in Order of Preference)**

| | Preferred[a] | Avoid (Reason) |
|---|---|---|
| Hypertensive encephalopathy | Labetalol<br>Trimethaphan<br>Nicardipine[b]<br>Nitroprusside<br>Phentolamine | Methyldopa (sedation)<br>Reserpine (sedation)<br>Diazoxide (fall in cerebral<br>  blood flow) |
| Acclerated-malignant hypertension | Labetalol<br>Enalaprilat<br>Nicardipine[b]<br>Nitroprusside | |
| Stroke or head injury | Labetalol<br>Trimethaphan<br>Phentolamine<br>Urapidil[b]<br>Esmolol | Methyldopa (sedation)<br>Reserpine (sedation)<br>Hydralazine (increase<br>  cerebral blood flow)<br>Diazoxide (decrease<br>  cerebral blood flow) |
| Left ventricular failure | Enalaprilat<br>Nitroglycerin<br>Nitroprusside<br>Nicardipine[b] | Labetalol, esmolol, and<br>  other beta-blockers<br>  (decrease cardiac<br>  output) |
| Coronary insufficiency | Nitroglycerin<br>Nitroprusside<br>Labetalol<br>Nicardipine[b]<br>Esmolol | Hydralazine (increase<br>  cardiac work)<br>Diazoxide (increase cardiac<br>  work) |
| Dissecting aortic aneurysm | Trimethaphan<br>Nitroprusside<br>Esmolol | Hydralazine (increase<br>  cardiac output)<br>Diazoxide (increase cardiac<br>  output) |
| Catecholamine excess | Phentolamine<br>Labetalol | All others (less specific) |
| Postoperative | Labetalol<br>Nitroglycerin<br>Esmolol<br>Nicardipine[b]<br>Hydralazine | Trimethaphan (bowel and<br>  bladder atony) |

[a]A loop diuretic will usually be needed, initially when fluid volume overload is present, or subsequently if reactive fluid retention occurs.
[b]Parenteral form not yet approved in United States.

## Nitroglycerin

Intravenous nitroglycerin is being used increasingly for coronary vasodilation in patients with myocardial ischemia with or without severe hypertension, as well as for controlled hypotension during neurosurgical anesthesia (Cottrell et al, 1978). Methemoglobin is formed during the administration of all organic nitrates, but its mean concentration in patients receiving nitroglycerin for 48 hours or longer averaged only 1.5%, with no clinical symptoms (Kaplan et al, 1985).

## Diazoxide

*Mechanism of Action.* A congener of the thiazide diuretics, diazoxide dilates the resistance arteries but not the capacitance veins. At the same time, it increases cardiac output and rate, even in the presence of beta-adrenergic blockade with propranolol (Mroczek et al, 1976).

Since it does not cross the blood-brain barrier, it has no effects on the cerebral circulation, but cerebral blood flow will fall if systemic pressure is reduced below the lower limit of autoregulation (Table 8.6).

*Clinical Use.* Diazoxide was initially given as a 300-mg bolus within 10 to 30 seconds to enhance its antihypertensive effect, but the immediate, rather precipitous 30% or greater fall in blood pressure induced some episodes of cerebral and myocardial ischemia (Kanada et al, 1976; Kumar et al, 1976; Henrich et al, 1977). The safer course is to give the drug either by slow infusion over 15 to 30 minutes (Garrett and Kaplan, 1982) or by smaller bolus doses, 75 to 100 mg intravenously, every 5 to 10 minutes (Ram and Kaplan, 1979).

*Side Effects and Cautions.* These include fluid retention, nausea, flushing, dizziness, and a propensity, with repeated doses, to hyperglycemia reflecting a direct suppression of insulin secretion (Greenwood et al, 1976).

## Hydralazine

The major advantage of this direct vasodilator as a parenteral drug is for the physician, since it can be given by repeated intramuscular injections as well as intravenously with a fairly slow onset and prolonged duration of action. Significant increases in cardiac output preclude its use as a sole agent except in very young patients, e.g., toxemia of pregnancy, who can handle the increased output without inducing ischemia, or very old patients who may not experience the reflex sympathetic discharge and consequent rise in cardiac output because of diminished baroreceptor activity.

## Trimethaphan

This agent has been popular with anesthesiologists, but, in addition to the problems of generalized autonomic nervous system blockade, it may rarely cause respiratory paralysis (Dale and Schroeder, 1976). Trimethaphan may be the drug of choice with dissecting aneurysms of the aorta (Palmer and Lasseter, 1976).

## Labetalol

The combined alpha-beta-blocker labetalol has been found to be both safe and effective when given intravenously either by repeated bolus (Wilson et al, 1983) (Fig. 8.5) or by continuous infusion (Wright et al, 1986). It starts acting within 5 minutes and lasts for 3 to 6 hours. The oral form can then be used to provide long-term control. Labetalol can likely be used in almost any situation requiring parenteral antihypertensive therapy such as postcoronary bypass surgery (Skrobic et al, 1989). Caution is needed to avoid postural hypotension if patients are allowed out of bed. Nausea, itching, and tingling of the skin and beta-blocker side effects may be noted.

Dilevalol, the stereoisomer of labetalol, is also an effective parenteral agent (Bursztyn et al, 1989).

## Esmolol

This relatively cardioselective beta-blocker is rapidly metabolized by blood esterases, thereby providing a very short (about 9-minute) half-life and total duration of action (about 30 minutes). Its effects begin almost immediately, and it has found particular use during anesthesia (Gold et al, 1989) and the postoperative period (Gibson et al, 1988).

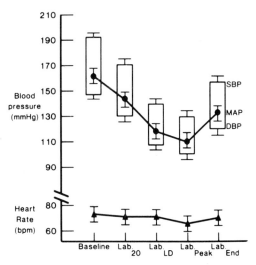

**Figure 8.5.** The effects of labetalol in 59 patients with initial BP > 200/125 mm Hg. The average blood pressure and heart rate are shown at baseline, after the first 20-mg minibolus of labetalol ($Lab_{20}$), after the last dose of labetalol ($Lab_{LD}$); the lowest blood pressures recorded after the last injection ($Lab_{PEAK}$); and the blood pressures and heart rate just prior to initiation of oral labetalol ($Lab_{END}$) for the total 59 patients in the study. (From Wilson DJ, Wallin JD, Vlachakis ND, et al: *Am J Med* 75:95, 1983.)

## Enalaprilat

This intravenous preparation of the active, free form of the prodrug enalapril will likely be used increasingly for treatment of hypertensive emergencies wherein ACE inhibition is thought to offer special advantages, such as congestive heart failure (Hornung and Hillis, 1987).

The previously noted, apparently unique effects of ACE inhibitors on cerebral autoregulation, resetting the autoregulatory curve to a lower pressure level, could protect against cerebral ischemia if pressure is lowered abruptly and markedly (Barry, 1989). On the other hand, the possibility of allowing greater hyperperfusion to occur if pressures stay high while the upper limit of autoregulation is reduced likely is not a real concern. As Barry (1989) states, "There is no evidence for a similar shift in the upper limit of autoregulation in awake humans. This is probably because most sudden increases in blood pressure are accompanied by sympathetic activation that counteracts the loss of angiotensin II-induced tone in the large brain vessels, enabling the patient to tolerate high blood pressure without loss of autoregulation."

## Nicardipine

When given by continuous infusion, the intravenous formulation of this dihydropyridine calcium entry blocker (CEB) produces a steady, progressive fall in blood pressure with a modest reflex tachycardia (Wallin et al, 1989). All CEBs may also increase cerebral blood flow, but one with a greater selectivity for cerebral vessels, nimodipine, has been approved for use to relieve the vasospasm that accompanies subarachnoid hemorrhage (Gelmers et al, 1988).

### Other Drugs

Parenteral *reserpine* and *methyldopa* have few advantages and many side effects. The alpha-blocker *phentolamine* is specifically indicated for pheochromocytoma or tyramine-induced catecholamine crisis.

## THERAPY OF HYPERTENSIVE URGENCIES

The hypertensive urgencies (Table 8.1) can usually be managed with oral therapy. This includes most patients with accelerated-malignant hypertension, except for those unable to swallow.

### Issue of Need

An even larger number of patients will be seen who are not true hypertensive urgencies but who simply have very high blood pressure, i.e., above 200/120 mm Hg. The prudent physician may prefer to ensure the patient's responsiveness to oral therapy before having the patient leave the office or emergency room with a prescription for one or more oral drugs. This holds true even for those patients who have been seen in similar circumstances many times before but who do not adhere to chronic treatment since they, too, may become truly resistant to therapy. Although most such patients could be safely started on one or more oral drugs and sent home to return in 24 or 48 hours for confirmation of their responsiveness, it may be preferable to observe them for a few hours after administration of an antihypertensive drug to ensure responsiveness. A group of such patients was first given 0.2 mg of clonidine and 25 mg chlorthalidone and then randomly assigned either to hourly clonidine until their diastolic blood pressures were below 105 mm Hg or to placebo (Zeller et al, 1989). When seen 24 hours later, their blood pressures were equally well controlled signifying that repeated loading therapy and prolonged observation are likely only rarely needed in asymptomatic patients with severe hypertension.

## Choice of Therapy

Virtually all oral antihypertensive agents have been tried and found to be effective in the treatment of severe hypertension (Opie, 1987). None is clearly better than the rest, and a combination will often be needed for long-term control. However, the three most widely used choices are nifedipine (and likely nicardipine), captopril, and clonidine (Table 8.8). Complete information about these oral drugs is provided in Chapter 7.

### Nifedipine

For years, this calcium entry blocker has been widely used for the treatment of hypertensive urgencies. Another oral dihydropyridine CEB, nicardipine, has been approved and likely more will soon become available.

Nifedipine will effectively and usually safely lower blood pressure after a single 5- to 10-mg oral dose. Results from one study of 25 consecutive patients with very high pressure given 10 to 20 mg by mouth are shown in Figure 7.30 (Bertel et al, 1983).

As might be expected with any drug that induces such a significant fall in blood pressure, occasional symptomatic hypotension can occur, but this has been quite rare when the drug is given in no more than a 10-mg initial dose (Friedman, 1987). The drug is effective even more quickly when the capsule is chewed and the contents swallowed as when it is squirted under the tongue (van Harten et al, 1987). For a slightly slower and probably safer effect, the sublingual route should be used.

### Captopril

This is the fastest acting of the three oral ACE inhibitors now available and it can also be used sublingually in patients who cannot swallow (Hauger-Klevene, 1986). As noted earlier in this chapter, captopril may be particularly attractive since it shifts the entire curve of cerebral autoregulation to the left, so cerebral blood flow should be well maintained as the systemic pressure falls (Barry, 1989).

Abrupt and marked first dose hypotension has been observed in patients with high renin status given an ACE inhibitor (Webster et al, 1985). Caution is advised in patients who have significant renal insufficiency or who are volume depleted.

### Clonidine

This central alpha-agonist has been widely used in repeated hourly doses to safely and effectively reduce very high blood pressure (An-

**Table 8.8. Oral Drugs for Hypertensive Urgencies**

| Drug | Class | Dose | Onset | Duration |
|------|-------|------|-------|----------|
| Nifedipine (Procardia; Adalat) | Calcium entry blocker | 5–10 mg sublingual or swallowed | 5–15 min | 3–5 hr |
| Captopril (Capoten) | Angiotensin converting enzyme inhibitor | 6.5–50 mg | 15 min | 4–6 hr |
| Clonidine (Catapres; others) | Central sympatholytic | 0.2 mg initial then 0.1 mg/hr, up to 0.8 mg total | ½–2 hr | 6–8 hr |

derson et al, 1981). It works slower than nifedipine but eventually brings the pressure down about as well (Jaker et al, 1989).

Significant sedation is the major side effect that contraindicates its use in patients with central nervous system involvement. Since it has a somewhat greater proclivity than other drugs to cause rebound hypertension if it is suddenly discontinued, caution is advised in its use among patients with severe hypertension who have shown themselves to be poorly compliant with therapy.

### Other Drugs

*Prazosin.* This alpha-blocker in a single oral dose of 2 mg produced a steady and significant fall in blood pressure, maximal by 2 hours (Yagil et al, 1983). The fall was slower than that seen with 10 mg of nifedipine but was eventually of a greater magnitude.

*Minoxidil.* Although too slow for use by itself in treatment of hypertensive urgencies, minoxidil in a dose of 20 mg was given 2 hours after a combination of 40 mg of oral propranolol and 40 mg of oral furosemide (Alpert and Bauer, 1982). The blood pressures fell smoothly and remained down for at least 24 hours thereafter.

*Beta-Blockers.* Other than intravenous esmolol, these drugs are also too slow for true hypertensive urgencies, but they will usually be equally effective as other oral drugs after 4 to 6 hours (Isles et al, 1986).

### Possible Danger of Salt Depletion

As with the use of parenteral drugs for hypertensive emergencies, diuretics, specifically large doses of furosemide or bumetanide intravenously, are often needed in patients with hypertensive urgencies, both to lower the blood pressure by getting rid of excess volume and to prevent the loss of potency from other antihypertensives because of their tendency to cause fluid retention. However, volume depletion may be overdone, particularly in those who start off with a shrunken fluid volume. Thereby renin secretion may be further increased, producing more intensive vasoconstriction and worsening the hypertension.

### Special Circumstances

The management of hypertensive emergencies and urgencies in a number of special circumstances is considered elsewhere. These include renal insufficiency (Chapter 9), toxemia of pregnancy (Chapter 11), pheochromocytoma (Chapter 12), and drug abuse (Chapter 15). The management of children and adolescents is covered in Chapter 16.

## MANAGEMENT AFTER THE EMERGENCY/URGENCY

### Evaluation for Secondary Causes

After the patient is out of danger, a careful search should continue for possible secondary causes, as delineated under Evaluation. Secondary causes are much more likely in patients with severe hypertension, in particular renovascular hypertension, which was present in one-third of the Vanderbilt series of patients with malignant hypertension (Davis et al, 1979).

### Chronic Therapy

Most patients will likely end up on multiple drug therapy. All of the guidelines delineated in Chapter 7 should be followed to ensure adherence to effective therapy.

Now that the background and therapy of primary hypertension and its rare end stage of accelerated-malignant hypertension have been covered, we will look in depth at the various secondary forms of hypertension, starting with the most common: renal parenchymal disease.

**References**

Ahmed MEK, Walker JM, Beevers DG, et al: *Br Med J* 292:235, 1986.
Alpert MA, Bauer JH: *Arch Intern Med* 142:2099, 1982.

Anderson RJ, Hart GR, Crumpler CP, et al: *JAMA* 246:848, 1981.
Baer L, Parra-Carrillo JZ, Radichevich I, et al: *Ann Intern Med* 86:257, 1977.

Bakir AA, Bazilinski N, Dunea G: *Am J Med* 80:172, 1986.
Barcenas CG, Gonzalez-Molina M, Hull AR: *Arch Intern Med* 138:1254, 1978.

Barnett AJ, Silberberg FG: *Med J Aust* 2:960, 1973.

Barry DI: *Am J Cardiol* 63:14C, 1989.

Bednarczyk EM, White WB, Munger MA, et al: *Am J Cardiol* 63:993, 1989.

Beilin LJ, Goldby FS: *Clin Sci Mol Med* 52:111, 1977.

Bennett NM, Shea S: *Am J Public Health* 78:636, 1988.

Bertel O, Conen D, Radu EW, et al: *Br Med J* 286:19, 1983.

Bing RF, Heagerty AM, Russell GI, et al: *J Hypertension* 4(Suppl 6):S42, 1986.

Britton M, de Faire U, Helmers C: *Acta Med Scand* 207:253, 1980.

Brott T, Reed RL: *Stroke* 24:1, 1989.

Bursztyn M, Gavras I, Blasucci DJ, et al: *J Cardiovasc Pharmacol* 13:799, 1989.

Byrom FB: *Prog Cardiovasc Dis* 17:31, 1974.

Cohn JN, Burke LP: *Ann Intern Med* 91:752, 1979.

Cottrell JE, Patel K, Turndorf H, et al: *J Neurosurg* 48:329, 1978.

Cottrell JE, Tundorf H: *Am Heart J* 96:550, 1978.

Cove DG, Seddon M, Fletcher RF, et al: *Br Med J* 2:245:1979.

Dale RC, Schroeder ET: *Arch Intern Med* 136:816, 1976.

De Sanctis RW, Doroghazi RM, Austen WG, et al: *N Engl J Med* 317:1060, 1987.

Davis BA, Crook JE, Vestal RE, et al: *N Engl J Med* 301:1273, 1979.

Dzau VJ, Siwek LG, Rosen S, et al: *Hypertension* 3(Suppl I):I-63, 1981.

Erbel R, Daniel W, Visser C, et al: *Lancet* 1:457, 1989.

Folkow B: *Am Heart J* 114:938, 1987.

Friedman CP: *Arch Intern Med* 147:1683, 1987.

Garg UC, Hassid A: *J Clin Invest* 83:1774, 1989.

Garrett BN, Kaplan NM: *Am Heart J* 103:390, 1982.

Gavras H, Brunner HR, Laragh JH, et al: *Circ Res* 36:300, 1975a.

Gavras H, Oliver N, Aitchison J, et al: *Kidney Int* 8:S-252, 1975b.

Gelmers HJ, Gorter K, de Weerdt CJ, et al: *N Engl J Med* 318:203, 1988.

Gibson BE, Black S, Maass L, et al: *Clin Pharmacol Ther* 44:650, 1988.

Giese J: *Acta Pathol Microbiol Scand* 62:497, 1964.

Gold MI, Sacks DJ, Grosnoff DB, et al: *Anesth Analg* 68:101, 1989.

Graham DI: *Am J Cardiol* 63:6C, 1989.

Greenwood RH, Mahler RF, Hales CN: *Lancet* 1:444, 1976.

Gross F, Dietz R, Mast GH, et al: *Clin Exp Pharmacol Physiol* 2:323, 1975.

Harrington M, Kincaid-Smith P, McMichael P: *Br Med J* 2:969, 1959.

Hauger-Klevene JH: *Lancet* 1:219, 1986.

Hauser RA, Lacey M, Knight MR: *Arch Neurol* 45:1078, 1988.

Hayreh SS, Servais GE, Virdi PS: *Ophthalmology* 92:60, 1985b.

Hayreh SS, Servais GE, Virdi PS, et al: *Ophthalmology* 92:45, 1985a.

Hayreh SS, Servais GE, Virdi PS: *Ophthalmology* 93:74, 1986.

Heistad DD: *Fed Proc* 43:205, 1984.

Henrich WL, Cronin R, Miller PD, et al: *JAMA* 237:264, 1977.

Hilme E, Herlitz H, Söderström T, et al: *J Hypertension* 7:91, 1989.

Hiwatari M, Abrahams JM, Saito T, et al: *Clin Sci* 70:191, 1986.

Hornung RS, Hillis WS: *Br J Clin Pharmacol* 23:29, 1987.

Hulse JA, Taylor DSI, Dillon MJ: *Lancet* 2:553, 1979.

Isles C, Brown JJ, Cumming AMM, et al: *Br Med J* 1:579, 1979.

Isles CG, Johnson AOC, Milne FJ: *Br J Clin Pharmacol* 21:377, 1986.

Isles CG, McLay A, Boulton Jones JM: *QJ Med* 53:439, 1984.

Jaker M, Atkin S, Soto M, et al: *Arch Intern Med* 149:260, 1989.

Johansson B, Strandgaard S, Lassen NA: *Circ Res* (Suppl I)34 and 35:I-167, 1974.

Jones DB: *Lab Invest* 13:303, 1974.

Jones JV: *Am J Cardiol* 63:10C, 1989.

Kanada SA, Kanada DJ, Hutchinson RA, et al: *Ann Intern Med* 84:696, 1976.

Kaplan KJ, Taber M, Teagarden JR, et al: *Am J Cardiol* 55:181, 1985.

Kaplan NM: *N Engl J Med* 269:1282, 1963.

Kawazoe N, Eto T, Abe I, et al: *Clin Cardiol* 10:513, 1987.

Kawazoe N, Eto T, Abe I, et al: *Clin Nephrol* 29:53, 1988.

Keith NM, Wagener HP, Barker NW: *Am J Med Sci* 197:332, 1939.

Kincaid-Smith P: *Am J Cardiol* 32:575, 1973.

Kincaid-Smith P: *Pharmacol Ther* 9:245, 1980.

Kontos HA, Wei EP, Dietrich WD, et al: *Am J Physiol* 240:H511, 1981.

Kumar GK, Dastoor FC, Robayo JR, et al: *JAMA* 235:275, 1976.

Laragh JH, Ulick S, Januszewicz W, et al: *J Clin Invest* 39:1091, 1960.

Lawton WJ: *Clin Nephrol* 17:277, 1982.

Ledingham JGG, Rajagopalan B: *Q J Med* 48:25, 1979.

Liu LX, Rustgi AK: *Am J Med* 82:1060, 1987.

MacKenzie ET, Strandgaard S, Graham DI, et al: *Circ Res* 39:33, 1976.

Mann T, Cohn PF, Holman BL, et al: *Circulation* 57:732, 1978.

Mayhan WG, Faraci FM, Siems JL, et al: *Circ Res* 64:658, 1989.

Meline LJ, Westenskow DR, Pace NL, et al: *Anesth Analg* 64:38, 1985.

Meyer JS, Teraura T, Marx P, et al: *Brain* 95:833, 1972.

Meyrier A, Laaban JP, Kanfer A: *Br Med J* 288:1045, 1984.

Möhring J: *Clin Sci Mol Med* 52:113, 1977.

Mroczek WJ, Lee WR, Davidov ME, et al: *Circulation* 53:985, 1976.

O'Connell MT, Kubrusly DB, Fournier AM: *Arch Intern Med* 145:265, 1985.

Opie LH: *Practical Cardiol* 13:110, 1987.

Padfield PL: *Br Med J* 3:353, 1975.

Palmer RF, Lasseter KC: *N Engl J Med* 292:294, 1975.

Palmer RF, Lasseter KC: *N Engl J Med* 394:1403, 1976.

Pentel P: *JAMA* 252:1898, 1984.

Rail DL, Perkin GD: *Arch Neurol* 37:310, 1980.

Ram CVS, Kaplan NM: *Am J Cardiol* 43:627, 1979.

Schroeder T, Sillesen H: *Eur J Clin Invest* 17:214, 1987.

Schulz V: *Clin Pharmacokinet* 9:239, 1984.

Shapiro LM, Beevers DG: *Br Heart J* 49:477, 1983.

Shepherd AMM, Irvine NA: *J Cardiovasc Pharmacol* 8:527, 1986.

Skrobic J, Cruise C, Webster R, et al: *Am J Hypertens* 2:74A, 1989 (abst).

Strandgaard S, MacKenzie ET, Jones JV, et al: *Stroke* 7:287, 1976.

Strandgaard S, Olesen J, Skinhj E, et al: *Br Med J* 1:507, 1973.

Strandgaard S, Paulson OB: *Am J Hypertens* 2:486, 1989.

van Harten J, Burggraaf K, Danhof M, et al: *Lancet* 1:1363, 1987.

Virmani R, Robinowitz M, Smialek JE, et al: *Am Heart J* 115:1068, 1988.

Wallin JD, Fletcher E, Ram CVS, et al: *Arch Intern Med* 149:2662, 1989.

Webster J, Newnham DM, Petrie JC: *Br Med J* 290:1623, 1985.

Wilson DJ, Wallin JD, Vlachakis ND, et al: *Am J Med* 75:95, 1983.

Wollner L, McCarthy ST, Soper NDW, et al: *Br Med J* 1:1117, 1979.

Wright JT, Wilson DJ, Goodman RP, et al: *J Clin Hypertens* 1:39, 1986.

Yagil Y, Kobrin I, Stessman J, et al: *Isr J Med Sci* 19:277, 1983.

Yu S-H, Whitworth JA, Kincaid-Smith PS: *Clin Exp Theory Practice* A8:1211, 1986.

Zeller KZ, Kuhnert LV, Matthews CA: *Arch Intern Med* 149:2186, 1989.

# 9 Renal Parenchymal Hypertension

## RELATIONSHIP BETWEEN THE KIDNEYS AND HYPERTENSION

In 1914, Volhard and Fahr proposed that all hypertension was secondary to renal disease. This view was widely accepted until the 1940s when Talbott and Smith showed that renal damage was the result, rather than the cause, of primary (essential) hypertension. Nevertheless, the kidney is of importance in most forms of hypertension. As described in Chapter 3, a defect in renal function is almost certainly involved in the pathogenesis of primary hypertension. Moreover, chronic renal disease is the most common cause of secondary hypertension. As shown in Table 1.11, chronic renal disease is the diagnosis in 2 to 5% of all hypertensive patients, ranking above renovascular disease and far above primary aldosteronism and pheochromocytoma. As evidence for the contribution of one form of chronic renal disease—pyelonephritis—as a cause of hypertension recedes, evidence for a major role of another—diabetic nephropathy—has risen.

More important than the fact that renal parenchymal disease is the most common cause of secondary hypertension is the fact that patients with primary hypertension almost always develop renal damage and thereby have a worse prognosis. Even patients with fairly mild hypertension and none of the usual findings of renal damage often have microalbuminuria and a blunted reserve of renal function (Losito et al, 1988). Most hypertensives, by 5 years after their diagnosis, have arteriographically demonstrable nephrosclerosis, even though the usual indices of renal function are normal (Hollenberg et al, 1969). The presence of even lesser degrees of renal damage that commonly occur in the course of primary hypertension is a powerful predictor of mortality, independent of other known risk factors. Among the 10,940 participants in the Hypertension Detection and Follow-up Program, baseline serum creatinine was closely related to 8-year mortality (Shulman et al, 1989) (Fig. 9.1). Even slightly elevated serum creatines clearly were associated with increased subsequent mortality, despite the fact that almost all of these patients were intensively treated and closely followed over the 8-year follow-up period.

When looked at from the other perspective—the contribution of various diseases to the incidence of end-stage renal disease (ESRD)—the role of hypertension looks even more ominous. In 1986, the number of people in the United States receiving therapy for ESRD reached 112,000, at a cost of $2.5 billion per year. The contributions of hypertension per se and of a process intimately associated with hypertension—diabetic nephropathy—have progressively increased (Whelton and Klag, 1989) (Fig. 9.2). In 1985, among all new ESRD patients diabetic nephropathy was the diagnosis in 30% and hypertension in 26% (Teutsch et al, 1989).

Thus, it is obvious that some degree of renal damage is common in hypertension and that hypertension is responsible for a large portion of

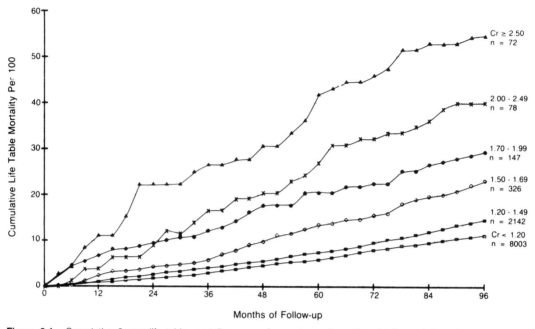

**Figure 9.1.** Cumulative 8-year life table mortality curves (percentage at months of follow-up) for selected strata of baseline serum creatinine. The sample size (*n*) and the creatinine stratum limits (mg/dl) are noted to the right of each curve. (From Shulman NB, Ford CE, Hall WD, et al: Prognostic value of serum creatinine and effect of treatment of hypertension on renal function. *Hypertension* 13(Suppl I):I-80, 1989 and by permission of the American Heart Association, Inc.)

renal failure so that the kidney is both the victim and the culprit. As described in Chapter 3, two models for extensive renal involvement in the pathogenesis of primary hypertension have considerable experimental support. Clinically, there is often a vicious cycle: Hypertension causes renal damage that causes more hypertension. The cycle can be broken by effective antihypertensive therapy if it is provided before the degree of renal damage is too extensive.

Usually, the role of the kidneys in the pathogenesis of hypertension is directed toward its *pressor* functions having gone awry, centered in the renin-angiotensin mechanism (see Chapter 3). However, the role of the kidneys may also involve a loss of *depressor* functions, as will be described before the varieties of renal disease are considered.

## VASODEPRESSORS OF RENAL ORIGIN

### Prostaglandins

Prostaglandins (PGs) were discovered in 1930 (Kurzrok and Lieb, 1930) and were shown to be vasodepressors soon thereafter (Goldblatt, 1933; von Euler, 1934). Their biosynthesis was worked out mainly by Bergstrom and Samuelsson in Sweden and Vane in England who also

discovered the inhibition of cyclooxygenase by aspirin (Vane, 1983).

The various PGs have different sites or origin and different effects on the blood pressure. Thromboxanes promote platelet aggregation, constrict vascular smooth muscle, and may inhibit sodium excretion. Prostacyclin, synthesized within the blood vessel wall, inhibits platelet aggregation, relaxes vascular smooth muscle, and by reducing renal vascular resistance may promote a natriuresis. $PGE_2$ is vasodilatory, $PGF_{2\alpha}$ vasoconstrictive.

### Prostaglandins and Primary Hypertension

There are numerous findings suggesting a role of PGs in primary hypertension, as summarized by Stoff (1986) (Table 9.1). The evidence, though it looks impressive, has actually added up to the general impression that PGs likely are not major players in primary hypertension although they clearly are important in circulatory control and thrombosis (Oates et al, 1988). This may be true because PGs are autocoids, i.e., they are synthesized to have a local (not systemic) effect. Their primary area of involvement in hypertension may be within the kidney.

*Renal Prostaglandins.* The kidney synthe-

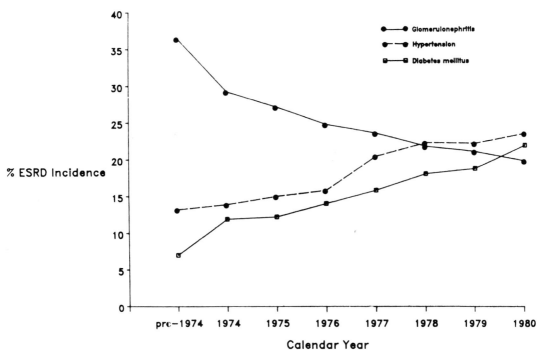

% ESRD Incidence

**Figure 9.2.** Plot of temporal trends in proportional incidence rates of provider-reported underlying cause of end stage renal disease (*ESRD*). (From Whelton PK, Klag MJ: *Hypertension* 13(Suppl I):I-19, 1989 [Adapted from Health Care Financing Administration, 1985].)

**Table 9.1. Evidence for the Role of Prostaglandins in Essential Hypertension[a]**

Decreased urinary excretion of prostaglandin $E_2$ and 6-keto-prostaglandin $F_{1\alpha}$
Increased urinary excretion of thromboxane $B_2$
Increased plasma prostaglandin $E_2$
Increased total peripheral resistance after indomethacin
Increased renal vascular resistance after indomethacin
Small increase in blood pressure in normotensive or untreated hypertensive patients after nonsteroidal antiinflammatory drug therapy
Increased blood pressure in patients treated with antihypertensive medications after nonsteroidal antiinflammatory drug therapy
Diets enriched in polyunsaturated fatty acids reduce blood pressure

[a]From Stoff JS: *Am J Med* 80(Suppl 1A): 56, 1986.

sizes several different PGs. Which of the PGs is physiologically important remains in question since considerable interconversion occurs between them, and most assays, until recently, have been nonspecific. Intrarenal vasodilatory PGs attenuate the renal response to various vasoconstrictor stimuli, including angiotensin, norepinephrine, and renal nerve stimulation (Olsen et al, 1987). Thus the major function of intrarenal prostaglandins is to sustain the renal circulation in the face of any situation wherein it is threatened.

## Effects of PG Inhibitors

Much of what is known about PGs in general and about their renal effects in particular come from studies after their synthesis is inhibited by aspirin and other nonsteroidal antiinflammatory drugs (NSAIDs). Multiple changes in renal function occur (Carmichael and Shankel, 1985) (Fig. 9.3).

*NSAIDs and Volume.* Under euvolemic circumstances, inhibition of the PG system by NSAIDs is without effect on the general circulation and the kidneys. However, when the PG system would normally be activated, either as a result of vasoconstrictor stimuli or in response to the actions of diuretics and other antihypertensive agents, the use of NSAIDs may result in fluid retention that may raise the blood pressure.

*NSAIDs and Antihypertensives.* NSAIDs may also interfere with the action of various antihypertensive drugs (Patrono and Dunn, 1987). Diuretics are the most commonly recognized (Patak et al, 1975), but beta-blockers (Beckmann et al, 1988) and ACE inhibitors (Salvetti et al, 1982) may also be affected.

*Aspirin and Sulindac.* Aspirin (in usual

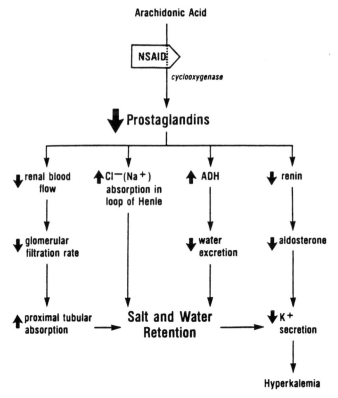

**Figure 9.3.** Changes in renal function following nonsteroidal antiinflammatory drugs (*NSAID*). *ADH*, antidiuretic hormone. (From Carmichael J, Shankel SW: *Am J Med* 78:992, 1985.)

doses) may not reduce renal PG synthesis because less is delivered to the kidney (de Gaetano et al, 1986); and sulindac (Clinoril) may produce less renal PG inhibition because the active sulfide metabolite is converted to an inactive metabolite by mixed function oxidases in the kidney (Patrono and Dunn, 1987). However, renal PG inhibition may be seen with any NSAID.

### PGs as Antihypertensives

Whether or not they are involved in the pathogenesis of hypertension, the vasodilatory and renal effects of PGs give them the potential to be attractive antihypertensive agents. An intravenous form of prostacyclin is available but must be given continuously, and it induces significant side effects. A stable, transdermally absorbed PGE$_2$ analogue, CL115.347, has been shown to lower blood pressure modestly but its effects were largely overcome by compensatory increases in vasoconstrictor hormones and sodium retention (Given et al, 1986). Another agent, cicletanine, which stimulates PGI$_2$ synthesis, may

have some effect when given orally (Hornych et al, 1988).

### Medullipin: The Renomedullary Vasodepressor Lipid

After 40 years of persistent work, Muirhead and coworkers (1989) seem to have documented both the existence and the role of a substance secreted from renal medullary cells. It appears to function as a counterbalance to the effects of angiotensin II, whose origin is from the action of renin, a substance secreted from renal cortical cells. The renomedullary hormone, called medullipin I, requires activation by the cytochrome P-450-dependent enzyme system of the liver into medullipin II.

The structure of this hormone remains unknown but its existence has been strongly inferred from multiple experiments, mainly involving rat kidneys. One set of these involve the effects of renal venous effluent collected after reversal of two-kidney, one-clip renovascular hypertension. The effluent induces vasodilation, reduced efferent renal sympathetic nerve activity, and natriuresis (Göthberg et al, 1982). These are identical to the effects of the reno-medullary lipid (Muirhead et al, 1989). Another study from Sweden has shown activation of a humoral antihypertensive system from a rat kidney exposed abruptly to a sharp rise in perfusion pressure (Karlström et al, 1988).

Thus, there appears to be a humoral renal vasodepressor substance in rats whose secretion is controlled by renal perfusion pressure. The actions of the renomedullary lipid are not inhibited by inhibition of both prostaglandins and kinins, pointing further to its separate status (Muirhead et al, 1989). Whether it functions under normal circumstances and is involved in various human hypertensive diseases remains to be seen.

### Platelet-Activating Factor

Another vasoactive lipid was discovered during the search for the renomedullary vasodepressors (Muirhead et al, 1983). This one was determined to be a glyceryl ether of phosphatidyl choline, which in turn was found to be the same as the platelet-activating factor (PAF) (Schlondorff and Neuwirth, 1986).

### Kallikrein-Kinin System

The fourth vasodepressor mechanism that could be involved in renoprival hypertension is the kallikrein-kinin system (Fig. 9.4). The kallikrein enzyme is of two forms: (1) plasma kallikrein, with a molecular weight of 100,000, is involved in coagulation and may be involved in blood pressure regulation; (2) glandular kallikrein, having a smaller molecular weight and found in multiple organs but in highest concentrations in the kidney where it is found close to the juxtaglomerular apparatus (Vio et al, 1988), suggesting possible interactions between the kinin and renin systems. The excretion of kallikrein into the urine is familial and those with the highest urinary levels tend to have normotensive parents (Berry et al, 1989). These investigators conclude that "a dominant allele expressed as high total urinary kallikrein excretion may be associated with decreased risk of essential hypertension."

Kallikrein acts upon the kininogen substrate to release bradykinins (Fig 9.4). These kinins may be involved in the control of blood flow, electrolyte excretion, and blood pressure (Carretero and Scicli, 1988). Although much is known about the genetic regulation of kallikrein and kininogen synthesis (Margolius, 1989), very little is known about the functions of the vasoactive products, the bradykinins. This is largely because they have been so difficult to measure, appearing to be mainly paracrine hormones with evanescent survival in the circulation.

Interest in the kinins has risen with the recognition that the peptidase that inactivates bradykinin, kininase II, is the same peptide that serves as the angiotensin-converting enzyme

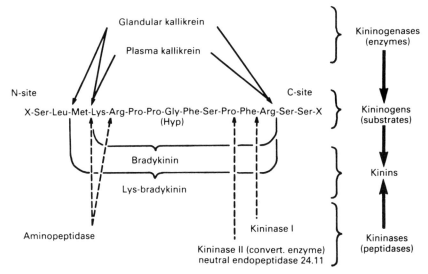

**Figure 9.4.** Site of kininogen cleavage (*solid arrows*) by the main kininogenases (glandular and plasma kallikrein). Site of kinin cleavage (*broken arrows*) by kininases (kininase I and II, neutral peptidase, and aminopeptidase). (From Carretero OA, Scicli AG: *Kidney Int* 34(Suppl 26):S-52, 1988 and reprinted from *Kidney International* with permission.)

(ACE) (Fig. 9.4). This is the enzyme inhibited by ACE inhibitors, which obviously would also block the inactivation of bradykinin. It may be that the rise in vasodepressor bradykinin after ACE inhibition is involved in the antihypertensive effect of the ACE inhibitors at least in part because bradykinin also stimulates synthesis of PGs (Carretero and Scicli, 1988).

### A Note of Caution About Intrarenal Vasodilators

Most of the effects of these intrarenal vasodilatory substances are likely autocrine or paracrine, exerted within or close to their sites of origin. The predominantly local effects of these hormones make it hazardous to assume that the findings of most studies done with them have pathophysiological meaning. Moreover, we have just begun to unravel what is likely a very complex set of interactions among these various local hormones.

We will now examine specific varieties of renal disease and how they relate to hypertension, starting from one extreme—the total absence of renal tissue—and going to the other—the presence of only unilateral renal involvement. Renovascular hypertension and renin-secreting tumors are covered in the next chapter.

## BLOOD PRESSURE IN THE ABSENCE OF KIDNEYS

### Experimental Studies

Starting in 1936, numerous short-term studies were performed on animals with both kidneys removed (Harrison et al, 1936). Only after perfecting the technique of peritoneal dialysis were Grollman and his coworkers (1949) able to keep nephrectomized dogs alive long enough to make prolonged observations. The cause of "renoprival hypertension" soon became a matter of controversy, with Grollman (1953) and Muirhead et al (1953) contending that it was secondary to the absence of some normal vasodepressor action in the kidney, and other investigators believing the blood pressure rose because the animals were volume expanded (Orbison et al, 1952).

### Clinical Studies

These experimental studies became applicable to humans in the early 1950s. Since then, using peritoneal dialysis and hemodialysis, it has been possible to keep people without renal tissue alive for years. Those who are hypertensive have an increased total peripheral resis-

tance. Since they are unable to excrete sodium and water, their hypertension likely develops in the pattern shown in the *top part* of Figure 9.5 involving first an increase in fluid volume that leads to a rise in cardiac output. Although studies in anephric animals by Coleman et al (1970) demonstrated a subsequent conversion to an increased peripheral resistance, presumably through whole body autoregulation, Kim et al (1980) found a number of different patterns when salt loads were given to four anephric humans and six with end stage renal disease who retained their own nonfunctioning kidneys.

Although excess volume may be the primary cause of hypertension in the anephric patient, other mechanisms are likely involved including the absence of vasodepressors of renal origin. During the postoperative course of eight bilaterally nephrectomized patients, hypertension was observed in three whose volumes were not thought to be overexpanded, in keeping with the concept of a "renoprival" hypertension (Lazarus et al, 1972).

### Effects of Bilateral Nephrectomy

A small number of patients with renal failure and severe hypertension, unresponsive to volume control during hemodialysis or drug therapy, may need bilateral nephrectomy as an emergency before a functioning homotransplant can be provided (Vertes et al, 1969; Sheinfeld et al, 1985). Fortunately, the availability of more effective antihypertensive drugs has diminished the need for this drastic step.

Immediately after bilateral nephrectomy the blood pressure usually becomes normal, but now volume homeostasis assumes an even greater role. Renin levels are markedly lower after nephrectomy, although some extrarenal renin may

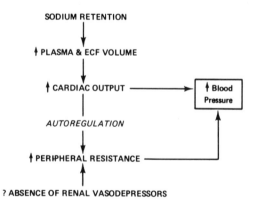

**Figure 9.5.** Probable mechanism for hypertension in the anephric state.

remain in the circulation and may contribute to inadequate blood pressure control (Taylor et al, 1986). Overall, volume is the predominant factor controlling the blood pressure in anephric patients. Neither the absence of renal vasodepressors nor the presence of extrarenal renin is likely very much involved.

## BLOOD PRESSURE DURING CHRONIC DIALYSIS

The blood pressure usually is quite variable in patients on chronic hemodialysis. With 24-hour ambulatory monitoring, the blood pressure of 10 ESRD hypertensive patients was found to be high during hemodialysis, to fall after and to remain low for the remainder of the 24-hours (Batlle et al, 1986). This is in keeping with the clinical observation that often no antihypertensive drugs are needed on the day after dialysis.

### Mechanisms of Hypertension

#### Responders

The usual fall in blood pressure after hemodialysis is attributable to a reduction in cardiac output from contraction of the blood volume, reflecting both external loss of volume, and an internal relocation to the interstitial compartment (Chaignon et al, 1981). In addition, plasma levels of norepinephrine and epinephrine, usually high before dialysis, may come down considerably, at least in part by simple removal by dialysis (Elias et al, 1985).

Continuous ambulatory peritoneal dialysis usually leads to easier control of hypertension, along with reversal of left ventricular hypertrophy (Leenen et al, 1985). This likely reflects the constancy of control of fluid volume, which is not given the chance to reaccumulate as between intermittent dialyses.

#### Nonresponders

Those who remain hypertensive often have high peripheral resistance that has been correlated with high levels of a circulating Na,K-ATPase pump inhibitor (Boero et al, 1988). In addition, patients on dialysis may have resistant hypertension because of the coexistence of renovascular stenosis (Olsen, 1983) or inadvertent hypercalcemia (Sica et al, 1984).

#### Overresponders

Sometimes hypotension during or immediately after dialysis may be clinically significant and may be of a magnitude greater than would be expected from simple volume shifts. This may reflect a number of factors including decreased cardiac reserve, autonomic insufficiency, too rapid a decline in plasma osmolality or too great a fall in fluid volume, and the use of acetate, which may act as a vasodilator (Henrich, 1986).

### Management of Hypertension

It is important to prevent hypertension in patients on chronic dialysis since it contributes to their risk of atherosclerosis (Rostand et al, 1982). Fortunately, the hypertension that is so common before institution of dialysis often disappears with control of fluid volume and various metabolic disturbances (Zucchelli et al, 1988).

In those patients whose hypertension is not controlled with dialysis, various antihypertensive drugs have been successfully used, sometimes only on the days between dialysis. The pharmacokinetics of some drugs may be altered both by the absence of renal function and variable clearance by dialysis. The reviews by Paton et al (1986) and Bennett (1988) provide data about the effects of various drugs. ACE inhibitors are being used increasingly, not only to control hypertension in those with increased renin secretion from their native kidneys (Ribstein et al, 1986) but also to ameliorate the marked thirst that drives some dialysis patients to maintain chronic fluid overload (Oldenburg et al, 1988).

Despite all attempts at treatment, the hypertension in a few patients with chronic renal failure on maintenance hemodialysis may be uncontrollable, except by means of bilateral nephrectomy.

## HYPERTENSION AFTER KIDNEY TRANSPLANTATION

More and more patients are receiving renal transplants. As more patients live longer after transplantation, hypertension has been recognized as a major complication, one that may, if uncontrolled, quickly destroy the transplant or add to the risk of accelerated atherosclerosis (Luke, 1987).

### Epidemiology

The prevalence of hypertension after successful renal transplantation has been reported to vary from 13% to as high as 86% (Rao et al, 1978; Kasiske, 1987). Hypertension becomes progressively more common during the first few months after transplantation and persists in about half of all patients. However, this is better than hemodialysis: In the study of Rao et al involving a series of 164 transplant recipients, 82% of the patients were hypertensive during prior maintenance hemodialysis, whereas only 49% of those whose transplant was functioning at 6 months were hypertensive.

Hypertension is more likely to occur after transplant in patients who were hypertensive pretransplant. In Rao's series, posttransplant hypertension was noted in 14% of those who had been normotensive but in 60% of those who had been hypertensive. The removal of one native kidney at the time of transplantation has been shown to reduce the prevalence of posttransplant hypertension (Abouna et al, 1989).

## Causes and Management

Beyond persistence of primary (essential) hypertension, a number of other causes of posttransplant hypertension have been documented (Table 9.2).

### Cyclosporine

Cyclosporine is a common cause (Mihatsch et al, 1988), much more likely than moderate doses of adrenal steroids (Luke, 1987). Hypertension may develop without overt renal damage, but, when cyclosporine is discontinued, even presumably "normal" renal function may improve (Curtis et al, 1986).

*Mechanism.* The mechanism of cyclosporine hypertension is uncertain (Bennett and Porter, 1988). The hypertension may be sodium dependent (Curtis et al, 1988), and it seems to be associated with both an inhibition of relaxation of peripheral resistance vessels (Richards et al, 1989) and enhanced vasoconstriction mediated by increased transmembrane calcium influx (Meyer-Lehnert and Schrier, 1989). In heart transplant recipients, cyclosporine was found to enhance sympathetic neural activity (Scherrer et al, 1988). It does not appear to stimulate renin

release in renal transplant patients (Bantle et al, 1987).

*Management.* If cyclosporine is continued, calcium entry blockers seem to be effective both in lowering the blood pressure and also in protecting renal function (Fcchally et al, 1987). Verapamil and diltiazem increase the plasma levels of cyclosporine, apparently by interfering with its hepatic metabolism (Robson et al, 1988). ACE inhibitors may also work but likely less well than CEBs (Bennett and Porter, 1988).

Conversion to azathioprine may at least relieve some of the renal dysfunction (Curtis et al, 1986). Obviously, the smallest possible doses of steroids and other immunosuppressive agents should be used.

### Posttransplant Stenosis

Renal artery stenosis may be detected by the following:

—the appearance of a new bruit (Whelton et al, 1979);
—the acute response to a single dose of captopril with a marked rise in plasma renin and a marked fall in glomerular filtration rate (GFR) assesed by renal scintigraphy (Luke, 1987);
—Doppler ultrasonography (Campieri et al, 1988);
—arteriography (Beachley et al, 1976).

If stenosis of the transplant artery is responsible, percutaneous transluminal dilation may be the first therapeutic intervention. It was technically successful in 10 of 12 patients and relieved the hypertension in nine of these (Sniderman et al, 1980). In patients with posttransplant stenosis, caution is needed in the use of ACE inhibitors that, by removal of the angiotensin II that maintains renal perfusion, may lead to rapid loss of graft function (Hricik, 1987).

### Native Kidney Hypertension

If graft stenosis and rejection have been excluded so that the hypertension appears to be arising from the host kidneys, medical management of the hypertension should be utilized. However, graft survival may be impaired in patients who are hypertensive after transplantation, even if the hypertension is apparently well controlled (Cheigh et al, 1989). If the hypertension cannot be controlled, bilateral nephrectomy may be effective (Curtis et al, 1985).

### Recurrent Primary Hypertension

The potential of transference of essential hypertension from the donor to the recipient is

**Table 9.2. Causes of Posttransplant Hypertension[a]**

Immunosuppressive therapy
  Steroids
  Cyclosporine
Allograft failure
  Chronic rejection
  Recurrent disease
Potentially surgically remediable causes
  Allograft renal artery stenosis
  Native kidneys
Speculative cause
  Recurrent essential hypertension
    As primary cause of ESRD
    From (pre-) hypertensive donor

[a]From Luke RG: *Kidney Int* 31:1024, 1987 and reprinted from *Kidney International* with permission.

suggested by the finding of more hypertension in recipients of a kidney from hypertensive donors (Guidi et al, 1985), including those who died of a subarachnoid hemorrhage (Strandgaard and Hansen, 1986).

## HYPERTENSION WITH CHRONIC RENAL DISEASE

Patients may start at either end of the spectrum: Hypertension without overt renal damage on the one end, severe renal insufficiency without hypertension on the other. Eventually, however, both groups move toward the middle—renal insufficiency with hypertension. Despite the reprieves available from dialysis and transplantation, hypertension remains a major risk factor for patients with chronic renal disease (CRD). For instance, among 288 patients with biopsy-proven chronic glomerulonephritis, renal function remained normal 5 years later in 92% who were initially normotensive but in only 47% of those who were hypertensive (Orofino et al, 1987). The development of renal insufficiency as a consequence of primary hypertension is described in Chapter 4. This chapter examines the development of hypertension as a secondary process to primary renal disease.

Before proceeding, three points should be remembered: First, even mild degrees of renal damage are a serious prognostic sign in the larger population with primary hypertension (Fig. 9.1) (Shulman et al, 1989); second, renal insufficiency may develop despite apparently good control of hypertension, particularly among blacks (Rostand et al, 1989); third, patients may present with refractory hypertension and renal insufficiency whose underlying problem is bilateral renovascular disease (Ying et al, 1984). The recognition of their renovascular etiology is critical since revascularization may relieve their hypertension and improve their renal function. More about this important group of patients is provided in the next chapter.

### Prevalence

Hypertension is usual in patients with overt renal insufficiency, as defined by a GFR below 50 ml/minute or a serum creatinine above 1.5 mg/dl. The prevalence of hypertension varies considerably even within the category of chronic glomerulonephritis, being most common with focal segmental sclerosis (Kincaid-Smith and Whitworth, 1988; Rambausek et al, 1989). Moreover, within each category of biopsy-proven chronic glomerulonephritis, the prevalence of hypertension varies considerably in different series. For example, hypertension has been reported in as few as 10% to as many as 52% of patients with mesangial IgA nephropathy (Berger's disease) (Beaman and Adu, 1988).

### Significance

The presence of hypertension is associated with a more rapid progression of renal damage no matter what the underlying renal disease. In a series of 86 patients initially seen with an average serum creatinine of 3.8 mg/dl, the rate of subsequent decline of renal function over an average of 33 months was twice as great in those whose diastolic blood pressure (DBP) remained above 90 mm Hg compared with those whose DBP remained below 90 (Brazy et al, 1989).

Most of what follows applies to the second most common mechanism for ESRD after hypertension—diabetes. However, since diabetic nephropathy has special features it will be considered separately.

### Hyperfiltration Mechanism of Renal Injury

The mechanism by which hypertension leads to progressive renal damage most likely involves glomerular hypertension, as championed by Brenner and coworkers (Anderson and Brenner, 1989) (Fig 9.6). Their hypothesis starts with any of a number of factors that increase glomerular capillary plasma flow rate or hydraulic pressure.

As shown in the *upper left* of Figure 9.6, systemic hypertension is one of these factors. The high systemic pressure may be transmitted into the glomerulus because afferent arteriolar resistance fails to increase adequately (Olson et al, 1986). The higher pressure and/or flow rate, in turn, damages glomerular cells and leads to progressive sclerosis, setting off a vicious cycle.

Other factors may be involved beyond glomerular hypertension and hyperfiltration including primary mesangial expansion induced by angiotensin (Keane and Raij, 1985), glomerular hypertrophy (Yoshida et al, 1989a), and loss of renal autoregulation (Bidani et al, 1987). However, at least in various rat models, the scheme shown in Figure 9.6 seems to explain best both the initiation and progression of renal damage.

### Secondary Mechanisms

If the progressive sclerosis of glomeruli is responsible for the usual progressive decline in renal function, the manner by which this in turn

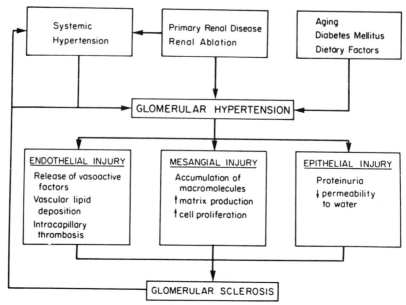

**Figure 9.6.** Pivotal role of glomerular hypertension in the initiation and progression of structural injury. (From Anderson S, Brenner BM: *Q J Med* 70:185, 1989.)

leads to or aggravates hypertension likely involves an inability of the reduced renal mass to excrete enough sodium and water. When renal mass is reduced, the blood pressure rises first because of volume expansion and an increased cardiac output, shifting later into an elevated peripheral resistance (Lombard et al, 1989).

Although measurements of both total extracellular fluid and blood volume may be normal in such patients (Boer et al, 1987), the hypertension is usually very responsive to manipulations of fluid volume (Vertes et al, 1969; Heyka and Vidt, 1989). In a small percentage, high renin levels may be responsible for "volume unresponsive" hypertension (Weidmann and Maxwell, 1975).

In addition to the simple loss of renal mass, sodium retention may also be caused by increased levels of a circulating $Na^+$, $K^+$-ATPase pump inhibitor, the putative natriuretic hormone (Boero et al, 1988). Moreover, the damaged kidneys may no longer make vasodilatory prostaglandins (Kishimoto et al, 1987) or may not be able to convert the potent salt-retaining cortisol to the relatively impotent metabolite cortisone (Stewart et al, 1988).

## Management of Hypertension

Many patients are seen only after significant renal insufficiency has developed, at which time all that can be done is to enter them into dialysis with the hope for transplantation. As noted earlier, the total number of ESRD patients on chronic dialysis in the United States is over 100,000, consuming a significant amount of money that could be far more effectively spent on prevention since the two most common causes of ESRD, nephrosclerosis related to hypertension and diabetic nephropathy, may be largely preventable.

Once renal insufficiency has developed, the goal is to slow its progress by interrupting the vicious cycle shown in Figure 9.6. As of now, the only means known to be effective are control of hypertension and decreasing the intake of dietary protein (Maschio et al, 1982; Bergström et al, 1986). Unfortunately in humans, unlike the rat, nothing has proven capable of stopping progression to ESRD once renal insufficiency has appeared (Dworkin and Benstein, 1989).

### Control of Hypertension

With both diuretics and other antihypertensive agents, transient falls in renal blood flow and glomerular filtration rate may accompany successful reduction of the blood pressure. Unless there is reason to believe that plasma volume is contracted too much or that there is drug-related nephrotoxicity, the best course is to proceed with control of the hypertension. In the long run, renal function may be preserved by tight control of the hypertension (Mroczek et al, 1969; Lee et al, 1989).

The major role of volume excess can be countered by adequate diuretic therapy if renal insufficiency is fairly mild and by removal of fluid via dialysis in overt renal failure.

*Diuretics.* All diuretics save spironolactone must gain entry to the tubular fluid and have access to the luminal side of the nephron to work (Brater, 1988). All diuretics save mannitol, being bound to serum proteins, are not filtered but reach the urine by secretion across the proximal tubule by way of organic acid or organic base secretory pathways. "Their entry to the urinary side of action can be compromised by anything that limits access to the secretory sites (e.g., diminished renal blood flow) or that blocks or competes for the secretory pump (endogenous organic acids or probenecid for acidic drugs and cimetidine for basic drugs)" (Brater, 1988).

Patients with chronic renal disease (CRD), then, are resistant to acidic diuretics such as thiazides and the loop diuretics both because of their reduced renal blood flow and because of the accumulation of organic acid end products of metabolism. To effect a diuresis, enough of the diuretic must be given to deliver adequate amounts of the agent to the tubular sites of action. This translates into a "sequential doubling of single doses until a ceiling dose is reached" (Brater, 1988), i.e., start with 40 mg of furosemide and, if little response is seen, give 80; if little response is seen, give 160 and so on up to a 400 mg maximum by mouth (200 mg intravenously). Once the ceiling dose is reached, that dose should be given as often as needed (usually once a day) as a maintenance dose.

As Brater (1988) points out, thiazides would probably work in many CRD patients if given in high enough doses. "However, such a strategy is still not worth pursuing due to the low intrinsic efficacy of these drugs compared to loop diuretics." Most do not try thiazides if the serum creatinine is above 2.0 mg/dl. On the other hand, in severely resistant patients, combining a loop diuretic with a thiazide may effect a response when neither is effective alone (Wollam et al, 1982).

In addition, metolazone may work as well as loop diuretics and, if control of hypertension requires most persistent volume control than provided by a once-a-day dose of a loop diuretic, it will provide a full 24-hour effect (Bennett and Porter, 1973).

Caution should be taken to avoid excessive diuresis with such potent diuretics on the one hand and interference with diuretic action by NSAIDs on the other.

Spironolactone, triamterene, and amiloride should be avoided in most patients with severe CRD since hyperkalemia may be induced particularly in diabetics who cannot secrete extra insulin to enhance transfer of potassium into cells and who may have low renin and aldosterone levels (Perez et al, 1977a). Similarly, CRD patients taking beta-blockers, who therefore cannot obtain the epinephrine-mediated transfer of potassium across cells, may be susceptible to hyperkalemia (Mitch and Wilcox, 1982).

*Sodium Restriction.* Patients with CRD may have a narrow range of sodium excretory capacity: If markedly restricted of dietary salt, they may not be able to conserve sodium and will become volume depleted; if given modest salt loads, they may be unable to excrete enough sodium to prevent volume expansion and hypertension. A very small number have severe salt-losing nephropathy, but few of them are hypertensive (Uribarri et al, 1983). Thus, sodium intake should be carefully monitored.

If $NaHCO_3$ is used to counter the metabolic acidosis, NaCl may have to be more severely restricted. In a practical manner, sodium restriction in the range of 1 to 2 g/day (44 to 88 mEq of sodium per day) is both feasible and necessary to control these patients' hypertension.

*Nondiuretic Antihypertensive Drugs.* The ongoing publications by W.M. Bennett (1988) provide the best data about the dosage of antihypertensive and other drugs in patients with varying degrees of CRD (Table 9.3).

*Minoxidil.* Those with refractory hypertension and renal insufficiency may be successfully treated with minoxidil (Keusch et al, 1978). Although renal function may continue to deteriorate, impressive improvement may be noted (Mitchell et al, 1980). As noted in Chapter 7, minoxidil is a potent vasodilator, and must be given with an adrenergic blocker (usually a beta-blocker) to prevent reflex cardiac stimulation and a diuretic (usually furosemide) to prevent fluid retention. The drug need be given only in a single daily dose as was done in a study of 55 patients with resistant hypertension, 12 of whom had CRD (mean serum creatinine of 2.5 mg/dl) (Spitalewitz et al, 1986) (Fig. 9.7). The beauty of these data is that they demonstrate

**Table 9.3. Guide to Drug Dosage in Renal Failure[a]**

| Drug | Elimination half-life ($t_{1/2}$) (adults) | | Excreted unchanged (%) | Normal dose interval (h) | Dose adjustment for renal failure creatinine clearance (ml/min) | | | Need for dose adjustment during dialysis[b] |
|---|---|---|---|---|---|---|---|---|
| | normal (h) | ESRD (h) | | | > 50 | 10–50 | < 10 | |
| **Beta-Adrenoceptor Antagonists** | | | | | | | | |
| Acebutolol | 7–9 | 7 | 55 | 12 or 24 | Unch[c] | 50% | 25% | No(H) |
| Atenolol | 6–9 | 15–35 | > 90 | 24 | Unch | 50% | 25% | Yes(H) No(P) |
| Labetalol | 3–8 | 3–8 | 0–5 | 12 | Unch | Unch | Unch | No(H) |
| Metoprolol | 2.5–4.5 | 2.5–4.5 | 5 | 12 | Unch | Unch | Unch | Yes(H) |
| Nadolol | 14–24 | 45 | 90 | 24 | Unch | 50% | 25% | Yes(H) |
| Pindolol | 2.5–4 | 3–4 | 40 | 12 | Unch | Unch | Unch | ? |
| Propranolol | 2–6 | 1–6 | < 5 | 6–12 | Unch | Unch | Unch | No(H) |
| Timolol | 2.5–4 | 4 | 15 | 8–12 | Unch | Unch | Unch | No(H) |
| **Other Antihypertensive Drugs** | | | | | | | | |
| Captopril | 1.9 | 21–32 | 50–70 | 12 | Unch | Unch | 50% | Yes(H) |
| Clonidine | 6–23 | 39–42 | 45 | 6–8 | Unch | Unch | Unch | No(H) |
| Guanabenz | 12–14 | ? | < 5 | 12 | Unch | Unch | Unch | ? |
| Guanethidine | 120–240 | ? | 25–50 | 24 | 24h | 24h | 24–36h | ? |
| Hydralazine | 2.0–2.5 | 7–16 | 25 | 8–12 | 8–12h | 8–12h | 8–16h 12–24h[d] | No(H,P) |
| α-Methyldopa | 1–1.7 | 7–16 | 20–60 | 6 | 6h | 9–18h | 12–24h | Yes(H,P) |
| Minoxidil | 2.8–4.2 | 2.8–4.2 | 15–20 | 8–12 | Unch | Unch | Unch | Yes(H) |
| Nitroprusside sodium | < 10 min | < 10 min | < 10 | Constant IV infusion | Unch | Unch | Unch | Yes(H) |
| Prazosin | 1.8–4.6 | ? | < 5 | 8–12 | Unch | Unch | Unch | No(H,P) |
| Reserpine | 46–168 | 87–323 | < 1 | 24 | Unch | Unch | Avoid | No(H,P) |

[a]From Bennett WM: *Clin Pharmacokinetics* 15:326, 1988.
[b]H, hemodialysis; P, peritoneal dialysis.
[c]Unch, Unchanged.
[d]Slow acetylators.

effective control of severe hypertension with once-a-day therapy and no deterioration of renal function.

*ACE Inhibitors.* In keeping with the hypothesis of Brenner et al, ACE Inhibitors (ACEIs) have been shown in rat models to provide better control of glomerular hypertension and preservation of renal function than other drugs that lower the blood pressure equally (Anderson et al, 1986). The observation is in keeping with a greater degree of efferent arteriolar vasodilation provided by blockade of intrarenal angiotensin II. By relieving this efferent constriction to a greater degree than affecting afferent resistance, ACEIs should reduce both pressure and flow within the glomeruli, thereby providing protection against progressive sclerosis.

Such is true for some rats but not for others (Yoshida et al, 1989b). In people, ACEIs clearly lower the blood pressure, likely reduce proteinuria (Heeg et al, 1987), and may preserve renal function. However, there are no adequate comparisons with other antihypertensive agents to know whether ACEIs are more protective than the others. Preservation of renal function has

been amply shown in patients with CRD using captopril (Vetter et al, 1984), enalapril (Bauer and Reams, 1988), or lisinopril (Donohoe et al, 1988). In patients with rapidly progressive renal failure from connective tissue disease, an ACEI may provide spectacular effects (Strongwater et al, 1989). On the other hand, some patients have progressive acute renal failure superimposed on chronic renal insufficiency when given an ACEI (in the absence of renovascular disease) (Verbeelen and De Boel, 1984). As noted in Table 9.3, the excretion of captopril is decreased in ESRD and a lower dose should be given. The same is true of enalapril and lisinopril (Kelly et al, 1988). All three are removed during dialysis.

*Calcium Entry Blockers.* These drugs are also effective in controlling the blood pressure and preserving already impaired renal function (Weidmann et al, 1989) perhaps even better than "standard" therapy (Eliahou et al, 1988). On theoretical grounds, the preferential vasodilation of afferent arterioles that is seen with calcium entry blockers (CEBs) in experimental models (Loutzenhiser and Epstein, 1989) would further increase glomerular hyperfiltration.

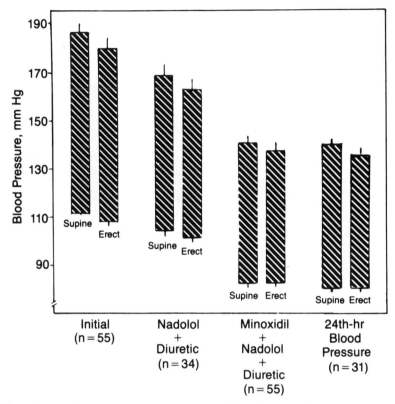

**Figure 9.7.** Effect of once-daily drug therapy on blood pressure. (From Spitalewitz S, Porush JG, Reiser IW: *Arch Intern Med* 146:882, 1986, Copyright 1986, American Medical Association.)

However, in clinical practice over fairly short intervals, CEBs have not been found to worsen renal function (Bauer and Reams, 1989).

**Restriction of Dietary Protein**

On theoretical and experimental grounds, a reduced protein intake should reduce glomerular hyperfiltration and slow hemodynamically mediated renal disease (Brenner et al, 1982). However, the usual progressive loss in renal function with aging occurs equally in life-long vegetarians on a long-term low-protein diet as in people on unrestricted protein intake (Blum et al, 1989). The effect of a diet restricted in protein (and phosphorus) on the progress of CRD is now under proper study, and hopefully definitive data will be available in 3 or 4 years (Klahr, 1989).

**Correction of Anemia**

As might have been predicted from data on correction of anemia by transfusion (Neff et al, 1971), the use of recombinant human erythropoietin to correct the anemia of CRD may raise the blood pressure rather markedly (Eschbach,

1989). This is related to the increase in blood viscosity and volume, so that the anemia should be corrected slowly and with close watch of the blood pressure (Raine, 1988).

**Renin-Dependent Hypertension**

A small number of patients with CRD and severe hypertension may have a highly activated renin-angiotensin system, hopefully from bilateral renal artery stenosis that can be relieved by revascularization (Ying et al, 1984), but more likely from diffuse intrarenal ischemia that can only be relieved by bilateral nephrectomy (Lazarus et al, 1974). Fortunately with better control of fluid volume and the use of ACEIs, the need for nephrectomies is less (Sheinfield et al, 1985), but they may relieve hypertension even if the hypertension preceded the renal failure (Curtis et al, 1983).

**Diabetic Nephropathy**

The progressive nephropathy seen with diabetes mellitus appears to represent another example of the deleterious effects of hyperfiltration.

## Pathology and Clinical Features

As delineated by Kimmelstiel and Wilson (1936), renal disease occurs among diabetics with a high incidence and with a particular glomerular pathology—nodular intercapillary glomerulosclerosis. The clinical description has been improved upon very little since their original paper:

The clinical picture appears . . . to be almost as characteristic as the histological one: the patients are relatively old; hypertension is present, usually of the benign type, and the kidneys frequently show signs of decompensation; there is a history of diabetes, usually of long standing; the presenting symptoms may be those of edema of the nephrotic type, renal decompensation or heart failure; the urine contains large amounts of albumin and there is usually impairment of concentrating power with or without nitrogen retention.''

The pathological specificity of the nodular glomerular lesion for diabetes has been upheld. The clinical description should be altered to include younger patients if they have been diabetic over 10 years, to involve hypertension in about 50 to 60% of patients, and to almost always be accompanied by retinal capillary microaneurysms.

## Epidemiology

As more diabetics are living longer, the number of patients with CRD related to diabetic nephropathy continues to increase (Fig. 9.2), with renal failure eventually developing in 30 to 50% of insulin-dependent diabetics and somewhat fewer of those with non-insulin-dependent diabetes (Noth et al, 1989). Compared with the general population, patients with diabetic nephropathy have a 37-fold greater mortality, both from coronary and renal disease, whereas diabetics without nephropathy have a 4.2-fold increased mortality rate (Borch-Johnsen and Kreiner, 1987).

The predisposition is genetic, particularly in those with poor glycemic control (Krolewski et al, 1988), and diabetic nephropathy occurs in familial clusters (Seaquist et al, 1989). Those who have nephropathy have higher sodium-lithium countertransport activity in red cells than found in those who do not have nephropathy (Mangili et al, 1988) so this may serve as a marker for the genetic predisposition both for the hypertension and the nephropathy in diabetic patients.

## Course

The rapidly progressive nature of diabetic nephropathy, usually advancing to renal failure within 10 years after onset of persistent proteinuria (Krolewski et al, 1985), appears to reflect some additional features to the overall scheme of the progression of glomerulosclerosis shown in Figure 9.6 that are unique to the diabetic state (Fig. 9.8) (Hostetter et al, 1982). Albuminuria is the first recognizable sign: The presence of microalbuminuria almost doubles the prevalence of hypertension, proliferative retinopathy, and neuropathy; the presence of macroalbuminuria doubles them again (Parving et al, 1988).

Hypertension is closely correlated with levels of albuminuria and is clearly related to the progress of renal insufficiency. Those with diabetic nephropathy that is responsible for their hypertension tend, on average, to have 100-fold more albuminuria than do diabetics with coincidental essential hypertension (Christensen et al, 1987). The hypertension is associated with expansion of plasma and extracellular fluid volume (Hommet et al, 1989). Plasma renin levels are inappropriately high for the degree of hypertension and volume expansion (O'Hare et al, 1985). High levels of both active renin (Paulsen et al, 1989) and pro-renin (Luetscher and Kraemer, 1988) may be predictive of the development of nephropathy.

## Management

*Glycemic Control.* All diabetics should be monitored at least once a year for microalbuminuria (Viberti, 1989). If it is present, tighter control of the diabetes is likely appropriate since poor glycemic control could produce vasodilation of renal afferent arterioles, exposing the glomeruli to systemic blood pressures (Fig. 9.8). In view of the evidence reviewed in Chapter 3 about the possible deleterious effects of hyperinsulinemia, there is concern about the use of increased amounts of exogenous insulin to achieve tighter control. Nonetheless, insulin-induced lowering of hyperglycemia will reverse glomerular capillary hypertension in diabetic rats (Scholey and Meyer, 1989), and a number of 1- to 4-year studies in humans have mostly shown a reduction in albuminuria and in GFR by tighter glycemic control (Mogensen, 1988; Chase et al, 1989).

*Antihypertensive Therapy.* The evidence is stronger for a slowing of the progression of di-

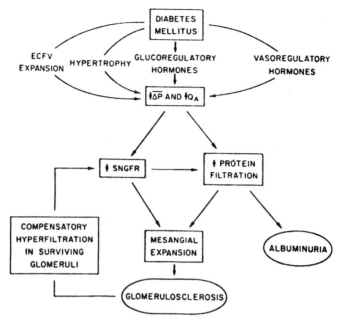

**Figure 9.8.** Hypothetical role of glomerular hyperfiltration in the initiation and progression of diabetic nephropathy. Hyperfiltration is stimulated by some feature(s) of the diabetic state such as extracellular fluid volume (*ECFV*) expansion due to hyperglycemia, renal hypertrophy, increased growth hormone and glucagon secretion, and/or altered levels of, or vascular responsiveness to, vasoactive hormones. Increases of the glomerular transcapillary hydraulic pressure gradient ($\Delta P$) and glomerular plasma flow rate ($Q_A$) are responsible for the hyperfiltration that increases transglomerular protein filtration leading to albuminuria and mesangial deposition of circulating proteins. The latter effect eventuates in mesangial expansion and ultimately glomerulosclerosis. This initial loss of functioning nephrons exerts a positive feedback stimulus to compensatory hyperfiltration in less affected surviving glomeruli, in turn contributing to their eventual destruction. *SNGFR*, single-nephron glomerular filtration rate. (From Hostetter TH, Rennke HG, Brenner BM: *Am J Med* 72:375, 1982.)

abetic nephropathy by reduction of elevated blood pressure than for any other therapy (Mogensen, 1988). The longest protective effect has been reported by Parving et al (1987) who followed nine insulin-dependent patients for 2 years before and 6 years after institution of effective antihypertensive therapy (Fig. 9.9). Note that this impressive reduction in the rate of decline of renal function was achieved by "traditional" antihypertensive therapy, i.e., without an ACEI.

Since Taguma et al (1985) reported a decrease in heavy proteinuria in six of 10 azotemic diabetics with captopril, a number of studies have documented in humans what has been seen in diabetic rats (Anderson et al, 1989): ACEIs have a special ability to reduce the proteinuria of diabetic nephropathy. This has been seen in both normotensive (Marre et al, 1988) and hypertensive (Parving et al, 1988) diabetics with nephropathy using either captopril or enalapril. The special effectiveness of ACEIs was suggested in a 6-week study wherein captopril reduced albuminuria in eight patients but nifedipine increased the level in another seven patients

(Mimran et al, 1988). Longer studies with ACEIs, examining their ability to mitigate the decline of renal function, are in process.

*Low Protein Diet.* A diet with 0.6 g/kg/day of high biological value protein given to 11 insulin-dependent diabetics for 2 years reduced the rate of decline in renal function (Evanoff et al, 1989).

*Platelet Inhibition.* Aspirin and dipyridamole daily for 3 months reduced albuminuria in seven of 28 patients (Donadio et al, 1988).

When all else fails, those who develop ESRD from diabetic nephropathy seem to respond well to the various therapies for renal failure including continuous ambulatory peritoneal dialysis (Amair et al, 1982) and renal transplantation (Sagalowsky et al, 1983). They have a high frequency of low renin hypertension, which may meld into a truly distinctive syndrome seen in CRD—hyporeninemic hypoaldosteronism. Whereas various forms of renal disease may be associated with the syndrome, elderly diabetics are more frequently affected (Perez et al, 1977b). Such diabetics, unable to mobilize either aldos-

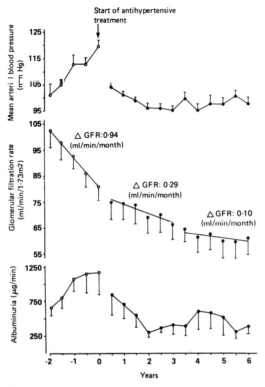

**Figure 9.9.** Average course of mean arterial blood pressure, glomerular filtration rate, and albuminuria before (o) and during (●) long-term effective antihypertensive treatment of nine insulin-dependent diabetic patients who had nephropathy. Therapy included furosemide, metoprolol, and hydralazine in most patients. (From Parving H-H, Andersen AR, Smidt UM, et al: *Br Med J* 294:1443, 1987.)

terone or insulin that are needed to transfer potassium out of the blood, are particularly vulnerable to hyperkalemia (Perez et al, 1977a).

## HYPERTENSION IN ACUTE RENAL DISEASE

Most acute severe insults to the kidney result in decreased urine formation, retention of salt and water, and hypertension. Acute renal failure with hypertension may result from bilateral renal artery occlusion, either by emboli or thromboses, or by removal of angiotensin II support of blood flow with ACEI therapy in the presence of bilateral renal artery disease (Diamond and Henrich, 1986), and cure may follow revascularization. Trauma to the kidney may cause hypertension that is renin mediated and quite variable in onset and severity (Watts and Hoffbrand, 1987). Rarely, a perirenal hematoma may so constrict the kidney as to cause persistent ischemia and hypertension (Hellebusch et al, 1970).

More about those syndromes that have a vascular component is given in the next chapter.

Extracorporeal shock wave lithotripsy for kidney stones may be followed by a transient rise in blood pressure in some patients (Toth et al, 1989) and the new onset of hypertension 1 to 4 years later in perhaps 8 to 20% (Williams and Thomas, 1989).

## Acute Glomerulonephritis

The classic syndrome is poststreptococcal (type-specific) nephritis occurring in a child with recent pharyngitis or impetigo who suddenly passes dark urine and develops facial edema. This syndrome, in which the renal injury represents the trapping of antibody-antigen complexes within the glomerular capillaries, has become less common. Nonetheless, it still occurs and it occurs sometimes in adults past middle age.

Typically, in the acute phase, patients are hypertensive and there is a close temporal relation between oliguria, edema, and hypertension. On occasion, hypertension of a severe, even malignant nature may be the overriding feature, with few urinary findings, although microscopic hematuria and red blood cell casts are almost always seen if the urinary sediment is properly examined (Grossman et al, 1973).

### Mechanism

The hypertension was thought to be secondary to fluid overload with an increased cardiac output, but a careful study of two patients revealed an increased peripheral resistance attributed to an inappropriately high renin level (Birkenhäger et al, 1970).

### Treatment and Course

The hypertension should be treated by salt and water restriction and, in mild cases, diuretics and other oral antihypertensives. In keeping with an apparent role of even low-normal levels of renin, ACEI (captopril) therapy was very effective in nine patients with acute glomerulonephritis (Parra et al, 1988). With more severe hypertension, dialysis may be needed in addition to parenteral antihypertensives (see Chapters 8 and 16).

In the classic disease, thought to be self-limited, the patient is free of edema and hypertension within days, of proteinuria within weeks, and of hematuria within months. With some exceptions (Schacht et al, 1979), most patients seem to recover from acute poststreptococcal glomerulonephritis, and most cases of chronic glomerulonephritis have no relation to prior streptococcal infection.

## Collagen Vascular Disease

Hypertension with renal damage is common with systemic lupus (Budman and Steinberg, 1976), polyarteritis nodosa (White and Schambelan, 1980), and scleroderma (progressive systemic sclerosis) (Eknoyan and Suki, 1985). All of these may enter into an acute, severe hypertensive phase, usually associated with markedly elevated plasma renin levels, likely reflecting intrarenal stenoses from multiple arteriolar lesions that can sometimes be rather remarkably reversed by ACEI therapy (Strongwater et al, 1989).

## Acute Renal Failure

A rapid decline in renal function may appear from various causes: prerenal, e.g., volume depletion; intrinsic, e.g., glomerulonephritis; or postrenal, e.g., obstructive uropathy (Diamond and Henrich, 1986).

Those with prerenal causes for acute renal failure usually have a disproportionate decrease in renal blood flow from intense renal vasoconstriction (Levinsky, 1977). Renin levels are high in these patients and are highest in the outer renal cortex, where the greatest reduction of blood flow occurs. The syndrome is seen most commonly in those clinical situations wherein renin levels are already high, such as pregnancy and cirrhosis with ascites.

With regard to hypertension, the important consideration is that fluid replacement be adequate but not excessive. Hypertension is rarely a problem, perhaps because peripheral vascular tone is decreased. Now that dialysis is so readily available, the management of such patients is much less difficult, and virtually complete recovery after prolonged oliguria is frequent.

## Acute Urinary Tract Obstruction

Hypertension may develop after unilateral (Wanner et al, 1987) or bilateral obstruction to the ureters (Savage et al, 1978). In most, the hypertension is fairly mild but high pressure chronic retention of urine with hydronephrosis and painless bladder distension may be associated with significant hypertension and enough volume retention to cause pedal and pulmonary edema (Jones et al, 1987). Catheter drainage of the residual urine may lead to rapid resolution of the hypertension and circulatory overload (Ghose and Harindra, 1989).

## HYPERTENSION WITH RENAL PARENCHYMAL DISEASE BUT WITHOUT RENAL INSUFFICIENCY

The hypertension seen with all of the preceding renal diseases seems appropriate to the extensive renal damage, with resultant defects in fluid excretion, renin secretion, or vasodepressor elaboration. Others of a more obvious vascular origin are covered in the next chapter. In some patients, however, hypertension is seen without enough overt renal damage or ischemia to explain the hypertension on any of these bases. This is particularly true in those with unilateral renal parenchymal disease whose hypertension is relieved by removal of the afflicted kidney.

## Hypertension in the Renal Donor

In normal humans, the removal of a kidney usually does not result in hypertension, likely because of downward adjustments in renin and aldosterone to maintain normal fluid volume (Gordon et al, 1975). The issue has been recently explored more thoroughly because of the theoretical possibility—in keeping with the hyperperfusion theory (Fig. 9.6)—that removal of one kidney would lead to progressive glomerulosclerosis in the other. The possibility does not seem to have been realized: In a long-term follow-up of over 8000 donor nephrectomies, mild, nonprogressive proteinuria was noted in about one-third and a diastolic blood pressure above 90 mm Hg in 25% (Bay and Hebert, 1987). However, both of these could also reflect familial renal disease and hypertension. It appears that only in the elderly, who have significantly less ability to modulate sodium excretion (Epstein and Hollenberg, 1976) and other functional defects (McLachlan, 1978), might removal of one kidney induce hypertension. Therefore, if unilateral renal disease causes hypertension, something must be happening in the presumably normal kidney as well.

## Chronic Pyelonephritis

Hypertension is found more frequently among patients with radiographic signs of chronic pyelonephritis, even if renal function is well preserved (Jacobson et al, 1988), and the pyelonephritis only affects one kidney (Siamopoulos et al, 1983). Hypertensive children are frequently found to have pyelonephritic scarring, usually resulting from vesicoureteric reflux and urinary tract infection in early childhood (Savage et al, 1978). Renal insufficiency and hypertension may not become manifest until middle-age (Jacobson et al, 1989).

The relationship between the pyelonephritis and the hypertension is uncertain, but an increased level of renin from the pyelonephritic kidney is usually noted in those whose hypertension is relieved by nephrectomy (Siamopoulos et al, 1983).

## Drug-Induced Renal Disease

Some patients thought to have chronic pyelonephritis have, instead, analgesic nephropathy from long-term, regular use of phenacetin or acetaminophen, a not uncommon cause of chronic renal failure in the United States (Sandler et al, 1989), England (Cove-Smith and Knapp, 1978), and Australia (Kincaid-Smith, 1980). Since renal salt wasting is frequent with this form of interstitial nephritis, hypertension may be relatively uncommon, but some instances of even malignant hypertension have been seen (Kincaid-Smith, 1980).

A number of other commonly used drugs and diagnostic agents may cause toxic nephropathy (Roxe, 1980). As noted earlier in this chapter, nonsteroidal antiinflammatory drugs have a propensity to induce both acute and chronic renal damage (Adams et al, 1986).

## Polycystic Kidney Disease

With autosomal dominant polycystic kidney disease, hypertension is usual, even without demonstrable renal insufficiency (Bell et al, 1988). The hypertension seems predominately volume dependent with an increased cardiac output and renal vascular resistance (Bell et al, 1988). Single cysts may induce segmental renal ischemia with renin-dependent hypertension (Hoard and O'Brien, 1976).

## Renal Tumors

As we shall see in the next chapter, renin-secreting tumors may cause severe hypertension. In addition to those rare tumors, hypertension may be seen with other renal tumors—nephroblastoma (Wilms' tumor), renal cell carcinoma, and hypernephroma (Dahl et al, 1981). Most appear to cause hypertension by activation of the renin system. Radiotherapy for Wilms' tumor may lead to hypertension 10 or more years later (Koskimies, 1982).

## Unilateral Renal Disease

In addition to these and other forms of renal disease, hypertension is not infrequently found in patients with a small kidney that is not secondary to obvious renal artery stenosis. After Goldblatt produced hypertension by unilateral renal ischemia, small kidneys were indiscriminately removed from hypertensive patients. Smith (1956) discouraged this practice by calling attention to a cure rate of only 26% in all reports published by 1956.

In most patients cured by unilateral nephrectomy, renovascular disease, not primary parenchymal disease, is probably the cause for both the atrophic kidney and the hypertension, presumably by means of the renin mechanism (Wesson, 1982). Renin levels are increased in the venous blood coming from many of those kidneys whose removal results in relief of hypertension (Gordon et al, 1986). Gifford et al (1965) found that arterial occlusive disease could explain the unilateral renal atrophy seen in 71% of 75 hypertensive patients, including a number with congenital hypoplasia.

On the other hand, there are reports of cure of hypertension by removal of kidneys thought to be atrophic because of parenchymal disease, usually pyelonephritis, and not because of vascular impairment (Eliahou et al, 1968).

In view of these questions concerning both the frequency and mechanism of unilateral parenchymal disease as a cause of hypertension, caution is advised before nephrectomy is performed in such patients. The cure rate with parenchymal atrophy is probably much less than that with vascular disease. Moreover, nephrectomy should never be done without prior knowledge of the normal functional state of the other kidney. Nephrectomy should probably be reserved for those with:

—severe hypertension;
—marked loss of renal function in the afflicted kidney that should be recognizable by renal scintigraphy. In practice, a renal size of less than 8.5 cm usually denotes an inability to salvage the kidney by revascularization.
—normal renal function in the other kidney.

A higher renin level from the abnormal side makes the likelihood of relief of the hypertension by nephrectomy more likely, but normal levels may be found in some whose hypertension recedes (Lamberton et al, 1981).

We will next turn to the disease in which surgical relief and renin are more closely connected, renovascular hypertension.

# References

Abouna GM, Samhan M, Kumar MSA, et al: *Transplant Proc* 21:2028, 1989.

Adams DH, Howie AJ, Michael J, et al: *Lancet* 1:57, 1986.

Amair P, Khanna R, Leibel B, et al: *N Engl J Med* 306:625, 1982.

Anderson S, Brenner BM: *Q J Med* 70:185, 1989.

Anderson S, Rennke HG, Brenner BM: *J Clin Invest* 77:1993, 1986.

Anderson S, Rennke HG, Garcia DL, et al: *Kidney Int* 36:526, 1989.

Bantle JP, Boudreau RJ, Ferris TF: *Am J Med* 83:59, 1987.

Batlle DC, von Riotte A, Lang G: *Am J Nephrol* 6:14, 1986.

Bauer JH, Reams GP: *Drugs* 35(Suppl 5):62, 1988.

Bauer JH, Reams GP: *Am J Hypertens* 2:173S, 1989.

Bay WH, Hebert LA: *Ann Intern Med* 106:719, 1987.

Beachley MC, Pierce JC, Boykin JV, et al: *Arch Surg* 111:134, 1976.

Bell PE, Hossack KF, Gabow PA, et al: *Kidney Int* 34:683, 1988.

Beaman M, Adu D: *J Hum Hypertens* 2:139, 1988.

Beckmann ML, Gerber JG, Byyny RL, et al: *Hypertension* 12:582, 1988.

Bennett WM: *Clin Pharmacokinetics* 15:326, 1988.

Bennett WM, Porter GA: *J Clin Pharmacol* 13:357, 1973.

Bennett WM, Porter GA: *Am J Med* 85:131, 1988.

Bergström J, Alvestrand A, Bucht H, et al: *Clin Nephrol* 25:1, 1986.

Berry TD, Hasstedt SJ, Hunt SC, et al: *Hypertension* 13:3, 1989.

Bidani AK, Schwartz MM, Lewis EJ: *Am J Physiol* 252:F1003, 1987.

Birkenhäger WH, Schalekamp MADH, Schalekamp-Kuyken PMA, et al: *Lancet* 1:1086, 1970.

Blum M, Averbuch M, Wolman Y, et al: *Arch Intern Med* 149:211, 1989.

Blumberg A, Hegstrom RM, Nelp WB, et al: *Lancet* 2:69, 1967.

Boer P, Koomans HA, Mees EJD: *Nephron* 45:7, 1987.

Boero R, Guarena C, Berto IM, et al: *Kidney Int* 34:691, 1988.

Borch-Johnsen K, Kreiner S: *Br Med J* 294:1651, 1987.

Brater DC: *Semin Nephrol* 8:333, 1988.

Brazy PC, Stead WW, Fitzwilliam JF: *Kidney Int* 35:670, 1989.

Brenner BM, Garcia DL, Anderson S: *Am J Hypertens* 1:335, 1988.

Brenner BM, Meyer TW, Hostetter TH: *N Engl J Med* 307:652, 1982.

Budman DR, Steinberg AD: *Arch Intern Med* 136:1003, 1976.

Campieri C, Mignani R, Prandi R, et al: *Nephron* 48:341, 1988.

Carmichael J, Shankel SW: *Am J Med* 78:992, 1985.

Carretero OA, Scicli AG: *Kidney Int* 34(Suppl 26):S-52, 1988.

Chaignon M, Chen WT, Tarazi RC, et al: *Hypertension* 3:327, 1981.

Chase HP, Jackson WE, Hoops SL, et al: *JAMA* 261:1155, 1989.

Cheigh JS, Haschemeyer RH, Wang JCL, et al: *Am J Hypertens* 2:341, 1989.

Christensen CK, Krusell LR, Mogensen CE: *Scand J Clin Lab Invest* 47:363, 1987.

Codde JP, Beilin LJ: *J Hypertension* 4:675, 1986.

Coleman TG, Bower JD, Langford HG, et al: *Circulation* 42:509, 1970.

Cove-Smith JR, Knapp MS: *Q J Med* 47:49, 1978.

Curtis JJ, Luke RG, Diethelm AG, et al: *Lancet* 2:739, 1985.

Curtis JJ, Luke RG, Dubovsky E, et al: *Lancet* 2:477, 1986.

Curtis JJ, Luke RG, Dustan HP, et al: *N Engl J Med* 309:1009, 1983.

Curtis JJ, Luke RG, Jones P, et al: *Am J Med* 85:134, 1988.

Dahl T, Eide I, Fryjordet A: *Acta Med Scand* 209:121, 1981.

de Gaetano G, Bucchi F, Gambino MC, et al: *Lancet* 1:736, 1986.

Diamond S, Henrich WL: *J Crit Illness* 1:37, 1986.

Donadio JV Jr, Ilstrup DM, Holley KE, et al: *Mayo Clin Proc* 63:3, 1988.

Donohoe JF, Kelly J, Laher MS: *Am J Med* 85(Suppl 3B):31, 1988.

Dworkin LD, Benstein JA: *Am J Hypertens* 2:162S, 1989.

Eknoyan G, Suki WN: *Semin Nephrol* 5:34, 1985.

Eliahou EH, Boner G, Rakowczick M: *J Urol* 99:379, 1968.

Eliahou HE, Cohen D, Ben-David A, et al: *Cardiovasc Drugs Ther* 1:523, 1988.

Elias AN, Vaziri ND, Maksy M: *Arch Intern Med* 145:1013, 1985.

Epstein M, Hollenberg NK: *J Lab Clin Med* 87:411, 1976.

Eschbach JW: *Kidney Int* 35:134, 1989.

Evanoff G, Thompson C, Brown J, et al: *Arch Intern Med* 149:1129, 1989.

Feehally J, Walls J, Mistry N, et al: *Br Med J* 295:310, 1987.

Ghose RR, Harindra V: *Br Med J* 298:1626, 1989.

Gifford RW Jr, McCormack LJ, Poutasse EF: *Mayo Clin Proc* 40:834, 1965.

Given BD, Vita NA, Black HR, et al: *Hypertension* 8:489, 1986.

Goldblatt H: *Urol Clin North Am* 2:219, 1975.

Goldblatt WA: *J Soc Chem Ind* (London) 52:1056, 1933.

Gordon RD, Thomas MJ, Thomas F, et al: *Clin Exp Pharmacol Physiol* (Suppl 2):109, 1975.

Gordon RD, Tunny TJ, Evans EB, et al: *Nephron* 44(Suppl 1):25, 1986.

Göthberg G, Lundin S, Folkow B, et al: *Acta Physiol Scand* 116:93, 1982.

Grollman A: *Am J Physiol* 173:364, 1953.

Grollman A, Muirhead EE, Vanatta J: *Am J Physiol* 157:21, 1949.

Grossman R, Ramanathan K, Fresco R: *Clin Pediatr* 12:250, 1973.

Guidi E, Bianchi G, Rivolta E, et al: *Nephron* 41:14, 1985.

Harrison TR, Mason MF, Resnick H, et al: *Trans Assoc Am Physiol* 51:280, 1936.

Health Care Financing Administration: End-Stage Renal Disease Program Highlights. Publication No. GPO 0-165-464. Washington, DC, US Government Printing Office, 1985.

Heeg JE, DeJong PE, van der Hem GK, et al: *Kidney Int* 32:78, 1987.

Hellebusch AA, Simmons JL, Holland N: *JAMA* 214:757, 1970.

Henrich WL: *Kidney Int* 30:605, 1986.

Heyka RJ, Vidt DG: *Cleve Clin J Med* 56:65, 1989.

Hoard TD, O'Brien DP III: *J Urol* 115:326, 1976.

Hollenberg NK, Epstein M, Basch RI, et al: *Am J Med* 47:845, 1969.

Hommel E, Mathiesen ER, Giese J, et al: *Scand J Clin Lab Invest* 49:537, 1989.

Hornych A, Boisson J, Gaschard JC: *J Hypertension* 6(Suppl 4):S721, 1988 (abst).

Hostetter TH, Rennke HG, Brenner BM: *Am J Med* 72:375, 1982.

Hricik DE: *Clin Nephrol* 27:250, 1987.

Jacobson SH, Eklöf O, Eriksson LG, et al: *Br Med J* 299:703, 1989.

Jacobson SH, Kjellstrand CM, Lins L-E: *Acta Med Scand* 224:47, 1988.

Jones DA, George NJR, O'Reilly PH, et al: *Lancet* 1:1052, 1987.

Karlström G, Arnman V, Folkow B, et al: *Hypertension* 11:597, 1988.

Kasiske BL: *Transplantation* 44:639, 1987.

Keane WF, Raij L: *Lab Invest* 52:599, 1985.

Keusch GW, Weidmann P, Campese V, et al: *Nephron* 21:1, 1978.

Kim KE, Onesti G, GelGuercio ET, et al: *Hypertension* 2:102, 1980.

Kimmelstiel P, Wilson C: *Am J Path* 12:83, 1936.

Kincaid-Smith P: *Kidney Int* 17:250, 1980.

Kincaid-Smith P, Whitworth JA: *Semin Nephrol* 8:155, 1988.

Kishimoto T, Terada T, Okahara T, et al: *Nephron* 47:49, 1987.

Klahr S: *N Engl J Med* 320:864, 1989.

Koskimies O: *Br Med J* 285:996, 1982.

Krolewski AS, Canessa M, Warram JH, et al: *N Engl J Med* 318:140, 1988.

Krolewski AS, Warram JH, Christlieb AR, et al: *Am J Med* 78:785, 1985.

Kurzrok R, Lieb C: *Proc Soc Exp Biol Med* 28:268, 1930.

Lamberton RP, Noth RH, Glickman M: *J Urol* 125L477, 1981.

Lazarus JM, Hampers CL, Bennett AH, et al: *Ann Intern Med* 76:733, 1972.

Lazarus JM, Hampers CL, Merrill JP: *Arch Intern Med* 133:1059, 1974.

Lee HC, Mitchell HC, Pettinger WA: *Clin Res* 37:396A, 1989 (abst).

Leenen FHH, Smith DL, Khanna R, et al: *Am Heart J* 110:102, 1985.

Levinsky NG: *N Engl J Med* 296:1453, 1977.

Lombard JH, Hinojosa-Laborde C, Cowley AW Jr: *Hypertension* 13:128, 1989.

Losito A, Fortunati F, Zampi I, et al: *Br Med J* 296:1562, 1988.

Loutzenhiser RD, Epstein M: *Am J Hypertens* 2:154S, 1989.

Luetscher JA, Kraemer FB: *Arch Intern Med* 148:937, 1988.

Luke RG: *Kidney Int* 31:1024, 1987.

Mangili R, Bending JJ, Scott G, et al: *N Engl J Med* 318:146, 1988.

Margolius HS: *Annu Rev Pharmacol Toxicol* 29:343, 1989.

Marre M, Chatellier G, Leblanc H, et al: *Br Med J* 297:1092, 1988.

Maschio G, Oldrizzi L, Tessitore N, et al: *Kidney Int* 22:371, 1982.

McLachlan MSF: *Lancet* 2:143, 1978.

Meyer-Lehnert H, Schrier RW: *Hypertension* 13:352, 1989.

Mihatsch MJ, Bach JF, Coovadia HM, et al: *Klin Wochenschr* 66:43, 1988.

Mimran A, Insua A, Ribstein J, et al: *J Hypertension* 6:919, 1988.

Mitch WE, Wilcox CS: *Am J Med* 72:536, 1982.

Mitchell HC, Graham RM, Pettinger WA: *Ann Intern Med* 93:676, 1980.

Mogensen CE: *Lancet* 1:867, 1988.

Mroczek WJ, Davidov M, Gavrilovich L, et al: *Circulation* 40:893, 1969.

Muirhead EE, Byers LW, Capdevila J, et al: *J Hypertension* 7:361, 1989.

Muirhead EE, Folkow B, Byers LW, et al: *Hypertension* 5(Suppl 1):112, 1983.

Muirhead EE, Jones F, Graham P: *Arch Pathol* 56:286, 1953.

Nath KA, Chmielewski DH, Hostetter TH: *Am J Physiol* 252:F829, 1987.

Neff MS, Kim KE, Persoff M, et al: *Circulation* 43:876, 1971.

Noth RH, Krolewski AS, Kaysen GA, et al: *Ann Intern Med* 110:795, 1989.

Oates JA, FitzGerald GA, Branch RA, et al: *N Engl J Med* 319:689, 1988.

O'Hare JA, Ferriss JB, Brady D, et al: *Hypertension* 7(Suppl II):II-43, 1985.

Oldenburg B, Macdonald GJ, Shelley S: *Br Med J* 296:1089, 1988.

Olsen ME: *Dan Med Bull* 30:343, 1983.

Olsen ME, Hall JE, Montani J-P, et al: *Clin Sci* 72:429, 1987.

Olson JL, Wilson SK, Heptinstall RH: *Kidney Int* 29:849, 1986.

Orbison JL, Christian CL, Peters E: *Arch Pathol* 54:185, 1952.

Orofino L, Quereda C, Lamas S, et al: *Nephron* 45:22, 1987.

Parra G, Rodriguez-Iturbe B, Colina-Chourio J, et al: *Clin Nephrol* 29:58, 1988.

Parving H-H, Andersen AR, Smidt UM, et al: *Br Med J* 294:1443, 1987.

Parving H-H, Hommel E, Smidt UM: *Br Med J* 297:1086, 1988.

Patak RV, Mookerjee BK, Bentzel CJ, et al: *Prostaglandins* 106:649, 1975.

Paton TW, Cornish WR, Manuel MA, et al: *Clin Pharmacokinet* 10:404, 1986.

Patrono C, Dunn MJ: *Kidney Int* 32:1, 1987.

Paulsen EP, Ayers CR, Seip RL, et al: *Hypertension* 13:781, 1989.

Perez G, Lespier L, Jacobi J, et al: *Arch Intern Med* 137:852, 1977b.

Perez G, Lespier L, Knowles R, et al: *Arch Intern Med* 137.1018, 1977a.

Raine AEG: *Lancet* 1:97, 1988.

Rambausek M, Rhein C, Waldherr R, et al: *Eur J Clin Invest* 19:176, 1989.

Rao TKS, Gupta SK, Butt KMH, et al: *Arch Intern Med* 138:1236, 1978.

Ribstein J, Mourad G, Mion C, et al: *J Hypertension* 4(Suppl 5):S255, 1986.

Richards NT, Poston L, Hilton PJ: *J Hypertension* 7:1, 1989.

Robson RA, Fraenkel M, Barratt LJ, et al: *Br J Clin Pharmac* 25:402, 1988.

Rodriguez-Iturbe B, Baggio B, Colina-Chourio J, et al: *Kidney Int* 19:445, 1981.

Rostand SG, Brown G, Kirk KA, et al: *N Engl J Med* 320:684, 1989.

Rostand SG, Kirk KA, Rutsky EA, et al: *Kidney Int* 22:304, 1982.

Roxe DM: *Am J Med* 69:759, 1980.

Sagalowsky AI, Gailunas P, Helderman JH, et al: *J Urol* 129:253, 1983.

Salvetti A, Pedrinelli A, Magagna A, et al: *Clin Sci* 63:261S, 1982.

Sandler DP, Smith JC, Weinberg CR, et al: *N Engl J Med* 320:1238, 1989.

Savage JM, Shah V, Dillon MJ, et al: *Lancet* 2:441, 1978.

Schacht RG, Gallo GR, Gluck MC, et al: *J Chronic Dis* 32:515, 1979.

Scherrer U, Vissing SF, Morgan BJ: *Hypertension* 12:342, 1988.

Schlondorff D, Neuwirth R: *Am J Physiol* 251:F1, 1986.

Scholey JW, Meyer TW: *J Clin Invest* 83:1384, 1989.

Sealey JE, Blumenfeld JD, Bell GM: *J Hypertension* 6:763, 1988.

Seaquist ER, Goetz FC, Rich S, et al: *N Engl J Med* 320:1161, 1989.

Sheinfeld J, Linke CL, Talley TE, et al: *J Urology* 133:379, 1985.

Shulman NB, Ford CE, Hall WD, et al: *Hypertension* 13(Suppl I):I-80, 1989.

Siamopoulos K, Sellars L, Mishra SC, et al: *Q J Med* 52:349, 1983.

Sica DA, Hartford AM, Zawada ET: *Clin Nephrol* 22:102, 1984.

Smith H: *J Urol* 86:685, 1956.

Sniderman KW, Sprayregen S, Sos TA, et al: *Transplantation* 30:440, 1980.

Spitalewitz S, Porush JG, Reiser IW: *Arch Intern Med* 146:882, 1986.

Stewart PM, Whitworth JA, Burt D, et al: *J Hypertension* 6:947, 1988 (abst).

Stoff JS: *Am J Med* 80(Suppl 1A):56, 1986.

Strandgaard S, Hansen U: *Br Med J* 292:1041, 1986.

Strongwater SL, Galvanek EG, Stoff JS: *Arch Intern Med* 149.582, 1989.

Taguma Y, Kitamoto Y, Futaki G, et al: *N Engl J Med* 313:1617, 1985.

Taylor GM, Carmichael DJS, Peart WS: *J Hypertension* 4:703, 1986.

Teutsch S, Newman J, Eggers P: *Am J Kid Dis* 13:11, 1989.

Toth PD, Woods JR, Lingeman JE, et al: *Am J Hypertens* 2:19A, 1989.

Uribarri J, Oh MS, Carroll HJ: *Am J Nephrol* 3:193, 1983.

Vane JR: *Br J Pharmacol* 79:821, 1983.

Verbeelen DL, De Boel S: *Br Med J* 289:20, 1984.

Vertes V, Cangiano JL, Berman LB, et al: *N Engl J Med* 289:978, 1969.

Vetter W, Wehling M, Foerster E-Ch, et al: *Klin Wochenschr* 62:731, 1984.

Viberti GC: *Am J Kid Dis* 13:41, 1989.

Vio CP, Figueroa CD, Caorsi I: *Am J Hypertens* 1:269, 1988.

von Euler US: *Arch Exp Pathol Pharmacol* 175:78, 1934.

Wanner C, Lüscher TF, Schollmeyer P, et al: *Nephron* 45:236, 1987.

Watnick TJ, Jenkins RR, Rackoff P, et al: *Transplantation* 45:59, 1988.

Watts RA, Hoffbrand BI: *J Hum Hypertens* 1:65, 1987.

Weidmann P, Gnädinger MP, Schohn D, et al: *Eur J Clin Pharmacol* 36:223, 1989.

Weidmann P, Maxwell MH: *Kidney Int* 8:S-219, 1975.

Wesson LG: *Nephron* 32:1, 1982.

Whelton PK, Klag MJ: *Hypertension* 13(Suppl I):I-19, 1989.

Whelton PK, Russell RP, Harrington DP, et al: *JAMA* 241:1128, 1979.

White RH, Schambelan M: *Ann Intern Med* 92:199, 1980.

Williams CM, Thomas WC Jr: *N Engl J Med* 321:1269, 1989.

Wollam GL, Tarazi RC, Bravo EL, et al: *Am J Med* 72:929, 1982.

Ying CY, Tifft CP, Gavrad H, et al: *N Engl J Med* 311:1070, 1984.

Yoshida Y, Fogo A, Ichikawa I, et al: *Kidney Int* 35:643, 1989a.

Yoshida Y, Kawamura T, Ikoma M, et al: *Kidney Int* 36:626, 1989b.

Zucchelli P, Santoro A, Zuccala A: *Semin Nephrol* 8:163, 1988.

# 10 Renal Vascular Hypertension

Renovascular disease is one of the more common causes of secondary hypertension, with reports of its frequency varying from less than 1% in unselected populations to as many as 20% of patients referred to special centers. Renovascular disease continues to attract great interest because of a confluence of these factors: (1) advances in our understanding of its pathogenesis; (2) availability of more accurate diagnostic tests; and (3) advent of improved therapy by drugs, surgery, and angioplasty.

## RENOVASCULAR DISEASE VERSUS RENOVASCULAR HYPERTENSION

*Renovascular hypertension* refers to hypertension caused by renal hypoperfusion. It is important to realize that *renovascular disease* may or may not cause sufficient hypoperfusion to set off the processes that lead to hypertension. The problem is simply that renovascular disease is much more common than is renovascular hypertension. For example, arteriography revealed some degree of renal artery stenosis in 32% of 304 normotensive patients and 67% of 193 hypertensives with an increasing prevalence the older the patients (Eyler et al, 1962) (Table 10.1).

**Table 10.1. Prevalence of Renal Arterial Lesions in Normotensive and Hypertensive Patients[a]**

| Age (Years) | Normotensive | | Hypertensive | |
|---|---|---|---|---|
| | Normal | Lesion | Normal | Lesion |
| 31–40 | 7 | 3 | 6 | 10 |
| 41–50 | 26 | 8 | 14 | 22 |
| 51–60 | 99 | 35 | 28 | 50 |
| Over 60 | 69 | 56 | 15 | 48 |

[a]Data from Eyler WR, Clark MD, Garman JE, et al: *Radiology* 78:879, 1962.

Note that almost half of normotensive patients over 60 had atherosclerotic lesions in their renal vessels.

Before procedures were available to prove the functional significance of stenotic lesions, surgery was frequently performed on hypertensive patients with a unilateral small kidney who did not have reversible renovascular hypertension. Homer Smith recognized this as early as 1948 as a misguided application of Goldblatt's experimental model of hypertension produced by clamping the renal artery of dogs. He found that only 25% of patients were relieved of their hypertension by nephrectomy and warned that only about 2% of all hypertensives probably could be helped by surgery (Smith, 1956).

## PREVALENCE

Smith's estimate of the true prevalence of renovascular hypertension may be right. The prevalence varies with the nature of the hypertensive population:

—In nonselected patient populations, the prevalence is less than 1% as noted in Table 1.11.

—Among patients referred for diagnostic studies, 2 to 4% have renovascular hypertension (Gifford, 1969; Ferguson, 1975).

—In patients with suggestive clinical features, the prevalence is higher. Horvath et al (1982) did arteriograms on 490 patients chosen because of severe, resistant, or rapidly progressive hypertension, particularly with rising serum creatinine or epigastric bruits. Renovascular hypertension was found in only one of the 152 who were below age 40 but in 50 of 338 (15%) of those over age 40, more often in those with poorly controlled hypertension, impaired renal function, or a history of analgesic abuse.

—Among patients with accelerated or malignant hypertension, the prevalence will be even higher. Of 123 adults with diastolic blood pressure (DBP) > 125 mm Hg and grade III or IV retinopathy, 4% of the blacks and 32% of the whites had renovascular hypertension (Davis et al, 1979). Similarly, those with severe hypertension and azotemia are more likely to have renovascular hypertension. Of 106 patients with severe hypertension, 39 (37%) had renovascular hypertension, whereas among the 21 of these 106 patients with serum creatinine > 1.5 mg/dl, 10 had this diagnosis (Ying et al, 1984). In another center, 14% of the patients with end stage renal disease had atherosclerotic renovascular disease as the cause (Scoble et al, 1989).

—Among black hypertensive patients the prevalence is lower. All published data support a lower frequency among black hypertensives: Keith (1982) found the disease in only 0.25% of 7200 unselected black hypertensives and in only 0.65% of those referred because of severe hypertension, abnormal intravenous pyelograms (IVP), or abdominal bruits.

—Diabetics have a higher prevalence of renovascular disease (Shapiro et al, 1965) but not of renovascular hypertension (Munichoodappa et al, 1979).

## MECHANISMS FOR HYPERTENSION

### Animal Models

A massive body of literature has appeared since Goldblatt and coworkers (1934) first induced hypertension in dogs by partially occluding one renal artery and removing the opposite kidney. Although an increased secretion of renin from the clipped kidney was demonstrated relatively early (Braun-Menendez et al, 1940), arguments arose about the role of renin versus the roles of renal retention of sodium or the absence of a normal renal depressor mechanism. Only during the past few years has the situation been sufficiently clarified to allow general agreement that *increased renin secretion is responsible for the hypertension caused by renal hypoperfusion* (Barger, 1979), whereas renal retention of sodium is the primary mechanism for hypertension resulting from loss of renal tissue (see Chapter 9).

### Original Goldblatt Experiment

The controversy started because Goldblatt and coworkers (1934), looking not for renovascular hypertension but for a renal cause for essential hypertension, put clamps on both renal arteries of their dogs. Fortunately, the clamps were inserted on separate occasions so that Goldblatt could observe the effect of unilateral obstruction (Fig. 10.1). However, with the modest degree of constriction that they used, unilateral clamping caused only transient hypertension. For permanent hypertension, both renal arteries had to be clamped, or one clamped and the contralateral kidney removed (Goldblatt, 1975). The sheep and rat have been found to be particularly susceptible to two-kidney, one-clip hypertension, so they are better models than dogs and rabbits for the human (Swales et al, 1983).

### Two-Kidney One-Clip Versus One-Kidney One-Clip

The experimental counterpart to renovascular hypertension in the human is unilateral clamping of the renal artery with the contralateral kidney untouched, i.e., "two-kidney one-clip Goldblatt hypertension." When one renal artery is

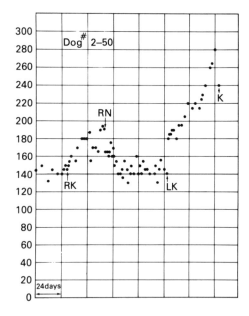

**Figure 10.1.** One of Goldblatt's original experiments. The graph shows the mean blood pressure of a dog whose right kidney was first moderately constricted (*RK*), with subsequent hypertension that was relieved after right nephrectomy (*RN*). After severe constriction of the left renal artery (*LK*), more severe hypertension occurred and the animal was sacrificed (*K*). (From Hoobler SW: In Stanley JC, Ernst CB, Fry WJ (eds). *Renovascular Hypertension.* Philadelphia: WB Saunders, 1984, 12–19.)

clipped and the other kidney removed, i.e., "one-kidney one-clip Goldblatt hypertension," a greater component of sodium retention is introduced, simply by the relative lack of functioning renal mass. This then is a model for renovascular hypertension plus chronic renal parenchymal disease.

An increase in renin release is responsible for the initial rise in blood pressure in both models. However, in the one-clip, one-kidney model, sodium retention from the AII stimulation of aldosterone becomes increasingly important (Swales et al, 1971). In the two-kidney one-clip model, sodium excretion is increased from the intact contralateral kidney as the pressure rises, i.e., pressure-natriuresis, so there is no sodium retention (Pickering, 1989).

Since the two-kidney, one-clip model is more appropriate to renovascular hypertension as seen in humans, only this model will be considered further.

**Time Course**

With a moderate stenosis, the relatively small increase in angiotensin II (AII) protects the stenotic kidney by restoring renal artery pressure distal to the stenosis, thereby maintaining renal perfusion with little effect on systemic blood pressure (Anderson et al, 1979). With a more severe stenosis, the course of experimental two-kidney one-clip hypertension can be divided into three phases (Brown et al, 1976) (Fig. 10.2). In Phase I the level of AII in the systemic circulation rises to such a high level that systemic arterial pressure is also increased, offering ad-

ditional protection to the stenotic kidney but at the cost of generalized hypertension via an increase in peripheral resistance. If the AII is removed, as during therapy with an angiotensin converting enzyme inhibitor (ACEI), renal perfusion beyond the stenosis will rapidly decrease (Bender et al, 1984).

During the next few days (phase II) while the hypertension and the renal hypoperfusion persist, the renin levels fall (Tagawa et al, 1974). However, the renin dependence of the hypertension is demonstrable by the fall in blood pressure when ACEIs are administered (Brunner et al, 1971; Wallace and Morton, 1984).

Although the levels of renin-angiotensin fall, they remain inappropriately high for the increased blood pressure and may still be responsible for the hemodynamic changes that characterize this phase (Maxwell et al, 1977a). Sodium and water are retained by the unclipped kidney, presumably from a combined effect of increased AII levels reaching it from the clipped kidney and neural effects mediated through renal nerves (Rademacher et al, 1986).

In phase III, removal of the clip will not relieve the hypertension, likely because of extensive arteriolar damage and glomerulosclerosis in the contralateral kidney.

**Mechanisms Beyond Renin and Volume**

Other factors may be involved that interrelate to these primary mechanisms including:

—activation of the sympathetic nervous system (Zimmerman et al, 1987);

—vasopressin (Ichikawa et al, 1983);

—endogenous opioid system: administration of an opioid antagonist attenuated development of hypertension in two-kidney, one-clip Goldbaltt rats (Chen et al, 1988);

—vasoconstrictive prostaglandins produced in the glomeruli of the clipped kidney (Stahl et al, 1984) or reduced vasodilatory prostaglandins from the nonclipped kidney (Machida et al, 1988). A role for renal prostaglandins is supported by the significant fall in blood pressure noted in patients with renovascular hypertension given aspirin (Imanishi et al, 1989).

**Mechanism in Humans**

As in the animal models, renovascular hypertension in humans is caused by increased renin release from the stenotic kidney (Barger, 1979; Pickering, 1989). An immediate release of renin has been measured in patients whose renal perfusion pressure was acutely reduced by

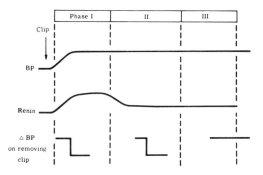

**Figure 10.2.** Sequential phases in experimental renovascular hypertension. After the clip is put on one main renal artery, with the contralateral kidney left untouched, blood pressure and renin secretion increase. In phase II, the blood pressure remains high, but renin secretion falls. In phase III, the blood pressure remains elevated despite removal of the clip, presumably reflecting vascular damage in the contralateral kidney. (From Brown JJ, Davies DL, Morton JJ, et al: *Lancet* 1:1219, 1976.)

a balloon-tipped catheter (Fiorentini et al, 1981). The high levels of AII increase renal vascular resistance, causing a shift in the pressure-natriuresis curve so that volume is maintained despite markedly elevated blood pressure (Kimura et al, 1987). Chronically, the stenotic kidney continues to secrete excess renin; fluid volume and peripheral resistance are both elevated (Tarazi and Dustan, 1973); the blood pressure falls when angiotensin antagonists are given; and, when the stenosis is relieved, hypertension recedes by a fall in peripheral resistance and fluid volume (Valvo et al, 1987). Sympathetic nervous overactivity likely plays a role in humans as well (Maslowski et al, 1983).

As in animal models, humans may enter into a third phase, wherein removal of the stenosis or the entire affected kidney will not relieve the hypertension because of widespread arteriolar damage and glomerulosclerosis in the contralateral kidney by prolonged exposure to high blood pressure and high levels of AII (London and Safar, 1989). This phenomenon is clinically relevant: The sooner an arterial lesion that is causing renovascular hypertension is removed, the more likely the chance for relief of the hypertension. Among 110 patients, corrective surgery for unilateral renovascular hypertension was successful in 78% of those with hypertension of less than 5 years' duration but in only 25% of those with a longer duration (Hughes et al, 1981).

Figure 10.3 represents a stepwise scheme for the hemodynamic and hormonal changes that underlie renovascular hypertension.

## CLASSIFICATION OF RENAL ARTERIAL LESIONS

The majority of renal arterial lesions are atherosclerotic; most of the rest are fibroplastic, but a number of other intrinsic and extrinsic

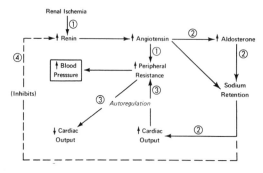

**Figure 10.3.** Hypertension with renovascular disease. Stepwise hemodynamic changes in the development of renovascular hypertension.

lesions can induce renovascular hypertension (Table 10.2). Among Japanese patients, 30% of renovascular hypertension is caused by progressive aortic arteritis (Takayasu's syndrome) (Hidai, 1975).

A classification of the fibrous and fibromuscular stenoses has been established by investigators from the Mayo Clinic (Lüscher et al, 1987) (Fig. 10.4). Of these, medial fibroplasia is the most common (Fig. 10.5). Focal fibroplastic lesions are most common in children (Stanley et al, 1978).

## Segmental Disease and Renal Infarction

Stenosis of only a small branch supplying a segment of one kidney may set off renovascular hypertension. Such segmental disease was found in 11% of one large series (Bookstein, 1968). Bookstein further recognized the presence of collateral vessels around areas of segmental stenoses with renal infarcts caused by thrombi or emboli. Presumably, if such collaterals are not adequate to relieve the hypoperfusion but the renal tissue remains viable, hypersecretion of renin from the partially infarcted tissue occurs and hypertension supervenes. After prolonged medical therapy, the hypertension may remit (Elkik et al, 1984).

## CLINICAL FEATURES

### General Features

The literature from 1940 through 1960 tends to characterize renovascular hypertension as a severe, rapidly accelerating disease of short duration, occurring mainly in those below 25 or over 50 years of age (Perera and Haelig, 1952). When techniques for recognition of the disease became more sensitive, it soon became obvious that most patients did not fit this pattern but rather had moderate hypertension of long duration, indistinguishable from essential hypertension (Page et al, 1959). The disease also occurs in neonates (Tapper et al, 1987) and children (Stanley et al, 1978) and may be discovered during pregnancy (Roach, 1973).

Attempts have been made to sharpen the clinical picture so as to provide some clues to the need for additional workup and guides for the decision concerning the need for surgical therapy. The most thorough was a cooperative study by 15 institutions involving 2442 hypertensive patients, 880 with renovascular disease (Maxwell et al, 1972). Of the 880, 502 had surgery;

**Table 10.2. Types of Lesions Associated with Renovascular Hypertension**

I. Intrinsic lesions
  A. Atherosclerosis
  B. Fibromuscular dysplasia
    1. Intimal
    2. Medial
      a. Dissection (Edwards et al: *May Clin Proc* 57:564, 1982)
      b. Segmental infarction (Elkik et al: *J Hypertens* 2:149, 1984)
    3. Periarterial or periadventitial
  C. Aneurysm (Martin et al: *J Vasc Surg* 9:26,1989)
  D. Emboli (Arakawa et al: *Arch Intern Med* 129:958, 1972
  E. Arteritis
    1. Polyarteritis nodosa (Dornfield et al: *JAMA* 215:1950, 1971)
    2. Takayasu's (Shelhamer et al: *Ann Intern Med* 103:121, 1985)
  F. Arteriovenous malformation (Ullian and Molitoris: *Clin Nephrol* 27:293, 1987)
  G. Angioma (Ferreras-Valenti et al: *Am J Med* 39:355, 1965)
  H. Neurofibromatosis (Pollard et al: *Postgrad Med J* 65:31, 1989)[a]
  I. Tumor thrombus (Jennings et al: *Br Med J* 2:1053, 1964)
  J. Rejection of renal transplant (Gunnels et al: *N Engl J Med* 274:543, 1966)
  K. Injury to the renal artery
    1. Thrombosis after umbilical artery cathterization (Plumer et al: *J Pediatr* 89:802, 1976)[a]
    2. Surgical ligation (McCormack et al: *Arch Surg* 108:220, 1974)
    3. Trauma (Monstrey et al: *J Trauma* 29:65, 1989)
    4. Radiation (Staab et al: *AJR* 126:634, 1976)
    5. Lithotripsy (Williams et al: *N Engl J Med* 320:739, 1989)
  L. Intrarenal cyst (Babka et al: *N Engl J Med* 291:343, 1974)
  M. Congenital unilateral renal hypoplasia (Ask-Upmark kidney) (Zezulka et al: *J Urol* 135:1000, 1986)
  N. Unilateral renal infection (Marks and Poutasse: *J Urol* 109:149, 1973)
II. Extrinsic lesions
  A. Pheochromocytoma (Brewster et al: *JAMA* 248:1094, 1982)
  B. Congenital fibrous band (Silver and Clements: *Ann Surg* 183:161, 1976)[a]
  C. Pressure from diaphragmatic crus (Martin: *Am J Surg* 121:351, 1971)[a]
  D. Metastatic tumors (Weidmann et al: *Am J Med* 47:528, 1969)
  E. Subcapsular or perirenal hematoma (Sterns et al: *Arch Intern Med* 145:169, 1985)
  F. Retroperitoneal fibrosis (Castle: *JAMA* 225:1085, 1973)
  G. Ptosis (de Zeeuw et al: *Lancet* 1:213, 1977)
  H. Ureteral obstruction (Nemoy et al: *JAMA* 225:512, 1973)
  I. Perirenal pseudocyst (Kato et al: *J Urol* 134:942, 1985)
  J. Stenosis of celiac axis with "steal" or renal blood flow (Alfidi et al: *Radiology* 102:545, 1972)

[a]More common in children.

of these, 60% had atherosclerotic lesions and 35% had fibromuscular disease.

Patients in this series with surgically cured renovascular disease were compared with a carefully matched group with essential hypertension (Table 10.3) (Simon et al, 1972). Of the features more common in patients with renovascular hypertension, only an abdominal bruit was of clear discriminatory value, heard in 46% of those with renovascular hypertension but only in 9% of those with essential hypertension. The bruit was heard over the flank in 12% of those with renovascular hypertension and only in 1% of those with essential hypertension. Many bruits heard in the epigastrium reflect stenosis within the celiac artery (McLoughlin et al, 1975), but the characteristics of the bruit provide useful information: A bruit that is high pitched, systolic and diastolic, and radiates laterally is strongly suggestive of functionally significant renal arterial stenosis; a diastolic bruit in a patient with fibrous disease usually indicates a favorable surgical result (Eipper et al, 1976).

Other clues suggestive of renovascular disease include these: onset of hypertension before age 25 or after age 60 (Anderson et al, 1988), headaches, cigarette smoking (Nicholson et al, 1983), white race, resistance to effective antihypertensive therapy on the one hand or an excellent response to angiotensin-converting enzyme (ACE) inhibitor therapy on the other (Vaughan, 1985).

Along with the last point, another criterion may now be added: Patients whose renal function rapidly deteriorates after treatment with an ACE inhibitor have a strong likelihood of bilateral renovascular disease or a stenosis in the artery to a solitary kidney (Bender et al, 1984). As noted earlier, the loss of renal function reflects a generalized loss of systemic vasoconstriction by angiotensin II that is needed to maintain adequate blood flow beyond the stenosis as well as a specific dilation of renal efferent arterioles that reduces glomerular filtration. A loss of renal function may also occur in the stenotic kidney of patients with unilateral renovascular disease and a normal contralateral kidney but can only be recognized by isotopic scan or other measures of renal perfusion (Wenting et al, 1984).

## Atherosclerotic Versus Fibromuscular Disease

The two major causes of renovascular hypertension—atherosclerosis and fibromuscular dysplasia—differ in numerous ways (Table 10.4).

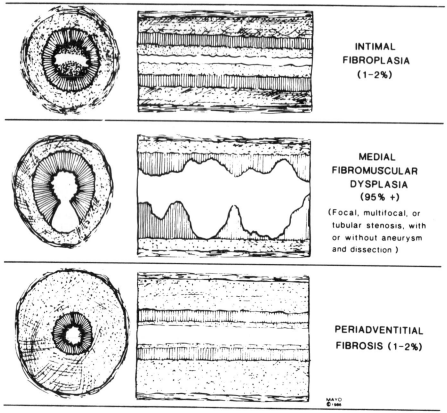

**Figure 10.4.** Histopathological classification of arterial fibromuscular dysplasia, based on predominant site of involvement of arterial wall intima (*top*), media (*middle*), and adventitia (*bottom*). (From Lüscher TF, Lie JT, Stanson AW, et al: *Mayo Clin Proc* 62:931, 1987.)

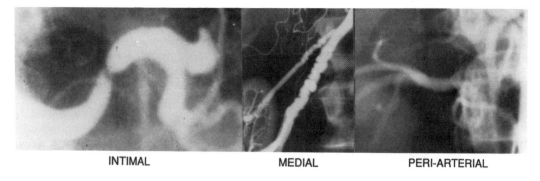

**Figure 10.5.** Representative x-rays of the three major types of fibromuscular dysplasia. (From Lüscher TF, Lie JT, Stanson AW, et al: *Mayo Clin Proc* 62:931, 1987.)

### Atherosclerotic Lesions

Patients with atherosclerotic renal artery disease are older and have more extensive renal damage, higher systolic pressure, and vascular disease elsewhere (Vidt, 1987). Their disease tends to progress if the stenoses are not relieved even if the hypertension is controlled. Progression has been noted in about half of 235 such

patients followed in three centers for 2 to 6 years (Wollenweber et al, 1968; Schreiber et al, 1981; Dean et al, 1981).

### Medial Fibroplasia

These lesions are usually noted in young women, the process often involving multiple arteries arising from the aorta, including the ca-

**Table 10.3. Clinical Characteristics of 131 Patients with Proved Renovascular Hypertension Compared with a Matched Group of Patients with Essential Hypertension**[a]

| | Essential Hypertension (%) | Renovascular Hypertension (%) |
|---|---|---|
| Duration of hypertension < 1 year | 12 | 24 |
| Age of onset after 50 | 9 | 15 |
| Family history of hypertension | 71 | 46 |
| Grade 3 or 4 funduscopic changes | 7 | 15 |
| Abdominal bruit | 9 | 46 |
| BUN > 20 mg/100 ml[b] | 8 | 15 |
| Serum K < 3.4 mEq/liter | 8 | 16 |
| Urinary casts | 9 | 20 |
| Proteinuria | 32 | 46 |

[a]From Simon N, Franklin SS, Bleifer KH, et al: *JAMA* 220:1209, 1972, Copyright 1972, American Medical Association.
[b]BUN, blood urea nitrogen.

rotid and celiac vessels (Lüscher et al, 1987). Half of patients with bilateral renal medial fibroplasia have extrarenal disease as well, which is rarely symptomatic. Compared with atherosclerotic disease, a progressive course may be somewhat less frequently seen with medial fibroplasia (Stewart et al, 1970). These features were found more commonly in 33 patients with fibromuscular dysplasia than in 61 subjects with normal renal arteries: cigarette smoking, HLA-DRw6 antigen, and a family history of cardiovascular disease (Sang et al, 1989). On the other hand, there was no association with oral contraceptive use, abnormal endogenous sex hormone levels, or increased renal mobility.

### Other Fibroplasias

Patients with the less common but more sharply localized fibroplastic lesions—intimal, perimedial, and periarterial—usually show rapid progression, so severe stenosis and hypertension

are frequently observed (Meaney et al, 1968; Pickering, 1989).

Based upon what we have learned about the natural history of the disease and the potential for sometimes acute and often progressive loss of renal function by medical therapy, repair of any form of functional renovascular disease seems indicated.

## Variants

### Bilateral Disease with Renal Failure

Renovascular disease, whether atherosclerotic or fibroplastic in origin, was bilateral in 25% of the patients in the Cooperative Study (Bookstein et al, 1972). Although the disease is usually predominant on one side, in some patients it may be sufficiently severe on both sides to induce renal insufficiency, i.e., ischemic renal disease (Jacobson, 1988). Such patients may be difficult to distinguish from the larger number with essential hypertension or primary renal parenchymal disease who progress into renal failure. The recognition is important since surgical repair or angioplasty may relieve both the hypertension and the renal failure (Morris et al, 1962; Ying et al, 1984; Kaylor et al, 1989).

The possibility of bilateral renovascular hypertension should be considered in:

—young women with severe hypertension, in whom fibroplastic disease is common;
—older patients with extensive atherosclerotic disease who suddenly have a worsening of hypertension or renal function;
—azotemic hypertensives who develop multiple episodes of acute pulmonary edema (Pickering et al, 1988);
—patients whose renal function quickly deteriorates after treatment with an ACEI (Bender et al, 1984) or other medical therapy;
—any hypertensive who develops rapidly pro-

**Table 10.4. Features of the Two Major Forms of Renal Artery Disease**

| Renal Artery Disease History | Incidence (%) | Age (yr) | Location of Lesion in Renal Artery | Natural |
|---|---|---|---|---|
| Atherosclerosis | 65 | > 50 | Proximal 2 cm; branch disease rare | Progression in 50%, often to total occlusion |
| Fibromuscular dysplasias | | | | |
| Intimal | 1–2 | Children, young adults | Mid main renal artery and/or branches | Progression in most cases; dissection and/or thrombosis common |
| Medial | 30 | 25–50 | Distal main renal artery and/or branches | Progression in 33%; dissection and/or thrombosis rare |
| Periarterial | 1–2 | 15–30 | Mid to distal main renal artery or branches | Progression in most cases, dissection and/or thrombosis common |

gressive oliguric renal failure without evidence of obstructive uropathy; the absence of marked proteinuria, red cells, and red blood cell casts in the urine further suggests that the process is not caused by an acute vasculitis or glomerulitis (Besarab et al, 1976).

Such patients should have arteriography to determine the presence of occlusive disease. Certain features on arteriography suggest viability of the renal tissue, including normal-sized kidneys, a nephrogram, and extensive collateral circulation, along with high renin levels from the renal veins.

In patients with these features, surgical repair or angioplasty should be considered since remarkable improvement may follow even in some whose renal function had deteriorated on medical therapy (Ying et al, 1984; Kaylor et al, 1989) (Fig. 10.6).

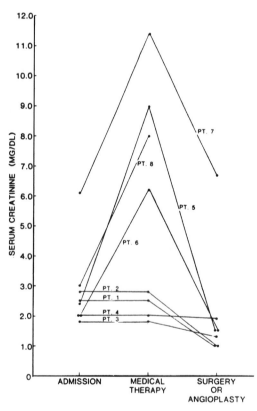

**Figure 10.6.** Effects of medical therapy and surgery or angioplasty on serum creatinine levels in eight patients with bilateral renovascular disease. Serum creatinine values represent the averages of three or more determinations. *Pt*, patient. (Reprinted with permission from Ying CY, Tifft CP, Gavras H, et al and *The New England Journal of Medicine* 311:1070, 1984.)

### Hypertension from Contralateral Ischemia

As described previously, hypertension may start with renal stenosis on one side but may persist because of damage to the nonstenotic kidney by the hypertension and high renin (Thal et al, 1963; Miller and Phillips, 1968; McAllister et al, 1972). The possibility should be considered if the renal vein renin level is paradoxically high from the nonstenotic kidney. In such cases, if repair of the stenosis does not relieve the hypertension, removal of the nonstenotic kidney should be considered.

### Hypertension After Renal Transplantation

As described in Chapter 9, patients who develop severe hypertension after successful renal transplantation should be evaluated for stenosis of the renal artery. These patients have the same propensity for marked loss of renal function if treated with an ACEI as do patients with bilateral renovascular disease.

### Hypertension and the Hypoplastic Kidney

As described in Chapter 9, most patients with a small kidney but without a stenotic lesion who respond to nephrectomy have increased plasma renin activity (PRA) from the venous blood draining the diseased kidney, suggesting a renovascular etiology (Stockigt et al, 1972). However, before making that conclusion and its logical corollary—only patients with a high renal vein PRA level should have nephrectomy—a word of caution is advised. In Gifford and associates' (1965) series from the Mayo Clinic the blood pressure of those patients with no evidence of vascular disease, most with unilateral pyelonephritis, had a *better* response to nephrectomy than did those with ischemic atrophy.

In another series, 57 of 174 patients with renovascular hypertension had a small, poorly perfused kidney with less than 25% of the total isotopic uptake (Geyskes et al, 1988). Revascularization, preferably by angioplasty, should always be considered since remarkable return on renal function may follow even when the kidney appears to be nonfunctioning. The continued secretion of renin into the renal vein is an indication of viability despite the absence of excretory function and the presence of severe tubular atrophy on biopsy.

Even with a unilateral small kidney, hypertension may arise from renovascular disease in the contralateral kidney. Such was the situation in eight young women with fibroplastic renovascular disease whose hypertension was relieved by relief of the stenosis without surgery on the small kidney (de Jong et al, 1989).

Total absence of one kidney, unilateral renal agenesis, occurs in one per 1500 people and should be recognized before evaluation and certainly before surgery upon the other kidney. In men, absence of the ipsilateral vas deferens is usually noted in those with renal agenesis (Donohue and Fauver, 1989).

### Nephroptosis

Although not observed in the 33 patients seen by Sang and associates (1989), increased mobility of the kidney (nephroptosis) has been associated with medial fibromuscular dysplasia (Derrick and Hanna, 1963). Ptosis of 7.5 cm or more was found on the affected side of 11 of 14 patients with fibromuscular dysplasia (de Zeeuw et al, 1977). The possibility that the repeated accordion-like movement of the renal artery results in the fibromuscular disease is an intriguing idea. Patients with hypertension that becomes worse when they stand or who have significant ptosis demonstrated on IVP should be considered for renin assays and angiography since nephropexy may relieve the hypertension (Clorius et al, 1978).

### Hyperaldosteronism

Occasional patients with renovascular hypertension have profound hypokalemia with excessive urinary potassium excretion and elevated aldosterone secretion—all reversed by nephrectomy (Goldberg and McCurdy, 1963).

### Nephrotic Syndrome

A small number of patients with renovascular hypertension have the nephrotic syndrome (Kumar and Shapiro, 1980). Although proteinuria was observed in 46% of the patients in the Cooperative Study (Table 10.3), the amount of protein wastage averaged only 0.5 g/day.

### Polycythemia

Polycythemia has occasionally been seen in patients with renovascular hypertension (Hudgson et al, 1967). Elevated peripheral and renal venous erythropoietin levels without polycythemia are much more common (Grützmacher et al, 1989).

## DIAGNOSTIC TESTS

A significant change in the recommendations for the screening and confirmation of the diagnosis of renovascular hypertension has oc-

curred. Whereas peripheral blood renin levels and intravenous pyelograms were frequently advocated as screening tests in the past, the recommendation now is to screen fewer patients—only those with suggestive clinical features—using selective renal arteriography (Fig. 10.7). Although the procedure is less definitive, a captopril challenge test utilizing peripheral blood PRA and isotonic renography after a single oral dose of captopril may be an acceptable screening test in those with less suggestive clinical features (Svetkey et al, 1989). As will be shown, more experience with this procedure is needed, but it may be used to rule out the disease in patients in whom renal arteriography is not thought to be indicated. Confirmation, if more is needed after arteriography, can be obtained by renal vein renin determinations.

This approach is predicated upon Bayes theorem and decision analysis as described in Chapter 2: the need for a test with few false-negatives to recognize a serious problem that requires special therapy. On the other hand, that test is acceptable if it gives rise to false-positive results but if additional studies (such as renal vein renins) are available to exclude those with renovascular disease that is not the cause of the hypertension.

Consider the routine isotopic renogram in this context: With a prevalence of 2% for renovascular hypertension in the overall hypertensive population and an 85% sensitivity and specificity for the test, an abnormal renogram will have a predictive value of only 10%. This increases the likelihood of renovascular hypertension 5-fold but hardly to the level that is adequate for a screening test. Moreover, 13 of the 15 abnormal renograms found in every 100 patients will turn out to be false-positives if the test is done routinely on unselected hypertensives who have at most a 2% prevalence of the disease.

The various tests now used to screen and diagnose renovascular disease will be described, not in the order shown in Figure 10.7 but grouped into those assessing renal perfusion, measuring renin levels, and visualizing the renal arteries.

## Tests Assessing Renal Perfusion

### Intravenous Pyelography

After Maxwell et al (1964) showed the advantages of the rapid-sequence IVP, this procedure became accepted as the best initial screening test for renovascular hypertension. However, extensive analyses of the costs and

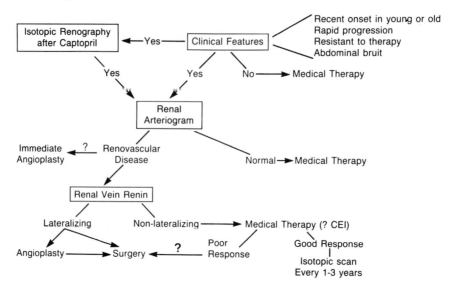

**Figure 10.7.** Scheme for the evaluation and management of renal vascular hypertension.

benefits of the procedure have shown that it is not a satisfactory screening test (Mushlin and Thornbury, 1989).

### Isotopic Scintigraphy

*Technique.* One of two radiolabeled agents, [131]iodohippurate or [99]technicium-diethylenetriamine pentaacetic acid (DTPA) can be used to evaluate renal function (Fine and Sarkar, 1989). About 80% of hippurate is removed from renal arterial blood during a single transit through the kidney, about 20% by glomerular filtration, the majority by extraction by proximal tubular cells, so that it can be used as a measure of renal blood flow. DTPA is excreted by glomerular filtration and is used as a measure of glomerular filtration rate.

The uptake of one or other of these radiolabeled compounds by the kidneys is measured during the first 1 to 3 minutes after intravenous injection to minimize interferences from renal pelvic accumulation and excretion. Simultaneous counting over both kidneys is usually done by a gamma camera interfaced with a computer. Sequential scintiphotos and renogram curves over computer-derived regions of interest are obtained.

### Captopril-Enhanced Scintigraphy

When used alone, isotopic renograms provided about 85% sensitivity and specificity for the diagnosis of renovascular hypertension, fig-

ures similar to those obtained with intravenous pyelography (Blaufox and Freeman, 1988).

The recognition that renal function in an ischemic kidney could abruptly be reduced further after a single dose of an angiotensin converting enzyme (ACE) inhibitor (Hricik et al, 1983) prompted the study of the effect of the most rapidly acting available ACE inhibitor, captopril, upon renal uptake of [99]Tc-DTPA (Majd et al, 1983; Wenting et al, 1984). The use of captopril before scintigraphy has markedly improved its accuracy with reports of over 80% sensitivity and 100% specificity (Geyskes et al, 1987; Fommei et al, 1987; Nally et al, 1988; Cuocolo et al, 1989; Dondi et al, 1989). Either a reduction of the uptake of DTPA or a slowing of the excretion of hippurate can be used to identify the effect of the ACE inhibitor in removing the protective actions of the high levels of angiotensin II upon the autoregulation of glomerular filtration and the maintenance of renal blood flow respectively (Fig. 10.8). Hippurate provides slightly better sensitivity and specificity than DTPA, particularly in patients with poor overall renal function (Sfakianakis et al, 1988; Kremer Hovinga et al, 1989).

Postcaptopril scintigraphy along with the measurement of peripheral blood renin activity as will be described later in this chapter now appears to be the best noninvasive screening test for renovascular hypertension (Wenting et al, 1988). Although it may give false-negative results in some patients with very small ischemic

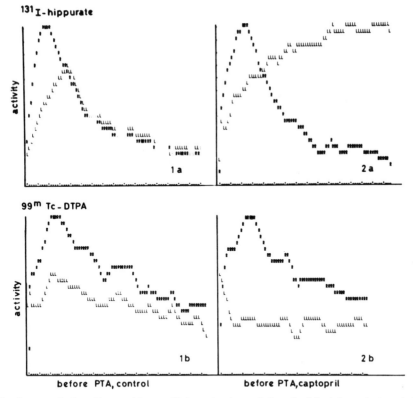

**Figure 10.8.** Renography in a 42-year-old man with hypertension and stenosis of the left renal artery. *L*, left kidney; *R*, right kidney. After percutaneous transluminal angioplasty (*PTA*), his hypertension was cured. The *upper half* of the figure shows [131]I-hippurate (*a*) and the *lower half* shows [99m]Tc-diethylenetriamine pentaacetic acid (*DTPA*) (*b*) time-activity curves in two different circumstances: (1) before PTA without any medication (control); (2) before PTA but with 25 mg of captopril taken orally 1 hour before the investigation. Before PTA, captopril slowed down the excretion of [131]-hippurate and reduced the uptake of [99m]Tc-DTPA only in the left kidney. After PTA this effect disappeared. (From Geyskes GG, Oei HY, Puylaert CBAJ, et al: Renovascular hypertension identified by captopril-induced changes in the renogram. *Hypertension* 9:451, 1987 and by permission of the American Heart Association, Inc.)

kidneys and false-positive results in some patients with chronic renal parenchymal disease (Fommei et al, 1988), I have inserted it into the flow diagram for the evaluation of renovascular hypertension (Fig. 10.8) as a possible first procedure.

## Tests Assessing Renin Release

Since hypersecretion of renin is the primary event in the pathogenesis of renovascular hypertension, it came as no surprise that increased peripheral plasma renin levels were found in patients with the disease after Helmer and Judson (1963) first described a practical method for its assay. However, subsequent experience with PRA assays in peripheral blood showed that many patients with curable disease did not have elevated levels, in keeping with the experimental evidence that secretion of renin from the clipped kidney falls to "normal" soon after renovas-

cular hypertension is induced, while at the same time renin release from the contralateral kidney is suppressed. Starting in 1967, reports of PRA assays on renal venous blood appeared, and the presence of an increased concentration of renin coming from the involved kidney became commonly used as a diagnostic and prognostic indicator. More recently, the dynamic effect of ACE inhibitors on renin release has been utilized to enhance the diagnostic accuracy of both peripheral and renal venous PRA assays. More about the control, variability, and measurement of PRA is given in Chapter 3.

### Peripheral Blood PRA

Elevated peripheral blood PRA is found in most patients with functionally significant renovascular hypertension. However, in the review of 24 published series by Rudnick and Maxwell (1984), the sensitivity of peripheral

PRA in renal vascular hypertension averaged only 57%, the specificity 66%. Of 326 patients with negative tests, 71% were improved by surgery; of 360 with positive tests, 86% were improved.

*Augmentation of Peripheral PRA.* In view of the discrepancies with peripheral PRA values obtained from patients while they were supine, various maneuvers have been used to augment PRA release in the hope that patients with curable disease would show a hyperresponsiveness and thereby improve the discriminatory value of peripheral levels. Most recently, the converting enzyme inhibitor captopril has been given orally in single 12.5- to 50-mg doses and peripheral blood obtained 60 to 120 minutes later (Case et al, 1979; Imai et al, 1980) (Fig. 10.9).

In the largest series using peripheral PRA after captopril, Muller et al (1986) established criteria for the performance and interpretation of the test (Table 10.5). Using these criteria, Muller et al found the test to identify all 56 patients in their series with renovascular hypertension and to give false-positive results in only two of 112 patients with essential hypertension and in six with secondary hypertension. They found the test to be neither as sensitive nor specific in the 46 patients in their series with renal insufficiency.

Since these criteria were published, most have found the test to provide excellent sensitivity but less specificity (Gaul et al, 1989) with overall predictive value of a positive test varying between 35% (Gosse et al, 1989) and 66% (Wilcox et al, 1988). Unfortunately, some authors use entirely different criteria that have not been validated and then report the test to be of no value (Idrissi et al, 1988). More prospective analyses are needed but, when they are done, they should either use the criteria of Muller et al or establish new ones.

At present, I believe the captopril test, combining the peripheral PRA response with a renogram, is a reasonable screening test to rule out renovascular disease in patients with relatively minimal clinical evidence for the diagnosis wherein an invasive procedure is not believed to be justified. But, if the patient has highly suggestive features or severe hypertension wherein renovascular hypertension should be ruled out with certainty, only a renal arteriogram will do so.

### Renal Vein Renin

In view of the poor sensitivity and specificity of measurements of peripheral PRA before the

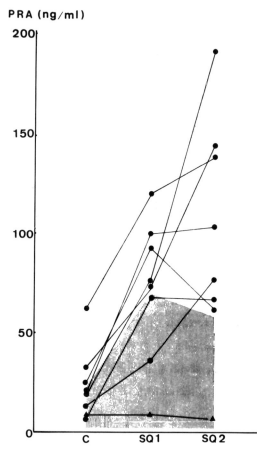

**PRA (ng/ml)**

**Figure 10.9.** Peripheral blood PRA response 1 hour (*SQ1*) and 2 hours (*SQ2*) after 50 mg of captopril in seven patients with unilateral renovascular hypertension (*solid circles*) and one patient with contralateral renal aplasia (*triangles*). Shaded area, the PRA response to captopril in normotensive subjects and essential hypertensive patients. The PRA assay utilized a 6-hour incubation, providing a normal range of 5 to 30 ng/ml, about 6 times higher than assays expressed in nanograms per milligrams per hour. (From Imai Y, Abe K, Otsuka Y, et al: *Jpn Heart J* 21:793, 1980.)

use of captopril challenge, most turned to comparison of renin levels from renal vein blood obtained by percutaneous catheterization as the most practical and definitive procedure to establish both the diagnosis and surgical curability of this disease. The initial success reported with this technique by Helmer and Judson (1960) has been amply confirmed.

The validity of the procedure is shown in Table 10.6, a compilation of the experience of numerous investigators from 1960 to 1983 compiled by Rudnick and Maxwell (1984). In most of these series, a ratio greater than 1.5 between the two renal vein PRA levels was considered abnormal. An abnormal ratio is 92% predictive of curability, and the 8% false-positives could

**Table 10.5. Criteria for the Captopril Screening Test**[a]

Method
  The patient should maintain a normal salt intake and receive no diuretics.
  If possible, all antihypertensive medications should be withdrawn 3 weeks prior to the test.
  The patient should be seated for at least 30 minutes; a venous blood sample is then drawn for measurement of baseline plasma renin activity.
  Captopril (50 mg diluted in 10 ml of water immediately before the test) is administered orally.
  At 60 minutes, a venous blood sample is drawn for measurement of stimulated plasma renin activity.
Interpretation: A positive test requires
  Stimulated plasma renin activity of 12 ng/ml/hour or more and;
  Absolute increase in plasma renin activity of 10 mg/ml/hour or more and;
  Increase in plasma renin activity of 150% or more, or 400% or more if baseline plasma renin activity is less than 3 ng/ml/hour.

[a]From Muller FB, Sealey JE, Case DB, et al: *Am J Med* 80:633, 1986.

represent errors in the renin test, surgical difficulties, or coincidental primary hypertension (Table 10.7).

*Nonlateralizing Ratio.* On the other hand, note that 65% of those whose ratio did not lateralize also were improved by surgery. These false-negatives may reflect problems with the technique or pathophysiological problems, particularly the presence of bilateral disease or the partial relief of ischemia by the development of extensive collateral circulation in the stenotic kidney (Table 10.7). The presence of collateral vessels is, in itself, indicative of a hemodynamically significant lesion, so the criteria of abnormality with renal vein renin levels should be lowered when collaterals are recognized by arteriography (Ernst et al, 1972).

As to the presence of bilateral disease, this can probably best be ascertained by looking for suppression of renin release from a nonischemic kidney (Stockigt et al, 1972). A renal/systemic

renin index should be calculated for both sides; the index = renal vein renin − systemic (infrarenal vena cava) renin ÷ systemic renin (Fig. 10.10). An index above 0.24 indicates that excess renin is being secreted from the kidney, whereas lower values indicate suppression (Vaughan, 1985). A "pure" unilateral lesion would show an index of zero from the nonischemic side and a ratio between the two renal veins above 1.5, i.e., lateralizing (Fig. 10.10).

The index or increment of renin for each renal vein over the level in the systemic vein (infrarenal vena cava) was found to be more sensitive and specific than the ratio between the two renal veins (Pickering et al, 1986b). With bilateral but asymmetric disease, the index would be above 0.24 on both sides, and the ratio between the two sides would be below 1.5, i.e., nonlateralizing. However, many patients with incomplete suppression from the contralateral kidney and a nonlateralizing renal vein ratio will improve after repair of the more ischemic kidney (Fig. 10.11). In this series from Michigan (Stanley and Fry, 1977), complete surgical cure was predicted by a high ratio and complete suppression in the contralateral kidney, i.e., index near zero. However, improvement was usual in those with bilateral renin secretion if the more ischemic side was repaired.

*What Ratio to Use.* Most of the series included in Table 10.6 used a ratio of 1.5 or higher to indicate lateralization. However, when the 95% confidence level is determined for the values obtained in patients without renovascular hypertension, i.e., in primary hypertensives, it is 1.63 (Sealey et al, 1973) to 2.0 (Maxwell et al, 1974).

The problem is the same as with all biological measurements used as diagnostic tests: The more specific it is made by using more rigid criteria for abnormality, the less sensitive it becomes.

**Table 10.6. Operative Results Versus Renal Vein Renin Ratios (RVRR) in Patients with Unilateral or Bilateral Renovascular Hypertension**[a]

| | Sensitivity RVRR+/Disease+ | Specificity RVRR−/Disease− | Surgical Improvement Improved/RVRR− | Improved/RVRR+ |
|---|---|---|---|---|
| All 58 series | 875/1097 (80%) | 120/193 (62%) | 222/342 (65%) | 875/948 (92%) |
| Bilateral RVHT (10 series) | 61/89 (68%) | 10/15 (67%) | 28/38 (74%) | 61/66 (92%) |
| Unilateral RVHT stimulated (16 series) | 300/377 (80%) | 24/45 (53%) | 77/101 (77%) | 300/321 (93%) |
| Simultaneous sampling (10 series) | 207/258 (80%) | 19/30 (63%) | 51/70 (73%) | 207/218 (95%) |

[a]Data from Rudnick MR, Maxwell MH: In Narins RG (ed): *Controversies in Nephrology and Hypertension.* New York, Churchill Livingston, 1984, p 123, by permission.

**Table 10.7. Causes of Problems with Renal Vein Renin Ratios**

False-negatives
  Errors of technique
    Improper positioning of catheters with admixtures of
      caval blood
    Nonsimultaneous sampling when renin secretion is
      changing
    Interference by contrast media
    Diuretic-induced increase in renin from nonstenotic
      kidney without increase from stenotic kidney
    Multiple renal veins (found in 25% on right, 2% on left)
    Errors in radioimmunoassay, particularly when renin
      levels are low
    Use of excessively high value for division between
      normal and abnormal
  Pathophysiological problems
    Bilateral disease of near equal degree
    Segmental disease (and failure to sample from
      segmental vein)
    Extensive collateral circulation
    Suppression of renin secretion by volume expansion,
      adrenergic blocking drugs, etc.
False-positives
  Nonsimultaneous sampling when renin secretion is
    changing
  Interference by contrast media
  Errors in radioimmunoassay, particularly when renin levels
    are low
  Asymmetric nephrosclerosis
  Inadequate surgical repair
  Use of excessively low value for division between normal
    and abnormal
  Coexisting primary (essential) hypertension

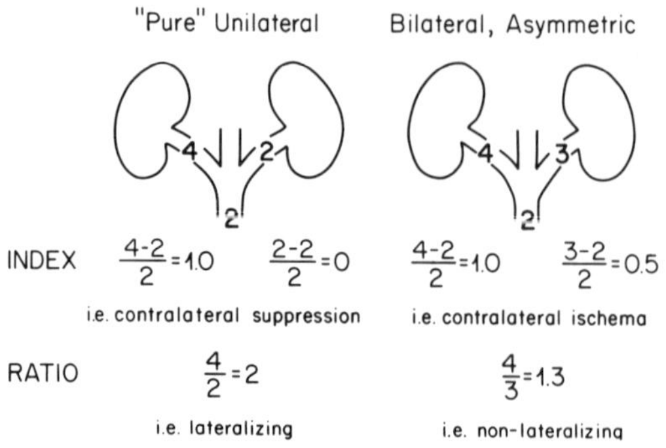

**Figure 10.10.** Representation of the renal vein renin levels in patients with "pure" unilateral renovascular hypertension (*left*) and bilateral but asymmetrical renovascular hypertension (*right*). *Index*, renal vein renin − systemic vein renin/systemic vein renin. *Ratio*, ischemic renal vein renin/contralateral renal vein renin.

With a ratio of 2.0, only 5% false-positives would be expected, but the number of false-negatives would be even higher than the 20% figure shown in Table 10.6 obtained mainly from series using a ratio of 1.5. Since there have been only 8% false-positives (lateralizing but unimproved by surgery) with the use of 1.5, that ratio should probably be used, with the recognition that a nonlateralizing ratio will be seen in many patients with correctable renovascular hypertension (Lüscher et al, 1986). Since other therapies are available, the main concern is to avoid unnecessary surgery. However, the use of a ratio of 2.0 would exclude curative surgery for a considerable number who would not be excluded by a ratio of 1.5 without significantly diminishing the number of false-positives who would have unnecessary surgery.

*Problems in Interpretation.* As noted in Table 10.7, many factors may give rise to false-negative or false-positive renal vein renin ratios. Despite these various problems, the data shown in Table 10.6 support the use of the test to establish the diagnosis and give a good indication of the likelihood of improvement by surgery or angioplasty (Pickering et al, 1986b). One could argue that the procedure is not needed after a lesion is seen by renal arteriography if angio-

plasty is the therapy to be used or if a marked renal artery stenosis is found in a patient with severe hypertension who likely should have either angioplasty or surgery regardless of the results of the renin assay.

*Bilateral and Segmental Disease.* Even though lesions are bilateral in 25% with renovascular hypertension, one side is usually responsible. Lateralization of renin secretion to one kidney has been found in about two-thirds of the small number of patients with bilateral renal arterial stenosis studied (Table 10.6). When lateralization is found, unilateral surgery will likely relieve the hypertension (Gittes and McLaughlin, 1974). Recall that the disease may start on one side, but the contralateral kidney may be damaged and become the predominant renin-secreting side (McAllister et al, 1972).

When a segmental or branch lesion is seen by arteriography, blood should be obtained under fluoroscopic control from the vein draining that segment to attempt to identify a significantly higher renin level (Korobkin et al, 1976).

## Tests Visualizing the Renal Arteries

The various tests described in the preceding sections are often recommended before renal arteriography. However, more and more experience seems to confirm the wisdom of Foster and Oates' statement made in 1975: "To identify renal artery stenosis one must look at the renal artery; the one adequate screening test for renovascular hypertension is therefore arteriography."

The reasons for choosing renal arteriography either as the initial study or before a renal vein renin study include:

1. Arteriography provides an immediate answer

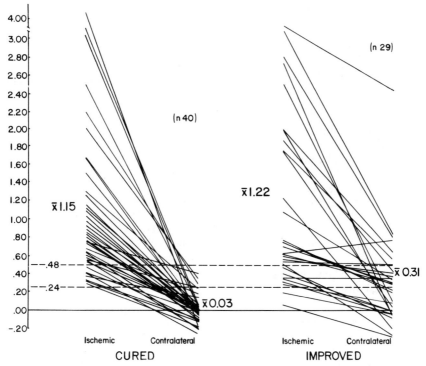

**Figure 10.11.** Renal vein renin/systemic vein renin index from the ischemic and contralateral sides in 40 patients who were cured (*left*) and 29 patients who were improved (*right*) after unilateral renal artery revascularization. (From Stanley JC, Fry WJ: *Arch Surg* 112:1291, 1977, Copyright 1977, American Medical Association.)

to the question: Is there renovascular disease that is potentially curable?

2. With digital subtraction techniques, small catheters and small quantities of dye are needed so that discomfort and danger for the patient are minimal (Hillman, 1989). Even with conventional arteriography using either nonionic or ionic contrast agents, the danger of contrast material-induced renal damage is small and can be further minimized by adequate hydration and avoidance of nonsteroidal antiinflammatory agents (Parfrey et al, 1989).

3. Knowledge of the renal vascular architecture is helpful before collection of renal vein renin samples. The recognition of branch or segmental vascular lesions, cysts, and tumors will indicate the need for selective venous sampling.

4. The development of extensive collateral flow to a kidney with a major vascular stenosis may diminish the hypersecretion of renin from the stenotic kidney so that the renal venous renin ratio no longer lateralizes.

5. The percentage of false-negative renin ratios is significant, so the absence of lateralization does not preclude the possibility of repair.

Therefore, renal arteriography should be considered on all patients with the clinical features suggestive of renovascular hypertension described earlier in this chapter (Carmichael et al, 1986; Pape et al, 1988).

**Intravenous Angiography**

For a brief time, digital subtraction *intravenous* angiography was recommended for both screening and confirmation (Hillman et al, 1982). Despite the superficial attractiveness of the "less invasive" venous angiographic procedure, arteriography will still be needed to visualize small, intrarenal vessels. The need to search carefully for such was shown by the Cooperative Study of Renovascular Hypertension (Bookstein et al, 1972). In those with atherosclerosis, stenoses were seen in segmental branches in 6.6%, and in those with fibromuscular disease, the lesions were seen most commonly in the mid- and distal third of the renal artery and in segmental branches in 5%. Therefore, the failure to visualize 10 to 20% of renal arteries with intravenous angiography and the multiple advantages of the intraarterial technique make arteriography the preferred procedure (Svetkey et al, 1988).

### Digital Subtraction Arteriography

This technique is likely to replace conventional arteriography (Hillman, 1989) even though it provides less definition of the renal vasculature. With digital video subtraction angiographic equipment, preexisting images are subtracted from films taken after injection of contrast media so that the renal arteries can be visualized with small quantities of diluted (15%) contrast material injected through a small catheter (Kaufman et al, 1984), making the procedure suitable for outpatient use even among children (Tonkin et al, 1988) with excellent safety (Saint-Georges and Aube, 1985).

### Prognostic Accuracy

Renal arteriography is almost always successful in diagnosing renal arterial *disease*. It is of relatively little value, however, in deciding upon surgical curability of renovascular *hypertension*. In the Cooperative Study, neither the degree of stenosis, the presence of poststenotic dilatation, nor the presence of collateral circulation was of significant discriminatory value in predicting success or failure of surgery (Bookstein et al, 1972). In patients with apparently totally occluded main renal arteries, the finding of a markedly delayed and reduced nephrogram is a useful indicator of irreversible renal damage that likely will not respond to revascularization (Feltrin et al, 1986).

There will be increasing temptation to proceed with transluminal balloon dilation at the time of arteriography. Some are doing so, but usually only after having obtained evidence for the presence of functionally significant renovascular hypertension by means of renin studies before the arteriogram (Pickering et al, 1984b).

### Ultrasound

The combination of duplex scanning and pulse echo imaging to evaluate ultrasound signals along with the simultaneous demonstration of the blood vessel lumen with the recording of Doppler shift signal may make duplex ultrasound a useful screening technique for renal artery stenosis (Robertson et al, 1988). Experience remains very limited and Doppler sonography is not now recommended (Hillman, 1989).

### Other Procedures

A number of other procedures have been used to diagnose renovascular hypertension but they are now outdated. These include:

—angiotensin infusion test (Kaplan and Silah, 1964);
—pressure gradient across the stenosis at surgery (Lupu et al, 1968);
—renal biopsy (Vertes et al, 1964);
—split renal function tests (Schaeffer and Stamey, 1975).

## THERAPY

Once a lesion is found and proved to be functionally significant, three choices are available for the treatment of renovascular hypertension: medical, surgical, and angioplasty. For each patient, the choice must be made individually, but for most patients chronic medical therapy is not the preferred choice. With increasing experience with and confidence in angioplasty, it has increasingly become the first choice. However, surgery remains the modality that is most certain to provide prolonged relief and, for a considerable number of patients, it is clearly the best choice. Parenthetically, if patients are clearly not candidates for surgery or angioplasty, there is no reason to subject them to the various procedures needed to make the diagnosis.

Formal decision analysis may be used to make the choice (Kopelman et al, 1988), but in most patients the decision is fairly simple: angioplasty if the lesion is amenable to balloon dilation, surgery if it is not or if angioplasty is unsuccessful.

The population of patients who are being operated upon has changed over the past 10 to 15 years, including more and more who have more complicated conditions including diffuse atherosclerotic disease, bilateral renal artery stenoses, totally occluded renal arteries, or azotemia (Libertino et al, 1988). Whereas more of the younger patients with less complicated disease are having angioplasty, more of the elderly with more severe disease are having surgery, increasingly to preserve renal function rather than to control the hypertension (Novick et al, 1987). Meanwhile, medical therapy, although it has become more effective, has been recognized to often lead to acute decreases in renal perfusion, occasionally to progressive loss of renal structure and function, and rarely to occlusion of stenotic renal arteries (Postma et al, 1989). Therefore, unless the patient is not suited to either surgery or angioplasty, medical therapy is usually given only for short intervals, often to prepare the patient for a reparative procedure. The response to chronic ACE inhibitor therapy is usually predictive of the response to angioplasty (Staessen et al, 1988) and likely to surgery as well.

In the following description of the results of the three forms of therapy, the terms established by the Cooperative Study (Foster et al, 1975) are used: "cure" is a diastolic blood pressure of 90 mm Hg or less without medication; "improved" is a 15% or greater decrease and a diastolic blood pressure between 90 and 110 mm Hg; "failure" is either a less than 15% decrease with a diastolic above 90 mm Hg or a diastolic greater than 110 mm Hg.

## Medical Therapy

The role of antihypertensive drug therapy in the long-term management of renovascular hypertension is shrinking, even as more effective agents have become available (Pickering, 1987). This shrinkage reflects the combination of improving results from surgery and angioplasty and concerns about the adverse long-term effects of medical therapy. However, if hypertension is well controlled and *renal function does not deteriorate* under careful surveillance, medical therapy may be continued indefinitely.

Renovascular hypertension in the neonate or young child may respond to medical therapy, reducing the need for early nephrectomy (Adelman et al, 1978).

### Medical Regimen

The most effective therapy is an angiotensin-converting enzyme inhibitor (ACEI). In the largest published series, captopril was effective for at least 3 months in over 80% of 269 patients with renovascular hypertension (Hollenberg, 1988). Similar good results have been noted with enalapril (Tillman et al, 1984) and lisinopril (Fyhrquist et al, 1987).

However, as noted earlier in this chapter, the use of an ACEI may cause a marked decrease of blood flow through the stenotic kidney and, if that is the only kidney or if there is bilateral renovascular disease, the result may be rapid though usually reversible renal failure. This is not unique to ACEIs (Textor et al, 1985) but is more likely to occur with their use because of their greater effectiveness, the removal of AII support of autoregulation, and the preferential dilation of renal efferent vessels that together lead to reduced glomerular filtration and renal perfusion. The recommendation has therefore been made that in patients who are candidates for operation, ACEI "be given for no more than 1 month before proceeding to corrective sur-

gery, to allow maximum blood pressure reduction without endangering the stenotic kidney for too long" (Tillman et al, 1984). Nonetheless, ACEIs may be successfully used for long-term therapy. In one series, only 20% of patients with unilateral renovascular hypertension had a significant fall in glomerular filtration rate after successful reduction of the blood pressure with enalapril plus hydrochlorothiazide (Franklin and Smith, 1985). Fortunately, return of renal function is usual when the ACEI is stopped, even after as long as 2 years (Salahudeen and Pingle, 1988). Nonetheless, numerous instances of complete occlusion of markedly stenotic renal arteries after ACEI therapy have been seen, particularly if the ACEI is given with a diuretic (Postma et al, 1989).

Calcium entry blockers such as nifedipine may provide equal control of hypertension and less impairment of renal function than ACEIs (Ribstein et al, 1988; Miyamori et al, 1988). Calcium entry blockers may maintain blood flow better because of their preferential preglomerular vasodilatory effect.

## Surgery

Pickering et al (1984a) have combined the results of published large series from single centers to provide a picture of the expected results from renovascular surgery (Table 10.8). The results with fibromuscular disease are better than with atherosclerotic.

Over the past 5 to 10 years, surgery has increasingly been performed on sicker and older patients with more extensive atherosclerotic disease, more to preserve renal function than to control hypertension (Novick et al, 1987). Surgical techniques have expanded with more aortic replacements and alternate bypass procedures and the use of microvascular and extracorporeal techniques for branch renal artery disease (Novick, 1986). Despite the inclusion of more difficult patients, results are as good as or better than those noted in Table 10.8 (Novick et al, 1987; Libertino et al, 1988; Tack and Sos, 1989; Lawrie et al, 1989).

### Long-term Follow-up

Long-term follow-up shows a progressive fall in the number of patients cured or improved, not surprising in view of the extensive vascular disease that most have at the time of surgery. In one series, the majority of patients operated upon for fibroplastic disease were alive and normotensive after 15 years, whereas only about

**Table 10.8. Results of Surgical Series for Treatment of Renovascular Hypertension[a]**

| | No. of Patients | Cured (%) | Improved (%) | Failed (%) | Deaths (%) | Nephrectomy (%) |
|---|---|---|---|---|---|---|
| Atheroma (all) | 969 | 38 | 42 | 20 | 3.9 | 14.9 |
| Focal | 382 | 42 | 46 | 13 | 0 | ? |
| Diffuse | 435 | 24 | 45 | 36 | 8.8 | 7.6 |
| Fibromuscular | 663 | 59 | 30 | 11 | <1 | ? |

[a]Data from Pickering TG, Sos TA, Laragh JH: *Am J Med* 77:61, 1984a.

half of those with atherosclerotic disease were alive after 10 years and only half of them were normotensive (Horvath et al, 1986).

### Results in Special Groups

In addition to these overall results, special consideration should be given to special groups and situations.

*Children.* Renovascular hypertension is usually severe and second only to coarctation as a surgically remediable form of hypertension among children. Results of surgical repair have been in general very good: Fry et al (1973) cured 19 of 22; Novick et al (1978) cured or improved 21 of 27; Berkowitz and O'Neill (1989) cured or improved 17 of 17.

*Elderly.* With their predominance of atherosclerotic disease, those over 65 might be expected to do worse. Nonetheless, in the Cleveland Clinic series, patients over 65 did better with surgery than with medical therapy or angioplasty (Vidt, 1987), and the surgical results were as good in those over 65 years of age as those obtained in those under 65 (Novick et al, 1987). Repair of coexistent significant carotid or coronary vascular disease should be considered before renovascular surgery.

*Nonfunctioning Kidneys.* Even after complete occlusion of the renal artery, revascularization may be successful, even if delayed for as long as 56 days (Libertino et al, 1980). Patients who suddenly become anuric should be considered for immediate angiography and, if a correctable vascular lesion is identified, revascularization should be performed (Williams et al, 1988).

*Bilateral Renovascular Disease.* In most patients with bilateral renal artery stenoses, one side is functionally most impaired, and its repair is usually indicated. Most such patients will be improved after unilateral surgery (Osada et al, 1978).

*Renal Insufficiency.* Patients with bilateral renovascular disease or disease in the artery to a solitary kidney may present with renal insuf-

ficiency (Ying et al, 1984; Scoble et al, 1989). In a review of four surgical series involving 268 patients with bilateral ischemic renal disease, Jacobson (1988) noted operative mortality ranged from 2 to 15% and the majority of patients showed improved renal function over 2- to 3-year follow-up.

Similarly good overall results were noted in 19 patients with a single, ischemic kidney (McCready et al, 1987) and in 18 patients with Takayasu's disease (Lagneau and Michel, 1985).

*Arterial Stenosis after Transplantation.* As discussed in Chapter 9, this is one of the more common causes of posttransplant hypertension. If a stenosis is responsible for difficult-to-control hypertension or a threat to preservation of renal function, operative intervention may be indicated (Dickerman et al, 1980) although angioplasty will usually be the first choice.

*Intrarenal Branch Lesions.* Microvascular techniques sometimes combined with ex vivo (i.e., extracorpeal) reconstruction may enable successful revascularization of lesions deep within the kidney, lesions that formerly required nephrectomy (Novick, 1986).

### Transluminal Angioplasty

Introduced in 1964 for repair of peripheral vascular disease, transluminal angioplasty became more widely used after Grüntzig developed a double-lumen, polyvinyl catheter in 1976. After the first report of successful treatment of renovascular hypertension by percutaneous transluminal dilation (Grüntzig et al, 1978), fairly extensive experience has been reported and the technical aspects have continually improved (Tack and Sos, 1989).

Results, overall, have been excellent for those in whom the procedure is technically feasible (Table 10.9). The experiences in one recently reported series of 100 patients with atherosclerotic renovascular hypertension (Canzanello et al, 1989) gives a representative view of current expectations: About 75% of patients can be successfully dilated and, of these, 60% experience

**Table 10.9. Results of Percutaneous Balloon Angioplasty for Renovascular Hypertension (4-Month to 4-Year Follow-up)**

| | No. of Patients | Cured (%) | Improved (%) | Failed (%) | Deaths (%) | Nephrectomy (%) |
|---|---|---|---|---|---|---|
| Geyskes et al, 1983 | 70 | 20 | 41 | 31 | 1 | 0 |
| Sos et al, 1983 | 82 | 28 | 24 | 48 | 0 | 2 |
| Tegtmeyer et al, 1984 | 98 | 26 | 67 | 7 | 1 | 0 |
| Miller et al, 1985 | 63 | 75 | | 12 | 2 | 2 |
| Kuhlman et al, 1985 | | | | | | |
|   Atherosclerotic | 35 | 29 | 48 | 23 | 0 | 0 |
|   Fibroplastic | 25 | 50 | 32 | 18 | 0 | 0 |
| Canzanello et al, 1989 (all atherosclerotic) | 100 | 59 | | 27 | 2 | 0 |

a sustained amelioration of hypertension; most failures occur with ostial lesions; transient worsening of renal function is common but sustained stability is usual thereafter; surgical intervention is needed in about 5% and mortality is about 2%. Results with fibroplastic disease are significantly better (Tack and Sos, 1989).

The follow-up in all currently published series is too short to ensure the long-term effectiveness of the procedure. Perhaps 30% of patients will restenose, almost always within the first year after successful angioplasty. They usually can be successfully redilated, with an excellent chance for at least immediate improvement (Tegtmeyer et al, 1984).

### Patients with Renal Insufficiency

Most series include a few patients with renovascular disease and renal insufficiency. Although some find that they are unlikely to respond to angioplasty (Luft et al, 1983), others report improvement in blood pressure and renal function in one-half or more (Pickering et al, 1986a). Even renal arteries that appear to be totally occluded may be dilated successfully (Sniderman and Sos, 1982). It is the procedure of choice when stenosis develops in a renal transplant (Greenstein et al, 1987), and it may safely be performed in patients with stenosis in a solitary kidney (McDonald et al, 1988).

### Complications

Complications occur in about 10% of patients (Table 10.10), the rate and severity almost always decreasing with increasing experience (Hayes et al, 1988). Since the balloon causes cracking and occasional separation of the intima from the media rather than compression of atherosclerotic plaques (Adams and Reidy, 1987), it is remarkable that so few complications have been observed. Rupture of the renal artery may occur as long as 9 days after the procedure (Olin

**Table 10.10. Complications of Transluminal Angioplasty of Renal Arteries**

| Major (3–10%) | Minor |
|---|---|
| 1. Rupture of renal artery | 1. Hemorrhage at puncture site |
| 2. Dissection of the renal or access artery | 2. Renal artery spasm |
| 3. Renal artery thrombosis | 3. Transient mild acute renal failure not requiring dialysis |
| 4. Contrast-induced ARF requiring dialysis | 4. Transient hypertension |
| 5. Embolism with segmental renal infarction | 5. Rupture of the balloon |
| 6. Peripheral artery embolization | |
| 7. Mortality | |

and Wholey, 1987), but serious complications are relatively rare. However, the ready availability of surgical backup for possible serious complications is considered mandatory before angioplasty is performed.

### Renal Embolization

In a few instances, percutaneous renal embolization by injection of ethanol into the renal artery has been successfully utilized to treat severe hypertension in patients with renovascular hypertension in whom neither surgery nor angioplasty was feasible and in whom medical therapy was unsuccessful (Iaccarino et al, 1989).

### Comparisons

There are no valid comparisons among the three major forms of therapy, and there likely never will be. In one uncontrolled series of 106 patients, those given each form did about as well as the others (Baer et al, 1985). However, for now, long-term medical therapy should be given only to a few too sick or unwilling to have repair. Surgery will continue to be the usual form of repair, but balloon angioplasty will be increasingly offered as the easiest and safest initial approach. If it fails, little will have been lost.

## RENIN-SECRETING TUMORS (PRIMARY RENINISM)

Since the recognition of the first case in 1967 (Robertson et al, 1967), more than 30 have been reported and the syndrome has been well described (Corvol et al, 1989). Most are relatively small and are comprised of juxtaglomerular cells that have been shown to make renin (Conn et al, 1972). In addition to these juxtaglomerular cell tumors or hemangiopericytomas, hypertension and high renin levels that revert to normal after nephrectomy have been reported in children with Wilms' tumor (Sheth et al, 1978), in patients with adenocarcinoma of the kidney (Lebel et al, 1977), and from tumors of various external sites including lung, ovary (Anderson et al, 1989), liver, pancreas, and epithelioid sarcoma (Chauveau et al, 1988). Large intrarenal tumors could also produce high renin hypertension by compressing renal vessels.

Most of these renin-secreting tumors of renal origin fit a rather typical pattern:

1. Severe hypertension appears in relatively young patients: the oldest reported has been 53 (Corvol et al, 1989) but most are below 25.
2. Very high prorenin and renin levels in the peripheral blood and even higher levels from the kidney harboring the tumor are found.

However, renal vein renin ratios of less than 1.5 have been seen (Brown et al, 1973). An attempt should be made to obtain blood from the segment draining the tumor, wherein very high renin levels should be found.

3. Secondary aldosteronism appears, manifested by hypokalemia.
4. The tumor should be recognizable by computed tomography (CT) scan or by selective angiography. The renal vascular tree should be normal.
5. The tumor is morphologically a hemangiopericytoma arising from the juxtaglomerular apparatus, and it contains large amounts of renin and prorenin.

Cure should be possible by removal of the tumor; if that is not possible, captopril should be used.

Primary reninism is not common, but clinicians should be alert to the possibility that hypertension with a high renal venous renin level from one kidney may not always represent renovascular hypertension.

Now that the renal causes of hypertension have been covered, we will turn to the only other common causes of secondary hypertension, those seen during pregnancy and with the use of oral contraceptives.

## References

Adelman RD, Merten D, Vogel J, et al: *Pediatrics* 62:71, 1978.

Adams CWM, Reidy J: *Atherosclerosis* 63:153, 1987.

Alfidi RJ, Tarar R, Fosmoe RJ, et al: *Radiology* 102:545, 1972.

Anderson GH Jr, Blakeman N, Streeten DHP: *AJH* 1:301, 1988.

Anderson PW, Macaulay L, Do YS, et al: *Medicine* (Baltimore) 68:257, 1989.

Anderson WP, Korner PI, Johnston CI: *Hypertension* 1:292, 1979.

Arakawa K, Torii S, Kikuchi Y, et al: *Arch Intern Med* 129:958, 1972.

Babka JC, Cohen MS, Sode J: *N Engl J Med* 291:343, 1974.

Baer L, Ricas RA, Williams GS: *Clin Res* 33:358A, 1985.

Barger AC: *Hypertension* 1:447, 1979.

Bender W, La France N, Walker WG: *Hypertension* 6 (Suppl I):I-193, 1984.

Berkowitz HD, O'Neill JA Jr: *J Vasc Surg* 9:46, 1989.

Besarab A, Brown RS, Rubin NT, et al: *JAMA* 235:2838, 1976.

Blaufox MD, Freeman LM: *Urol Radiol* 10:35, 1988.

Bookstein JJ: *Radiology* 90:1073, 1968.

Bookstein JJ, Abrams HL, Buenger RE, et al: *JAMA* 221:368, 1972.

Braun-Menendez E, Fasciolo JC, Leloir FL, et al: *J Physiol* 98:283, 1940.

Brewster DC, Jensen SR, Novelline RA: *JAMA* 248:1094, 1982.

Brown JJ, Davies DL, Morton JJ, et al: *Lancet* 1:1219, 1976.

Brown JJ, Lever AF, Robertson JIS, et al: *Lancet* 2:1228, 1973.

Brunner HR, Kirshman JD, Sealey JE, et al: *Science* (Wash DC) 174:1344, 1971.

Canzanello VJ, Millan BG, Spiegel JE, et al: *Hypertension* 13:163, 1989.

Carmichael DJS, Snell ME, Mathias CJ, et al: *Lancet* 1:667, 1986.

Case AB, Atlas SA, Laragh JH: *Clin Sci* 57:313S, 1979.

Castle CH: *JAMA* 225:1085, 1973.

Chauveau D, Julien J, Pagny J-Y, et al: *J Hum Hypertens* 2:261, 1988.

Chen M, Lee J, Malvin RL, et al: *Am J Physiol* 255:E839, 1988.

Clorius JH, Kjelle-Schweigler M, Ostertag H, et al: *J Nucl Med* 19:343, 1978.

Conn JW, Cohen EL, Lucas CP, et al: *Arch Intern Med* 130:682, 1972.

Corvol P, Pinet F, Galen FX, et al: In: Laragh JH, Brenner BM, Kaplan NM (eds): *Perspectives in Hypertension, Vol 2: Endocrine Mechanisms in Hypertension.* New York: Raven Press, 1989: 189–199.

Cuocolo A, Esposito S, Volpe M, et al: *J Nucl Med* 30:51, 1989.

Davis BA, Crook JE, Vestal RE, et al: *N Engl J Med* 301:1273, 1979.

Dean R, Kieffer R, Smith B, et al: *Arch Surg* 116:1408, 1981.

Derrick JR, Hanna E: *Am J Surg* 106:673, 1963.

de Jong PE, van Bockel JH, de Zeeuw D: *Ann Intern Med* 110:437, 1989.

de Zeeuw D, Donker AJM, Burema J, et al: *Lancet* 1:213, 1977.

Dickerman RM, Peters PC, Hull AR, et al: *Ann Surg* 192:639, 1980.

Dondi M, Franchi R, Levorato M, et al: *J Nucl Med* 30:615, 1989.

Donohue RE, Fauver HE: *JAMA* 261:1180, 1989.

Dornfield L, Lecky JW, Peter JB: *JAMA* 215:1950, 1971.

Edwards BS, Stanson AW, Holley KE, et al: *Mayo Clin Proc* 57:564, 1982.

Eipper DF, Gifford RW Jr, Stewart BH, et al: *Am J Cardiol* 37:48, 1976.

Elkik F, Corvol P, Idatte J-M, et al: *J Hypertens* 2:149, 1984.

Ernst CB, Bookstein JJ, Montie J, et al: *Arch Surg* 104:496, 1972.

Eyler WR, Clark MD, Garman JE, et al: *Radiology* 78:879, 1962.

Feltrin GP, Rossi GP, Talenti E, et al: *Hypertension* 8:962, 1986.

Ferguson RK: *Ann Intern Med* 82:761, 1975.

Ferreras-Valenti P, Rozman C, Jurado-Grau J: *Am J Med* 39:355, 1965.

Fine EJ, Sarkar S: *Semin Nucl Med* 19:101, 1989.

Fiorentini C, Guazzi MD, Olivari MT, et al: *Circulation* 63:973, 1981.

Fommei E, Ghione S, Palla L, et al: *Hypertension* 10:212, 1987.

Fommei E, Ghione S, Palla L, et al: *AJH* 1:77A, 1988 (abstr).

Foster JH, Maxwell MH, Franklin SS, et al: *JAMA* 231:1043, 1975.

Foster JH, Oates JA: *Hosp Prac* 10:61, 1975.

Franklin SS, Smith R: *Am J Med* 79 (Suppl 3C):14, 1985.

Fry WJ, Ernst CB, Stanley JC, et al: *Arch Surg* 107:692, 1973.

Fyhrquist F, Grönhagen-Riska C, Tikkanen I, et al: *J Cardiovasc Pharmacol* 9 (Suppl 3):S61, 1987.

Gaul MK, Linn WD, Mulrow CD: *AJH* 2:335, 1989.

Geyskes GG, Oei HY, Klinge J, et al: *Q J Med* 251:203, 1988.

Geyskes GG, Oei HY, Puylaert CBAJ, et al: *Hypertension* 9:451, 1987.

Gifford RW Jr: *Milbank Mem Fund Q* 47:170, 1969.

Gifford RW Jr, McCormack LJ, Poutasse EF: *Mayo Clin Proc* 40:834, 1965.

Gittes RF, McLaughlin AP III: *J Urol* 111:292, 1974.

Goldberg M, McCurdy DK: *Ann Intern Med* 59:24, 1963.

Goldblatt H: *Urol Clin North Am* 2:219, 1975.

Goldblatt J, Lynch J, Hanzal RD, et al: *J Exp Med* 59:347, 1934.

Gosse Ph, Dupas JY, Reynaud P, et al: *AJH* 2:191, 1989.

Greenstein SM, Verstandid A, McLean GK, et al: *Transplantation* 43:29, 1987.

Grüntzig A, Vetter W, Meier B, et al: *Lancet* 1:801, 1978.

Grützmacher P, Radtke HW, Stahl RAK, et al: *Kidney Int* 35:326, 1989.

Gunnels JC Jr, Stickel DL, Robinson RR: *N Engl J Med* 274:543, 1966.

Hayes JM, Risius B, Novick AC, et al: *J Urol* 139:488, 1988.

Helmer OM, Judson WE: *Hypertension* 8:38, 1960.

Helmer OM, Judson WE: *Circulation* 27:1050, 1963.

Hidai H: *Urol Int* 30:445, 1975.

Hillman BJ: *AJR* 153:5, 1989.

Hillman BJ, Ovitt TW, Capp MP, et al: *Radiology* 142:577, 1982.

Hollenberg NK: *Cardiovasc Rev Rep* 4:852, 1983.

Hollenberg NK: *AJH* 1:338S, 1988.

Hoobler SW: In Stanley JC, Ernst CB, Fry WJ (eds): *Renovascular Hypertension*. Philadelphia: W.B. Saunders, 1984: 12–19.

Horvath JS, Fischer WE, May J: *J Hypertens* 4 (Suppl 6):S688, 1986.

Horvath JS, Waugh RC, Tiller DJ, et al: *Q J Med* 51:139, 1982.

Hricik DE, Browning PJ, Kopelman R, et al: *N Engl J Med* 308:373, 1983.

Hudson P, Pearce JMS, Yeates WK: *Br Med J* 1:18, 1967.

Hughes JS, Dove HG, Gifford RW Jr, et al: *Am Heart J* 101:408, 1981.

Hunt JC, Strong CG: *Am J Cardiol* 32:562, 1973.

Iaccarino B, Russo D, Niola R, et al: *Br J Radiol* 62:593, 1989.

Ichikawa I, Ferrone RA, Duchin KL, et al: *Circ Res* 53:592, 1983.

Idrissi A, Fournier A, Renaud H, et al: *Kidney Int* 34 (Suppl 25):S-138, 1988.

Imai Y, Abe K, Otsuka Y, et al: *Jpn Heart J* 21:793, 1980.

Imanishi M, Kawamura M, Akabane S, et al: *Hypertension* 14:461, 1989.

Jacobson HR: *Kidney Int* 34:729, 1988.

Jennings RC, Shaikh VA, Allen WM: *Br Med J* 2:1053, 1964.

Kaplan NM, Silah JH: *J Clin Invest* 43:659, 1964.

Kato K, Takashi M, Narita H, et al: *J Urol* 134:942, 1985.

Kaufman SL, Chang R, Kadir S, et al: *Radiology* 151:323, 1984.

Kaylor WM, Novick AC, Ziegelbaum M, et al: *J Urology* 141:486, 1989.

Keith TA III: *Hypertension* 4:438, 1982.

Kimura G, Saito F, Kojima S, et al: *Hypertension* 10:11, 1987.

Kopelman RI, McNutt RA, Pauker SG: *Hypertension* 12:611, 1988.

Korobkin M, Glickman MG, Schambelan M: *Radiology* 118:307, 1976.

Kremer Hovinga TK, de Jong PE, Piers DA, et al: *J Nucl Med* 30:605, 1989.

Kumar A, Shapiro AP: *Arch Intern Med* 140:1631, 1980.

Lagneau P, Michel JB: *J Urol* 134:876, 1985.

Lawrie GM, Morris GC Jr, Glaeser DH, et al: *Am J Cardiol* 63:1085, 1989.

Lebel M, Talbot J, Grose J, et al: *J Urol* 118:923, 1977.

Libertino JA, Flam TA, Zinman LN, et al: *Arch Intern Med* 148:357, 1988.

Libertino JA, Zinman L, Breslin DJ, et al: *JAMA* 244:1340, 1980.

London GM, Safar ME: *Am J Hypertens* 2:244, 1989.

Luft FC, Grim CE, Weinberger MH: *J Urol* 130:654, 1983.

Lupu AN, Laufman JJ, Maxwell MH: *Ann Surg* 167:246, 1968.

Lüscher TF, Greminger P, Kuhlmann U, et al: *Nephron* 44 (Suppl 1):17, 1986.

Lüscher TF, Lie JT, Stanson AW, et al: *Mayo Clin Proc* 62:931, 1987.

Machida J, Ueda S, Yoshida M, et al: *Nephron* 49:74, 1988.

Majd M, Potter BM, Guzzetta PC, et al: *J Nucl Med* 24:P23, 1983 (abstr).

Marks LS and Poutasse EF: *J Urol* 109:149, 1973.

Martin DC Jr: *Am J Surg* 121:351, 1971.

Martin RS III, Meacham PW, Ditesheim JA, et al: *J Vasc Surg* 9:26, 1989.

Maslowski AH, Nicholls MG, Espiner EA, et al: *Hypertension* 5:597, 1983.

Maxwell MH, Bleifer KH, Franklin SS, et al: *JAMA* 220:1195, 1972.

Maxwell MH, Gonick HC, Wilta R, et al: *N Engl J Med* 270:213, 1964.

Maxwell MH, Lupu AN, Visokoper RJ, et al: *Circ Res* 40 (Suppl 1):1–24, 1977a.

Maxwell MH, Marks LS, Varady PD: *J Lab Clin Med* 86:901, 1974.

McAllister RG Jr, Michelakis AM, Oates JA, et al: *JAMA* 221:865, 1972.

McCormack JL, Bain AC, Kenny GM, et al: *Arch Surg* 108:220, 1974.

McCready RA, Daugherty ME, Nighbert EJ, et al: *J Vasc Surg* 6:185, 1987.

McDonald DN, Smith DC, Maloney MD: *AJR* 151:1041, 1988.

McLoughlin MJ, Colapinto RJ, Hobbs BB: *JAMA* 232:1238, 1975.

Meaney TF, Dustan HP, McCormack LJ: *Radiology* 91:881, 1968.

Miller HC, Phillips CE: *Surg Gynecol Obstet* 127:1274, 1968.

Miyamori I, Yasuhara S, Matsubara T, et al: *AJM* 1:359, 1988.

Monstrey SJM, Beerthuizen GIJM, vander Werken CHR, et al: *J Trauma* 29:65, 1989.

Morris GC Jr, DeBakey ME, Cooley DA: *JAMA* 182:609, 1962.

Muller FB, Sealey JE, Case DB, et al: *Am J Med* 80:633, 1986.

Munichoodappa C, D'Elia JA, Libertino JA, et al: *J Urol* 121:555, 1979.

Mushlin AI, Thornbury JR: *Ann Intern Med* 111:58, 1989.

Nally JV, Gupta BK, Clarke HS Jr, et al: *Cleve Clin J Med* 55:311, 1988.

Nemoy NJ, Fichman MP, Sellers A: *JAMA* 225:512, 1973.

Nicholson JP, Alderman MH, Pickering TG, et al: *Lancet* 2:765, 1983.

Novick AC: *Nephron* 44 (Suppl 1):40, 1986.

Novick AC: In Kaplan NM, Brenner BM, Laragh JH (eds): *Perspectives in Hypertension, Vol 1: The Kidney in Hypertension.* New York: Raven Press, 1987: 225–237.

Novick AC, Straffon RA, Stewart BH, et al: *J Urol* 119:794, 1978.

Novick AC, Ziegelbaum M, Vidt DG, et al: *JAMA* 257:498, 1987.

Olin JW, Wholey M: *JAMA* 257:518, 1987.

Osada Y, Amano T, Momose S, et al: *J Urol* 120:537, 1978.

Page IH, Duston HP, Poutasse EF: *Ann Intern Med* 51:196, 1959.

Pape JF, Gudmundsen TE, Pedersen HK: *Scand J Urol Nephrol* 22:41, 1988.

Parfrey PS, Griffiths SM, Barrett BJ, et al: *N Engl J Med* 320:143, 1989.

Perera GA, Haelig AW: *Circulation* 6:549, 1952.

Pickering TG: *Semin Nucl Med* 19:79, 1989.

Pickering TG: In Kaplan NM, Brenner BM, Laragh JH (eds): *Perspectives in Hypertension, Vol 1: The Kidney in Hypertension.* New York: Raven Press, 1987: 213–223.

Pickering TG, Devereux RB, James GD, et al: *Lancet* 2:551, 1988.

Pickering TG, Sos TA, Laragh JH: *Am J Med* 77:61, 1984a.

Pickering TG, Sos TA, Saddekni S, et al: *J Hypertens* 4 (Suppl 6):S667, 1986a.

Pickering TG, Sos TA, Vaughan ED Jr, et al: *Am J Med* 76:398, 1984b.

Pickering TG, Sos TA, Vaughan ED Jr, et al: *Nephron* 44 (Suppl 1):8, 1986b.

Plumer LB, Kaplan GW, Mendoza SA: *J Pediatr* 89:802, 1976.

Pollard SG, Hornick P, Macfarlane R, et al: *Postgrad Med J* 65:31, 1989.

Postma CT, Hoefnagels WHL, Barentsz JO, et al: *J Hum Hypertension* 3:185, 1989.

Rademacher R, Berecek KH, Ploth DW: *Hypertension* 8:1127, 1986.

Ribstein J, Mourad G, Mimran A: *AJH* 1:239, 1988.

Roach CJ: *Obstet Gynecol* 42:856, 1973.

Robertson PW, Klidjian A, Harding LK, et al: *Am J Med* 43:963, 1967.

Robertson R, Murphy A, Dubbins PA: *Br J Radiol* 61:196, 1988.

Rudnick MR, Maxwell MH: In: Narins RG (ed): *Controversies in Nephrology and Hypertension.* New York: Churchill Livingstone, 1984: 123.

Saint-Georges G, Aube M: *AJR* 144:235, 1985.

Salahudeen AK, Pingle A: *J Hum Hypertens* 2:57, 1988.

Sang CN, Whelton PK, Hamper UM, et al: *Hypertension* 14:472, 1989.

Schaeffer AJ, Stamey TA: *Urol Clin North Am* 2:327, 1975.

Schreiber MJ, Novick AC, Pohl MA: *Kidney Int* 19:175, 1981.

Scoble JE, Maher ER, Hamilton G, et al: *Clin Nephrol* 31:119, 1989.

Sealey JE, Bühler FR, Laragh JH, et al: *Am J Med* 55:391, 1973.

Sellars L, Shore AC, Wilkinson R: *J Hypertens* 3:177, 1985.

Sfakianakis GN, Jaffe DJ, Bourgoignie JJ: *Kidney Int* 34 (Suppl 25):S-142, 1988.

Shapiro AP, Perez-Stable E, Moutos SE: *JAMA* 192:813, 1965.

Shelhamer JH, Volkman DJ, Parrillo JE, et al: *Ann Intern Med* 103:121, 1985.

Sheth KJ, Tang TT, Blaedel ME, et al: *J Pediatr* 92:921, 1978.

Silver D, Clements JB: *Ann Surg* 183:161, 1976.

Simon N, Franklin SS, Bleifer KH, et al: *JAMA* 220:1209, 1972.

Smith H: *J Urol* 76:685, 1956.

Sniderman KW, Sos TA: *Radiology* 142:607, 1982.

Staab GE, Tegtmeyer CJ, Constable WC: *AJR* 126:634, 1976.

Staessen J, Wilms G, Baert A, et al: *AJH* 1:208, 1988.

Stahl RAK, Helmchen U, Paravicini M, et al: *Am J Physiol* 247:F975, 1984.

Stanley JC, Fry WJ: *Arch Surg* 112:1291, 1977.

Stanley P, Gyepes MT, Olson DL, et al: *Radiology* 129:123, 1978.

Sterns RH, Rabinowitz R, Segal AJ, et al: *Arch Intern Med* 145:169, 1985.

Stewart BH, Dustan HP, Kiser WS, et al: *J Urol* 104:231, 1970.

Stockigt JR, Collins RD, Noakes CA, et al: *Lancet* 1:1194, 1972.

Svetkey LP, Dunnick NR, Coffman TM, et al: *Transplantation* 45:56, 1988.

Svetkey LP, Himmelstein SI, Dunnick RN, et al: *Hypertension* 14:247, 1989.

Swales JD, Bing RF, Russell GI, et al: *Clin Exp Pharmacol Physiol* 10:239, 1983.

Swales JD, Queiroz FP, Thurston H, et al: *Lancet* 2:1181, 1971.

Tack C, Sos TA: *Semin Nucl Med* 19:89, 1989.

Tagawa H, Gutmann FD, Haber E, et al: *Proc Soc Exp Biol Med* 146:975, 1974.

Tapper D, Brand T, Hickman R: *Am J Surg* 153:495, 1987.

Tarazi RC, Dustan HP: *Clin Sci* 44:197, 1973.

Tegtmeyer CJ, Kellum CD, Ayers C: *Radiology* 153:77, 1984.

Textor SC, Novick AC, Tarazi RC, et al: *Ann Intern Med* 102:308, 1985.

Thal AP, Grage TB, Vernier RL: *Circulation* 27:36, 1963.

Tillman DM, Malatino LS, Cumming AMM, et al: *J Hypertens* 2 (Suppl 2):93, 1984.

Tonkin IL, Stapleton FB, Roy S III: *Pediatrics* 81:150, 1988.

Ullian ME, Molitoris BA: *Clin Nephrol* 27:293, 1987.

Valvo E, Bedogna V, Gammaro L, et al: *J Hypertens* 5:629, 1987.

Vaughan ED Jr: *Kidney Int* 27:811, 1985.

Vensel LA, Devereux RB, Pickering TG, et al: *Am J Cardiol* 58:575, 1986.

Vertes V, Grauel JA, Goldblatt H: *N Engl J Med* 270:656, 1964.

Vidt DG: *Geriatrics* 42:59, 1987.

Wallace ECH, Morton JJ: *J Hypertens* 2:285, 1984.

Weidmann P, Siegenthaler W, Ziegler WH, et al: *Am J Med* 47:528, 1969.

Wenting GJ, Tan-Tjiong HL, Derkx FHM, et al: *Br Med J* 288:886, 1984.

Wenting GJ, Tan-Tjiong HL, Derkx FHM, et al: Abstract 12th International Society of Hypertension Meeting, June 1988. Kyoto, Japan, Abstract #0951.

Wilcox CS, Williams CM, Smith TB, et al: *AJH* 1:344S, 1988.

Williams B, Feehally J, Attard AR, et al: *Br Med J* 296:1591, 1988.

Williams CM, Thomas WC Jr, Newman RC, et al: *N Engl J Med* 320:739, 1989.

Wollenweber J, Sheps SG, Davis GD: *Am J Cardiol* 21:60:1968.

Ying CY, Tifft CP, Gavras H, et al: *N Engl J Med* 311:1070, 1984.

Zezulka AV, Arkell DG, Veebers DG: *J Urol* 135:1000, 1986.

Zimmerman JB, Robertson D, Jackson EK: *J Clin Invest* 80:443, 1987.

# 11 Hypertension with Pregnancy and the Pill

Hypertension occurs in over 5% of all pregnancies and in 5% of women who take oral contraceptives for 5 years. Gestational proteinuric hypertension (preeclampsia) is responsible for one-sixth of all maternal deaths (Kaunitz et al, 1985) and doubles perinatal mortality (Taylor, 1988). Although maternal mortality from preeclampsia has fallen markedly over the past 30 years (Sachs et al, 1987), eclampsia remains the cause of a considerable number of avoidable deaths (Redman, 1988). Hypertension associated with the use of oral contraceptives may rapidly accelerate or more slowly cause vascular damage. The causes of neither gestational nor pill-induced hypertension are known. However, if recognized early and handled appropriately, the morbidity and mortality they cause can be largely prevented.

## TYPES OF HYPERTENSION DURING PREGNANCY

Hypertension has been reported in as few as 1.5% (Andersch et al, 1984) to as many as 25% of pregnancies (Rubin, 1983). These differences reflect differences in the definition of what is hypertension, the level of surveillance, racial and socioeconomic makeup of the population, as well as age and parity.

In this chapter, Davey and MacGillivray's (1988) classification (Table 11.1) will be followed since it has been approved by the International Society for the Study of Hypertension in Pregnancy. Most of this chapter relates to "pregnancy-induced hypertension" or PIH, shown in the footnote to Table 11.1 as the term reserved by Davey and MacGillivray for

. . . that form of hypertension that commonly but not exclusively occurs in primigravida women and is primarily caused by an abnormality of pregnancy, which if it is severe or progresses is associated with the development of proteinuria and other features of "preeclampsia."

For convenience, the terms PIH or preeclampsia will be used throughout this chapter rather than the more cumbersome "gestational proteinuric hypertension."

There is more than academic interest in correctly categorizing hypertension during pregnancy into gestational or chronic. The management of both the hypertension and the pregnancy, as well as the prognosis for future pregnancies, varies with the diagnosis. To approach these problems, an understanding of the profound changes in hemodynamics and the hormonal milieu that occur during normal pregnancy is needed.

## CIRCULATION IN NORMAL PREGNANCY

### Blood Pressure

In measuring the blood pressure (BP), two changes in technique should be made to account for the effects of pregnancy. First, the BP is usually lower in the left lateral recumbent position, and that should be used to make the diagnosis of hypertension if the BP in the sitting position is found to be high (Svensson, 1988). Second, the hyperdynamic circulation may cause Korotkoff sounds to remain audible much below the true diastolic BP; if so, the 4th phase (muffling) should be used (Wichman and Ryden, 1986).

**Table 11.1. Clinical Classification of Hypertensive Disorders of Pregnancy**[a]

A. Gestational hypertension and/or proteinuria: Hypertension and/or proteinuria developing during pregnancy, labor, or the puerperium in a previously normotensive nonproteinuric woman subdivided into
   1. Gestational hypertension[b]: DBP > 110 once or > 90 twice, 4 hours apart
   2. Gestational proteinuria: > 300 mg/24 hours or two clean voided specimens 4 hours apart with 2+ reagent strip (1 g/liter)
   3. Gestational proteinuric hypertension (preeclampsia)
B. Chronic hypertension and chronic renal disease: Hypertension and/or proteinuria at the first visit before the 20th week of pregnancy or the presence of chronic hypertension or chronic renal disease diagnosed before, during, or after pregnancy
C. Unclassified hypertension and/or proteinuria: Hypertension and/or proteinuria found either
   1. At first examination after 20 weeks (140 days) in a woman without known chronic hypertension or chronic renal disease
      or
   2. During pregnancy, labor, or the puerperium when information is insufficient to permit classification is regarded as unclassified during pregnancy and is subdivided into
      1. Hypertension (without proteinuria)
      2. Proteinuria (without hypertension)
      3. Proteinuric hypertension
D. Eclampsia: The occurrence of generalized convulsions during pregnancy, during labor, or within 7 days of delivery and not caused by epilepsy or other convulsive disorders

[a](Adapted from Davey DA, MacGillivray I: *Am J Obstet Gynecol* 158:892, 1988.)
[b]"Gestational hypertension" is often regarded as synonymous with "pregnancy-induced hypertension," but the term pregnancy-induced hypertension is reserved in this classification for that form of hypertension that commonly but not exclusively occurs in primigravid women and is primarily caused by an abnormality of pregnancy, which if it is severe or progresses is associated with the development of proteinuria and other features of "preeclampsia."

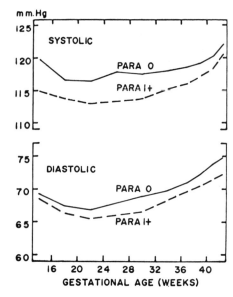

**Figure 11.1.** Mean blood pressure by gestational age and parity for white gravidas 25 to 34 years of age who delivered single live term births. 1046 primigravidas (*para 0*) and 2227 multigravidas (*para 1+*) were examined. (From Christianson RE: *Am J Obstet Gynecol* 125:511, 1976.)

BP is low during the early and mid portions of normal pregnancy with a gradual return toward nonpregnancy levels during the third trimester (Christianson, 1976) (Fig. 11.1). The somewhat higher readings in the 1046 nulliparous women compared with the 2227 multiparas were partly attributable to the higher rate of PIH among the nulliparas.

The lower diastolic BPs of normal pregnancy suggest that criteria for what is high BP should be set lower in pregnancy. In a prospective study on the course of pregnancy involving over 38,000 women, an increased rate of fetal mortality was noted when the diastolic BP rose above 84 mm Hg at any gestational age (Friedman and Neff, 1978) (Fig. 11.2). An even steeper rise in mortality was seen when proteinuria accompanied the elevated BP.

Those destined to develop gestational hypertension may have slightly elevated BP well before they become overtly hypertensive. Among 808 primigravida women seen throughout pregnancy, the 46 who developed PIH had significantly higher BP at 9 to 12 weeks, although the levels rose into an overtly hypertensive range only after 33 weeks (Moutquin et al, 1985) (Fig. 11.3). A greater chance of developing PIH has been noted among those with BP above 110/75 at 17 to 20 weeks' gestation (Gallery et al, 1977) or with a mean BP of 85 mm Hg or higher at 20 weeks (Ales et al, 1989).

## Hemodynamic Changes

Normal pregnancy is associated with a progressive increase in plasma and extracellular fluid volume and a rise in cardiac output (Robson et al, 1989), which are likely adaptations (via renal sodium retention) to progressive vasodilation induced by the hormonal milieu (Mashini et al, 1987). Since sequential invasive measurements are not possible in humans, Phippard et al (1986) studied eight baboon pregnancies. By 4 weeks' gestation, they observed reductions in systemic arterial pressure accompanied by falls in vascular resistance and right atrial pressure despite increases in stroke volume and cardiac output. Although plasma renin activity and aldosterone

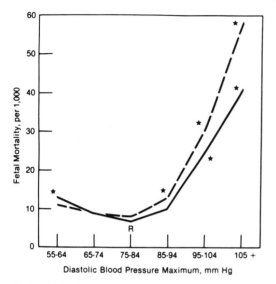

**Figure 11.2.** Fetal mortality in relation to the maximal diastolic blood pressure recorded during 38,636 pregnancies by the Collaborative Perinatal Project. *Solid line*, total series; *broken line*, patients with concomitant proteinuria. *Stars*, mortality rates significantly higher than in patients with normal maximal diastolic values (*R*). (From Friedman EA, Neff RK: *JAMA* 239:2249, 1978, Copyright 1978, American Medical Association.)

levels were elevated by 4 weeks, plasma volume did not expand until 12 weeks. Since cardiac filling pressures were never increased, they conclude that "pregnancy is a state of reduced ef-

fective blood volume associated with vasodilation from the early weeks."

A host of causes for vasodilation are present: The placenta imposes an arteriovenous shunt on the maternal circulation, the endothelial cells make more vasodilatory prostaglandins, and high levels of progesterone and estrogen may contribute (Schrier, 1988). As a result of these vasodilatory forces, the pressor response to exogenous angiotensin II becomes progressively less (Abdul-Karim and Assali, 1961).

Plasma levels of atrial natriuretic factor are normal (Bond et al, 1989), further evidence that despite an increased fluid volume, the central circulation is not overexpanded.

Despite the reduced effective blood volume, peripheral edema is common, but this often arises from interference of venous return by the enlarged uterus. Thomson et al (1967) found significant edema in 35% of women who remained normotensive throughout their pregnancy; the edema was generalized in 15% and pedal in 20%.

## Sodium Transport

As noted in Chapter 3, various measures of sodium transport in blood cells are altered in patients with primary hypertension. The following changes have been reported in *normotensive* pregnancy:

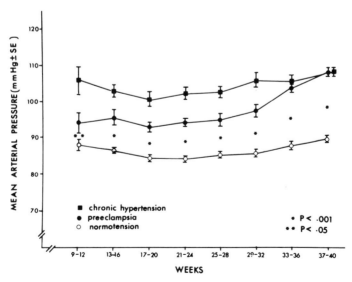

**Figure 11.3.** Average mean arterial blood pressures (± 1 SE) in 710 women who remained normotensive throughout pregnancy, in 46 who developed preeclampsia, and in 37 with chronic hypertension (From Moutquin JM, Rainville C, Giroux L, et al: *Am J Obstet Gynecol* 151:191, 1985).

—increased white blood cell (WBC) and red blood cell (RBC) sodium content (Seon and Forrester, 1989);

—increased RBC rubidium uptake, a measure of $Na^+,K^+$-ATPase activity (Gallery et al, 1988b);

—increased number of RBC ouabain binding sites, measured as $Na^+,K^+$-ATPase units (Gallery et al, 1988b);

—increased RBC sodium-lithium countertransport (Worley et al, 1982);

—increased RBC $Na^+,K^+$-cotransport (Gallery et al, 1988a);

—increased RBC sodium efflux rates and sodium permeability (Weissberg et al, 1983).

These various indices of increased sodium transport across cells are accompanied by high plasma levels of a digoxin- or ouabain-like factor that is thought to inhibit the membrane $Na^+,K^+$-ATPase pump (Delva et al, 1989). The presence of this factor, which may arise in the placenta, could lead to the synthesis of more pump units (ouabain binding sites).

### Renal Function

Renal blood flow and glomerular filtration are increased by about 50% early in pregnancy, with a gradual return to nonpregnant levels toward the end of gestation (Davison, 1984) (Fig. 11.4). The supernormal renal function and plasma volume expansion of pregnancy cause the normal blood urea, creatinine, and uric acid levels to be less than the nonpregnant normal. The normal range of serum creatinine during pregnancy

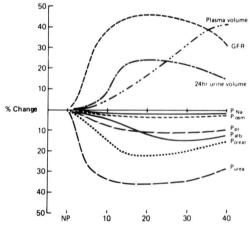

**Figure 11.4.** Percentage of change in various blood and urinary measurements throughout pregnancy in reference to nonpregnant baseline. (From Davison JM: *Scand J Clin Lab Invest* 44(Suppl 169):15, 1984.)

is 0.46 + 0.06 mg/100 mol as opposed to 0.67 + 0.07 in nonpregnant women. Normal pregnant women appear to handle sodium and water loads as do normal nonpregnant women but retain more administered sodium in late pregnancy (Brown et al, 1988).

### Renin-Angiotensin-Aldosterone System

Plasma renin levels, both active and inactive, and substrate are all increased in normal pregnancy (Brown et al, 1963). The levels of renin activity and concentration are elevated, in part, as a consequence of the estrogen-induced stimulation of renin substrate, which increases about sixfold. When active plasma renin activity (PRA) values were normalized to the nonpregnant renin substrate concentrations, about half of the increase in PRA during pregnancy was attributable to the increase in substrate, the other half to increases in the concentration of renin in the blood (Sealey et al, 1982).

Two other factors contribute: first, the various hemodynamic and renal changes described above, which tend to activate the release of renin, and second, the contribution of renin synthesized both in the trophoblastic cells of the chorion (Craven et al, 1983) and in the epithelial cells of the amnion (Poisner et al, 1982). Most of the high levels of prorenin in the maternal circulation come from the ovary (Derkx et al, 1987).

The probable importance of these high levels of active renin and angiotensin II (AII) in maintaining blood pressure and uterine blood flow during normal pregnancy is supported by the finding that when the action of endogenous AII is blocked by the angiotensin-converting enzyme inhibitor (ACEI) captopril, the mean BP of normal pregnant women fell from 78 to 64 mm Hg (Taufield et al, 1988). This is reminiscent of the effects of ACEI in pregnant rabbits wherein BP fell 20 mm Hg and uterine blood flow fell from 32 to 21 ml/min (Ferris and Weir, 1983).

The increased levels of AII in the maternal circulation increase the secretion of aldosterone (Stevens et al, 1989), presumably to compensate for the various salt-losing features of pregnancy. When its secretion is inhibited, salt wastage occurs (Ehrlich, 1971). Along with increased aldosterone the plasma concentration of deoxycorticosterone (DOC) is increased (Brown et al, 1972), apparently from extraadrenal 21-hydroxylation of plasma progesterone (Winkel et al, 1980).

At the same time as various forces raise levels

of renin-angiotensin-aldosterone, normal pregnancy brings forth numerous mechanisms to protect the circulations of both mother and fetus from the intense vasoconstriction, volume retention, and potassium wastage that high AII and aldosterone levels would ordinarily engender.

## Responsiveness to Angiotensin and Aldosterone

Pregnant women are relatively resistant to the pressor effects of exogenous AII (Abdul-Karim and Assali, 1961), but they have a normal pressor response to exogenous norepinephrine (Lumbers, 1970). Pregnant women also have a blunted renal response to AII, with a lesser inhibition of salt and water excretion than nonpregnant subjects (Chesley et al, 1963). The resistance to AII is not altered by volume expansion even though levels of plasma renin activity are thereby reduced (Matsuura et al, 1981).

Studies in pregnant sheep have shown that the placenta is less responsive to AII than most nonreproductive tissues, which results in a preferential maintenance of perfusion through the uteroplacental bed, protecting the fetus from the high levels of AII present during normal pregnancy (Rosenfeld and Naden, 1989).

The large amounts of potent mineralocorticoids present during pregnancy would be expected to maintain sodium balance at the cost of progressive renal wastage of potassium, yet pregnant women are normokalemic. This appears to be due to a high level of progesterone, which acts as an aldosterone antagonist (Brown et al, 1986). This makes pregnant women virtually refractory to the potassium-wasting action of mineralocorticoids (Ehrlich and Lindheimer, 1972) and explains why the hypokalemia in a woman with primary aldosteronism was ameliorated during her pregnancy (Biglieri and Slaton, 1967).

## Increased Prostaglandin Synthesis

The resistance to angiotensin may also be caused by the vasodilatory action of increased levels of prostaglandins produced in the uterus (Mitchell et al, 1978; Gerber et al, 1981) and present in the plasma (Lewis et al, 1980). Exogenous prostacyclin further attenuated the pressor response to AII in normotensive women in the second trimester of pregnancy while inducing a small fall in BP (Broughton Pipkin et al, 1989). When normal pregnant women were

given inhibitors of prostaglandin synthesis (indomethacin or aspirin), they lost their refractoriness (Everett et al, 1978a). These same investigators found that a metabolite of progesterone, 5α-dihydroprogesterone, restored the refractoriness of such patients and they suggested that this steroid may be involved, perhaps in concert with prostaglandins, in the vascular refractoriness to AII seen in normal pregnancy (Everett et al, 1978b).

The prostaglandin-mediated protection against AII-induced vasoconstriction may not apply to all vascular beds: In near-term pregnant sheep infused with AII, prostacyclin blunted AII vasoconstriction in the renal and intestinal circulations of the fetus but did not reverse the vasoconstriction in the placental bed (Parisi and Walsh, 1989).

Nonetheless, the increased production of prostacyclin in normal pregnancy may account for many of the hemodynamic changes that are seen in addition to the resistance to AII (Friedman, 1988) and, as we shall see, alterations in prostaglandins may be involved in the pathogenesis of gestational hypertension.

## Other Hormones

Plasma concentrations of all maternal glucocorticoids and their precursors are high throughout pregnancy, reflecting increased amounts of corticosteroid-binding globulin and increased maternal adrenocortical secretion as well as steroid production from the feto-placental unit (Dörr et al, 1989). Plasma ACTH is lower than the levels in nonpregnant women but rises slowly during pregnancy (Carr et al, 1981). Plasma corticotropin-releasing hormone levels are increased but are of placental origin and appear not to control maternal pituitary-adrenal function (Campbell et al, 1987). Plasma catechols are unchanged (Lindheimer et al, 1980), though amniotic catechols are increased from mid- to late gestation (Divers et al, 1981).

## Overview of the Circulation in Normal Pregnancy

Normal pregnancy, then, is a low BP state associated with marked vasodilation that reduces peripheral resistance but an expanded fluid volume that increases cardiac output. Renal blood flow is markedly increased, a state of hyperperfusion that, as we shall see, could be involved in the pathophysiology of pregnancy-induced hypertension.

## PREGNANCY-INDUCED HYPERTENSION

### Hemodynamic Changes

All of the preceding is a prologue to our understanding of pregnancy-induced hypertension. Almost all of these various hemodynamic, renal, and renin-angiotensin-aldosterone changes of normal pregnancy are altered in PIH (Table 11.2).

The basic abnormality appears to be a widespread and often intense vasospasm, a phenomenon recognized in 1918 by Volhard and later amply confirmed by various studies on both structure and function (Chesley, 1978). This spasm can be seen in the nail beds, retinas, and coronary arteries (Bauer et al, 1982). The hypoxia resulting from the vasospasm is responsible for the various changes in tissue structure and function. Beyond spasm, structural alterations with increased thickness of the media relative to lumen diameter were found in omental resistance vessels from women with PIH (Aalkjaer et al, 1984). Deposition of fibrin products is also widespread and may play a role in the diminution of blood flow.

Unfortunately, most of the data on the hemodynamics of PIH have been obtained in women with severe disease relatively late in its course. In such patients, plasma volume is reduced by 10 to 40%, cardiac output is low, and peripheral resistance is increased (Wallenburg, 1988) (Fig.

11.5). However, in women with less severe PIH, the hemodynamic findings are more heterogeneous, with some having high cardiac output and low peripheral resistance (Easterling and Benedetti, 1989).

Since changes in blood flow (Pickles et al, 1989a) and vascular sensitivity (Gant et al, 1973) are known to precede the rise in blood pressure in those destined to develop PIH, Easterling and Benedetti (1989) offer this scheme for the hemodynamic changes:

If preeclampsia is characterized by high cardiac output before the onset of severe disease, then a fundamental change in hemodynamics must occur in some patients late in the course of the disease to account for the clinical observations of some patients with high vascular resistance. Such a "crossover" of hemodynamics from high cardiac output state to high resistance with progression of the disease is not without precedence. Such a model has been advanced for the changes observed in nonpregnant persons with chronic hypertension. As such, the process that we hypothesize for preeclampsia may parallel, at a more rapid pace, the disease process of essential hypertension.

Easterling and Benedetti (1989) carry their "hyperdynamic model" one step further, suggesting that renal hyperperfusion mediates the development of hypertension and proteinuria, in keeping with the hypothesis proposed by Brenner (1983) presented in Chapter 9 as the basic mechanism for progressive glomerulosclerosis

**Table 11.2. Changes in Normal Pregnancy and Preeclampsia**

| | Normal Pregnancy | Changes Occurring with Preeclampsia[a] |
|---|---|---|
| Hemodynamics | | |
| Plasma volume | Expanded | Decrease |
| Exchangeable sodium | Increased | Increase |
| Cardiac output | Increased | Decrease |
| Peripheral resistance | Reduced | Increase |
| Vascular reactivity | | |
| To norepinephrine | Unchanged | Increase |
| To angiotensin | Reduced | Increase |
| Uterine blood flow | | Decrease |
| Renal function | | |
| Blood flow | Increased | Decrease |
| Glomerular filtration | Increased | Decrease |
| Plasma uric acid | Decreased | Increase |
| Excretion of sodium load | Normal | Unchanged |
| Hormonal changes | | |
| Plasma renin substrate | Increased | Unchanged |
| Plasma renin activity | Increased | Decrease |
| Plasma renin concentration | Increased | Decrease |
| Plasma angiotensin II | Increased | Decrease |
| Plasma aldosterone | Increased | Decrease |
| Plasma deoxycorticosterone | Increased | Decrease |
| Atrial natriuretic factor | Normal | Increase |

[a]These changes are relative, as compared with those seen in normal pregnancy, and are not compared with those seen in nonpregnant women.

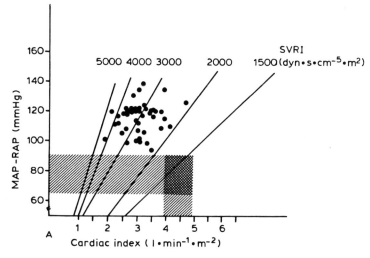

**Figure 11.5.** Relationship between systemic perfusion pressure, cardiac index, and systemic vascular resistance index in 44 untreated nulliparous preeclamptic patients. Values for normotensive pregnant women fall within the *crosshatched area*. (From Wallenburg HCS: In: Rubin PC (ed). *Handbook of Hypertension*, Vol 10: *Hypertension in Pregnancy*. Amsterdam: Elsevier Science Publishers, 1988:66.)

in various forms of renal disease and in Chapter 3 as a possible mechanism for essential hypertension.

Despite the attractiveness of this hyperperfusion model, we are left with no explanation of what happens in those women who develop PIH to start the process.

## Pathogenesis of PIH

The cause of PIH must explain these features, as delineated by Chesley (1978; 1985):

1. It occurs almost exclusively during the first pregnancy: nulliparas are from 6 to 8 times more susceptible than are multiparas.
2. It occurs more frequently in the young and in those with multiple fetuses, hydatidiform mole, or diabetes.
3. It rapidly disappears when the pregnancy is terminated.
4. The incidence increases as term approaches; it is unusual before the end of the second trimester.
5. The features of the syndrome are hypertension, edema, proteinuria, and, when advanced, convulsions and coma.
6. There is characteristic renal and hepatic pathology.
7. The syndrome has an hereditary tendency. In the families of women who had PIH, the syndrome developed in 25% of their daughters and granddaughters, but only in 6% of their daughters-in-law Chesley (1980).

It should be noted that clinical observations suggest that all PIH is not the same disease. Women who developed hypertension with heavy proteinuria before 34 weeks gestation more frequently had PIH during a previous pregnancy, a history of infertility, headaches, and an elevated serum alpha-fetoprotein concentration, as well as a higher perinatal morbidity and mortality experience than did those with late onset disease (Moore and Redman, 1983).

### Uteroplacental Hypoperfusion

The scheme portrayed in Figure 11.6 is a unified hypothesis of the pathogenesis of PIH that centers on a decreased fetoplacental production of prostacyclin as a consequence of suboptimal uteroplacental perfusion (Friedman, 1988). The decreased perfusion may, in turn, arise when placental mass is relatively large, e.g., multiple pregnancy and hydatidiform mole, or when uterine blood flow is compromised, e.g., diabetes and preexisting hypertensive disease. The problem in otherwise normal but young primigravidas can only be conjectured: Either the placenta is relatively large, or uterine blood flow is relatively poor.

The evidence for uteroplacental hypoperfusion includes these findings:

—Robertson and coworkers have shown that, at about 16 weeks during normal pregnancy, the spiral arteries in the placental bed progressively lose musculoelastic tissue from their

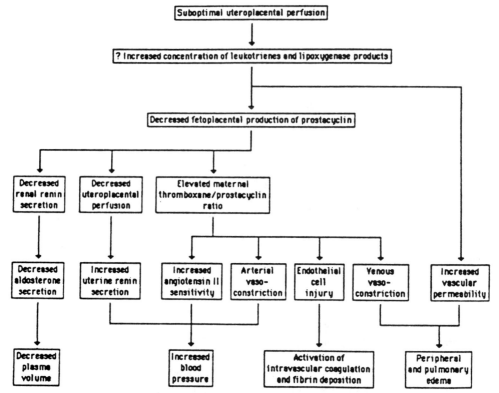

**Figure 11.6.** Proposed model to explain the pathophysiology of preeclampsia. (The consequences of the activation of intravascular coagulation and fibrin deposition are shown in Fig. 11.8). [From Friedman SA and reprinted with permission from The American College of Obstetricians and Gynecologists. (*Obstetrics and Gynecology*, 71, 1988, 122.)]

walls and widen, thereby allowing for the 10-fold increase in blood supply required by the pregnant uterus. In PIH, these changes do not occur in some decidual segments of spiral arteries, leaving a constricting segment of the artery (Khong et al, 1986).

—Some features of PIH can be induced by chronic uterine ischemia in various experimental animals (Phippard and Horvath, 1988).

—Uterine arteriography shows a much poorer blood flow (Bieniarz et al, 1969).

—Uteroplacental blood flow, measured by an isotopic accumulation curve, is decreased (Lunell et al, 1982).

—By using the clearance of steroid precursors used in the synthesis of estrogens by the placenta, Everett et al (1980) found a marked fall in placental perfusion after hypertension develops.

**Prostaglandin Imbalance**

As originally suggested by Speroff in 1973, PIH appears to represent defective prostaglandin production. As reviewed by Friedman (1988), the evidence continues to mount that PIH represents an imbalance in the production of the two major prostaglandins, less of the vasodilatory prostacyclin and too much of the vasoconstrictor thromboxane. Decreased levels of prostacyclin have been demonstrated in maternal urine (Fitzgerald et al, 1985), and decreased production of prostacyclin has been measured in maternal vascular endothelium (Bussolini et al, 1980) and fetal vessels (Ylikorkala and Mäkilä, 1985). Thromboxane excess has been measured in placenta (Walsh, 1985; Ylikorkala and Mäkilä, 1985) and platelets (Wallenburg and Rotmans, 1982; Fitzgerald et al, 1987b).

These alterations have been shown to precede the onset of PIH and to be related to uteroplacental blood flow (Fitzgerald et al, 1987a). The reduced levels of prostacyclin may be related to the increased production of progesterone in the preeclamptic placenta since progesterone inhibits placental prostacyclin synthesis (Walsh, 1988).

*Low-Dose Aspirin.* The hypothesis that an imbalance between prostacyclin and thromboxane is responsible for PIH suggests that the administration of small doses of aspirin that block platelet synthesis of thromboxane but do not interfere with endothelial synthesis of prostacyclin would be beneficial. Crandon and Isherwood (1979) had noted a lower incidence of PIH in women who took aspirin during pregnancy. Beaufils et al (1985) found that aspirin prevented recurrent PIH. In the first randomized, placebo-controlled, double-blind trial, Wallenburg et al (1986) reported that 60 mg a day of aspirin, started at 28 weeks' gestation, reduced significantly the frequency of PIH in women judged to be at high risk because of their increased sensitivity to angiotensin infusion. Two more prospective randomized trials have confirmed the benefit of low-dose aspirin. Schiff et al (1989) found a decrease in the incidence of PIH from 35% among 31 women given placebo to 12% of 34 women given 100 mg of aspirin daily during the third trimester. Benigni et al (1989) showed that the women at high risk for PIH who took 60 mg of aspirin daily from the 12th week of gestation had a longer pregnancy and increased weight of their newborns compared with the 16 similar women given placebo. In both Schiff and associates' and Benigni and associates' studies, decreased thromboxane and unaltered prostacyclin levels were measured in those given these low doses of aspirin.

Concerns about possible adverse effects of aspirin on the fetus have been voiced (Rennie, 1986), but no effects on neonatal platelet aggregation or pulmonary circulation were found with 60 or 80 mg per day started during the third trimester (Sibai et al, 1989). Uncertainty remains as to when during pregnancy aspirin should be started, some believing late (Thornton et al, 1986), others early (Goodlin, 1986). Obviously, larger controlled clinical trials are needed. But, in the meantime, the evidence for a prostaglandin imbalance as an important factor in the pathogenesis of PIH and the ability of low doses of aspirin to improve the imbalance looks increasingly impressive (Thorp et al, 1988; Cunningham and Gant, 1989).

### Increased Vascular Reactivity

Whether from lower levels of prostacyclin, increased thromboxane, or other unidentified mechanisms, women with PIH have an increased pressor responsiveness to various stimuli, even before their BP rises. Gant et al (1973) demonstrated that women destined to develop PIH have an increased pressor sensitivity to exogenous AII as early as the 22nd week of ges-

tation, often 10 to 15 weeks before hypertension appears (Fig. 11.7).

This hypersensitivity is thought to reflect an increased vascular responsiveness and not a better filled vascular bed since volume expansion with normal saline or high-hematocrit blood did not decrease the resistance of normotensive women near term to that seen in those women destined to develop PIH (Cunningham et al, 1975).

The pressor responsiveness to AII is reduced by low doses of aspirin (Spitz et al, 1988), supporting a major role for increased thromboxane in the increased sensitivity noted in PIH. In addition, subtle changes in the renin-aldosterone mechanism may be demonstrable in women destined to develop PIH (Brown et al, 1988).

### Other Theories

A host of other theories have been proposed for the pathogenesis of PIH. Some are supported by various types of evidence, but none seems to fulfill all of the requirements needed to explain the syndrome better than the theory of uteroplacental hypoperfusion. Among these theories, one is based on intravascular coagulation, another on immunological injury. In addition, abnormalities in sodium transport and other associations have been described.

### Genetic Susceptibility

Whatever else is responsible, there is clearly a familial factor that appears to be inherited from

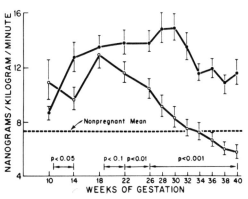

**Figure 11.7.** Comparison of the mean angiotensin II doses (ng/kg/min) required to evoke a pressor response in 120 primigravidas who remained normotensive (●——●) and 72 primigravidas who ultimately developed pregnancy-induced hypertension (○——○). The *nonpregnant mean* is shown as a *dashed line*. The *vertical bars* represent the SEM. The difference between the two groups became significant after Week 23, and the two groups continued to diverge widely after the 26th week. (From Gant N: *J Clin Invest* 52:2682, 1973.)

the mother since PIH is more frequent in the mothers but not the mothers-in-law of women with PIH (Sutherland et al, 1981). Moreover, the frequency of eclampsia is increased in the daughters of women who had eclampsia (Cooper et al, 1988). From their pedigree analysis, Cooper et al favor an autosomal recessive mechanism with a gene frequency of the abnormal gene of about 0.25. They also find a suggestion that the fetal genotype can contribute to susceptibility to eclampsia in the mother.

### Intravascular Coagulation

As noted in Figure 11.8, activation of intravascular coagulation and fibrin deposition are likely responsible for much of the specific organ damage seen in severe PIH. The fibrinolytic system may be involved since increased maternal levels of total plasminogen activator inhibitor are found (de Boer et al, 1988). Increased release of serotonin from platelets has been hypothesized to be a contributor to various features of severe preeclampsia (Weiner, 1987).

As noted, the release of thromboxane from platelets may play a primary role in the etiology of PIH, but the various features of slow intravascular coagulation including thrombocytopenia (Romero et al, 1989) that are seen in severe PIH are almost certainly secondary (Pritchard et al, 1976).

### Immunological Injury

The trophoblast must normally perform a major role in preventing immunological rejection of the fetus. As described by Serhal and Craft (1987):

Immunological tolerance between two genetically dissimilar tissues (maternal and fetal) is needed for successful reproduction. The fetus is said to be protected from maternal rejection by the low-grade antigenicity of the trophoblastic tissue, by the masking of trophoblast antigens by surface coat sialomucin, and by "blocking antibodies." It has been suggested that in pregnancy maternal exposure to allelic antigens in the fetus normally induces blocking antibodies which block reactivity to paternal antigens. However, in pre-eclampsia, when paternal and maternal HLA or other antigens are similar, the antigenic stimulus for production of blocking antibodies may be inadequate.

An immunological mechanism is supported by the decreased incidence of PIH in women who have had prior term pregnancy (Campbell et al, 1985) or blood transfusion (Feeney et al, 1977) and by the increased risk for users of contraceptives that prevent exposure to sperm (Klonoff-Cohen et al, 1989), suggesting that the disease is related to initial exposure of the patient to foreign antigens. The risk of PIH is increased 1.9-fold when the parents are of different races with greater genetic dissimilarity (Alderman et al, 1986). Moreover, when multiparas develop PIH, it is often in association with a new father (Ikedife, 1980), further suggesting an inadequate immune response to different fetal antigens.

Beer (1989) proposes that "the focus of the immune attack . . . appears to be the placental cytotrophoblastic component of the arterioles . . . and the resulting immune vasculitis results in the well-defined consequences that are typical of preeclampsia."

### Alterations in Sodium Transport

Some, but not all, of the alterations in sodium transport across cell membranes seen in normal

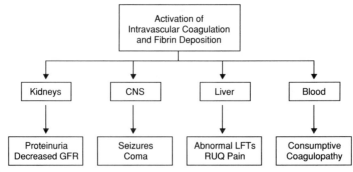

**Figure 11.8.** Proposed model to explain the consequences of activation of intravascular coagulation and fibrin deposition in the pathophysiology of preeclampsia. *CNS*, central nervous system; *GFR*, glomerular filtration rate; *LFT*, liver function test; *RUQ*, right upper quadrant. [From Friedman SA and reprinted with permission from The American College of Obstetricians and Gynecologists. (*Obstetrics and Gynecology*, 71, 1988, 122.)]

pregnancy may be accentuated during PIH. These include:

—a further increase in sodium permeability across red cells (Weissberg et al, 1983);
—an increase in intracellular sodium (Forrester and Alleyne, 1980);
—a decrease in RBC Na$^+$,K$^+$-ATPase activity (Testa et al, 1988; Tranquilli et al, 1988);
—although increased levels of a ouabain-like sodium pump inhibitor in amniotic fluid of hypertensive pregnant women were reported (Graves and Williams, 1984), no increase in maternal serum levels of a digoxin-like immunoreactive substance has been found (Phelps et al, 1988; Jakobi et al, 1989).

The plasma levels of atrial natriuretic factor (ANF) are increased in women with preeclampsia (Bond et al, 1989). These high levels are seen despite a reduction in plasma volume and low central venous and capillary wedge pressures, suggesting another mechanism for the release of ANF than atrial pressure (Thomsen et al, 1987).

## Other Associations

*Plasma Volume Contraction.* The incidence of hypertension and perinatal complications among 54,382 singleton pregnancies were strikingly related to the initial hemoglobin concentration, usually obtained before the 20th week (Murphy et al, 1986). The authors propose that "the adverse findings among the high Hb group may reflect some failure in plasma-volume expansion." They note that Blekta et al (1970) and Gallery et al (1979a) had previously observed plasma volume contraction *before* the onset of preeclampsia. Such contraction, perhaps related to vasoconstriction that has not yet raised the systemic blood pressure, could increase viscosity and reduce uteroplacental perfusion.

*Hyperinsulinemia.* Among 16 women with nonproteinuric hypertension in the third trimester, eight had marked hyperinsulinemia (but normal plasma glucose levels) in response to an oral glucose load (Bauman et al, 1988). As described in Chapter 3, hyperinsulinemia may be involved in the pathogenesis of primary hypertension.

*Sympathetic Nervous System Activity.* In one study, plasma catecholamines were no different between women who did or did not develop PIH (Rubin et al, 1986), whereas, in another small group of women, those with preeclampsia had

significantly higher arterial epinephrine and norepinephrine levels (Øian et al, 1986). Obviously, more data are needed to resolve the different findings.

## Diagnosis of PIH

Whatever its pathogenesis, hypertension developing after the 20th week of gestation with proteinuria and edema in a young nullipara is probably PIH, particularly if she has a positive family history for the syndrome. If convulsions and coma supervene, the diagnosis is almost certainly eclampsia, although other hypertensive disorders may produce a similar picture if they enter an accelerated or malignant phase during the latter stages of pregnancy.

### Hypertension

The blood pressure should be 140/90 or higher, with the systolic having risen 30 mm Hg or more and the diastolic 15 mm Hg or more over prior levels to meet the official criteria. These pressures should be recorded on at least two occasions, 6 hours or more apart. Obviously, there is not sufficient time, as there is with nonpregnant patients, to reconfirm the pressure levels over longer intervals.

Despite the greater overall perinatal mortality with even such transient elevations in pressure, as noted earlier in this chapter, for the individual patient there is a significant chance of overdiagnosing PIH on the basis of a midtrimester DBP > 90 or a third trimester increase of 30/15 mm Hg on two occasions 6 hours apart. These values were found to have only a 23 to 33% positive predictive value and a 81 to 85% negative predictive value (Villar and Sibai, 1989). Obviously, multiple readings and careful follow-up are needed for those who display such findings in the absence of any other suggestive features before making the diagnosis or instituting therapy. Short-term variability is as marked with PIH as with primary hypertension (Sawyer et al, 1981).

On the other hand, the level of pressure may not be inordinately high for it to have serious consequences: Women may convulse with pressures of only 160/110. This may well reflect the relatively low pressure at which the breakthrough of cerebral blood flow occurs in previously normotensive patients, as described by Strandgaard et al and detailed in Chapter 8. Since women with PIH are usually young and, by definition, previously normotensive, their blood vessels would be particularly susceptible to the pressure-induced marked breakthrough vaso-dilation that leads to encephalopathy. More-over, the usual fall in blood pressure seen during sleep, even in severe primary hypertension, may be blunted in women with PIH (Beilin et al, 1982).

### Proteinuria

The urine should contain more than 300 mg of protein in a 24-hour collection or 1 g per liter in two random, cleanly voided specimens collected at least 4 hours apart. Proteinuria usually appears after hypertension and edema and is a serious omen when superimposed on the other two features. The proteinuria may be so great as to lead to the nephrotic syndrome (Fisher et al, 1977).

### Edema

Sudden and excessive weight gain of more than 2 lb in 1 week is usually the earliest warning sign that PIH is developing, and it is detectable before edema. Since some pedal edema is common in normal pregnancy, the edema must be generalized before it is accepted as part of the syndrome.

Patients usually are not bothered by the three main features of PIH—hypertension, protein-uria, and edema. Obviously, prenatal care is needed to detect these features early and thereby prevent the dangerous sequelae of the fully developed syndrome.

### Other Features: Mild Versus Severe (Table 11.3)

Headache is rare in mild cases but may be a forerunner of eclampsia. Epigastric pain is another late and serious symptom. Visual blurring probably reflects retinal arteriolar spasm, ischemia, and edema. Sequential constriction of the retinal arterioles is the first change and is present in most patients. Retinal edema may follow severe arteriolar narrowing and often gives the retina a sheen. Hemorrhages and exudates are rare with PIH and, if present, suggest underlying chronic hypertension.

### Errors in Making the Diagnosis

Among those who have onset of preeclampsia before the 37th week of gestation there is a greater likelihood of another disease—usually chronic essential hypertension or chronic renal disease—rather than PIH as the mechanism (Ihle et al, 1987; Lindheimer and Chesley, 1987). Although rarely indicated, renal biopsy findings are most discriminatory: Those with "pure" PIH have subendothelial deposits in capillary loops (which soon disappear after delivery) and endothelial cell swelling (which persists longer) (Packham et al, 1988). Those with underlying chronic hypertension display nephrosclerosis; those with chronic renal disease, findings specific for various forms of glomerulonephritis. In one recent series of 23 patients with no known history of chronic hypertension or renal disease, 45% turned out to have features of underlying renal disease on biopsy (Hill et al, 1988).

The error can be minimized by recognition of these features, which favor the diagnosis of chronic hypertension more than of PIH:

—onset of hypertension before 20 weeks of gestation;
—hypertension in a previous pregnancy;
—failure to develop hypertension during the first pregnancy but its appearance in subsequent ones;
—absence of proteinuria and edema;
—evidence of sustained and severe hypertension (systolic pressure of 200 mm Hg) with

**Table 11.3. Indicators of Severity of PIH[a]**

| Abnormality | Mild | Severe |
|---|---|---|
| Diastolic blood pressure | < 100 mm Hg | 110 mm Hg or higher |
| Proteinuria | Trace to 1 + | Persistent 2 + or more |
| Headache | Absent | Present |
| Visual disturbances | Absent | Present |
| Upper abdominal pain | Absent | Present |
| Oliguria | Absent | Present |
| Convulsions | Absent | Present |
| Serum creatinine | Normal | Elevated |
| Thrombocytopenia | Absent | Present |
| Hyperbilirubinemia | Absent | Present |
| Liver enzyme elevation | Minimal | Marked |
| Fetal growth retardation | Absent | Obvious |

[a]From Cunningham FG, Leveno KJ: In: Rubin PC (ed). *Handbook of Hypertension*, Vol 10: *Hypertension in Pregnancy*. Amsterdam: Elsevier Science Publishers, 1988:290.

retinal hemorrhages and exudates or left ventricular hypertrophy (Thompson et al, 1986);

—age of 30 years or more.

The only laboratory procedure that has proved to be of practical value in the diagnosis of PIH is an elevated serum uric acid (McFadyen et al, 1986). A number of other laboratory tests have been used in an attempt to recognize preeclampsia before it develops and to differentiate it from chronic hypertension. As Sibai (1988) notes: "More than 100 clinical, biophysical, and biochemical tests have been recommended to predict the future development of the disease. Results of the pooled data and the wide scatter therein suggest that none of these tests is sufficiently sensitive or specific for use as a screening test in clinical practice." The search, nonetheless, continues: Fibronectin, a glycoprotein found in the uterine muscle, has been reported to be increased in the plasma weeks before preeclampsia appears (Lazarchick et al, 1986). Another possibility is 24-hour urine calcium excretion, which was reduced during the third trimester in 12 women with preeclampsia and seven with chronic hypertension and superimposed preeclampsia compared with the levels in 10 normotensive and 11 nonpreeclamptic hypertensive pregnant women (Taufield et al, 1987).

### Early Detection

Women with the following features should be closely watched because they have a higher likelihood of developing PIH: (1) young primigravidas; (2) a family history of PIH; (3) multiple fetuses; (4) black race; (5) preexisting hypertension, heart or renal disease; and (6) hydatidiform mole (Guzick et al, 1987). In addition, those whose weight increased more than 35% above their nonpregnant weight were found to have a 4-fold greater risk of developing preeclampsia (Shepard et al, 1986).

*Rollover Test.* In addition to careful attention to even small rises in blood pressure, one simple clinical test has been claimed to recognize the predisposition to PIH—the rollover test (Gant et al, 1974), performed as follows:

1. The woman lies on her left side until the blood pressure is stable.
2. She is put flat on her back.
3. The blood pressure is recorded in the right arm immediately and after 5 minutes.
4. A positive test is a 20-mm Hg or greater rise in diastolic blood pressure.

Initial results with the test were closely correlated with sensitivity to exogenous angiotensin, previously found to be an index of susceptibility to PIH, and with the subsequent course of the blood pressure. Subsequent experience with the rollover test has shown it to have less specificity and sensitivity than originally claimed (Kassar et al, 1980; Tunbridge et al, 1983). Another technique, the blood pressure response to an isometric contraction (Degani et al, 1985), has been advocated as a more accurate predictor. Neither of these tests nor a positive cold pressor test was found to be a predictor of the development of PIH (Eneroth-Grimfors et al, 1988).

### Management of PIH

A succinct overview of the management of hypertension in pregnancy is provided by Svensson (1988):

The purpose of treating the hypertensive pregnant woman is dual; to protect the mother from the acute complications of high blood pressure and to diminish the risk of fetal/neonatal morbidity and mortality. Occasionally, these two objectives are incompatible. . . .

Following delivery, blood pressure will generally be normalized very rapidly. If pharmacological treatment is necessary, the possible negative effects on the fetus have to be considered before delivery, but post partum this is not the case. Therefore, delivery is the treatment of choice in pregnancy-induced hypertensive disease. With the progress in neonatal care made in recent years, it is possible to deliver hypertensive women as early as in the 32nd gestational week with very good results.

If the blood pressure is elevated in early pregnancy, rest is the initial treatment in most cases. If the blood pressure is very high, or remains elevated in spite of rest, pharmacological treatment will be necessary. Blood pressure ≥ 160/110 mm Hg should be reduced, but there is no general agreement on how to treat women with [systolic] blood pressure ≥ 140 [and < 160] mm Hg. Some authorities advocate the use of antihypertensive drugs, but most are reluctant to use drugs in this situation. In none of the relatively small, adequately controlled studies of drug treatment in mild-to-moderate hypertension in pregnancy has a reduction of perinatal death rate been observed.

As reviewed by Fletcher and Bulpitt (1988), there is a paucity of randomized clinical trials of sufficient size to provide guidelines for the treatment of hypertension during pregnancy. They conclude, "We are uncertain as to the place of diuretic and hydralazine treatment. Nor do we know whether methyldopa is to be preferred to beta-adrenoceptor-blocking drugs or calcium-channel-blocking drugs. All that appears established is that lowering blood pressure reduced fetal mortality and the incidence of pre-eclampsia."

The overall plan prepared by Lubbe (1984) is in keeping with recommendations of most experts (Fig. 11.9).

*Modified Bed Rest.* Once the blood pressure has been found to be high, the patient should be kept on limited activity, preferably in a high-risk obstetrical unit. Although most advocate bed rest, the only randomized, controlled trial of *complete* bed rest showed no benefit over "ambulation as desired" (Mathews et al, 1982). Nonetheless, simply relaxing in a low-key hospital setting while consuming a regular diet and no medication but iron tablets has been enough for 85% of women admitted with PIH to diurese and normalize their blood pressure (Gant and Pritchard, 1984).

Sibai et al (1987a) randomly allocated half of 200 primigravidas with mild preeclampsia to hospitalization alone or to hospitalization combined with labetalol. The addition of the drug

made no difference in perinatal outcome but was associated with *more* fetal growth retardation (19 versus 9%).

For some with mild PIH, home management may be feasible with visits by nurses (Feeney, 1984) and self-monitoring of blood pressure (Rayburn et al, 1985). Programmed relaxation with or without biofeedback may help (Little et al, 1984).

*Sodium and Volume.* For many years, obstetricians have warned against sodium restriction in pregnancy even in the presence of significant hypertension (Robinson, 1958; Mengert and Tacchi, 1961). More recently, Millar (1988) has suggested that "Oral salt supplementation might improve the haemodynamic abnormalities and prognosis in pre-eclampsia by increasing plasma volume and suppressing production of angiotensin II." Gallery and associates (1984) have reported significant falls in blood pressure after the administration of plasma expanders, particularly when given after vasodilator therapy (Belfort et al, 1989).

*Antihypertensive Therapy.* Most now ad-

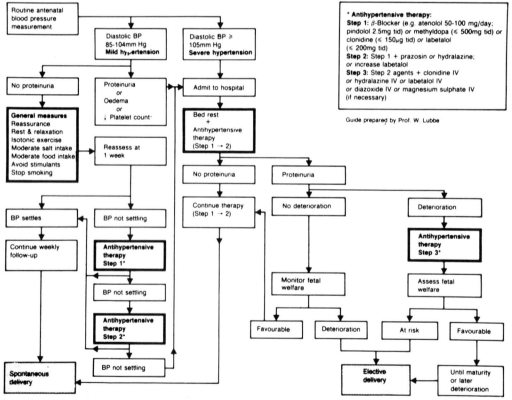

**Figure 11.9.** A plan of management for hypertension during pregnancy. (From Lubbe WF: *Drugs* 28:170, 1984.)

vise antihypertensive drug therapy only if the diastolic blood pressure is above 105 mm Hg and does not fall on modified bed rest. Such caution may be appropriate since uteroplacental perfusion, measured by the metabolic clearance rate of dehydroisoandrosterone sulfate ($MCR_{DS}$), was shown to fall after intravenous furosemide, oral thiazides, or hydralazine (Gant et al, 1976). However, using an isotopic uptake-disappearance technique, uteroplacental blood flow has been found not to fall despite significant reduction of systemic blood pressure with these drugs: hydralazine, labetalol (Lunell et al, 1984); nifedipine (Lindow et al, 1988); and pindolol (Nylund and Lunell, 1988).

There are no good data on the relative effectiveness and safety of various antihypertensives in pregnant women, and most of the limited trials that have been done admixed women with PIH and chronic hypertension. The data that are available involve these drugs:

—methyldopa. Leather et al (1968) and Redman et al (1976) showed that its use reduced the number of midtrimester abortions and perinatal deaths. Cockburn et al (1982) followed 195 children born to the women treated with methyldopa in the trial of Redman and associates for 7½ years and found no evidence of physical or mental developmental difficulty.

—clonidine. This drug worked as well as methyldopa (Henderson-Smart et al, 1984).

—Beta-blockers. Atenolol was more effective than placebo in one of the few randomized, double-blind prospective studies done, with no adverse effects on mother or baby (Rubin et al, 1984). Metoprolol was safe but did not prevent the development of albuminuria (Wichman et al, 1984).

In the conclusion of a review on the use of beta-blockers in pregnancy, Frishman and Chesner (1988) suggest these guidelines:

(1) Avoid, whenever possible, the use of beta-blocker therapy during the first trimester of pregnancy. (2) Use the lowest possible beta-blocker dose. (3) If possible, discontinue beta-blocker therapy at least 2 to 3 days prior to delivery, both as a way of limiting the effects of beta-blockers on uterine contractility and for preventing possible neonatal complications secondary to beta-blockade. (4) Use of beta-blockers with $beta_1$-selectivity, intrinsic sympathetic activity, or alpha-blocking activity may be preferable in that these agents would be less likely to interfere with beta$_2$-mediated uterine relaxation and peripheral vasodilation.

—alpha-blockers. Prazosin was effective in a group of eight women (Rubin et al, 1983).

—combined alpha- and beta-blockers. Labetalol has been successfully used in a number of trials. In a study involving 56 women, it caused less fetal growth retardation than atenolol (Lardoux et al, 1983). In other studies, it protected the fetus as well as methyldopa (Plouin et al, 1988) and better than placebo (Pickles et al, 1989b).

—calcium entry blockers. Good results have been reported with the dihydropyridines nifedipine (Walters and Redman, 1984) and nitrendipine (Allen et al, 1987) and with verapamil (Orlandi et al, 1986).

—diuretics. In keeping with the concerns about sodium restriction, the use of diuretics has been denigrated. However, when Collins et al (1985) combined the results of nine trials using diuretics in 7000 women, there was a suggested improvement in perinatal mortality. Regardless, de Swiet (1985) concludes that "the overall lack of efficacy of diuretics in controlling blood pressure in pregnancy, the associated reduction in circulating blood volume, and the rise in urate concentration militate against their use."

—ACEIs. Captopril is lethal to sheep and rabbit fetuses, and the use of ACEIs is contraindicated in pregnancy. In a survey of 22 patients given captopril and nine given enalapril, mostly because other drugs had failed, there were increased numbers of neonatal renal failure and patent ductus arteriosus (Kreft-Jais et al, 1988).

*Timing of Delivery.* Gestation is allowed to continue until spontaneous labor ensues or the cervix becomes favorable for induction of labor at or near term. Delivery before term is considered in patients with persistent or recurrent hypertension and one or more of the following:

—rapid weight gain;
—decrease in creatinine clearance;
—appearance of significant proteinuria;
—clinical or sonographic evidence of fetal growth retardation;
—development of severe headache, scotomata, or right upper quadrant pain.

With the use of such a conservative approach, more than 3000 nulliparas with PIH have been managed on the high-risk antepartum unit at

Parkland Memorial Hospital (Cunningham and Leveno, 1988). The results have been remarkable: Among the first 545 who remained until delivery, there were no maternal deaths and a perinatal mortality rate of only nine per 1000, much lower than the 24 per 1000 among the general obstetric population of the same hospital (Gilstrap et al, 1978). Among the 31 patients who left the high-risk unit against medical advice, the perinatal mortality rate was 129 per 1000.

**Therapy of Severe PIH**

Those with the manifestations of severe PIH shown in Table 11.3 who do not improve after a few days of bed rest and antihypertensive therapy will likely require termination of pregnancy, i.e., "elective delivery" as diagrammed in Figure 11.9. An attempt should be made to induce labor by use of oxytocin. If that is unsuccessful, cesarean delivery may be indicated.

The clinical course may be complicated by pulmonary edema (Sibai et al, 1987b) or the HELLP syndrome of hemolysis (H), elevated liver enzymes (EL), and low platelets (LP) that is often associated with disseminated intravascular coagulation (Van Dam et al, 1989).

*Antihypertensive Therapy.* To protect the mother from cerebral hemorrhage and from encephalopathy, the blood pressure should be reduced, usually with a parenteral drug (Van Assche et al, 1989). However, caution is needed to prevent abrupt and marked falls in maternal BP that could cause fetal distress. Hydralazine is preferred by most, but labetalol seems to work well (Mabie et al, 1987) as may nifedipine (Waisman et al, 1988). Nitroprusside (Shoemaker and Meyers, 1984) or diazoxide (Dudley, 1985) will lower the blood pressure, but the potential for fetal cyanide toxicity with the former and the interference with uterine contractions with the latter make them less attractive.

*Magnesium Sulfate.* This agent is widely used in the United States to prevent convulsions in patients with severe preeclampsia (Pritchard, 1984). The Pritchard protocol utilizes 4 g intravenously followed by 5 g intramuscularly immediately and every 4 hours thereafter, if patellar reflexes are present, respirations are not depressed, and urine output is adequate (Gant and Pritchard, 1984). Neuromuscular transmission can be altered (Ramanathan et al, 1988), but when used with appropriate care, magnesium sulfate has been remarkably safe and effective

in preventing convulsions (Cunningham and Leveno, 1988).

In addition, magnesium sulfate may lower the blood pressure particularly during contractions (Bhatia et al, 1987), overcome spasms of umbilical and placental vessels (Altura et al, 1983), enhance production of prostacyclin in endothelial cells (Watson et al, 1986), and reduce plasma renin activity (Sipes et al, 1989).

*Other Therapies.* Glucocorticoids have been used in an attempt to induce fetal pulmonary maturity (Ruvinsky et al, 1984). Prostacyclin (Fidler et al, 1980) and prostaglandin $A_1$ (Toppozada et al, 1983) have been given intravenously but remain purely investigational. Caution has been advised to limit the amount of parenteral fluids so as not to reduce further plasma colloid osmotic pressure (Zinaman et al, 1985).

*Outcome.* Despite everything, the fetal salvage for midtrimester severe PIH was only 13% of 60 pregnancies (Sibai et al, 1985). The same investigators reported 100% fetal survival when the disease developed after 36 weeks of gestation (Sibai et al, 1984).

Fortunately, the developmental status of children born to women with preeclampsia is usually excellent. As Ounsted (1988) says: "These fetuses and newborn babies either die, or survive, intact."

## ECLAMPSIA

When PIH is not recognized or treated, a few women develop eclampsia, manifested by repeated, generalized tonic-clonic convulsions followed by coma. This serious complication is becoming less common as better prenatal care is given, with the present incidence in the United States estimated to be about one in every 2000 deliveries. However, where prenatal care is neglected, eclampsia remains both common and deadly (Lopez-Llera, 1982) and, even where prenatal care is readily available, "eclampsia still kills" (Redman, 1988).

### Clinical Features

Eclampsia is a form of hypertensive encephalopathy (Redman, 1988). The convulsions that signify eclampsia almost always are preceded by the clinical manifestations of PIH. Chesley (1978) estimated that one-half of the cases develop antepartum, one-quarter of them during delivery, and another one-quarter after delivery. The postpartum cases usually occur within 24 hours after delivery, although rare instances have been reported up to 6 days later. As with PIH, the frequency of eclampsia is higher in patients with twin pregnancies, hydramnios, and hydatidiform mole.

### Convulsions

Although patients may have preceding auras, epigastric pain, apprehension, and hyperreflexia, the convulsions often begin with little or no warning. After the intense tonic-clonic convulsion, patients become stuporous and usually comatose. Coma may persist for days and is often followed by a period of semiconsciousness and amnesia. In about 5% of eclamptics, an acute psychosis may follow the coma and may last for 1 to 2 weeks.

Computed tomography of the head reveals abnormalities in half or more, but the procedure is not indicated in most patients since the findings seldom alter management (Brown et al, 1988).

### Other Features

Hypertension may be severe, although some patients may have only minimal pressure elevations. Proteinuria is frequently pronounced. Oliguria is invariable, and anuria may supervene if adequate fluid intake is not maintained (Turney et al, 1989). Edema is variable and occasionally massive. Pulmonary edema is common in fatal cases and probably represents direct damage to the capillary bed, as well as heart failure. Blindness, usually from retinal edema but sometimes from retinal detachment, rarely is noted.

These and other features reflect widespread vascular damage, the etiology of which is as enigmatic as the cause of PIH. The process may simply reflect more intense vasospasm than occurs with PIH, with secondary hypoxic damage to vessels and the organ they supply. Evidence of intravascular coagulation is prominent and probably secondary to the widespread vascular damage (Pritchard et al, 1976).

### Differential Diagnosis

The usual picture of a young woman, near term, normal during the first two-thirds of pregnancy, who develops PIH and then convulsions, should present no difficulty in diagnosis. Other causes of convulsions should be considered, including epilepsy, central nervous system infection, brain tumor, and cerebrovascular accident. Rarely, a pheochromocytoma may masquerade as eclampsia.

### Management

For over 200 years, eclampsia has been known to be caused by pregnancy and to be relieved by delivery. Delivery is delayed until convulsions are stopped, the blood pressure is controlled, and reasonable fluid and electrolyte balance have been established. With the following standardized treatment of 245 consecutive cases of eclampsia, only one maternal death occurred, and all but one of the fetuses survived who were alive when treatment was started and who weighed 1800 g or more at birth (Pritchard et al, 1984):

1. Magnesium sulfate to control convulsions
2. Control of severe hypertension (DBP > 110 mm Hg) with intermittent intravenous injections of hydralazine
3. Avoidance of diuretics and hyperosmotic agents
4. Limitation of fluid intake unless fluid loss was excessive
5. Delivery once convulsions were arrested and consciousness regained.

### Consequences

Considering the seriousness of eclampsia, many physicians have advised affected women that they should not become pregnant again. However, Chesley (1980) found that in 466 later pregnancies in 189 women who had had eclampsia, only 25% had recurrent hypertension, and only four had a second episode of eclampsia. Fetal salvage was 76% overall and 93% in those carrying beyond 28 weeks.

In a 22- to 44-year follow-up of these women, the remote prognosis for those who had eclampsia during their first pregnancy was excellent (Chesley et al, 1976). The distribution of their blood pressures was identical to those of the general population. In white women having eclampsia as primigravidas, the remote mortality rate was not increased; in white women having eclampsia as multiparas and in all black women, the remote mortality was from 2 to 5 times that expected. This probably reflects the likelihood that many of these women had underlying but unrecognized chronic hypertension.

### PREVENTION OF PIH

As noted earlier, there is strong evidence that PIH involves an imbalance of uteroplacental vascular prostacyclin and platelet thromboxane production. Low doses of aspirin may correct this imbalance and preliminary trials support this effect (Wallenburg and Rotmans, 1988; Schiff et al, 1989). However, a large controlled trial is needed for documentation.

In the meantime, the only sure preventive measure beyond abstinence is prevention of teenage pregnancies. Adequate nutrition, with at least 2200 calories per day so that a 25-lb weight gain occurs, may diminish the incidence (Primrose and Higgins, 1971). Increased levels of leisure time physical activity may also, in some manner, be protective (Marcoux et al, 1989).

Women with PIH may have a lower calcium intake even though they do not have lower serum total or ionized calcium levels than normotensive pregnant women (Belizán et al, 1988). These same investigators have shown a fall in blood pressure with 1 to 2 g/day of calcium supplementation in normotensive pregnant women (Villar et al, 1987), a fall that may be predicted by initial low serum calcium and plasma renin levels (Repke et al, 1989). In another randomized, double-blind, controlled trial, the 49 nulliparas who took 2 g of calcium per day from the 24th week had a lower rate (4%) of PIH than did the 43 women given placebo (28%) (Lopez-Jaramillo et al, 1989). A much larger experience will be needed to document a prophylactic effect from calcium supplements.

Both diuretics and sodium restriction have been proposed for prophylaxis against PIH. As noted earlier, neither is indicated in the treatment of established gestational hypertension, and there is no reason to believe that either would be prophylactic.

## CHRONIC HYPERTENSION AND PREGNANCY

Pregnant women may have any of the other types of hypertension listed in Chapter 1. Because the blood pressure usually falls during the first half of pregnancy, their preexisting hypertension may not be recognized if they are first seen at that time. If their chronic pressures *are* high then, however, they almost certainly have chronic hypertension and not PIH.

Pregnancy seems to bring out latent essential hypertension in certain women whose pressures return to normal between pregnancies but eventually remain elevated. Young women found to have arteriolar nephrosclerosis on renal biopsy during pregnancy presumably fit that category (Smythe et al, 1964). In addition, renal biopsies have shown an unexpected high percentage of young pregnant hypertensives to have chronic renal parenchymal disease (McCartney, 1964; Hill et al, 1988).

To elucidate the true mechanism of hypertension seen during a pregnancy, it is usually necessary to follow the patient postpartum. By 3 months, complete resolution of the various changes seen in pregnancy will have occurred so that, if indicated, further studies can be obtained (Gallery, 1988).

### Primary Hypertension During Pregnancy

The frequency of primary (essential) hypertension is higher in older women and multiparas. They may suffer no noticeable effects from their mild to moderate hypertension, and if other adverse factors are not present, the perinatal mortality of their infants is not increased (Walters, 1966). However, if the pressures are high and evidence of organ damage (retinopathy, cardiomegaly, renal impairment) already exists, infant mortality is increased perhaps 3-fold (Silverstone et al, 1980).

### Management of Chronic Hypertension During Pregnancy

Women with severe hypertension should be advised not to become pregnant, particularly if they have had PIH superimposed (see below) during previous pregnancies.

Women with mild to moderate hypertension should be watched more closely, warned about signs of early PIH, and delivered at 37 weeks of gestation. A program of bed rest, avoidance of diuretics, and judicious use of hydralazine if the diastolic BP (DBP) was above 110 mm Hg resulted in a halving of perinatal mortality in 66 patients with chronic hypertension cared for during 72 pregnancies (Curet and Olson, 1979). Antihypertensive therapy may protect the mother and may improve the chances for successful outcome to the pregnancy (Gallery, 1988).

On the other hand, many may be able to discontinue therapy used before pregnancy: Of 211 pregnant women with mild chronic hypertension who stopped their medications at the first prenatal visit, only 13% required reinstitution of therapy and only 10% had superimposed PIH (Sibai et al, 1983). Among the 190 without superimposed PIH, only 5.3% had small-for-age infants, and there was only one perinatal death.

## PIH Superimposed on Chronic Hypertension

The superimposition of PIH on chronic hypertension introduces a greater hazard to both mother and fetus (Sibai et al, 1983), and this happens with a higher frequency in women already hypertensive than in previously normotensive women, with the figures varying from as low as 10% to as high as 50% (Chesley, 1978). The diagnosis is usually based on the appearance of proteinuria, edema, and aggravation of the hypertension. About 1% of these women develop eclampsia, and they are prone to redevelop PIH with subsequent pregnancies: Chesley (1978) found a 71% recurrence rate of superimposed PIH.

## POSTPARTUM SYNDROMES

All antihypertensive drugs taken by mothers enter their breast milk. Most are present in very low concentration, with the apparent exception of beta-blockers (except propranolol) (White, 1984) and calcium entry blockers (Penny and Lewis, 1989), which are excreted in concentrations similar to those present in maternal plasma.

### Postpartum Hypertension

Cardiac output remains elevated for at least 48 hours after normal delivery (Robson et al, 1987). In one study, 12% of all women had a DBP above 110 mm Hg over the first 4 days after delivery (Walters et al, 1986). In women who were preeclamptic, the hypertension may worsen during those first few days postpartum (Crawford et al, 1987).

A certain percentage of women, varying in published series from 4 to 17%, are found to have hypertension when seen at their 6-week postpartum visit, even though they were not hypertensive during the prior pregnancy or the first few days after delivery. Of those followed by Stout (1934), 91% had become normotensive again after 1 year. Few have significant abnormalities on follow-up (Piver et al, 1967). This may represent the uncovering of early primary hypertension hidden by the hemodynamic and hormonal changes of pregnancy.

### Postpartum Heart Failure

Homans (1985) reviewed 347 cases of cardiomyopathy presenting in the last month of pregnancy or the first 6 months after delivery, without other identifiable causes. The incidence in the United States is around one in 3000 deliveries, mostly among blacks. The cause in most is attributable to chronic underlying hypertension or valvular disease (Cummingham et al, 1986).

### Postpartum Nephrosclerosis

At least 40 cases of postpartum nephrosclerosis, a catastrophic syndrome, have been reported since it was first recognized (Strauss and Alexander, 1976). Typically, women who were seemingly normal during their previous pregnancy develop a nonspecific flu-like illness 1 to 10 weeks postpartum and rapidly progress into oliguric renal failure and die unless dialysis or renal transplantation is performed. Hypertension, although initially often minimal, becomes severe.

The cause of this syndrome is unknown. Similar cases have been reported in women taking oral contraceptives (Hauglustaine et al, 1981).

## HYPERTENSION WITH ORAL CONTRACEPTIVES

Oral contraceptives, i.e., "the pill," have been used by millions of women since the early 1960s. Current estimates are that 64 million women throughout the world (Rosenfield, 1989) and 13 million in the United States (Mishell, 1989) used the pill for contraception.

Nonetheless, there remains a great need for temporary contraception. Worldwide, approximately 57% of the 880 million married couples of reproductive age are unprotected (Rosenfield, 1989). With an earlier menarche and a relaxation of social inhibitions, more and more teenage girls are sexually active, with two-thirds having had intercourse by age 19 (Zelnik and Kantner, 1980). Only about one of three sexually active teenage girls uses contraception, and the use of the pill among them has been decreasing (Harvey, 1980), so that the rate of unwanted teenage pregnancies in the United States has increased (Freeman and Rickels, 1979).

Acceptance of the pill has been hampered by recognition of various cardiovascular risks that are increased with its use (Rosenfield, 1989). These risks, although real, have been overemphasized in the medical literature and exaggerated in the public's perception. The problem revolves around the very definite, statistically significant increase in risk associated with pill use, on the one hand, but the failure to recognize that the absolute number of people afflicted is quite small, on the other, and that the risk is

**344** / *Clinical Hypertension*

not equal for all who use the pill, being quite small for its primary audience.

Thus, in a large prospective study in England, a 40% higher death rate was found among women who used the pill (Royal College study, 1981). Virtually all of the excess mortality was due to cardiovascular disease, with a 4-fold greater risk of ischemic heart disease and subarachnoid hemorrhage. However, when the actual number of pill users who would suffer a vascular complication is calculated (the attributable risk), the 4-fold excess turns out to be a relatively small number—about two deaths per 10,000 women per year (Stadel, 1981). Furthermore, the risk was concentrated in women 35 years or older and in smokers. In the large Royal College of General Practitioners' study, current use of the pill increased the risk for acute myocardial infarction only among women who also smoked (Croft and Hannaford, 1989).

It should be further noted that the pill used today is safer than that used 5 to 10 years ago. Smaller amounts of estrogen and progestogen are associated with fewer cardiovascular complications (Rosenberg and Rosenthal, 1987).

To put the dangers of the pill in proper perspective, its use in women aged 15 to 34 who do not smoke is associated with less risk of death than most other contraceptive methods, particularly when its lower rate of failure to prevent pregnancy is considered (Ory, 1983). Only the condom, plus abortion if it fails, is safer and more effective than the pill. Nonetheless there are hazards, and hypertension is a major component of the increased risk for cardiovascular disease associated with the use of the pill (Prentice, 1988).

Although past users were thought to maintain excess cardiovascular risk, both the Royal College study and the massive Nurses' Health Study (Stampfer et al, 1988) show no excess risk among former pill users.

## Incidence of Hypertension

The blood pressure rises a little in most women who take estrogen-containing oral contraceptives (Woods, 1988). The rise is enough to push the pressure beyond 140/90 in about 5% over a 5-year period of pill use (Royal College, 1974). In a very small number, the rise will be so abrupt and severe as to cause accelerated or malignant hypertension (Lim et al, 1987).

Though the first report of pill-induced hypertension appeared a few years after its introduction (Brownrigg, 1962), the association was

not clearly defined until 1967 (Laragh et al, 1967; Woods, 1967). Not until a prospective study was begun in Glasgow did it become apparent that the blood pressure rose in *most* women who started oral contraceptives. Among 186 women who took estrogen-containing oral contraceptives for 2 years, systolic pressure rose in 164 and diastolic in 150 (Weir, 1982) (Fig. 11.10). Of these, eight had increases in systolic pressure greater than 25 mm Hg, and two had diastolic pressure increases of 24 to 34 mm Hg.

Despite some exceptions (Blumenstein et al, 1980), the majority of careful studies document an increase of incidence of hypertension with estrogen-containing oral contraceptives (Woods, 1988). The incidence may be less with present day, lower dose formulations containing only 30 to 35 $\mu$g of estrogen (Malatino et al, 1988).

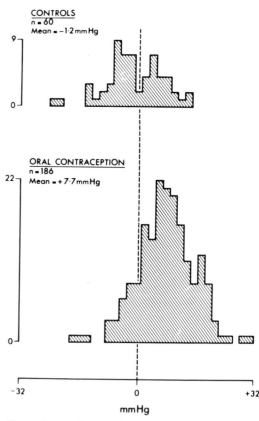

**Figure 11.10.** Changes in systolic blood pressure after 2 years in women taking oestrogen-progestagen oral contraceptives and in controls. (From Weir RJ: In: Amery A (ed). *Hypertensive Cardiovascular Disease: Pathophysiology and Treatment.* The Hague: Martinus Nijhoff Publishers, 1982:612.)

When eight women who had developed hypertension on 50-$\mu$g estrogen, 1- to 3-mg progestogen pills were switched to ones containing 30 $\mu$g of estrogen and 150 to 250 $\mu$g levonorgestrel, a lesser rise in pressure developed (Weir, 1979).

Although, as we shall see, the estrogen has been incriminated as the cause of pill-induced hypertension, the progestogen component may also be involved. When used alone as a "minipill," progestogens do not appear to raise the blood pressure (Spellacy and Birk, 1972), but when given with estrogens, they may potentiate the problem (Meade, 1988). Whether these synthetic progestogens, which have mineralocorticoid effects in contrast to the natriuretic effects of natural progesterone, are implicated in the hypertension or not, they appear to significantly increase the potential for cardiovascular complications from the pill (Meade, 1988). Therefore, the lowest effective dose of both estrogen and progestogen seems safest.

## Clinical Features and Predisposing Factors

Older age and obesity are the only known predisposing factors to pill-induced hypertension. Women over age 35 are particularly susceptible. A positive family history of hypertension is noted in about half of those with pill-induced hypertension, but there seems to be little added likelihood for it to develop in women with prior pregnancy-induced hypertension. Only nine of 180 women who had had hypertension during pregnancy had a rise in diastolic pressure beyond 90 after 6 months to 2 years of pill use (Pritchard and Pritchard, 1977). Similarly, women with preexisting hypertension do not appear to be particularly more susceptible (Spellacy and Birk, 1974).

In most who develop hypertension, the disease is mild, and in more than half, the pressure returns to normal when the pill is stopped (Crane et al, 1971; Weir, 1978). Whether the pill is causing hypertension de novo or simply uncovering the propensity toward primary hypertension that would eventually appear spontaneously is unknown. Among 14 women whose pressures returned to normal after the pill was stopped, seven developed spontaneous hypertension during the ensuing 6 years (Woods et al, 1972). The incidence of hypertension among women who previously used the pill is similar to that seen among women who have never used the pill (Fisch and Frank, 1977).

In a few, the hypertension is severe, rapidly accelerating into a malignant phase and causing irreversible renal damage (Lim et al, 1987). Even in those with reversible hypertension, considerable renal damage may be found by means of arteriography and renal biopsy (Boyd et al, 1975). A hemolytic uremic syndrome may also follow pill use (Hauglustaine et al, 1981).

## Mechanism

The manner in which oral contraceptives induced hypertension is unknown, though hemodynamic changes have been measured in a few, and alterations in the renin-angiotensin-aldosterone mechanism have been examined in many. As noted, the estrogen in the pill appears to be the culprit, but the progestogen may also play a role.

### Hemodynamic Changes

Many women gain weight when put on the pill. Though a direct relation between weight gain and hypertension has not been observed, Walters and Lim (1969) and Lehtovirta (1974) found that body weight, plasma volume, and cardiac output were significantly increased in previously normal women after 2 to 3 months of pill intake. Thus, the hemodynamics suggest a volume-overload type of hypertension.

Crane and Harris (1973) found a 100- to 200-mEq increase in total body exchangeable sodium after 3 weeks' intake of stilbestrol, conjugated estrogens, estradiol, or mestranol. They also found that some of the progestogens used in the oral contraceptives—norethindrone, ethynodiol diacetate, chlormadinone—caused comparable sodium retention when given to normal subjects.

### Renin-Angiotensin-Aldosterone Changes

Estrogens increase the hepatic synthesis of renin substrate (Helmer and Judson, 1967). The increase in substrate is accompanied by an increase in total renin activity but a fall in the concentration of renin (Derkx et al, 1986). This is thought to result from the sequences shown in Figure 11.11.

Whether these changes in the renin-angiotensin-aldosterone mechanism are responsible for the hypertension is uncertain. With few exceptions (Saruta et al, 1970), most have noted no significant differences in the direction or degree of these changes in the renin-aldosterone mechanism between the majority of women who remain normotensive and the minority who become

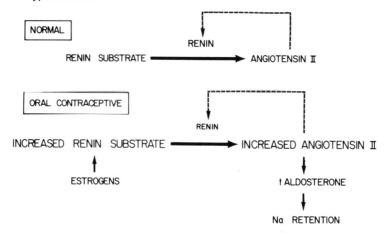

**Figure 11.11.** Schematic representation of the changes in the renin-angiotensin system induced by oral contraceptives containing estrogen. The *dashed lines* show the feedback suppression of renin release by angiotensin II.

hypertensive. Cain et al (1971) suggest that, though all are susceptible, only those with underlying renal disease that prevents the full expression of various compensatory mechanisms may develop hypertension. In most women on the pill, the renal vasculature responds to the higher levels of AII with a reduction in renal blood flow (Hollenberg et al, 1976). Though the mean fall was 25%, in some it was as high as 50%. Perhaps those with the greatest renal vasoconstriction develop sodium retention and hypertension.

Among other possible mechanisms, insulin resistance and higher plasma insulin levels after an oral glucose load have been found in women on a low-dose oral contraceptive pill for 3 months (Kasdorf and Kalkhoff, 1988). The levels tended to become more normal after 6 months of pill use.

### The Pill in Perspective

The pill is safe for most women for temporary contraception. However, the BP will increase in most, and hypertension will appear in 5% of those taking it for 5 years. Along with the changes in clotting, the rise in triglycerides and low-density lipoprotein (LDL)-cholesterol (Burkman et al, 1988), and the abnormalities in glucose tolerance, hypertension may be an important risk factor, responsible for various cardiovascular problems that occur with increased frequency with pill use.

However, the availability and use of the pill has been the major reason for the progressive fall in unwanted, unplanned pregnancies accomplished over the past 25 years. Since neither the progestogen-only "mini-pill" nor the intrauter-

ine device (IUD) has proved to be an ideal contraceptive, the combination oral contraceptive will continue to be needed.

When it is used, however, the following precautions should be taken:

—The lowest effective dose of estrogen and progestogen should be dispensed.
—No more than a 6-month supply should be provided at one time.
—The blood pressure should be taken every 6 months or whenever the woman feels ill.
—If the blood pressure rises significantly, the pill should be stopped and another form of contraceptive provided.
—If the blood pressure does not become normal within 3 months, appropriate workup and therapy should be provided.
—If the pill must be continued, antihypertensive therapy may be needed to control the blood pressure. Caution is advised with the increasing use of nonsteroidal antiinflammatory drugs (NSAIDs) to treat primary dysmenorrhea in women on antihypertensives; NSAIDs may antagonize the antihypertensive effects of diuretics and beta-blockers.

## POSTMENOPAUSAL ESTROGEN REPLACEMENT

Although hypertension may rarely occur with postmenopausal estrogen use (Crane et al, 1971), a prospective analysis of a large group of women aged 52 to 87 found that the use of oral estrogens for an average of 5 months did not alter the level or lability of the blood pressure (Pfeffer et al, 1979). In fact, lower blood pressures among postmenopausal estrogen users have been reported (Barrett-Connor et al, 1989; Hassager et al, 1987). Moreover, multiple case-control studies have found a significantly lower death rate from ischemic heart disease among postmenopausal estrogen users than nonusers (Beaglehole, 1988; McFarland et al, 1989). A smaller number of studies have also reported a lower death rate from stroke (Paganini-Hill et al, 1988; Ross et al, 1989; Thompson et al, 1989). Thus, though postmenopausal estrogens may cause other problems, they do not appear to cause hypertension, and they protect against coronary disease and stroke.

## References

Aalkjaer C, Johannesen P, Petersen EB, et al: *J Hypertens* 2(Suppl 3):183, 1984.

Adbul-Karim R, Assali NS: *Am J Obstet Gynecol* 82:246, 1961.

Alderman BW, Sperling RS, Daling JR: *Br Med J* 292:372, 1986.

Ales KL, Norton ME, Druzin ML: *Obstet Gynecol* 73:928, 1989.

Allen J, Maigaard S, Forman A, et al: *Br J Obstet Gynaecol* 94:222, 1987.

Altura BM, Altura BT, Carella A: *Science* (Wash DC) 221:376, 1983.

Andersch B, Svensson A, Hansson L: *Acta Obstet Gynecol Scand* 118(Suppl):33, 1984.

Barrett-Connor E, Wingard DL, Criqui MH: *JAMA* 261:2095, 1989.

Bauer TW, Moore GW, Hutchins GM: *Circulation* 65:255, 1982.

Bauman WA, Maimen M, Langer O: *Am J Obstet Gynecol* 159:446, 1988.

Beaglehole R: *Br Med J* 297:571, 1988.

Beaufils M, Uzan S, Donsimon R, et al: *Lancet* 1:840, 1985.

Beer AE: *JAMA* 262:3184, 1989.

Beilin LJ, Deacon J, Michael CA, et al: *Clin Exp Pharmacol Physiol* 9:321, 1982.

Belfort M, Uys P, Dommisse R, et al: *Br J Obstet Gynecol* 96:634, 1989.

Belizán JM, Villar J, Repke J: *Am J Obstet Gynecol* 158:898, 1988.

Benigni A, Gregorini G, Frusca T, et al: *N Engl J Med* 321:357, 1989.

Bhatia RK, Bottoms SF, Sokol RJ: *Am J Perinatol* 4:352, 1987.

Bieniarz J, Yoshida T, Robero-Salinas G, et al: *Am J Obstet Gynecol* 103:19, 1969.

Biglieri EG, Slaton PE Jr: *J Clin Endocrinol Metab* 27:1628, 1967.

Blekta M, Hlavaty V, Trnkova M, et al: *Am J Obstet Gynecol* 106:10, 1970.

Blumenstein BA, Douglas MB, Hall WD: *Am J Epidemiol* 112:539, 1980.

Bond AL, August P, Druzin ML, et al: *Am J Obstet Gynecol* 160:1112, 1989.

Boyd WN, Burden RP, Aber GM: *Q J Med* 44:415, 1975.

Brenner BM: *Kidney Int* 23:647, 1983.

Brown CEL, Purdy P, Cunningham FG: *Am J Obstet Gynecol* 159:915, 1988.

Brown JJ, Davies DL, Doak PB, et al: *Lancet* 2:900, 1963.

Brown RD, Strott CA, Liddle GW: *J Clin Endocrinol Metab* 35:736, 1972.

Brownrigg GM: *Can Med Assoc J* 87:408, 1962.

Broughton Pipkin F, Morrison R, O'Brien PMS: *Clin Sci* 76:529, 1989.

Brown MA, Nicholson E, Gallery EDM: *Br J Obstet Gynaecol* 95:1237, 1988.

Brown MA, Sinosich MJ, Saunders DM, et al: *Am J Obstet Gynecol* 155:349, 1986.

Burkman RT, Robinson JC, Kruszon-Moran D, et al: *Obstet Gynecol* 71:33, 1988.

Bussolino F, Benedetto C, Massobrio M, et al: *Lancet* 2:702, 1980.

Cain MD, Walters WA, Catt KJ: *J Clin Endocrinol Metab* 33:671, 1971.

Campbell EA, Linton EA, Wolfe CDA, et al: *J Clin Endocrinol Metab* 64:1054, 1987.

Carr BR, Parker CR Jr, Madden JD, et al: *Am J Obstet Gynecol* 139:416, 1981.

Chesley LC: In: Hellman LM, Pritchard JA (eds). *Hypertensive Disorders in Pregnancy*. New York: Appleton-Century-Crofts, 1978.

Chesley LC: *Kidney Int* 18:234, 1980.

Chesley LC: *Obstet Gynecol* 65:423, 1985.

Chesley LC, Annitto JE, Cosgrove RA: *Am J Obstet Gynecol* 124:446, 1976.

Chesley LC, Wynn RM, Silverman NI: *Circ Res* 13:232, 1963.

Christianson RE: *Am J Obstet Gynecol* 125:511, 1976.

Cockburn J, Moar VA, Ounsted M, et al: *Lancet* 1:647, 1982.

Collins R, Yusuf S, Peto R: *Br Med J* 290:17, 1985.

Cooper DW, Hill JA, Chesley LC, et al: *Br J Obstet Gynaecol* 95:644, 1988.

Crandon AJ, Isherwood DM: *Lancet* 1:1356, 1979.

Crane MG, Harris JJ: In: Fregly MJ (ed). *Oral Contraceptives and High Blood Pressure*. Gainesville, FL: Dolphin Press, 1973.

Crane MG, Harris JJ, Winsor W III: *Ann Intern Med* 74:13, 1971.

Crawford JS, Lewis M, Weaver JB: *Lancet* 2:693, 1987.

Croft P, Hannaford PC: *Br Med J* 298:165, 1989.

Cunningham FG, Cox K, Gant NF: *Obstet Gynecol* 46:581, 1975.

Cunningham FG, Gant NF: *N Engl J Med* 321:606, 1989.

Cunningham FG, Leveno KJ: In: Rubin PC (ed). *Handbook of Hypertension, Vol 10: Hypertension in Pregnancy*. Amsterdam: Elsevier Science Publishers, 1988:290.

Cunningham FG, Pritchard JA, Hankins DGV, et al: *Obstet Gynecol* 67:157, 1986.

Curet LB, Olson RW: *Obstet Gynecol* 53:336, 1979.

Davey DA, MacGillivray I: *Am J Obstet Gynecol* 158:892, 1988.

Davison JM: *Scand J Clin Lab Invest* 44(Suppl 169):15, 1984.

de Boer K, Lecander I, ten Cate JW, et al: *Am J Obstet Gynecol* 158:518, 1988.

Degani S, Abinader E, Eibschitz I, et al: *Obstet Gynecol* 65:652, 1985.

Delva P, Capra C, Degan M, et al: *Eur J Clin Invest* 19:95, 1989.

Derkx FHM, Alberda AT, De Jong FH, et al: *J Clin Endocrinol Metab* 65:349, 1987.

de Swiet M: *Br Med J* 291:365, 1985.

Divers WA Jr, Wilkes MM, Babaknia A, et al: *Am J Obstet Gynecol* 139:483, 1981.

Dörr HG, Heller A, Versmold HT, et al: *J Clin Endocrinol Metab* 68:863, 1989.

Dudley DKL: *Am J Obstet Gynecol* 151:196, 1985.

Easterling TR, Benedetti TJ: *Am J Obstet Gynecol* 160:1447, 1989.

Ehrlich EN: *Am J Obstet Gynecol* 109:963, 1971.

Ehrlich EN, Lindheimer MD: *J Clin Invest* 51:1301, 1972.

Eneroth-Grimfors E, Bevegard S, Nilsson BA: *Acta Obstet Gynecol Scand* 67:109, 1988.

Everett RB, Worley RJ, MacDonald PC, et al: *J Clin Endocrinol Metab* 46:1007, 1978a.

Everett RB, Worley RJ, MacDonald PC, et al: *Am J Obstet Gynecol* 131:352, 1978b.

Everett RB, Porter JC, MacDonald PC, et al: *Am J Obstet Gynecol* 136:435, 1980.

Feeney JG: *Br Med J* 288:1046, 1984.

Feeney JG, Tovery LAD, Scott JS: *Lancet* 1:874, 1977.

Ferris TF, Weir EK: *J Clin Invest* 71:809, 1983.

Fidler J, Bennett MJ, DeSwiet M, et al: *Lancet* 2:31, 1980.

Fisch IR, Frank J: *JAMA* 237:2499, 1977.

Fisher KA, Ahuja S, Luger A, et al: *Am J Obstet Gynecol* 129:643, 1977.

Fitzgerald DJ, Entman SS, Mulloy K, et al: *Clin Res* 33:361A, 1985.

Fitzgerald DJ, Entman SS, Mulloy K, et al: *Circulation* 75:956, 1987a.

Fitzgerald DJ, Mayo G, Catella F, et al: *Am J Obstet Gynecol* 157:325, 1987b.

Fletcher AE, Bulpitt CJ: In: Rubin PC (ed). *Handbook of Hypertension, Vol 10: Hypertension in Pregnancy*. Amsterdam: Elsevier Science Publishers, 1988:186.

Forrester TE, Alleyne GAO: *Clin Sci* 59:199s, 1980.

Freeman EW, Rickels K: *Obstet Gynecol* 53:388, 1979.

Friedman EA, Neff RK: *JAMA* 239:2249, 1978.

Friedman SA: *Obstet Gynecol* 71:122, 1988.

Frishman WH, Chesner M: *Am Heart J* 115:147, 1988.

Gallery E: In: Rubin PC (ed). *Handbook of Hypertension, Vol 10: Hypertension in Pregnancy*. Amsterdam: Elsevier Science Publishers, 1988:202.

Gallery EDM, Esber RP, Brown MA, et al: *J Hypertension* 6:153, 1988a.

Gallery EDM, Hunyor SN, Gyory AZ: *Q J Med* 192:593, 1979a.

Gallery EDM, Hunyor SN, Ross M, et al: *Lancet* 1:1273, 1977.

Gallery EDM, Mitchell MDM, Redman CWG: *J Hypertension* 2:177, 1984.

Gallery EDM, Rowe J, Brown MA, et al: *Clin Sci* 74:145, 1988b.

Gant N: *J Clin Invest* 52:2682, 1973.

Gant NF, Chand S, Worley RJ, et al: *Am J Obstet Gynecol* 120:1, 1974.

Gant NF, Daley GL, Chand S, et al: *J Clin Invest* 52:2682, 1973.

Gant NF, Madden JD, Siiteri PK, et al: *Am J Obstet Gynecol* 124:143, 1976.

Gant NF, Pritchard JA: *Semin Nephrol* 4:260, 1984.

Gerber JG, Payne NA, Murphy RC, et al. *J Clin Invest* 67:632, 1981.

Gilstrap LC III, Cunningham FG, Whalley PJ: *Semin Perinatol* 2:73, 1978.

Goodlin RC: *Lancet* 1:329, 1986.

Graves SW, Williams GH: *J Clin Endocrinol Metab* 59:1070, 1984.

Guzick DS, Klein VR, Tyson JE, et al: *Clin Exp Hyper* B6:281, 1987.

Harvey SM: *Fam Plann Perspect* 12:301, 1980.

Hassager C, Riis BJ, Strom V, et al: *Circulation* 76:753, 1987.

Hauglustaine D, Van Damme B, Vanrenterghem Y, et al: *Clin Nephrol* 15:148, 1981.

Helmer OM, Judson WE: *Am J Obstet Gynecol* 99:9, 1967.

Henderson-Smart DJ, Horvath JS, Phippard A, et al: *Clin Exp Pharmacol Physiol* 11:351, 1984.

Hill PA, Zimmerman M, Fairley KF, et al: *Clin Exper Hyper* B7:343, 1988.

Hollenberg NK, Williams GH, Burger B, et al: *Circ Res* 38:35, 1976.

Homans DC: *N Engl J Med* 312:1432, 1985.

Ihle BU, Long P, Oats J: *Br Med J* 294:79, 1987.

Ikedife D: *Br Med J* 1:985, 1980.

Jakobi P, Krivoy N, Weissman A, et al: *Obstet Gynecol* 74:29, 1989.

Kasdorf G, Kalkhoff RK: *J Clin Endocrinol Metab* 66:846, 1988.

Kassar NS, Aldridge J, Quirk B: *Obstet Gynecol* 55:411, 1980.

Kaunitz AM, Hughes JM, Grimes DA, et al: *Obstet Gynecol* 65:605, 1985.

Khong TY, De Wolf F, Robertson WB, et al: *Br J Obstet Gynaecol* 93:1049, 1986.

Klonoff-Cohen HS, Savitz DA, Cefalo RC, et al: *JAMA* 262:3143, 1989.

Kreft-Jais C, Pouin P-F, Tchobroutsky C, et al: *Br J Obstet Gynaecol* 95:420, 1988.

Laragh JG, Sealey JE, Ledingham JGG, et al: *JAMA* 201:198, 1967.

Lardoux H, Gerard J, Blazquet G, et al: *Eur Heart J* 4(Suppl G):35, 1983.

Lazarchick J, Stubbs TM, Romein L, et al: *Am J Obstet Gynecol* 154:1050, 1986.

Leather HM, Humphreys DM, Baker P, et al: *Lancet* 2:488, 1968.

Lehtovirta P: *J Obstet Gynaecol Br Commonw* 81:517, 1974.

Lewis PJ, Boylan P, Friedman LA, et al: *Br Med J* 280:1581, 1980.

Lim KG, Isles CG, Hodsman GP, et al: *Br Med J* 294:1057, 1987.

Lindheimer MD, Chesley LC: *Br Med J* 294:1547, 1987.

Lindheimer MD, Fisher KA, Katz AI: *Contrib Nephrol* 23:125, 1980.

Lindow SW, Davies N, Davey DA, et al: *Br J Obstet Gynaecol* 95:1276, 1988.

Little BC, Benson P, Beard RW, et al: *Lancet* 1:865, 1984.

Lopez-Jaramillo P, Narvaez M, Weigel RM, et al: *Br J Obstet Gynecol* 96:648, 1989.

Lopez-Llera M: *Am J Obstet Gynecol* 142:28, 1982.

Lubbe WF: *Drugs* 28:170, 1984.

Lumbers ER: *Aust J Exp Biol Med Sci* 48:493, 1970.

Lunell NO, Lewander R, Mamoun I, et al: *Scand J Clin Lab Invest* 44(Suppl 169):28, 1984.

Lunell NO, Nylund LE, Lewander R, et al: *Clin Exp Hypertens* B1:105, 1982.

Mabie WC, Gonzalez AR, Sibai BM, et al: *Obstet Gynecol* 70:328, 1987.

Malatino LS, Glen L, Wilson ESB: *Curr Ther Res* 43:743, 1988.

Marcoux S, Brisson J, Fabia J: *J Epidemiol Comm Health* 43:147, 1989.

Mashini IS, Albazzaz SJ, Fadel HE, et al: *Am J Obstet Gynecol* 156:1208, 1987.

Mathews DD, Agarwal V, Shuttleworth TP, et al: *Br J Obstet Gynecol* 89:128, 1982.

Matsuura S, Naden RP, Gant NF Jr, et al: *Am J Physiol* 140:H908, 1981.

McCartney CP: *Circ Res* 29 and 30(Suppl 2):37, 1964.

McFadyen IR, Greenhouse P, Price AB, et al: *Br J Obstet Gynaecol* 93:482, 1986.

McFarland KF, Boniface ME, Hornung CA, et al: *Am Heart J* 117:1209, 1989.

Meade TW: *Am J Obstet Gynecol* 158:1646, 1988.

Mengert WF, Tacchi DA: *Am J Obstet Gynecol* 81:601, 1961.

Millar JA: *Lancet* 2:514, 1988.

Mishell DR Jr: *N Engl J Med* 320:777, 1989.

Mitchell MM, Bibby JG, Hicks BR, et al: *Prostaglandins* 16:931, 1978.

Moore MP, Redman CWG: *Br Med J* 287:580, 1983.

Moutquin JM, Rainville C, Giroux L, et al: *Am J Obstet Gynecol* 151:191, 1985.

Murphy JG, O'Riodan J, Newcombe RG, et al: *Lancet* 1:992, 1986.

Nylund L, Lunell N-O: *Am J Obstet Gynecol* 158:440, 1988.

Øian P, Lande K, Kjeldsen SE, et al: *Br J Obstet Gynaecol* 93:548, 1986.

Orlandi C, Marlettini MG, Cassani A, et al: *Curr Ther Res* 39:884, 1986.

Ory HW: *Fam Plan Perspect* 15:57, 1983.

Ounsted M: In: Rubin PC (ed). *Handbook of Hypertension, Vol 10: Hypertension in Pregnancy*. Amsterdam: Elsevier Science Publishers, 1988:341.

Packham DK, Mathews DC, Fairley KF, et al: *Kidney Int* 34:704, 1988.

Paganini-Hill A, Ross RK, Henderson BE: *Br Med J* 297:519, 1988.

Parisi VM, Walsh SW: *Am J Physiol* 257:E102, 1989.

Penny WJ, Lewis MJ: *Eur J Clin Pharmacol* 36:427, 1989.

Pfeffer RI, Kurosaki TT, Charlton SK: *Am J Epidemiol* 110:469, 1979.

Phelps SJ, Cochran EB, Gonzalez-Ruiz A, et al: *Am J Obstet Gynecol* 158:34, 1988.

Phippard AF, Horvath JS: In: Rubin PC (ed). *Handbook of Hypertension, Vol 10: Hypertension in Pregnancy*. Amsterdam: Elsevier Science Publishers, 1988:168.

Phippard AF, Horvath JS, Glynn EM, et al: *J Hypertension* 4:773, 1986.

Pickles CJ, Brinkman CR, Stainer K, et al: *Am J Obstet Gynecol* 160:678, 1989a.

Pickles CJ, Symonds EM, Broughton Pipkin F: *Br J Obstet Gynaecol* 96:38, 1989b.

Piver MS, Corson SL, Folognese RJ: *Obstet Gynecol* 30:238, 1967.

Plouin P-F, Breart G, Maillard F, et al: *Br J Obstet Gynaecol* 95:868, 1988.

Poisner AM, Wood GW, Poisner R, et al: *Proc Soc Exp Biol Med* 169:4, 1982.

Pollack VE, Nettles JB: *Medicine* (Baltimore) 39:469, 1960.

Prentice RL: *Am J Epidemiol* 127:213, 1988.

Primrose T, Higgins A: *J Reprod Med* 7:257, 1971.

Pritchard JA, Cunningham FG, Mason RA: *Am J Obstet Gynecol* 124:855, 1976.

Pritchard JA, Cunningham FG, Pritchard SA: *Am J Obstet Gynecol* 148:951, 1984.

Pritchard JA, Pritchard SA: *Am J Obstet Gynecol* 129:733, 1977.

Ramanathan J, Sibai BM, Pillai R, et al: *Am J Obstet Gynecol* 158:40, 1988.

Rayburn WF, Piehl EJ, Compton AA: *Clin Exp Hyper* B4:63, 1985.

Redman CWG: *Br Med J* 296:1209, 1988.

Redman CWG, Beilin LJ, Bonnar J, et al: *Lancet* 1:753, 1976.

Rennie J: *Lancet* 1:328, 1986.

Repke JT, Villar J, Anderson C, et al: *Am J Obstet Gynecol* 160:684, 1989.

Robinson M: *Lancet* 1:178, 1958.

Robson SC, Dunlop W, Hunter S: *Br Med J* 294:1065, 1987.

Robson SC, Hunter S, Boys RJ, et al: *Am J Physiol* 256:H1060, 1989.

Romero R, Mazor M, Lockwood CJ, et al: *Am J Perinatol* 6:32, 1989.

Rosenberg MJ, Rosenthal SM: *Am J Public Health* 77:833, 1987.

Rosenfeld CR, Naden RP: *Am J Physiol* 257:H17, 1989.

Rosenfield A: *Ann Rev Pub Health* 10:385, 1989.

Ross RK, Pike MC, Henderson BE, et al: *Lancet* 1:505, 1989.

Royal College of General Practitioners. In: *Oral Contraceptives and Health*. New York: Pitman Publishing, 1974:37.

Royal College of General Practitioners: *Lancet* 1:541, 1981.

Rubin PC: In: Robertson JIS (ed). *Handbook of Hypertension, Clinical Aspects of Secondary Hypertension*, Vol 2. Amsterdam: Elsevier Science Publishers, 1983:304.

Rubin PC, Butters L, Clark D, et al: *Am J Obstet Gynecol* 150:389, 1984.

Rubin PC, Butters L, Low RA, et al: *Br J Clin Pharmacol* 16:543, 1983.

Rubin PC, Butters L, McCabe R, et al: *Clin Sci* 71:111, 1986.

Ruvinsky ED, Douvas SG, Roberts WE, et al: *Am J Obstet Gynecol* 149:722, 1984.

Sachs BP, Brown DAJ, Driscoll SG, et al: *N Engl J Med* 316:667, 1987.

Saruta T, Saade GA, Kaplan NM: *Arch Intern Med* 127:621, 1970.

Sawyer MM, Lipshitz J, Anderson GD, et al: *Obstet Gynecol* 58:29, 1981.

Schiff E, Peleg E, Goldenberg M, et al: *N Engl J Med* 321:351, 1989.

Schrier RW: *N Engl J Med* 319:1127, 1988.

Sealey JE, Wilson M, Morganti AA, et al: *Clin Exp Hypertens Theory Pract* A4(11 and 12):2379, 1982.

Seon R, Forrester T: *Clin Sci* 76:199, 1989.

Serhal PF, Craft I: *Lancet* 2:744, 1987.

Shepard MJ, Hellenbrand KG, Bracken MB: *Am J Obstet Gynecol* 155:947, 1986.

Shoemaker CT, Meyers M: *Am J Obstet Gynecol* 149:171, 1984.

Sibai BM: *Am J Obstet Gynecol* 159:1, 1988.

Sibai BM, Abdella TN, Anderson GD: *Obstet Gynecol* 61:571, 1983.

Sibai BM, Gonzalez AR, Mabie WC, et al: *Obstet Gynecol* 70:323, 1987a.

Sibai BM, Mabie BC, Harvey CJ, et al: *Am J Obstet Gynecol* 156:1174, 1987b.

Sibai BM, Mirro R, Chesney CM, et al: *Obstet Gynecol* 74:551, 1989.

Sibai BM, Spinnato JA, Watson DL, et al: *Obstet Gynecol* 64:319, 1984.

Sibai BM, Taslimi M, Abdella TN, et al: *Am J Obstet Gynecol* 152:32, 1985.

Silverstone A, Trudinger BJ, Lewis PJ, et al: *Br J Obstet Gynecol* 87:457, 1980.

Sipes SL, Weiner CP, Gellhaus TM, et al: *Obstet Gynecol* 73:934, 1989.

Skinner SL, Cran EJ, Gibson R, et al: *Am J Obstet Gynecol* 121:626, 1975.

Smythe CM, Bradham WS, Dennis EJ, et al: *J Lab Clin Med* 63:562, 1964.

Spellacy WN, Birk SA: *Am J Obstet Gynecol* 112:912, 1972.

Spellacy WN, Birk SA: *Fertil Steril* 25:467, 1974.

Speroff L: *Prostaglandins* 3:721, 1973.

Spitz B, Magness RR, Cox SM, et al: *Am J Obstet Gynecol* 159:1035, 1988.

Stadel BV: *N Engl J Med* 305:672, 1981.

Stampfer MJ, Willett WC, Colditz GA, et al: *N Engl J Med* 319:1313, 1988.

Stevens KJ, Paintin DB, Few JD: *Br J Obstet Gynaecol* 96:80, 1989.

Stout ML: *Am J Obstet Gynecol* 27:730, 1934.

Strauss RG, Alexander RW: *Obstet Gynecol* 47:169, 1976.

Sutherland A, Cooper DW, Howie PW, et al: *Br J Obstet Gynaecol* 88:785, 1981.

Svensson A: In: Hansson L (ed). *ISH 1988 Hypertension Annual*. London: Gower Academic Journals Ltd, 1988:33.

Taufield PA, Ales KL, Resnick LM, et al: *N Engl J Med* 316:715, 1987.

Taufield PA, Mueller FB, Edersheim TG, et al: *Clin Res* 36:433A, 1988.

Taylor DJ: In: Rubin PC (ed). *Handbook of Hypertension, Vol 10: Hypertension in Pregnancy*. Amsterdam: Elsevier Science Publishers, 1988:223.

Testa I, Rabini A, Danieli G, et al: *Scand J Clin Lab Invest* 48:7, 1988.

Thompson JA, Hays PM, Sagar KB, et al: *Am J Obstet Gynecol* 155:994, 1986.

Thompson SG, Meade TW, Greenberg G: *J Epidemiol Commun Health* 43:173, 1989.

Thomsen JK, Strom TL, Thamsborg G, et al: *Br Med J* 294:1508, 1987.

Thomson AM, Hytten FE, Billewicz WZ: *J Obstet Gynaecol* 74:1, 1967.

Thorp JA, Walsh SW, Brath PC: *Am J Obstet Gynecol* 159:1381, 1988.

Thorton JG, Hughes R, Davies JA, et al: *Lancet* 1:329, 1986.

Toppozada MK, Shaala SA, Moussa HA: *Clin Exp Hypertens* B2:217, 1983.

Tranquilli AL, Mazzanti L, Bertoli E, et al: *Obstet Gynecol* 71:627, 1988.

Tunbridge RDG, Donnai P: *Br J Obstet Gynecol* 90:1027, 1983.

Turney JH, Ellis CM, Parsons FM: *Br J Obstet Gynecol* 96:679, 1989.

Van Assche FA, Spitz B, Vansteelant L: *Am J Cardiol* 63:22C, 1989.

Van Dam PA, Renier M, Baekelandt M, et al: *Obstet Gynecol* 73:97, 1989.

Villar J, Repke J, Belizan JM, et al: *Obstet Gynecol* 70:317, 1987.

Villar MA, Sibai BM: *Am J Obstet Gynecol* 160:419, 1989.

Waisman GD, Mayorga LM, Camera MI, et al: *Am J Obstet Gynecol* 159:308, 1988.

Wallenburg HCS: In: Rubin PC (ed). *Handbook of Hypertension, Vol 10: Hypertension in Pregnancy*. Amsterdam: Elsevier Science Publishers, 1988:66.

Wallenburg HCS, Dekker GA, Makovitz JW, et al: *Lancet* 1:1, 1986.

Wallenburg HCS, Rotmans N: *Am J Obstet Gynecol* 144:523, 1982.

Wallenburg HCS, Rotmans N: *Lancet* 1:939, 1988.

Walsh SW: *Am J Obstet Gynecol* 152:335, 1985.

Walsh SW: *Obstet Gynecol* 71:222, 1988.

Walters BNJ, Thompson ME, Lee A, et al: *Clin Sci* 71:589, 1986.

Walters BNJ, Redman CWG: *Br J Obstet Gynecol* 91:330, 1984.

Walters WAW: *Lancet* 2:1214, 1966.

Walters WAW, Lim YL: *Lancet* 2:879, 1969.

Wasserstrum N, Kirshon B, Rossavik IK, et al: *Obstet Gynecol* 74:34, 1989.

Watson KV, Moldow CF, Ogburn PL, et al: *Proc Natl Acad Sci* 83:1075, 1986.

Weiner CP: *Am J Obstet Gynecol* 156:885, 1987.

Weir RJ: *Drugs* 16:522, 1978.

Weir RJ: In: Yamori Y et al (eds). *Reduced Hypertensive Risks of Low Dose Contraceptive Steroids*. New York: Raven Press, 1979.

Weir RJ: In: Amery A (ed). *Hypertensive Cardiovascular Disease: Pathophysiology and Treatment*. The Hague: Martinus Nijhoff Publishers, 1982:612.

Weissberg PL, Weaver J, Woods KL, et al: *Br Med J* 287:709, 1983.

White WB: *Hypertension* 6:297, 1984.

Wichman K, Ryden G: *Acta Obstet Gynecol Scand* 65:561, 1986.

Wichman K, Ryden G, Karlberg BE: *Scand J Clin Lab Invest* 44(Suppl 169):90, 1984.

Winkel CA, Milewich L, Parker CR Jr, et al: *J Clin Invest* 66:803, 1980.

Woods JW: *Lancet* 2:653, 1967.

Woods JW: *Hypertension* 11(Suppl II):II-11, 1988.

Woods JW, Algary WA, Stier FM: *Circulation* 45 and 46(Suppl 2):82, 1972 (abst).

Worley RJ, Hentschel WM, Cormier C, et al: *N Engl J Med* 307:412, 1982.

Ylikorkala O, Mäkilä U-M: *Am J Obstet Gynecol* 152:318, 1985.

Zelnik M, Kantner JF: *Fam Plan Perspect* 12:230, 1980.

Zinaman M, Rubin J, Lindheimer MD: *Lancet* 1:1245, 1985.

# 12

# Pheochromocytoma (with a Preface About Incidental Adrenal Masses)

## INCIDENTAL ADRENAL MASS

Before considering adrenal causes of hypertension in this and the subsequent two chapters, the management of incidentally discovered adrenal masses will be covered. Such masses are being found increasingly during abdominal computed tomography (CT) and magnetic resonance imaging (MRI), and they must be evaluated both because they may be functionally active and because they may be malignant.

### Incidence

Nonfunctioning adrenal masses have long been known to be present in many people at autopsy: In one series, adrenal masses from 2 mm to 4 cm in size were found in 8.7% of 739 autopsies and in 12.4% of the patients known to have been hypertensive (Hedeland et al, 1968). Such masses are rarely functional (Kaplan, 1967) and have been usually disregarded by pathologists.

With the increasing use of CT scans and MRIs, these previously unrecognized masses are now being recognized in many patients who have no clinical evidence of adrenal hyperfunction. As the resolution of these procedures continues to improve and as they are increasingly performed for various reasons, more and more of the incidental adrenal masses present in up to 10% of all people will be recognized. Thus, there is the potential for a tremendous amount of unnecessary work-up and surgery, in addition to a great deal of anxiety induced by the knowledge of the presence of a possible cancer. To reduce the potential mischief, CT scans and MRI should be done only in those whose clinical features

and laboratory tests are suggestive of adrenal pathology, not as the initial diagnostic procedure. However, in the course of searching for unrelated abdominal pathology, adrenal masses will continue to be discovered incidentally. Therefore, guidelines for the subsequent management of such patients are needed.

### Evaluation of the Incidentally Discovered Adrenal Mass

The first concern is to rule out adrenocortical cancers that, though very rare, represent the major reason for surgery in those with no clinical evidence of a hormonally active tumor. Since most adrenocortical cancers are larger than 6 cm and most benign lesions are considerably smaller, most of those larger than 6 cm are thought to require surgery (Copeland, 1983). According to Copeland's recommendations, biochemical assessment is the first step in evaluation of those that are smaller than 6 cm. As will be described in considerable detail in the remainder of the following three chapters, the assessment need not go beyond the search for suggestive clinical features and abnormalities in the laboratory screening tests shown in Table 12.1. For the majority, the absence of both clinical features and laboratory abnormalities will be adequate to rule out an active tumor. Those with suggestive clinical features or abnormal screening tests will require additional testing, as will be described in the subsequent coverage of each specific diagnosis.

According to Copeland's approach, if the mass is less than 6 cm and is inactive and solid, sur-

**Table 12.1.** **Evaluation of Incidental Adrenal Masses**

| Diagnosis | Suggestive Clinical Features | Laboratory Screening Tests |
|---|---|---|
| Pheochromocytoma | Paroxysmal hypertension<br>Spells of sweating, headache, palpitations | Spot-urine metanephrine<br>Normal: <1 $\mu$g or 5.5 $\mu$mol/mg of creatinine |
| Cushing's syndrome | Trunkal obesity<br>Thin skin<br>Muscle weakness | 8 AM plasma cortisol after 1 mg of dexamethasone at bedtime<br>Normal: <5 mg/dl (140 nmol/L) |
| Primary aldosteronism | Hypokalemia | Urine potassium excretion<br>Normal: <30 mmol/24 hour urine in presence of hypokalemia |
| Adrenocortical carcinoma | Virilization or feminization | Urine 17-ketosteroids<br>Normal:<br>  Men: 6–20 mg or<br>       20–70 $\mu$mol/24 hours<br>  Women: 6–17 mg or<br>       20–60 $\mu$mol/24 hours<br>Plasma androgens or estrogens |

gery is not indicated but repeat CT scans are recommended in 2, 6, and 18 months; if it is cystic, puncture of the cyst is recommended.

Others have questioned the validity of using a size of 6 cm as the major indication for surgery (Seddon et al, 1985; Belldegrun et al, 1986). These investigators argue that adrenal cancers obviously must start as smaller masses and the fact that most are only recognized when they are larger than 6 cm indicates the inability to do so before the availability of CT scans. However, as Copeland points out, many more deaths would likely result from surgery if all incidental adrenal masses smaller than 6 cm were removed than would occur from unremoved cancers if they were all left alone.

The increasing availability of adrenal scintigraphy with an iodinated cholesterol derivative (NP-59) that localizes in functioning adrenal cortical tissue but not in most malignant adrenal masses has offered a rational way to handle the dilemma. As described by Gross et al (1988) on the basis of 119 euadrenal patients with unilateral masses found on CT scans, those adrenals that take up the NP-59, i.e., lateralized or concordant, are almost certainly benign; those that do not take up the NP-59, i.e., nonlateralized or discordant, are mostly malignant, either metastatic or primary.

The scheme shown in Figure 12.1 may provide a reasonable approach that would identify those predictably few patients with smaller than 6-cm tumors that are malignant without subjecting more to unnecessary surgery. Moreover, the patient should be reassured by the normal NP-59 scan that the incidental mass is almost certainly not malignant.

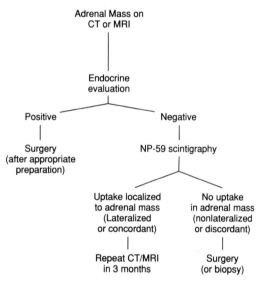

**Figure 12.1.** Scheme for the management of an adrenal mass incidentally discovered by CT or MRI. The endocrine evaluation is shown in Table 12.1.

With MRI, tissue characterization may be possible that will accurately predict the histological type of the adrenal tumor. However, eight of 38 such tumors could not be differentiated (Reinig et al, 1986), so the use of NP-59 scintigraphy likely is the better approach for now. On the other hand, if the adrenal mass has a uniform configuration on CT indicative of a high fat content, the diagnosis of myelolipoma can be reasonably assured and no further work-up performed save a test to rule out a pheochromocytoma (Brinker et al, 1988).

A few adrenal masses discovered incidentally turn out to be functional but at a level below that identifiable by routine, baseline studies. Patients have been reported to have normal basal plasma and urine cortisol levels but evidence of autonomous secretion at levels too low to completely suppress the pituitary-adrenal axis (Beyer and Doe, 1986; Huiras et al, 1989; Virkkala et al, 1989). The danger is that removal of the subclinically functioning tumor may expose the patient to adrenal insufficiency from the prolonged suppression of the other gland. A dexamethasone suppression test should be part of the evaluation (Table 12.1), and if it fails to show suppression, indicating autonomous hypersecretion from the adrenal mass, steroid support should be provided postoperatively.

## PHEOCHROMOCYTOMA

Beyond the need to evaluate patients with incidentally discovered adrenal masses, consideration of an adrenal cause for hypertension is much more commonly needed than the low prevalence—less than 0.5%—of these causes would suggest. The presence of one or another form of adrenal hyperfunction is often considered in the evaluation of hypertensive patients because many of the symptoms and signs of adrenal hyperfunction are nonspecific and are encountered in patients whose adrenal function is normal. Recurrent ''spells'' suggestive of pheochromocytoma, hypokalemia pointing to primary aldosteronism, and cushingoid features are all encountered in many more patients than the relatively few who turn out to have these diseases. Of all of these, consideration of a pheochromocytoma is likely most important.

## INCIDENCE

The presence of a pheochromocytoma (pheo) should be considered in all hypertensives since, if not recognized, it may provoke fatal hypertensive crises during anesthesia and other stresses. In the past, it has frequently been missed. At the Mayo Clinic from 1928 to 1977, of 54 pheos found at autopsy, only 13 had been diagnosed during life (Lie et al, 1980). Of the 41 previously unrecognized, death was related to the manifestations of the tumor in 30 patients. This experience with unrecognized pheos should be contrasted to the excellent results obtained at the Mayo Clinic on 138 patients proved to have a pheo and operated upon during these years: The survival curve of those with a benign tumor was similar to that of the normal population (ReMine et al, 1974).

Of further interest, the incidence of pheos,

diagnosed during life or at autopsy, among the residents of Rochester, Minnesota, the location of the Mayo Clinic, was found to be 0.95 cases per 100,000 person-years (Beard et al, 1983). This figure, the most accurate estimate of the incidence of the tumor now available, suggests that, if 15% of the adult population is hypertensive, only about six pheos would be expected to be found among 100,000 hypertensives each year. Even lower rates, approximately two cases per million people per year, have been estimated in Japan (Takeda et al, 1986), Sweden (Stenström and Svärdsudd, 1986), and Denmark (Andersen et al, 1988).

## PATHOPHYSIOLOGY

### Development

The cells of the sympathetic nervous system arise from the primitive neural crest as primordial stem cells, called sympathogonia (Fig. 12.2). These cells have the biochemical machinery to synthesize a variety of amines and peptides including neuropeptide Y (Tischler et al, 1985); galanin (Bauer et al, 1986); opioid peptides (Bostwick et al, 1987); and somatostatin (Morice et al, 1989). These secretions may give rise to a host of ancillary syndromes along with those related to catecholamines including acromegaly (Roth et al, 1986), watery diarrhea (Salmi et al, 1988), and flushing (Sheps et al, 1988). The secretion of somatostatin may have suppressed release of catechols from a pheo in a patient whose blood and urine catechol levels were repeatedly normal despite frequent hypertensive paroxysms that were relieved by removal of the tumor (Morice et al, 1989).

The sympathogonia migrate out of the central nervous system to occupy a place behind the aorta. These stem cells may differentiate into either sympathoblasts, which give rise to sympathetic ganglion cells, or pheochromoblasts, which give rise to chromaffin cells. As seen in

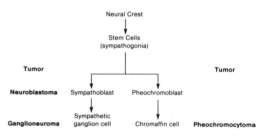

**Figure 12.2.** Developmental pathway for sympathetic ganglion and chromaffin cells and the tumors that may arise from them.

Figure 12.1, tumors may arise from each of these cell lines, often sharing histological and biochemical characteristics. These include highly malignant neuroblastomas, arising from sympathoblasts, and ganglioneuromas, which are usually more benign. These tumors are rarely seen after adolescence and usually are recognized by the excretion of large amounts of homovanillic acid (HVA), the urinary metabolite of dopamine, which is the immediate precursor of norepinephrine.

The chromaffin cells, which have the capacity to synthesize and store catecholamines and therefore stain brown on treatment with chromium, are found mainly in the adrenal medulla. They also appear in the sympathetic ganglia and paraganglia that lie along the sympathetic chain and organ of Zuckerkandl, located anteriorly at the bifurcation of the aorta. In a developmental sense, the adrenal medulla may be considered as a sympathetic ganglion that lacks postsynaptic fibers. In a functional sense, its chromaffin cells differ from the rest by having the capacity to convert norepinephrine to epinephrine (Fig. 12.3). The methylation requires the enzyme phenylethanolamine *N*-methyltransferase. The increased activity of this enzyme within the adrenal medulla reflects stimulation by adrenocortical glucocorticoids (cortisol) and suggests that the adrenal medulla is located next to the adrenal cortex to enhance this capacity for secreting epinephrine, one of the body's defenses against stress (Wurtman and Axelrod, 1965).

## Location and Tumor Nomenclature

Chromaffin cell tumors, i.e., pheochromocytomas, can arise wherever these cells are found. Almost 90% are found in one or both adrenal glands (Table 12.2), but they may be located anywhere along the sympathetic chain and, rarely, in aberrant sites. Those functioning tumors arising outside the adrenal medulla are best termed extraadrenal pheochromocytomas whereas those nonsecreting extraadrenal tumors are termed *paragangliomas* (Shapiro and Fig, 1989). Those paragangliomas that arise from the specialized chemoreceptor tissue in the carotid body, glomus jugulare, and aortic body have been separately classified as *chemodectomas*. Glomus jugular tumors are fairly common in the middle ear and temporal bone, and they may secrete catecholamines (Kremer et al, 1989).

Among the most frequent sites of extraadrenal pheos are the organ of Zuckerkandl (Glenn and Gray, 1976) and the urinary bladder (Raper et

al, 1977). However, they may arise wherever there are paraganglion cells, even within the interatrial septum (Hodgson et al, 1984) or prostate (Dennis et al, 1989). Rarely, extraadrenal pheos may be multiple (Reinholdt and Pedersen, 1988) or familial (Glowniak et al, 1985).

A total of 5 to 15% of all pheos are malignant, with metastases found in paraaortic lymph nodes, liver, lungs, and skeleton. These metastases may be functional. On the other hand, benign tumors may invade their capsule. Since histological differentiation is of little value, the only valid criterion of malignancy is the presence of distant metastases (Manger et al, 1985).

## Chromaffin Cell Secretion

The chromaffin cells synthesize catecholamines from the dietary amino acid tyrosine (Fig 12.3), with norepinephrine the end product, except in the adrenal medulla, where over 75% is methylated into epinephrine. Most adrenal medullary pheochromocytomas secrete some epinephrine, but a few, usually small in size and having a rapid turnover of catecholamines, secrete only norepinephrine (Crout and Sjöerdsma, 1964). On the other hand, with rare exceptions (Mannix et al, 1972), extraadrenal pheos do not secrete epinephrine.

When catecholamines are released by exocytosis from adrenal storage vesicles, there is a coupled, proportional release of the enzyme dopamine beta-hydroxylase and the soluble protein, chromogranin A. Plasma chromogranin A levels are elevated in patients with pheos and other endocrine tumors (O'Connor and Deftos, 1986).

## Patterns of Catechol Secretion

Secretion from pheos varies considerably. Small pheos tend to secrete larger proportions of active catecholamines; larger pheos, having the capacity to store and metabolize large quantities of catecholamines, tend to secrete less of their content, and most of that may be secreted in inactive forms.

The frequency and severity of symptoms and signs likely relate to the secretory pattern of the pheo: Those that are continuously releasing large amounts of catecholamines may induce sustained hypertension with few paroxysms since the adrenergic receptors become desensitized after prolonged exposure to their agonists (Valet et al, 1988); those that are less active but cyclically release their catecholamine stores may induce striking paroxysms of hypertension with

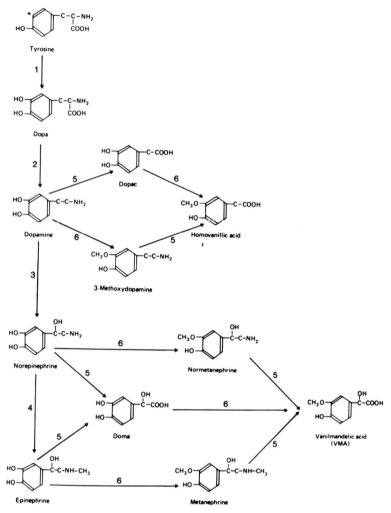

**Figure 12.3.** Pathways and enzymes of catecholamine metabolism. *1*, tyrosine hydroxylase; *2*, aromatic amino acid decarboxylase; *3*, phenylamine beta-hydroxylase; *4*, phenylethanolamine N-methyltransferase; *5*, monamine oxidase plus aldehyde dehydrogenase; and *6*, catechol 0-methyltransferase. (From Sheps SG, Jiang N-S, Klee GG: *Endocrinol Metab Clin North Am* 17:397, 1988.)

the classical symptoms of a pheo since the receptors are more responsive.

The nature of the signs and symptoms also reflects the predominant catecholamine that is secreted: NE produces more alpha-mediated vasoconstriction, Epi more beta-mediated cardiac stimulation. Those patients whose pheos mainly secrete Epi (almost always arising in the adrenal) tend to have predominantly systolic hypertension, tachycardia, sweating, flushing, and tremulousness. On occasion they may present with *hypotension* to the point of shock (Page et al, 1969), from vasodilation by beta-adrenergic stimulation in the presence of a shrunken vascular volume.

Those with a pheo secreting mainly NE (either adrenal or extraadrenal in location) tend to have both diastolic and systolic hypertension, less tachycardia, and fewer paroxysms of anxiety and palpitation.

Variability of clinical features may also reflect varying degrees of inactivation of circulating catechols by means of conjugation (Kuchel et al, 1986a).

*Dopa and Dopamine.* Two normotensive patients had a pheo that secreted large amounts of the precursors dopa and dopamine in addition to Epi and NE (Louis et al, 1972). Since the hypotensive action of dopa and dopamine may protect against the hypertensive action of the

**Table 12.2. Location of Pheochromocytoma**

| Location | % |
|---|---|
| Intraabdominal | 97–99 |
| Single adrenal tumor | 50–70 |
| Single extraadrenal tumor[a] | 10–20 |
| Multiple tumors[b] | 15–40 |
| Bilateral adrenal tumors | 5–25 |
| Multiple extraadrenal tumors | 5–15 |
| Outside abdomen | 1–3 |
| Intrathoracic[c] | 2 |
| In neck | <1 |

[a]Sites: along the sympathetic chain—lumbar, paravertebral, epigastrium, bladder.
[b]More common in children and in familial syndrome with medullary thyroid cancer.
[c]Usually in the posterior mediastinum.

**Table 12.3. Symptoms and Signs of Pheochromocytoma[a]**

Common (more than one-third of patients)
  Hypertension—probably over 90%
    Intermittent only—2 to 50%
    Sustained—50 to 60%
    Paroxysms superimposed—about 50%
  Hypotension, orthostatic—50 to 70%
  Headache—40 to 80%
  Sweating—40 to 70%
  Palpitations and tachycardia—45 to 70%
  Pallor—40 to 45%
  Anxiety and nervousness—35 to 40%
  Nausea and vomiting—10 to 50%
  Funduscopic changes—50 to 70%
  Weight loss—80%
Less Common (fewer than one-third)
  Tremor
  Anxiety
  Abdominal pain
  Chest pain
  Polydipsia, polyuria
  Acrocyanosis, cold extremities
  Flushing
  Dyspnea
  Dizziness
  Convulsions
  Bradycardia
  Fever (Kirby et al, 1983)
  Thyroid swelling (Buchels et al, 1983)

[a]Data from Hume DM: *Am J Surg* 99:458, 1960; Stackpole RH, Melicow MM, Uson AC: *J Pediatr* 63:315, 1963; Hermann H, Mornex R: *Human Tumors Secreting Catecholamines*. New York: Pergamon Press, 1964; Moorhead EL, Caldwell JR, Kelly AR, et al: *JAMA* 196:1107, 1966; Manger WM: *Arch Intern Med* 145:229, 1985; Ross EJ, Griffith DNW: *Q J Med* 71:485, 1989.

catecholamines, a similar mechanism could explain the rarity of symptoms in patients with neuroblastomas and in some with malignant pheos who also hypersecrete dopa and dopamine (Goldstein et al, 1986).

*Other Secretion.* As noted above, various peptide hormones may be released concomitantly with catecholamines from pheos, and their secretion may be associated with various clinical manifestations.

### Hemodynamics

The hemodynamics in 24 patients with a pheo were little different from those in age- sex- and weight-matched patients with essential hypertension despite the 10-fold higher plasma NE levels in the pheo patients (Bravo et al, 1989). The major finding in both was an increased peripheral resistance, whereas the pheo patients had lower blood volumes. Heart rate is usually around 90 beats per minute, even when the blood pressure is not high, but cardiac output is usually normal, except during surges of Epi release.

## CLINICAL FEATURES

The symptoms and signs of catecholamine excess are varied and often dramatic (Table 12.3). Most patients have either headache, sweating, or palpitations, and many have all three occurring in paroxysms.

### Symptoms

#### Paroxysms

The paroxysms represent the classic picture of the disease, but true paroxysmal hypertension with intervening normotension is relatively uncommon, and more than 50% of patients have sustained hypertension. In those with paroxysms, the spell can be brought on in multiple ways, including exercise, bending over, urina-

tion, defecation, taking an enema, induction of anesthesia, smoking, dipping snuff, palpation of the abdomen, or pressure from an enlarging uterus during pregnancy. Episodes may follow use of multiple drugs that either increase catecholamine release, e.g., histamine, opiates, or nicotine (McPhaul et al, 1984); or antagonize dopamine, e.g., droperidol (Montiel et al, 1986); or inhibit catechol reuptake, e.g., tricyclic antidepressants (Achong and Keane, 1981).

Wide episodic fluctuations of blood pressure (BP) may occur spontaneously (Ganguly et al, 1984). Considerable falls in pressure have been noted during sleep with ambulatory monitoring (Imai et al, 1988).

The spells vary in frequency, duration, and severity. They may occur many times per day or only every few months, but most patients experience at least one episode per week. Their features may suggest other conditions (Table 12.4). Patients are often considered psychoneurotic, particularly when they describe a sensation of tightness starting in the abdomen and rising into the chest and head, anxiety, tremors, sweating, and palpitations, followed by marked weakness (Manger, 1985). Overt psychiatric

**Table 12.4. Conditions That May Simulate Pheochromocytoma**

Cardiovascular
  Hyperdynamic, labile hypertension
  Paroxysmal tachycardia
  Angina, coronary insufficiency
  Acute pulmonary odema
  Eclampsia
  Hypertensive crisis during or after surgery
  Hypertensive crisis with MAO inhibitors
  Rebound hypertension after abrupt cessation of
    clonidine and other antihypertensives
Psychoneurological
  Anxiety with hyperventilation
  Panic attacks
  Migraine and cluster headaches
  Brain tumor
  Basilar artery aneurysm
  Stroke
  Diencephallic seizures
  Porphyria
  Lead poisoning
  Familial dysautonomia
  Acrodynia
  Autonomic hyperreflexia, as with quadriplegia
Endocrinological
  Menopausal symptoms
  Thyrotoxicosis
  Diabetes mellitus
  Hypoglycemia
  Carcinoid
  Mastocytosis
Factitious: ingestion of sympathomimetics

disturbances may rarely be found (Medvei and Cattell, 1988).

These episodes, sometimes with BP above 250/150, may lead to angina (Goldbaum et al, 1986), cardiomyopathy with acute congestive heart failure (Scott et al, 1988), or noncardiogenic pulmonary edema (de Leeuw et al, 1986). Rarely, the presentation may be as an acute abdomen (Jones and Durning, 1985), sudden death after minor abdominal trauma (Primhak et al, 1986), lactic acidosis (Bornemann et al, 1986), or high fever and encephalopathy (Newell et al, 1988). Tumors arising in the wall of the bladder may cause symptoms only with micturition and, in about half, produce painless hematuria (Raper et al, 1977).

In those patients with predominant Epi secretion, beta-blockers can raise the blood pressure by blocking the beta$_2$-mediated vasodilator action of Epi, leaving the alpha-mediated vasoconstrictor action unopposed (Prichard and Ross, 1966). Those with NE producing pheos likely will not have a pressor response to betablockers since NE has little action on vasodilatory beta$_2$-receptors (Plouin et al, 1979).

Be alert to recurrent spells precipitated by certain activities that begin abruptly, advance explosively, and subside within minutes. On the other hand, rare patients may be virtually asymptomatic despite having high levels of circulating catecholamines (Taubman et al, 1974).

Although many patients have lost some weight, eight of 22 cases in one series were 10% or more overweight, with four being definitely obese (Lee and Rousseau, 1967).

**Hypotension**

As noted, patients with a pheo secreting predominantly Epi may, rarely, have profound hypotension and go into shock. Sweating, fever, and ventricular arrhythmias may accompany the periods of hypotension. Prolonged hypotension may also occur in patients with a pheo by spontaneous necrosis of the tumor (Atuk et al, 1977) or after administration of a phenothiazine (Lund-Johansen, 1962). Much more commonly, patients have modest falls in blood pressure with standing, associated with dizziness. The presence of postural hypotension in an untreated hypertensive may be a valuable lead to the diagnosis.

**Pheochromocytoma During Pregnancy**

The association may be greater than by chance: More than 180 cases have been reported (Harper et al, 1989). When not recognized before delivery, the maternal mortality is about 40% and the infant mortality about 30%. Patients are usually thought to have preeclampsia, but their features and laboratory tests are fairly typical of pheo. When recognized and treated properly, the disease should pose no great problems.

**Pheochromocytoma in Children**

The younger the patient, the more likely it is that the syndrome is familial, the pheos multiple and extraadrenal, and the hypertension persistent (Stackpole et al, 1963; Hodgkinson et al, 1980). The clinical manifestations are generally more severe in children, and not infrequently grade 3 or 4 funduscopic changes are present along with a history of convulsions. The youngest patient in Stackpole's series was only 1 month old. Catecholamine-induced hypertension is also seen in about 20% of children with neurogenic tumors (Weinblatt et al, 1983).

**Familial Syndromes (Table 12.5)**

The familial incidence of pheo is almost certainly higher than the 6% reported by Hermann and Mornex in their 1964 survey of 507 cases. Often the search for the disease in other family members is either not made or not reported.

**Table 12.5. Types of Pheochromocytoma**

| | Usual Age of Diagnosis | Bilateral Tumors (%) |
|---|---|---|
| Nonfamilial | 40 | 0[a] |
| Familial | | |
|   Simple | 20 | 45 |
|   Multiple endocrine neoplasia, 2a and 2b | 30–35 | 80 |
| Neurofibromatosis | 40–45 | 12 |

[a]Hume (1960) reported 5% of nonfamilial tumors to be bilateral, but Knudson and Strong (1972) argue that such patients almost certainly represent unrecognized familial cases.

Knowledge of the family history is obviously important since, if the disease is familial, inheritance is by a dominant gene that will cause a pheo in approximately 90% of the half of the offspring who inherit it (Knudson and Strong, 1972).

Of the familial cases, most become manifest by the fourth decade, and the average age of diagnosis is 20. The clinical features are similar to those of the sporadic, nonfamilial cases. There is a much greater tendency for bilateral adrenal tumors: Fewer than 5% of sporadic cases are bilateral; 45% of familial cases are bilateral, with the locations often similar in the affected individuals.

**Simple Familial Syndromes**

About 60% of familial pheos occur without other glandular dysfunction. They occur in young people, usually before age 20, and at least 40% of childhood cases represent the familial form. The simple familial gene is dominant with almost 100% penetrance. The child may be diagnosed before the parent.

**Multiple Endocrine Neoplasia**

The two most common combinations of multiple, familial endocrine tumors are:

1. multiple endocrine neoplasia (MEN), type 1 (Wermer's syndrome) with tumors of the pituitary, pancreatic islet cells, parathyroids, carcinoids of the gastrointestinal tract and lung, frequently with fulminant peptic ulcer disease, i.e., Zollinger-Ellison syndrome (Marx et al, 1988);
2. multiple endocrine neoplasia, type 2a (Sipple's syndrome) with medullary carcinoma of the thyroid, pheo, parathyroid hyperplasia or adenoma, and, less frequently, bilateral adrenocortical hyperplasia with Cushing's syndrome.

A variant of MEN 2 has been identified with mucosal neuromas, bumpy lips, hypertrophied corneal nerves, and, less commonly, skeletal defects and gastrointestinal abnormalities (Gorlin et al, 1968) and characterized as an apparently distinct entity (MEN 2b) (Fig. 12.4) (Khairi et al, 1975).

Both MEN 2a and 2b are inherited as autosomal dominant traits. The gene for MEN 2a has been mapped to chromosome 10 (Mathew et al, 1987). The majority, as many as 75%, of patients with medullary thyroid cancer have the sporadic form that is not associated with pheochromocytomas or other components of MEN 2a or 2b (Ponder et al, 1988). However, since penetrance of the MEN 2 gene is incomplete, only 50% of carriers will have presented with symptoms before age 55 (Ponder et al, 1988). Therefore, all members of families with medullary thyroid cancer should have plasma calcitonin and urine catecholamine measurements frequently, and any who become hypertensive should be carefully evaluated for a pheo. [131]MIBG scintigraphy may depict adrenal involvement early but may give false-negative readings (Turner et al, 1986).

Most of the pheos that are seen in the MEN 2a and 2b syndromes are bilateral (Lips et al,

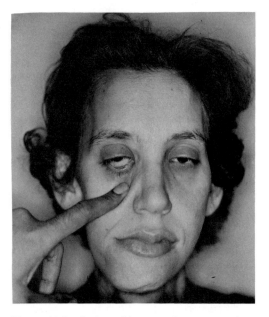

**Figure 12.4.** Patient with mucosal neuromas, pheochromocytoma, and medullary thyroid carcinoma (MEN 2b). She has the typical facies, "bumpy" lips, and neuroma on the right lower eyelid. [From Khairi MRA, Dexter RN, Burzynski NJ, et al: Mucosal neuroma, pheochromocytoma and medullary thyroid carcinoma: Multiple endocrine neoplasia type 3. *Medicine* (Baltimore) 54:89, Copyright by Williams & Wilkins, 1975.]

1981), and there is increasing evidence that diffuse hyperplasia may precede the development of tumors (Carney et al, 1976). The hypertension in patients with MEN 2a or 2b is almost always paroxysmal, reflecting the predominant secretion of epinephrine demonstrable by urinary epinephrine levels above 20 μg per 24 hours (Hamilton et al, 1978).

### Other Neurocutaneous Syndromes

About 1% of patients with multiple neurofibromatosis and café-au-lait spots (von Recklinghausen's disease) will have a pheo, comprising about 5% of all pheos (Kalff et al, 1982). About 10% of the pheos are bilateral. The average age of onset of pheo symptoms is 40 to 45. Other family members may have neurofibromatosis, but no cases of familial pheos have been reported among them (Knudson and Strong, 1972). Other endocrine tumors have been reported in patients with neurofibromatosis and pheo, including duodenal carcinoids (Griffiths et al, 1983), somatostatinoma (Cantor et al, 1982), and multiple paragangliomas (DeAngelis et al, 1987).

### Other Associated Diseases

*Cholelithiasis* was found in 15 to 76 of patients (Manger and Gifford, 1977).

*Diabetes*, with fasting glucose levels above 125 mg/dl, was present in 14 of 60 patients (Stenström et al, 1984).

*Polycythemia* has been ascribed to erythropoietin production (Waldmann and Bradley, 1961), but the more likely cause of a patient's high hematocrit would be a shrunken plasma volume.

*Renovascular hypertension* may occur concurrently by compression of the renal artery by a pheo (Ishibashi et al, 1975) or may be iatrogenically induced when the pheo is removed (Brooks et al, 1969). Confusion may arise from high renin levels often seen in patients with a pheo (Plouin et al, 1988).

*Adrenocortical Hyperfunction.* A patient had a pheo in one adrenal and a cortisol-secreting adenoma in the other, both discovered incidentally (Ooi and Dardick, 1988).

*Adrenocortical insufficiency* has been recognized in rare patients preoperatively and has been implicated in postoperative hypotension (Mulrow et al, 1959). A hypertensive crisis may be precipitated by the administration of adrenocorticotropin (ACTH) in evaluation of patients for adrenocortical involvement in MEN syndromes (Moorhead et al, 1966). Presumably, the cortisol secreted in response to ACTH increases catecholamine synthesis in the tumor.

### Malignant Pheochromocytoma

As many as 10% of pheos are malignant (Manger et al, 1985). To be classified as malignant, metastases must be found where aberrant chromaffin tissue does not occur, since benign pheos often show dysplasia and invasion of vessels. Most metastases are to skeleton, lymph nodes, liver, and lungs. Many secrete large amounts of dopamine, recognized from its metabolite homovanillic acid in the urine. Tumor growth is often slow, and long survival is possible, likely enhanced by aggressive medical and surgical therapy, as will be described at the end of this chapter. The extent of metastatic disease may be determined by scintigraphy with [131I]metaiodobenzylguanidine (Shapiro and Fig, 1989).

### Death from Pheochromocytoma

Most deaths are related to the failure to consider the disease in patients undergoing severe stress such as surgery or delivery. Many deaths are unexpected and sudden, likely related to catecholamine-induced damage to the cardiac muscle and conduction system, even in young patients (Primhak et al, 1986). At least seven deaths have followed acute hemorrhagic necrosis of a pheo, most of them after phentolamine administration (Van Way et al, 1976).

### Conditions Simulating a Pheo (Table 12.4)

Most patients with hypertension and one or more of the manifestations of pheo turn out *not* to have that diagnosis. Some patients with highly suggestive symptoms have been found to have surges of dopamine or a decreased rate of inactivation of catecholamines, leading to increased free levels in the circulation that might account for their symptoms (Kuchel et al, 1986b). A few patients with severe hypertensive paroxysms have baroreceptor dysfunction (Kuchel et al, 1987) or prostaglandin-mediated catechol surges (Sato et al, 1988).

Clinical confusion arises mostly from neurotic patients with hyperkinetic circulation. Patients having angina may have sudden rises in blood pressure, possibly as a reflex from reduction of coronary blood flow (Sjöerdsma et al, 1966). Various central nervous system lesions—tumors (Gabriel and Harrison, 1974), strokes (Mazey et al, 1974), and trauma (Wortsman et al, 1980)—may activate the sympathoadrenal pathway, produce neurogenic hypertension, and closely mimic pheo.

Perhaps as common as the clinical confusion is that arising from the use of inaccurate urinary vanillylmandelic acid (VMA) screening tests and interference by various medications with one or another laboratory test, problems considered in the next few pages.

## LABORATORY CONFIRMATION

Routine laboratory screening for pheochromocytoma in the workup of every hypertensive is *not* recommended. Testing should be reserved for those with features suggestive of pheo (Table 12.3) or those with incidentally found adrenal masses.

### Making the Diagnosis

The simplest screening procedure is a metanephrine assay of a single voided (spot) urine specimen, preferably obtained while the patient is on no medication. The spot-urine metanephrine level was 0.35 ± 0.35 (2 SD) with a range of 0.06 to 1.18 μg per milligram of creatinine in 500 patients diagnosed as having essential hypertension (Kaplan et al, 1977). Results with the single-voided specimen correlated closely to those found with 24-hour urine specimens.

In addition to urine metanephrine, assays of other catecholamines and their metabolites in urine and plasma are available (Table 12.6). In patients with a pheo, the levels of all of these are almost always elevated, although a rare patient with infrequent paroxysms may have high levels only for awhile after an episode. Such patients should be given a bottle with a few drops of HCl as a preservative and asked to collect a urine sample during and for a few hours after the next episode. The finding of normal blood and urine catecholamines during a paroxysm of hypertension almost certainly excludes pheo even in the very rare instance of a pheo that also secretes somatostatin that may inhibit the release of catechols most of the time (Morice et al, 1989). Plasma catecholamines assays, though increasingly available, should not be used for screening purposes, since they are so frequently false-positive, either because of nonspecific stimulation of catechol release by numerous activities or because of interference with the excretion of catechols as seen when the glomerular filtration rate is below 20 ml/min (Laederach and Weidmann, 1987).

A common and difficult current problem is the interference from metabolites of the antihypertensive drug labetalol, the combined alpha- and beta-blocker, particularly with more severe forms of hypertension in which the drug is likely to be used and where pheo may be more likely looked for. The labetalol metabolites cause falsely high levels of urinary excretion of epinephrine by fluorometry, norepinephrine by radioenzymatic or fluorometric assays, and metanephrine by spectrophotometry or high-pressure liquid chromatography (HPLC) (Feldman, 1987) as well as plasma catechol assays by HPLC (Bouloux and Perrett, 1985). Fortunately, these metabolites do not interfere with measurements of urine VMA or plasma catechols by radioenzymatic assay (Feldman, 1987). Samples should be collected before labetalol is used or 3 days after it is discontinued.

### Urine Tests

Assays are available for each of the three urinary products of catecholamine metabolism: free catecholamines, metanephrines, and VMA (Fig 12.3). Patients with small, active tumors may excrete mainly free catecholamines; those

**Table 12.6. Normal Values for Catecholamines and Their Metabolites**

| | Present Units | Conversion Factor | SI Units |
|---|---|---|---|
| Plasma | | | |
| Dopamine | <100 pg/ml | | |
| Epinephrine | 31–95 pg/ml | 5.5 | 170–520 pmol/L |
| Norepinephrine | 15–475 pg/ml | 5.9 | 90–2800 pmol/L |
| | | | (0.09–2.8 nmol/L) |
| Urine | | | |
| Homovanillic acid | <8 mg/d | 5.5 | <45 μmol/d |
| Vanillylmandelic acid | <8.8 mg/d | 5.0 | <35 μmol/d |
| 3,4-Dihydroxy-phenylglycol | 1.3–4.3 mg/d | 5.5 | <1.0 μmol/d |
| Metanephrines | <1.3 mg/d | 5.5 | <7.5 μmol/d |
| Epinephrine | <10 μg/d | 5.5 | <55 nmol/L |
| Norepinephrine | <100 μg/d | 5.9 | <590 nmol/d |
| Catecholamines, total | <120 μg/d | 5.9 | <675 nmol/d |

with large, indolent tumors may excrete predominantly VMA. In most patients, excretion of all will be elevated, but normal values of one of the urinary products may be found in patients with proved tumors: In one series, 18 of 43 had normal urinary VMA, and nine of 43 had normal urinary metanephrine (Bravo and Gifford, 1984).

A compilation of the findings in nine of the larger series reported in the recent past documents the greater sensitivity of the urine metanephrine procedure (Table 12.7). In a disease so rare and with such varied manifestations, diagnostic tests should give few false-negatives. False-negatives with the urine metanephrine assay may be attributable to the collection of the specimen soon after various x-ray procedures using the contrast medium methylglucamine (McPhaul et al, 1984). This chemical reacts with the reagent needed to convert metanephrine to vanillin, the end product that is analyzed in the spectrophotometric assay. The interference can be removed by chromatography, but the better course is to obtain the urine before x-ray procedures are done. False-negative metanephrine assays by the Pisano procedure may also be caused by a 4-hydroxy metabolite of propranolol in the urine that, by producing a high blank level, spuriously decreases the level of the measured metanephrine (Chou et al, 1980).

The specificity of all three tests in the multiple series shown in Table 12.7 was 99%, so very few false-positives are to be expected with any of them. The few false-positives seen with the urine metanephrine assay may be related to drug intake (Table 12.8). An even longer list of factors that have been purported, sometimes with little validation, to interfere with these assays has been compiled by Young et al (1975).

Remember that patients under considerable stress, e.g., perioperative, acute myocardial infarction, or severe congestive heart failure, may have high catechols, and they should be tested only after the stress has subsided for 5 to 7 days (Thomas and Marks, 1978).

Children excrete more of these metabolites per milligram of creatinine, and their levels should be compared with those given in Table 12.9 (Gitlow et al, 1968).

## Plasma Tests

Elevated basal plasma levels of both NE and Epi have been found in most patients with a pheo, sometimes with fewer false-negatives than either urinary VMA or metanephrine assays (Bravo and Gifford, 1984). However, most published series report 10 to 30% of patients to have falsely normal values (Cryer, 1980; Plouin et al, 1981; Brown et al, 1981; Duncan et al, 1988). As previously noted, there are too many false-positive plasma NE and Epi levels to use plasma assays for screening purposes.

To improve the diagnostic accuracy of plasma assays, various maneuvers have been utilized, including:

—fractionating the Epi from the NE, with the finding that small tumors secrete relatively more Epi; moreover, in patients without a pheo, Epi levels are more likely normal than are NE levels (Brown et al, 1981).

—measuring a metabolite of NE, 3,4-dihydroxyphenylglycol (DHPG), which mainly reflects release of NE from sympathetic nerves; most of those with a pheo have more NE than DHPG; those without a pheo have more DHPG than NE (Duncan et al, 1988).

—measuring the catecholamine content of platelets, wherein catechols are concentrated, which therefore tend to reflect more accurately the longer-term circulating levels (Zweifler and Julius, 1982).

**Table 12.7. Urinary Tests for Pheochromocytoma[a]**

| Compound | Urinary Excretion (mg/day or μg/mg of creatinine) | | No. of Patients with Pheo | % of Patients with Pheochromocytoma Correctly Identified |
|---|---|---|---|---|
| | Normal Adults | Pheochromocytoma | | |
| Free catecholamines | <0.1 | 0.1–10.0 | 179 | 85 |
| Metanephrine + normetanephrine | <1.2 | 1.0–100.0 | 282 | 96 |
| Vanillylmandelic acid | <6.5 | 5–600 | 294 | 84 |

[a]Data from Sjöerdsma A, Engelman K, Waldmann TA, et al: *Ann Intern Med* 65:1302, 1966; Gitlow SE, Mendlowitz M, Bertani LM: *Am J Cardiol* 26:70, 1970; ReMine WH, Chong GC, Van Heerden JA, et al: *Ann Surg* 179:740, 1974; DeOreo GA Jr, Stewart GH, Tarazi RC, et al: *J Urol* 111:715, 1974; Bravo EL, Tarazi RC, Gifford RW, et al: *N Engl J Med* 301:682, 1979; Stewart GH, Bravo EL, Meaney TF: *J Urol* 122:579, 1979; Jones DH, Redi JL, Hamilton CA, et al: *Q J Med* 49:341, 1980; Plouin P-F, Duclos JM, Menard J, et al: *Br Med J* 281:853, 1981; van Heerden JA, Sheps SG, Hamberger B, et al: *Surgery* 91:367, 1982; as collated by Manu P, Runge LA: *Am J Epidemiol* 120:788, 1984.

**Table 12.8. Factors That Interfere with Urine Tests for Catecholamines and Metabolites**

| Assay | Factors That Interfere | |
|---|---|---|
| | Increase | Decrease |
| Catecholamines | Pharmacological<br>  Exogenous catecholamines<br>  L-dopa, methyldopa<br>  Theophylline<br>Analytical<br>  Tetracycline, erythromycin<br>  Quinine, quinidine<br>  Chloral hydrate<br>  Chlorpromazine<br>  Labetalol | Pharmacological<br>  Sympathetic nervous inhibitors,<br>    e.g., clonidine<br>  Fenfluramine |
| Metanephrines | Pharmacological<br>  Exogenous catecholamines<br>  MAO inhibitors<br>  Rapid withdrawal or sympathetic<br>    inhibitors<br>Analytical<br>  Acetaminophen<br>  Benzodiazepines<br>  Triamterene<br>  Labetalol<br>  Sotalol | Analytical<br>  Methylglucamine (x-ray)<br>    contrast)<br>  Propranolol |
| VMA | Pharmacological<br>  Exogenous catecholamines<br>  L-dopa<br><br><br>Analytical<br>  Nalidixic acid | Pharmacological<br>  MAO inhibitors<br>  Methyldopa<br>  Ethanol<br>  Dietary phenolic acids, e.g.,<br>    vanilla, bananas, coffee<br>Analytical<br>  Clofibrate<br>  Disulfiram |

**Table 12.9. Urinary Excretion of VMA, HVA, and Total Metanephrines in Children[a]**

| Age (yr) | VMA | | HVA | | Total Metanephrines | |
|---|---|---|---|---|---|---|
| | Mean | SD | Mean | SD | Mean | SD |
| <1 | 6.9[b] | 3.2 | 12.9 | 9.6 | 1.6 | 1.3 |
| 1–2 | 4.6 | 2.2 | 12.6 | 6.3 | 1.7 | 1.1 |
| 2–5 | 3.9 | 1.7 | 7.6 | 3.6 | 1.2 | 0.8 |
| 5–10 | 3.3 | 1.4 | 4.7 | 2.7 | 1.1 | 0.8 |
| 10–15 | 1.9 | 0.8 | 2.5 | 2.4 | 0.6 | 0.5 |
| 15–18 | 1.3 | 0.6 | 1.0 | 0.6 | 0.2 | 0.2 |

[a]From Gitlow SE, Mendlowitz M, Wilk EK, et al: *J Lab Clin Med* 72:612, 1968.
[b]All values are given as micrograms per milligram of creatinine.

—using changes in plasma levels in response to pharmacological manipulations, as will be described below.

The use of plasma assays requires careful attention to the patient's circumstances: Upright posture, sodium deprivation, exercise, fasting, and smoking will all elevate plasma catecholamines. The patient should be supine for 1 hour after placement of an indwelling venous catheter. Blood should be immediately chilled and the plasma separated quickly and frozen at −90°C until assayed. Antihypertensive drugs may affect plasma catechols: Some lower them (e.g.,

clonidine), whereas others raise them slightly, either by setting off reflex sympathetic activity (e.g., diuretics, vasodilators) or by blocking adrenergic receptors with "overflow" of catechols into the circulation (e.g., beta-blockers). Cimetidine may raise plasma levels, presumably by a decrease in hepatic clearance (Feely et al, 1982). Recall again the false-positive values from labetalol. Plasma levels may be elevated in patients with renal insufficiency and falls are usually noted after hemodialysis (Musso et al, 1989).

## Pharmacological Tests

In view of the availability of accurate urinary assays, there is little need to subject patients to the discomfort and hazard of either provocative (histamine, tyramine, glucagon) or suppression (Regitine) tests. Moreover, they give both false-positive and false-negative results (Sheps and Maher, 1968; White et al, 1973).

*Provocative Tests.* The only rational use of the best of these provocative procedures, the glucagon stimulation test, would be to identify bilateral medullary hyperplasia in patients with medullary carcinoma of the thyroid whose control urine metanephrine assays are normal, or to diagnose a pheo in the extremely rare patient with normal plasma and urine catecholamine levels. The specificity of the glucagon test is increased by use of plasma NE assays (Bravo and Gifford, 1984). The safety of glucagon testing is improved by pretreatment with an alpha-blocker that does not block the rise in plasma catecholamines (Elliott et al, 1989).

*Suppression Tests.* Two suppression tests measuring plasma catecholamine levels have been described, which by nature seem more physiological and are likely safer than provocative tests.The first suppression test uses a 2.5-mg intravenous dose of the preganglionic blocking agent pentolinium (Brown et al, 1981). Pheos do not have preganglionic nerve supply, and therefore pentolinium should not suppress their autonomous catechol secretion. The test was correct in separating all 18 patients with a pheo who did not suppress their plasma Epi or NE levels from 20 patients with intermittently elevated plasma catechols who did.

The second and more widely used test uses the effect of the centrally acting sympathetic inhibitor clonidine upon plasma catechols (Bravo et al, 1981). Plasma NE levels are measured before and 2 and 3 hours after a single oral 0.3-mg dose of clonidine; the NE levels fall to below the normal range in those without a pheo but remain high in those with a pheo. The authors found a normal response, i.e., an absolute fall of plasma NE to below 500 pg/ml and a relative fall of at least 40% from the basal level in all 70 nonpheo hypertensives but in only one of 32 patients with a pheo (Fig. 12.5) (Bravo and Gifford, 1984). The 2-hour sample almost always gives the best discrimination. To save money, the 3-hour sample can be frozen and analyzed only if the 2-hour sample is equivocal.

The test has performed well in most investigators' experience (Gross et al, 1987; Mannelli et al, 1987). A few false-positives have been reported because of diuretic therapy (Hui et al, 1986) or use of a radioimmunoassay that also measures slowly turned over conjugated catechols in plasma (Aron et al, 1983). More bothersome but even rarer false-negatives have been reported (Taylor et al, 1986).

Results as good as those with the plasma response have been reported with an overnight clonidine suppression test measuring urine catecholamines in urine collected from 2100 to 0700 hours after 0.3 mg of clonidine at 2100 (Macdougall et al, 1988).

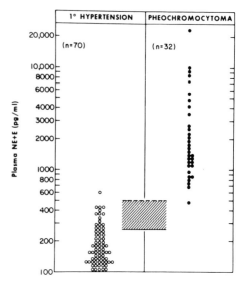

**Figure 12.5.** Plasma catecholamine (*NE* + *E*) levels in 32 patients with and 70 patients without a pheochromocytoma before and 2 or 3 hours after a single oral dose of clonidine, 0.3 mg. *Hatched area*, mean values obtained from 60 healthy adult subjects (+2 SD). (From Bravo EL, Gifford RW and by permission of *The New England Journal of Medicine* 311:1298, 1984.)

## Summary of Confirmatory Testing

In summary, these guidelines should simplify the laboratory confirmation of pheo:

1. Obtain a metanephrine assay on a single-voided urine specimen on all patients with suggestive features, preferably while they are taking no medications. If the patient is on therapy with antihypertensive drugs, recall that falsely low values have been found in patients on propranolol and falsely high values with triamterene and labetalol.

   If the urine tests are normal, the diagnosis has been excluded with a specificity of over 99%. However, if the patient has only paroxysmal symptoms, collect a urine sample during and after a hypertensive paroxysm and measure free catecholamines.

2. If the urinary metanephrine assay is abnormal, confirm the diagnosis by measuring metanephrine and total catecholamines in a 24-hour urine specimen and a plasma catechol obtained after the patient has been supine for 1 hour.

3. If the urine assays are borderline, a clonidine suppression test may prove useful if the patient is hypertensive, or a glucagon provocative test if normotensive. It may simply be better to repeat the evaluation in 3 to 6 months

while protecting the patient with oral anti-hypertensive agents preferably starting with an alpha-blocker.

## Localizing the Tumor

Computer tomography (CT) of the abdomen has simplified greatly the localization of pheochromocytomas (Fig. 12.6). Most are big enough, larger than 2 cm, to be easily identified. CT can identify extraadrenal tumors (Shapiro and Fig, 1989) and metastatic disease (Thomas et al, 1980) and has been of considerable help in evaluating those with the MEN syndrome who may be normotensive and difficult to assess by biochemical tests (Thomas and Bernardino, 1981).

The most accurate way to localize a pheo is by a combination of CT with scintigraphy using an analogue of guanethidine (MIBG) labeled with $^{131}$I, which concentrates in adrenergic vesicles and has been found to be taken up preferentially by pheos (Sisson et al, 1981). At the University of Michigan, of 562 patients among whom 26% had a pheo, the $^{131}$I-MIBG scan has provided 88% sensitivity and 99% specificity, which translate into a 95% predictive accuracy of a positive scan and a 98% predictive accuracy of a negative scan (Shapiro and Fig, 1989). The isotope is now available through the Nuclear Medicine Pharmacy of the University of Michigan, and the scintigraphy equipment is widely available so the procedure should be performed in any patient with equivocal findings on a CT scan.

With the widespread availability of CT, other procedures are rarely indicated. In a few cases, selective sampling of venous blood from multiple sites for plasma NE and Epi levels may be required (Allison et al, 1983).

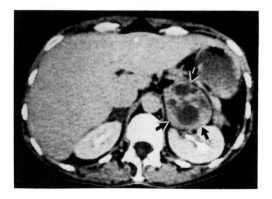

**Figure 12.6.** Computerized tomography scan of a 40-year-old woman with a large left adrenal pheochromocytoma. Note the multiple cystic areas within the tumor.

The few extraabdominal tumors can be localized by palpation of the neck, routine X-rays of the chest and thoracic spine, and, perhaps, by CT.

## THERAPY FOR BENIGN PHEOS

The symptoms of pheo can be controlled medically but, if possible, surgery should be done with the expectation that all symptoms will be relieved in the majority of patients who have benign tumors and in the hope that metastatic spread will be limited in the minority with malignant ones.

Before surgery, the patient should be treated medically for at least 1 week, preferably until hypertension and spells are controlled. In those who cannot be cured by surgery, medical therapy can be used chronically.

### Medical Therapy

#### Acute

In the face of a hypertensive crisis, the patient should be put in bed with the head elevated and given the alpha-adrenergic blocker phentolamine (Regitine) intravenously, 2 to 5 mg every 5 minutes, until the blood pressure is controlled. If serious tachycardia or arrhythmias are present, propranolol may also be given intravenously, 1 to 2 mg over a 5- to 10-minute period. Once the patient is over the crisis, control should be maintained by oral therapy until the patient is ready for surgery. Recall the potential for hemorrhagic necrosis of the tumor with alpha-blockers (van Way et al, 1976).

#### Chronic

A number of drugs that act in different ways can be used to prepare a patient for surgery or, lacking that, to manage the disease in the long term (Shapiro and Fig, 1989) (Table 12.10).

In preparation for surgery, the effects of catecholamine excess can almost always be controlled by alpha- and beta-blockers. The alpha-blockade relieves the hypertension mediated by alpha-adrenergic vasoconstriction. The beta-blockade prevents the tachycardia and arrhythmias caused by the action of catecholamines on the heart. However, the beta-blocker should be used only after alpha-blockade.

*Alpha-Blockers.* Oral *phenoxybenzamine* (Dibenzyline) is preferred since it has a smoother and more prolonged action, requiring only one or two doses daily. The alpha-receptor blockade is irreversible and persists even longer than 24 hours, so the effects of daily administration are

**Table 12.10. Pharmacotherapy of Pheochromocytoma**[a]

| | |
|---|---|
| Blockade of hormone receptor | Alpha-adrenergic blockers: Alpha$_1$ and alpha$_2$—phentolamine Alpha$_1$—prazosin Beta adrenergic blocker |
| Inhibition of hormone release | Calcium-entry blockers |
| Inhibition of hormone synthesis | Alpha-methyl-para-tyrosine |
| Nonspecific cytotoxins | Chemotherapy: cyclophosphamide, vincristine, dacarbazine |
| Tissue specific cytotoxins | 6-OH-dopamine (not clinically applicable) |

[a]Adapted from Shapiro B, Fig LM: *Endocrinol Metab Clin North Am* 18:443, 1989.

cumulative for up to 1 week. The dose should be started at 10 mg once daily and increased slowly until the pressure is at the desired level. Side effects—postural hypotension, nasal stuffiness, and inhibition of ejaculation—are rarely bothersome. Since the presynaptic alpha$_2$-receptor is also blocked by this drug, the release of NE from adrenergic neurons may increase, leading to tachycardia, which may call for the use of a beta-blocker.

*Prazosin* may be useful since it will preferentially block the postsynaptic alpha$_1$-receptors on the vessel wall but will leave the presynaptic alpha$_2$-receptors on the neuronal surface open. Thereby, the feedback inhibition of neuronal release of NE is preserved, unlike the situation with phenoxybenzamine. Tachycardia should be less of a problem, so that a beta-blocker may not be needed. In patients with a pheo, prazosin may provide a dramatic and prolonged lowering of the blood pressure, but additional phentolamine may be needed during surgery (Havlik et al, 1988).

*Doxazosin.* This longer acting selective alpha-blocker will provide similar effects to prazosin (Miura and Yoshinaga, 1988).

*Beta-Blockers.* Beta-blockers may be given to control tachycardia and arrhythmias but only after alpha-blockers have been started. If inadvertently used alone, beta-blockers may cause either a pressor response, since the beta-blockade of the beta$_2$-mediated vasodilator actions of epinephrine leaves the alpha-mediated vasoconstrictor actions unopposed, or pulmonary edema, presumably by removal of beta-adrenergic drive to the heart (Sloand and Thompson, 1984). Moreover, beta-blockade decreases the clearance of catecholamines from the circulation (Cryer et al, 1980). Not all who receive beta-blockers alone will get into trouble, probably because

their tumors secrete mainly norepinephrine which has little action on vasodilatory beta$_2$-receptors (Plouin et al, 1979).

The combined alpha- and beta-blocking drug labetalol has been used with good results (Reach et al, 1980). However, since it causes more beta-blockage than alpha-blockade, a rise in blood pressure may be seen, so it should be used with great caution (Feek and Earnshaw, 1980). And recall the false-positive catecholamine assays from labetalol.

Rare patients cannot be controlled on any alpha-blocker (Hauptman et al, 1983), whereas a few cases have been reported to respond well to a calcium-entry blocker (Chari et al, 1988) or a converting enzyme inhibitor (Blum, 1987).

*Alpha-Methyltyrosine.* An inhibitor of catecholamine synthesis, *alpha*-methyl-*p*-tyrosine, or metyrosine, is now available (Demser; Merck, Sharp and Dohme). Though effective, it may cause sedation, diarrhea, and other side effects, so its primary use is for those whose tumors are inoperable. It should not be used without concomitant use of an alpha-blocker (Ram et al, 1985).

## Surgical Therapy

These patients, susceptible to extreme swings in blood pressure, malignant arrhythmias, and profound postoperative shock, should be managed by physicians who are knowledgeable about the problems. Patients with a pheo who are not under adequate control are at high risk during surgery, with mortality rates as high as 50%. With adequate preoperative control and intraoperative management, the risks should be little more than with other major surgical procedures. The details are well delineated by Shapiro and Fig (1989).

### Preoperative Management

With the medical therapy previously described, the blood pressure and symptoms can be controlled, the shrunken blood volume restored, and swings of pressure during surgery minimized.

### Anesthesia

Various anesthetic agents have been advocated because they tend not to cause a release of catecholamines or to sensitize the myocardium. However, in the extensive experience of Desmonts and Marty (1984), the type of anesthetic agent was of secondary importance to the control of operative hypotension by replacement of fluid volume. Neuromuscular relaxants, e.g., atracurium, should be avoided because they can cause severe hypertension (Amaranath et al, 1988).

## Surgical Procedure

Most surgeons prefer an upper abdominal incision long enough to expose both adrenals, the entire periaortic sympathetic chain, and the urinary bladder. Although only one pheo may be found, exploration must be thorough since as many as 20% of patients have multiple pheos. In familial cases multiple pheos are almost always present. Rises in pressure during palpation may help locate small tumors.

After removal of the pheo, the blood pressure may fall precipitously for one or more reasons (Fig. 12.7). The major factor seems to be the shrunken blood volume, which is no longer supported by intense vasoconstriction.

## Postoperative Care

Patients may become hypoglycemic in the immediate postoperative period, presumably because the sudden decrease in catecholamines leads to an increase in insulin secretion while simultaneously decreasing the formation of glucose from glycogen and fat. Therefore, adequate glucose should be infused and the blood level monitored.

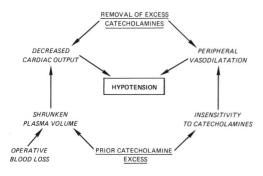

**Figure 12.7.** Possible causes of hypotension after removal of a pheochromocytoma.

If the pressure remains high, some of the tumor may have been inadvertently left behind; less commonly, a renal artery may have been damaged, with induction of renovascular hypertension. The presence of residual tumor can be checked by the response to intravenous phentolamine, but reexploration should await repeated collection of urines for catecholamines and appropriate CT or scintigraphy.

## Long-Term Follow-up

The prognosis is usually excellent for benign pheos. If the pheo is not totally resectable or the patient is a high surgical risk, long-term medical therapy can provide excellent control of all pheo manifestations (Pelegri et al, 1989). If the patient has a familial syndrome, repeated assays in conjunction with blood calcitonin levels and palpation of the neck for medullary thyroid cancer should be continued for life.

## THERAPY FOR MALIGNANT PHEOS

The prognosis is obviously not as good for those with inaccessible metastases. As much tumor mass as can be reached should be resected, and medical therapy should be provided to shrink the tumor and control the symptoms. Shrinkage of tumor mass has been reported with metyrosine (Serri et al, 1984), streptozocin (Feldman, 1983), and [$^{131}$I]MIBG (Sisson et al, 1984), and skeletal metastases may respond to irradiation (Scott et al, 1982). The best response has been reported with chemotherapy combining cyclophosphamide, vincristine, and dacarbazine (Averbuch et al, 1988). Long-term control of symptoms is possible with alpha- and beta-blockers and metyrosine. With such aggressive therapy, long-term survival is possible.

We will next examine primary aldosteronism, another uncommon but fascinating adrenal cause of hypertension.

### References

Achong MR, Keane PM: *Ann Intern Med* 94:358, 1981.
Allison DJ, Brown MJ, Jones DH, et al: *Br Med J* 286:1122, 1983.
Amaranath L, Zanettin GG, Bravo EL, et al: *Anesth Analg* 67:1127, 1988.
Andersen GS, Toftdahl DB, Lund JO, et al: *J Hum Hypertens* 2:187, 1988.
Aron DC, Bravo EL, Kapcala LP: *Ann Intern Med* 98:1023, 1983.
Atuk NO, Teja K, Mondzelewski JP, et al: *Arch Intern Med* 137:1073, 1977.
Averbuch SD, Steakley CS, Young RC, et al: *Ann Intern Med* 109:267, 1988.

Bauer FE, Hacker GW, Terenchi G, et al: *J Clin Endocrinol Metab* 63:1372, 1986.
Beard CM, Sheps SG, Kurland LT, et al: *Mayo Clin Proc* 58:802, 1983.
Belldegrun A, Hussain S, Seltzer SE, et al: *Surg Gynecol Obstet* 163:203, 1986.
Beyer HS, Doe RP: *J Clin Endocrinol Metab* 62:1317, 1986.
Blum R: *Ann Intern Med* 106:326, 1987.
Bornemann M, Hill SC, Kidd GS II: *Ann Intern Med* 105:880, 1986.
Bostwick DG, Null WE, Holmes D, et al: *N Engl J Med* 317:1439, 1987.

Bouloux P-MG, Perrett D: *Clin Chim Acta* 150:111, 1985.
Bravo EL, Fouad-Tarazi FM, Rossi GP, et al: *Hypertension* 13:527, 1989 (abst).
Bravo EL, Gifford RW Jr: *N Engl J Med* 311:1298, 1984.
Bravo EL, Tarazi RC, Fouad FM, et al: *N Engl J Med* 305:623, 1981.
Bravo EL, Tarazi RC, Gifford RW, et al: *N Engl J Med* 301:682, 1979.
Brinker M, Bailey S, Kraus SD, et al: *South Med J* 81:92, 1988.
Brooks MH, Guha A, Danforth E Jr, et al: *Metabolism* 18:445, 1969.

Brown MJ, Allison DR, Jenner DA, et al: *Lancet* 1:174, 1981.

Cantor AM, Rigby CC, Beck PR, et al: *Br Med J* 285:1618, 1982.

Carney JA, Sizemore GW, Sheps SG: *Am J Clin Pathol* 66:279, 1976.

Chari P, Katariya RN, Venkataraman RK, et al: *Anaesthesia* 43:791, 1988.

Chou D, Tsuru M, Holtzman JL, et al: *Clin Chem* 26:776, 1980.

Copeland PM: *Ann Intern Med* 98:940, 1983.

Crout JR, Sjöersdma A: *J Clin Invest* 43:94, 1964.

Cryer PE, Rizza RA, Haymond WM, et al: *Metabolism* 29:1114, 1980.

DeAngelis LM, Kelleher MB, Post KD, et al: *Neurology* 37:129, 1987.

de Leeuw PW, Waltman FL, Birkenhäger WH: *Hypertension* 8:810, 1986.

DeOreo GA Jr, Stewart GH, Tarazi RC, et al: *J Urol* 111:715, 1974.

Dennis PJ, Lewandowski AE, Rohner TJ, Jr, et al: *J Urol* 141:130, 1989.

Desmonts JM, Marty J: *Br J Anaesth* 56:781, 1984.

Duncan MW, Compton P, Lazarus L, et al: *N Engl J Med* 319:136, 1988.

Elliott WJ, Murphy MB, Straus FH II, et al: *Arch Intern Med* 149:214, 1989.

Feek CM, Earnshaw PM: *Br Med J* 2:387, 1980.

Feely J, Robertson D, Island DP: *N Engl J Med* 306:1054, 1982.

Feldman JM: *J Clin Pharmacol* 27:288, 1987.

Gabriel R, Harrison BDW: *Br Med J* 2:312, 1974.

Ganguly A, Grim CE, Weinberger MH, et al: *Hypertension* 6:281, 1984.

Gitlow SE, Mendlowitz M, Bertani LM: *Am J Cardiol* 26:70, 1970.

Gitlow SE, Mendlowitz M, Wilk ED, et al: *J Lab Clin Med* 72:612, 1968.

Glenn F, Gray GF: *Ann Surg* 183:578, 1976.

Goldbaum TS, Henochowicz S, Mustafa M, et al: *Am J Med* 81:921, 1986.

Gorlin RJ, Sedano HO, Vickers RA, et al: *Cancer* (Phila) 22:293, 1968.

Goldstein DS, Stull R, Eisenhofer G, et al: *Ann Intern Med* 105:887, 1986.

Griffiths DFR, Williams GT, Williams ED: *Br Med J* 287:1341, 1983.

Gross MD, Shapiro B, Bouffard JA, et al: *Ann Intern Med* 109:613, 1988.

Gross MD, Shapiro B, Sisson JC, et al: *J Endocrinol Invest* 10:359, 1987.

Hamilton BP, Landsberg L, Levine RJ: *Am J Med* 65:1027, 1978.

Harper MA, Murnaghan GA, Kennedy L, et al: *Br J Obstet Gynaecol* 96:594, 1989.

Hauptman JB, Modlinger RS, Ertel NH: *Arch Intern Med* 143:2321, 1983.

Havlik RJ, Cahow E, Kinder BK: *Arch Surg* 123:626, 1988.

Hedeland H, Östberg G, Hökfelt B: *Acta Med Scand* 184:211, 1968.

Hermann H, Mornex R: *Human Tumors Secreting Catecholamines*. New York: Pergamon Press, 1964.

Hodgkinson DJ, Telander RL, Sheps SG, et al: *Mayo Clin Proc* 55:271, 1980.

Hodgson SF, Sheps SG, Subramanian R, et al: *Am J Med* 77:157, 1984.

Hui TP, Krakoff LR, Felton K, et al: *Hypertension* 8:272, 1986.

Huiras CM, Pehling GB, Caplan RH: *JAMA* 261:894, 1989.

Hume DM: *Am J Surg* 99:458, 1960.

Imai Y, Abe K, Miura Y, et al: *J Hypertension* 6:9, 1988.

Ishibashi M, Takeuchi A, Yokoyama S, et al: *Jpn Heart J* 16:741, 1975.

Jones DH, Reid JL, Hamilton CA, et al: *Q J Med* 49:341, 1980.

Jones DJ, Durning P: *Br Med J* 291:1267, 1985.

Kalff V, Shapiro B, Lloyd R, et al: *Arch Intern Med* 142:2092, 1982.

Kaplan NM: *J Clin Invest* 46:728, 1967.

Kaplan NM, Kramer NJ, Holland OB, et al: *Arch Intern Med* 137:190, 1977.

Khairi MRA, Dexter RN, Burzynski NJ, et al: *Medicine* (Baltimore) 54:89, 1975.

Knudson AG Jr, Strong LC: *Am J Hum Genet* 24:514, 1972.

Kremer R, Michel RP, Posner B, et al: *Am J Med Sci* 297:46, 1989.

Kuchel O, Buu NT, Racz K, et al: *Fed Proc* 45:2254, 1986a.

Kuchel O, Cusson JR, Larochelle P, et al: *J Hypertension* 5:277, 1987.

Kuchel O, Buu NT, Larochelle P, et al: *Arch Intern Med* 146:1315, 1986b.

Laederach K, Weidmann P: *Kidney Int* 31:107, 1987.

Lee RE, Rousseau P: *J Clin Endocrinol Metab* 27:1050, 1967.

Lie JT, Olney BA, Spittel JA: *Am Heart J* 100:716, 1980.

Lips KJM, Veer JVDS, Struyvenberg A, et al: *Am J Med* 70:1051, 1981.

Louis WJ, Doyle AE, Heath WC, et al: *Br Med J* 4:325, 1972.

Lund-Johansen P: *Acta Med Scand* 172:525, 1962.

Macdougall IC, Isles CG, Stewart H, et al: *Am J Med* 84:993, 1988.

Manger WM: *Arch Intern Med* 145:229, 1985.

Manger WM, Gifford RW Jr: *Pheochromocytoma*. New York: Springer-Verlag, 1977.

Manger WM, Gifford RW, Hoffman BB: In: Hickery RC, Clark RL (eds). *Current Problems in Cancer*, Vol IX: *Pheochromocytoma: A Clinical and Experimental Overview*. Chicago: Year Book Medical Publishers, 1985.

Mannelli M, De Feo ML, Maggi M, et al: *J Endocrinol Invest* 10:377, 1987.

Mannix H Jr, O'Grady WP, Gitlow SE: *Arch Surg* 104:216, 1972.

Manu P, Runge LA: *Am J Epidemiol* 120:788, 1984.

Marx SJ, Sakaguchi K, Green J III, et al: *J Clin Endocrinol Metab* 67:149, 1988.

Mathew CGP, Chin KS, Easton DF, et al: *Nature* (Lond) 328:527, 1987.

Mazey RM, Kotchen TA, Ernst CB: *JAMA* 230:575, 1974.

McPhaul M, Punzi HA, Sandy A, et al: *JAMA* 252:2860, 1984.

Medvei VC, Cattell WR: *J R Soc Med* 81:550, 1988.

Miura Y, Yoshinaga K: *Am Heart J* 116:1785, 1988.

Montiel C, Artalejo AR, Bermejo PM, et al: *Anesthesiology* 65:474, 1986.

Moorhead EL, Caldwell JR, Kelly AR, et al: *JAMA* 196:1107, 1966.

Morice AH, Price JS, Ashby MJ, et al: *Br Med J* 298:1358, 1989.

Mulrow PJ, Cohn GL, Yesner R: *Yale J Biol Med* 31:363, 1959.

Musso NR, Deferrari G, Pende A, et al: *Nephron* 51:344, 1989.

Newell K, Prinz RA, Braithwaite S, et al: *Am J Hypertens* 1:189S, 1988.

O'Connor DT, Deftos LJ: *N Engl J Med* 314:1145, 1986.

Ooi TC, Dardick I: *CMAJ* 139:869, 1988.

Page LB, Raker JW, Berberich FR: *Am J Med* 47:648, 1969.

Pearce AGE: *J Histochem Cytochem* 17:303, 1969.

Pelegri A, Romero R, Reguant M, et al: *J Hum Hypertens* 3:145, 1989.

Plouin P-F, Chatelleri G, Rougeot M-A, et al: *J Hypertension* 6:579, 1988.

Plouin P-F, Duclos JM, Menard J, et al: *Br Med J* 281:853, 1981.

Plouin P-F, Menard J, Corvol P: *Br Heart J* 42:359, 1979.

Ponder BAJ, Ponder MA, Coffey R, et al: *Lancet* 1:397, 1988.

Primhak RA, Spicer RD, Variend S: *Br Med J* 292:95, 1986.

Pritchard BNC, Ross EJ: *Am J Cardiol* 18:394, 1966.

Pullertis J, Ein S, Balfe JW: *Can J Anaesth* 35:526, 1988.

Ram CVS, Meese R, Hill SC: *Arch Intern Med* 145:2114, 1985.

Raper AJ, Jessee EF, Texter JH Jr, et al: *Am J Cardiol* 40:820, 1977.

Reach G, Thibonnier M, Chevillard C, et al: *Br Med J* 280:1300, 1980.

Reinholdt S, Pedersen KE: *Acta Med Scand* 223:285, 1988.

Reinig JW, Doppman JL, Dwyer AJ, et al: *AJR* 147:493, 1986.

ReMine WH, Chong GC, Van Heerden JA, et al: *Ann Surg* 179:740, 1974.

Ross EJ, Griffith DNW: *Q J Med* 71:485, 1989.

Roth KA, Wilson DM, Eberwine J, et al: *J Clin Endocrinol* 63:1421, 1986.

Salmi J, Pelto-Huikko M, Auvinen O, et al: *Acta Med Scand* 224:403, 1988.

Sato T, Igarashi N, Minami S, et al: *Acta Endocrinol* (Copenh) 117:189, 1988.

Scott HW, Reynolds V, Green N, et al: *Surg Gynecol Obstet* 154:801, 1982.

Scott I, Parkes R, Cameron DP: *Med J Aust* 148:94, 1988.

Seddon JM, Baranetsky N, Van Boxel PJ: *Urology* 25:1, 1985.

Serri O, Comtois R, Bettez P, et al: *N Engl J Med* 310:1264, 1984.

Shapiro B, Fig LM: *Endocrinol Metab Clin of North Am* 18:443, 1989.

Sheps SG, Jiang N-S, Klee GG: *Endocrinol Metab Clin North Am* 17:397, 1988.

Sheps SG, Maher FT: *JAMA* 205:895, 1968.

Sisson JC, Frager MS, Valk TW, et al: *N Engl J Med* 305:12, 1981.

Sisson JC, Shapiro B, Beierwaltes WH, et al: *J Nucl Med* 25:197, 1984.

Sjöersdma A, Engelman K, Waldmann TA, et al: *Ann Intern Med* 65:1302, 1966.

Sloand EM, Thompson BT: *Arch Intern Med* 144:173, 1984.

Stackpole RH, Melicow MM, Uson AC: *J Pediatr* 63:315, 1963.

Stenström G, Sjöström, Smith U: *Acta Endocrinol* 106:511, 1984.

Stenström G, Svärdsudd K: *Acta Med Scand* 220:225, 1986.

Stewart GH, Bravo EL, Meaney TF: *J Urol* 122:579, 1979.

Takeda R, Yashuhara S, Miyamori I, et al: *J Hypertension* 4(Suppl 5):S397, 1986.

Taubman I, Pearson OH, Anton AH: *Am J Med* 57:953, 1974.

Taylor HC, Mayes D, Anton AH: *J Clin Endocrinol Metab* 63:238, 1986.

Thomas JA, Marks BH: *Am J Cardiol* 41:233, 1978.

Thomas JL, Bernardino ME: *JAMA* 245:1467, 1981.

Thomas JL, Bernardino ME, Samaan NA: *AJR* 135:477, 1980.

Tischler AS, Allen JM, Costopoulos D, et al: *J Clin Endocrinol Metab* 61:303, 1985.

Tokioka H, Takahashi T, Kosogabe Y, et al: *Br J Anaesth* 60:582, 1988.

Turner MC, DeQuattro V, Flak R, et al: *Hypertension* 8:851, 1986.

Valet P, Damase-Michel C, Chamontin B, et al: *Eur J Clin Invest* 18:481, 1988.

van Heerden JA, Sheps SG, Hamberger B, et al: *Surgery* 91:367, 1982.

van Way CE III, Faraci RP, Cleveland HC, et al: *Ann Surg* 184:26, 1976.

Virkkala A, Välimäki M, Pelkonen R, et al: *Acta Endocrinol* 121:67, 1989.

Waldmann T, Bradley JE: *Proc Soc Exp Biol Med* 108:425, 1961.

Weinblatt ME, Heisel MA, Siegel SE: *Pediatrics* 71:947, 1983.

White LW, Levy RP, Anton AH: *Res Commun Chem Pathol Pharmacol* 5:252, 1973.

Wortsman J, Brns G, Van Beek AL, et al: *JAMA* 243:1459, 1980.

Wurtman RJ, Axelrod J: *Science* (Wash DC) 150:1464, 1965.

Young DS, Pestaner LC, Gibberman V: *Clin Chem* 21:246D, 1975

Zweifler AJ, Julius S: *N Engl J Med* 306:890, 1982.

# 13  Primary Aldosteronism

## INCIDENCE

Although relatively rare as a cause of hypertension, primary aldosteronism has received a great deal of attention since it was first recognized in 1954. The recognition of the disease in a relatively high proportion—2 to 10%—of referred populations (Conn, 1968; Grim et al, 1977; Streeten et al, 1979) led to the expectation that it would be found commonly among unselected patients as well. However, in most series of unselected patients, it is found in fewer than 0.5% of hypertensives (Gifford, 1969; Beevers et al, 1974; Berglund et al, 1976). Throughout Denmark from 1977 to 1981, only 19 cases were identified, corresponding to 0.8 cases per million people per year (Andersen et al, 1988). During the same interval, 47 cases of pheochromocytoma were identified.

Regardless of its rarity, primary aldosteronism is a fascinating disease—protean in its manifestations, logical in its pathophysiology, and straightforward in its diagnosis and treatment.

## DEFINITION

*Primary aldosteronism* is the syndrome resulting from the secretion of excessive amounts of aldosterone caused by autonomous hyperfunction of the adrenal cortex, usually by a solitary adenoma. Confusion arises because most aldosteronism seen in clinical practice is *secondary* to an increase in renin-angiotensin activity and many patients with the syndrome turn out to have bilateral adrenal hyperplasia rather than a tumor.

A classification of the various forms of secondary aldosteronism, by mechanism, is given in Table 13.1, which is virtually the same as the *right side* of Table 3.6, Clinical Conditions with Increased PRA. Some of these conditions may be easily confused with primary aldosteronism in that the classical features of this disease—hypertension and hypokalemia—are also present. Diuretic therapy of hypertension is the most common. In a few instances, renovascular hypertension or malignant hypertension may be the most difficult to differentiate. Most of these, however, should present no problem, particularly when the patient is edematous, taking estrogens, or not hypertensive. The ability to measure plasma renin activity (PRA) has made the differentiation much easier.

## CLINICAL FEATURES

The disease is usually seen in patients between the ages of 30 and 50, though cases have been found in patients from age 3 to 75, and in women more frequently than in men.

The clinical features of classical primary aldosteronism are hypertension, hypokalemia, excessive urinary potassium excretion, hypernatremia, and metabolic alkalosis. The reason that each of these features is usually present will become obvious when we examine the pathophysiology of aldosterone excess.

## PATHOPHYSIOLOGY

### Sources of Aldosterone Excess

#### Aldosterone-Producing Adenomas (Conn's Syndrome)

Solitary benign adenomas (Fig. 13.1) are present in most patients with classical primary aldosteronism. The tumor is almost always unilateral. Some refer to these tumors as "aldosterone-producing adenomas" with the abbreviation APA. I will refer to them simply as "adenomas."

**Table 13.1. Secondary Aldosteronism**

I. Renin-angiotensin excess
  A. Decreased pressure at the juxtaglomerular apparatus
    1. Shrunken effective blood volume
      a. Volume depletion
        Low sodium intake
        Hemorrhage
        Renal losses
          Diuretic therapy
          Salt-wasting nephritis
          Decreased chloride reabsorption (Bartter's syndrome)
          Gastrointestinal losses
      b. Edematous states
        Cirrhosis with ascites
        Nephrotic syndrome
        Congestive heart failure
        Idiopathic edema
    2. Decreased renal perfusion pressure
      a. Peripheral vasodilator therapy
      b. Obstruction to renal blood flow
        Renovascular hypertension
        Accelerated-malignant hypertension
        Chronic renal disease with renin-dependent hypertension
  B. Decreased sodium at the macula densa
  C. Increased sympathetic stimulation
    1. Pheochromocytoma
    2. Severe stress
  D. Increased renin substrate
    1. Estrogen therapy
    2. Pregnancy
  E. Renin-secreting renal tumor
II. Adrenocorticotropin (ACTH) excess
  A. Exogenous administration (transient)
  B. Non-salt-losing congenital adrenal hyperplasia
III. Potassium excess

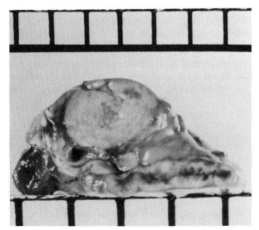

**Figure 13.1.** Solitary adrenal adenoma with diffuse hyperplasia removed from a patient with primary aldosteronism.

Most adenomas are small, weighing less than 6 g and measuring less than 3 cm in diameter. Histologically, most adenomas are composed of lipid-laden cells arranged in small acini or cords, similar in appearance and arrangement to the normal zona fasciculata, the middle zone of the adrenal cortex. These cells, however, usually possess ultrastructural features characteristic of cells of the zona glomerulosa, the outer layer of the adrenal cortex wherein aldosterone is normally synthesized (Reidbord and Fisher, 1969).

Somewhat surprisingly, focal or diffuse hyperplasia of the zona glomerulosa as seen in Figure 13.1 is present in both the remainder of the adrenal with the adenoma and the contralateral glands (Neville and Symington, 1966).

**Bilateral Adrenal Hyperplasia**

In the early 1970s, reports of hyperaldosteronism with no adenoma but only with bilateral adrenal hyperplasia began to appear (George et al, 1970; Biglieri et al, 1970; Baer et al, 1970). This has been referred to as "idiopathic hyperaldosteronism," abbreviated as IHA, but I will simply use the term "hyperplasia."

Overall, such cases represent about one-quarter of all cases of primary aldosteronism (Table 13.2). These patients tend to have milder biochemical and hormonal abnormalities that are less obvious than those seen with adenomas. The need for more detailed investigations to recognize hyperplasia could explain what appears to be an increasing prevalence of this form in more recently collected series (Table 13.2) since the necessary tests are now much easier to obtain. At the Mayo Clinic, adenoma was found in 70% of cases before 1978 but in only 54% from 1978 to 1987 (Young and Klee, 1988).

The clear separation between adenoma and hyperplasia has been blurred by the recognition that, in response to suppression or stimulation tests, a few with a solitary adenoma behave as if they had bilateral hyperplasia (Gordon et al, 1987) whereas a few with bilateral hyperplasia mimic the responses seen with a solitary adenoma (Biglieri et al, 1989).

*Evidence that Hyperplasia is Secondary.* The presence of bilateral hyperplasia suggests a secondary response to some stimulatory mechanism rather than a primary neoplastic

**Table 13.2. Pathology of Primary Aldosteronism**

| Series | Adenoma No. (%) | Hyperplasia No. (%) |
|---|---|---|
| Conn, 1966 | 22 (100) | 0 (0) |
| Priestly, 1968 | 48 (96) | 2 (4) |
| Hunt, 1975 | 66 (86) | 11 (14) |
| Ferris, 1983a | 62 (78) | 17 (22) |
| Bravo, 1983 | 70 (87) | 10 (13) |
| Melby, 1984 | 151 (71) | 60 (29) |
| Biglieri, 1989 | 98 (65) | 52 (35) |

growth. Two aldosterone-stimulating sub-stances have been identified in a few patients with hyperplasia, a glycoprotein found in human pituitary glands (Sen et al, 1983) and a factor that seems related to pro-gamma-melanotropin (Griffing et al, 1985).

### Variants of Bilateral Hyperplasia

*Unilateral Hyperplasia.* Even more difficult to explain than the presence of bilateral hyperplasia are the few cases of hyperaldosteronism that apparently are caused by hyperplasia of only one adrenal gland (Ganguly et al, 1983; Oberfield et al, 1984).

*Glucocorticoid-Suppressible Hyperplasia.* A few more cases have been reported of familial hyperaldosteronism with bilateral hyperplasia that are glucocorticoid suppressible and have an autosomal dominant mode of inheritance (Sutherland et al, 1966; Gill and Bartter, 1981). This syndrome may reflect a supersensitivity to ACTH (Ganguly et al, 1984). These patients secrete large amounts of 18-oxocortisol and 18-hydroxycortisol indicating a disorder of hybrid, transitional cells that also produce aldosterone (Gomez-Sanchez et al, 1988).

*Hyperplasia with DOC Excess.* A few patients with the features of mineralocorticoid hypertension have an excess of desoxycorticosterone (DOC) rather than aldosterone. These include patients with DOC-secreting tumors or congenital adrenal hyperplasia (Biglieri, 1988), described in Chapter 14.

### Carcinoma

Aldosterone-producing carcinomas are rare. Most are associated with concomitant hypersecretion of other adrenal hormones, but some may hypersecrete only aldosterone (Lüscher et al, 1984; Arteaga et al, 1984).

### Associated Conditions

A few patients have been reported with primary aldosteronism caused by an adrenal adenoma and coexisting acromegaly (Dluhy and Williams, 1969) or primary hyperparathyroidism (Ferriss et al, 1983a). Single ectopic aldosterone-producing tumors have been found in the lower pole of the right kidney (Flanagan and McDonald, 1967) and in an ovary (Jackson et al, 1986).

### Effects of Aldosterone Excess

Virtually all of the features of primary aldosteronism were well delineated in the first case found and proved to be caused by an ad-

renal tumor (Mader and Iseri, 1955). Figure 13.2 outlines the manner in which aldosterone excess produces the two classic features—hypertension and hypokalemia.

### Hypertension

Almost all patients recognized with primary aldosteronism have been hypertensive. Five normotensive cases have been reported, mostly from Japan (Matsunaga et al, 1983). The blood pressure may be quite high—the mean in one series of 136 patients was 205/123 (Ferriss et al, 1978b). In another series of 140 patients, 28 had severe, resistant hypertension (Bravo et al, 1988). More than a dozen cases have had malignant hypertension (Kaplan, 1963; Beevers et al, 1976). In the MRC series, 31 of 136 patients with primary aldosteronism had either a stroke or myocardial infarction (Kloppenborg et al, 1974). Significant renal damage may be present (Danforth et al, 1977) along with considerable left ventricular enlargement and increased end-diastolic internal dimension index (Suzuki et al, 1988).

*Hemodynamics.* The hypertension is hemodynamically characterized by an increased peripheral resistance, a slightly expanded plasma volume (Tarazi et al, 1973), and an increased total body and exchangeable sodium content (Williams et al, 1984). When 10 patients with primary aldosteronism, previously well controlled on spironolactone, were studied 2 weeks after the drug was stopped and the hypertension reappeared, cardiac output and sodium content (both plasma volume and total exchangeable sodium) rose initially (Wenting et al, 1982) (Fig. 13.3). Between weeks 2 and 6, the hemody-

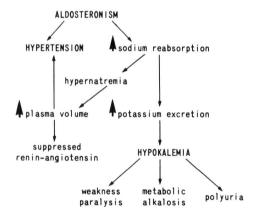

**Figure 13.2.** Pathophysiology of primary aldosteronism. (From Kaplan NM: In: Astwood EB, Cassidy CE (eds): *Clinical Endocrinology*, vol 2. New York: Grune & Stratton, 1968:468).

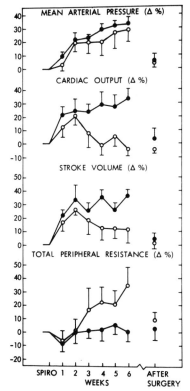

**Figure 13.3.** Changes (mean ± SEM) in systemic hemodynamics after discontinuation of spironolactone treatment (*spiro*) and after surgery in 10 patients with primary aldosteronism. Note the fall of stroke volume and cardiac output after 2 weeks in the five patients with "high-resistance" hypertension (*open circles*), as compared with the five with "high-flow" hypertension (*closed circles*). (Reprinted from Wenting GJ, Man in't Veld AJ, Schalekamp MADH: *Clin Exp Hypertens Theory Pract* A4:1727, 1982, by courtesy of Marcel Dekker, Inc.)

namic patterns separated into two types: In five of the patients, the hypertension was maintained through increased cardiac output; in the other five, cardiac output and blood volume returned to their initial values, but total peripheral resistance rose markedly. Total body sodium space remained expanded in both groups, though more so in those with increased cardiac output who tended to preferentially expand their intravascular compartment (Man in't Veld et al, 1984). After surgery, the cardiac output fell in the "high flow" patients, and the peripheral resistance fell in the "high resistance" patients.

*Mechanism of Sodium Retention.* The hypertensinogenic actions of aldosterone are generally related to its effects on sodium retention via its action on mineralocorticoid receptors. The human kidney mineralocorticoid receptor has been cloned, sequenced, and expressed (Ar-

riza et al, 1987), which will likely lead to a much greater understanding of its functions and control. Even before that signal achievement, the mystery was solved of how relatively small concentrations of aldosterone could be bound to the mineralocorticoid receptor in the face of much higher concentrations of glucocorticoids (mainly cortisol) that have equal affinity for the mineralocorticoid receptor.

The answer came from studies with licorice, which had long been known to cause sodium retention, presumably by a direct mineralocorticoid effect of its major component, glycyrrhetinic acid (Card et al, 1953). Stewart, Edwards, and coworkers (Stewart et al, 1987; Edwards et al, 1988) found that licorice inhibited the 11-beta-hydroxysteroid dehydrogenase (11-beta-OHSD) enzyme in the kidney that is responsible for the renal conversion of cortisol (which has potent mineralocorticoid effects) into cortisone (which is impotent). Thus, under normal circumstances, aldosterone is able to reach its receptor because little competing steroid is around. In the presence of either a congenital deficiency of 11-beta-OHSD (the syndrome of apparent mineralocorticoid excess) or an acquired deficiency (induced by licorice), cortisol is now provided access to the mineralocorticoid receptor, inducing major sodium retention, hypokalemia, and hypertension. More about this fascinating revelation of physiology from a quirk of nature will be covered later in this chapter. For now, it is fascinating to understand how so little aldosterone (0.1 mg/day from normal glands, 0.3 to 1.0 mg/day from aldosterone-producing adenomas) can produce such profound effects.

With excess mineralocorticoid, sodium reabsorption in the distal tubule is increased, leading to volume expansion and a decrease in sodium reabsorption in the proximal tubule, so that renal retention of sodium "escapes." The escape from progressive renal sodium retention despite the continued presence of aldosterone excess involves an increase in renal perfusion pressure and an increase in atrial natriuretic factor (Gonzalez-Campoy et al, 1989).

Aldosterone's actions, moreover, are not limited to renal sodium retention. Others include:

—direct hypertensive effects when administered into the brain, increasing total peripheral resistance without increasing fluid volume or cardiac output (Kageyama and Bravo, 1988);
—an increase in sodium influx into vascular smooth muscle (Menard and Friedman, 1985)

and an increase in sodium efflux (Moura et al, 1988);

—an increase in the number of cardiac calcium channels (Fukuda et al, 1988);

—an enhancement of vasopressin effects in the kidney (Jeffries et al, 1988).

### Hypokalemia

*Incidence.* Although a few patients have been recognized who are persistently normokalemic (Conn et al, 1965; Bravo et al, 1983), the overwhelming majority have had hypokalemia. In the MRC series, hypokalemia occurred in all 62 patients with a proved adenoma and was persistent in 53; among the 17 with hyperplasia, plasma potassium was persistently normal in three (Ferriss et al, 1983b). Similarly, hypokalemia was present in all eight patients with an adenoma but in only seven of 14 with hyperplasia (Streeten et al, 1979). On the other hand, some patients with an adenoma are normokalemic on presentation, five of 40 in a series from Indiana (Weinberger et al, 1979), 17 of 70 in a series from the Cleveland Clinic (Bravo et al, 1983).

*Significance.* Thus, persistent normokalemia is rare in patients with adenoma but more frequent in those with hyperplasia. Since it is probably unnecessary to identify those with hyperplasia, the search for primary aldosteronism should only be undertaken in those with hypokalemia. The few who might initially be missed because of a normal potassium will almost certainly show up subsequently with diuretic-induced or spontaneous hypokalemia. In the interim, a few may have had a delay in their diagnosis, but many more will be saved the expense and discomfort of unnecessary workups.

*Mechanism.* Considering the effects of persistent aldosterone excess, hypokalemia is certainly to be expected. Whereas with continued exposure to excessive mineralocorticoids the renal retention of sodium "escapes," the renal wastage of potassium is unrelenting. This has been aptly demonstrated experimentally. When progressively larger amounts of aldosterone were infused into adrenalectomized dogs for 13 weeks, the blood pressure rose rather quickly by some 20 mm Hg and remained at that level; plasma potassium continued to fall, from 4.0 to 2.5 mEq/l, throughout the experiment (Young and Guyton, 1977).

The aldosterone-driven increase in potassium secretion also involves an exchange of hydrogen for sodium so that metabolic alkalosis is generated; increased proximal and distal reabsorption of bicarbonate maintains the alkalosis, the

severity being related to the degree of hypokalemia (Seldin and Rector, 1972). Other effects of hypokalemia include muscular weakness and easy fatigability, loss of renal concentrating ability with polyuria, impaired insulin secretion with decreased carbohydrate tolerance, decreased aldosterone synthesis even from presumably autonomous adenomas (Kaplan, 1967), and blunting of circulatory reflexes with postural falls in pressure without compensatory tachycardia (Biglieri and McIllroy, 1966).

### Suppression of Renin Release

As a consequence of the initial expansion of vascular volume and the elevated blood pressure, the baroreceptor mechanism in the walls of the renal afferent arterioles suppresses the release of renin (Conn et al, 1964). Patients with primary aldosteronism usually have low levels of PRA that respond poorly to upright posture and diuretics, two maneuvers that usually raise PRA (Fig. 13.4).

The presence of suppressed PRA is only suggestive and not diagnostic of primary aldosteronism since, as detailed in Chapter 3, many more hypertensives have low PRA than the relatively few who have primary aldosteronism.

### Other Effects

*Hypernatremia* is usual. In most forms of edematous secondary aldosteronism, the sodium concentration is low since intravascular volume is decreased and antidiuretic hormone levels are stimulated to reabsorb water.

*Hypomagnesemia* from excessive renal excretion of magnesium may produce tetany.

*Sodium retention* and *potassium wastage* may be demonstrable wherever such exchange is affected by aldosterone: sweat, saliva, and stool can usually be shown to have less sodium and more potassium than normal.

*Atrial natriuretic factor* (ANF) levels are appropriately elevated for a state of volume expansion (Tunny and Gordon, 1986).

### DIAGNOSIS*

The diagnosis of primary aldosteronism should be easy to make in patients with unprovoked

---

*Conversion of laboratory values from traditional units to SI units can be performed as follows:

Plasma aldosterone from nanograms per deciliter to picomoles per liter: multiply by 27.7;

Urine aldosterone from micrograms per day to nanomoles per day: multiply by 2.77;

Plasma renin activity from nanograms per milligram per hour to nanograms per liter: multiply by 0.278.

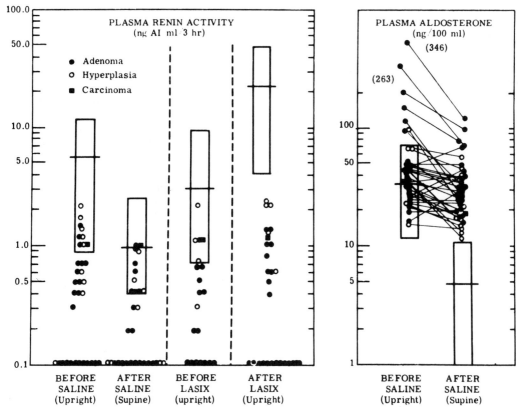

**Figure 13.4.** Responses of plasma renin activity (*left panel*) and plasma aldosterone (*right panel*) to suppressive and stimulating maneuvers. Scales are logarithmic to accommodate the range of values. Normal values (114 subjects) are represented as mean (*bars*) ±95% confidence limits (*boxes*). Values for patients with primary aldosteronism are indicated by symbols (see *key*); connecting lines for plasma aldosterone represent values of a given patient. AI, angiotensin I. (From Weinberger MH, Grim CE, Hollifield JW, et al: *Ann Intern Med* 90:386, 1979.)

hypokalemia and other manifestations of the fully expressed syndrome. It can be much more difficult in patients with minimal findings. The milder form of the disease may be more common, but, as we have seen, surgery is rarely indicated for such cases, and they can be treated medically without having to go through an extensive workup. The decision to perform a diagnostic workup is based upon the attitude that the less wrong with the patient, the less need for a prolonged and expensive evaluation. The need for evaluation is based upon this characterization of patients: (1) the normokalemic hypertensive, (2) the hypertensive who becomes hypokalemic on thiazide diuretics, and (3) the hypertensive with unprovoked hypokalemia.

## Normokalemic Hypertension

Such patients need not be screened for the very unlikely presence of primary aldosteronism. No instances of primary aldosteronism were found among 400 patients with uncomplicated hypertension carefully evaluated in three centers (Kaplan, 1967; Ledingham et al, 1967; Beevers et al, 1974). In the Syracuse series of 1028 patients referred for study, only eight cases of adenomatous hyperaldosteronism were found (Streeten et al, 1979).

### Potassium Measurements

Caution should be used to ensure that hypokalemia is not inadvertently missed. Care should be used in the timing and performance of blood potassium measurements: (1) a very low sodium diet will stop renal potassium wastage and blood potassium levels will rise; (2) if difficulty is encountered in obtaining the blood, requiring the patient to close and open the fist repeatedly, potassium may enter the blood from the exercised muscles; (3) even the slightest degree of hemolysis will raise the plasma level; (4) blood potassium levels increase on changing from the supine to the upright position (Sonkodi et al, 1981). On the other hand, the level of potassium that should be considered abnormally low is at least 0.2 mmol/l lower in plasma, which is usually used for automated chemistry analyses, than in serum (Hyman and Kaplan, 1985); the normal plasma level is probably 3.2 mmol/l or higher.

### Screening by Plasma Aldosterone:Renin Ratio

If a screening procedure is deemed necessary, the best and easiest is to look for the combination of a high plasma aldosterone and a low plasma renin in a peripheral venous blood sample obtained while the patient is on no antihypertensive drugs and without prior manipulation of diet (Hiramatsu et al, 1981). The values are put into a ratio, dividing the plasma aldosterone (normal 5 to 20 ng/dl) by the plasma renin activity (normal 1 to 3 ng/ml/hour). The normal ratio would be around 10, whereas patients with primary aldosterone are usually well above 20. This simple procedure that requires one blood sample and no special conditions has proved to be quite useful as a screening study (Hamlet et al, 1985; Lins and Adamson, 1986) and should be performed *before any therapy is given* to any patient suspected of having primary aldosteronism.

### Hypertension with Thiazide-Induced Hypokalemia

As many as 25% of patients given chronic diuretic therapy develop hypokalemia. Very few of them have primary aldosteronism (Kaplan, 1967), but some patients with the disease may become hypokalemic only after diuretic therapy. Therefore, it is essential that every patient have a potassium level determined *before* the start of the diuretic therapy. If normal, the level should be rechecked a few weeks after therapy is started. If it is then low, moderate salt restriction and increased potassium intake should be tried. If it remains low, the following should be done:

1. Stop the diuretic since hypokalemia may be difficult to correct if the diuretic is continued even with 60 to 80 mmol daily of supplemental potassium.
2. During the first week off the diuretic, have the patient on a normal sodium intake. At the end of this time, collect a 24-hour urine specimen for sodium and potassium content and repeat the plasma potassium.
   —If the patient is *normokalemic*, the measurement of urine potassium will not be

needed since normokalemic patients will excrete whatever potassium they ingest so the urine could have well over 30 mEq of potassium. No further workup is needed unless hypokalemia recurs.
   —*If the patient is still hypokalemic* and the urine has less than 30 mmol of potassium in the presence of at least 100 mEq of sodium, it is very unlikely that aldosteronism is present (Fig. 13.5), and the workup can be considered complete with virtual certainty that the hypokalemia was thiazide induced.
   —If the patient is hypokalemic and the urine has over 30 mmol of potassium, further workup is needed since aldosteronism or other diseases causing renal wastage of potassium (Table 13.3) may be present.
3. If the urinary potassium level is above 30

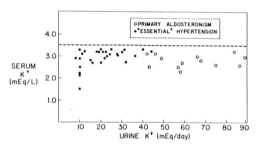

**Figure 13.5.** Urinary potassium excretion in patients with primary aldosteronism was uniformly above 30 mEq/day, whereas most patients with essential hypertension and comparable hypokalemia (mostly secondary to prior thiazide therapy) had less than 30 mEq of potassium in the 24-hour urine specimen. (From Kaplan NM: *Ann Intern Med* 66:1079, 1967.)

**Table 13.3. Causes of Renal Loss of Potassium**

1. Diuretic therapy
2. Osmotic diuresis: glucose, nonreabsorbable anions
3. Primary renal disease
   a. Renal tubular disease
   b. Fanconi syndrome
   c. $K^+$-wasting renal disease
      1. With hypomagnesemia
      2. With $Na^+$ conservation
      3. Bartter's syndrome
4. Metabolic alkalosis
5. Hypercalcemia
6. Adrenocortical hormone excess
   a. Exogenous cortisol
   b. Cushing's syndrome
   c. Primary aldosteronism
   d. Excess DOC or other mineralocorticoid
   e. Secondary aldosteronism
      1. Accelerated hypertension
      2. Renovascular hypertension
      3. Renin-secreting humor

mmol/day while the patient is hypokalemic, give supplemental potassium, preferably as potassium chloride (KCl), for as long as it takes to restore body potassium deficits. Remember that at least 200 mmol is lost for each 1-mmol fall in plasma potassium, and despite marked deficits, all of the supplemental potassium is not retained. Months of daily therapy with 60 to 80 mmol of potassium may be needed to restore the level to normal. Restricting the patient's daily sodium intake to 2 g (88 mmol) hastens the return by diminishing renal potassium losses.

4. After a suitable interval—perhaps 3 weeks for most patients with relatively mild hypokalemia—stop the supplemental potassium for at least 3 days and recheck the plasma potassium level. Plasma potassium levels may be normal while the patient is taking supplemental potassium only to fall again if the deficit has not been replenished. Even with marked deficits, some of the supplemental possium is excreted, so the urinary measurements are uninterpretable. If the plasma potassium level is normal, perform the plasma renin and either plasma or urinary aldosterone measurements detailed below. If the plasma potassium is low, resume repletion until normokalemia is established.

If hypokalemia persists for more than 6 to 8 weeks despite supplemental potassium, the workup may need to proceed but the renin and aldosterone tests are best *not* done while the patient is hypokalemic since renin levels may be elevated and aldosterone levels depressed by hypokalemia. Patients with primary aldosteronism may have "normal" urinary aldosterone excretion while hypokalemic so that a borderline aldosterone level may be abnormally high in the presence of severe hypokalemia (Kaplan, 1967).

## Hypertension with Unprovoked Hypokalemia

As opposed to the rarity of the disease in those who are normokalemic, about half of the hypertensives seen with unprovoked hypokalemia turn out to have primary aldosteronism. They certainly deserve a thorough workup, particularly since surgery is probably indicated if they have an adenoma causing aldosteronism. Obviously, patients may have other causes for "unprovoked" hypokalemia (Table 13.4), which are either not recognizable, or more likely, not looked for. Thus, chronic laxative use may provoke severe hypokalemia and,

**Table 13.4. Causes of Hypokalemia**

A. Cellular shifts
  1. Rapid changes in cell mass
  2. Alkalosis
  3. Hormones: insulin, beta-agonists
  4. Periodic paralysis
B. Decreased intake: starvation
C. Increased loss
  1. Gastrointestinal
    a. Vomiting and drainage
    b. Diarrhea and laxatives
  2. Skin
    a. Sweating
    b. Burns
  3. Renal
    a. Diuretic therapy
    b. Osmotic diuresis
    c. Primary renal disease
    d. Metabolic alkalosis (subsequent to acid loss)
    e. Hypercalcemia
    f. Adrenocortical hormone excess
    g. Licorice ingestion

by depleting body fluid volume, secondary aldosteronism (Wolff et al, 1968). Surreptitious vomiting or diuretic intake may be denied by neurotic patients, and few people who eat large amounts of licorice consider it worth mentioning to their physicians if not asked. Having sought and not found these causes for hypokalemia, the following workup is indicated (Fig. 13.6):

1. Obtain a blood sample for immediate determination of the plasma aldosterone:renin ratio.

2. Determine the 24-hour *urinary potassium and sodium* level before starting potassium replacement therapy. Few patients are endangered by 1 more day of a hypokalemic state that may have been present for years.

3. If the urinary potassium is above 30 mmol/day, proceed with *replacement therapy* as outlined above under Hypertension with Thiazide-Induced Hypokalemia. Antihypertensive agents other than diuretics can be given during the period of potassium replacement with caution about the hyperkalemic potential of ACE inhibitors used along with supplemental potassium. If after 6 to 8 weeks or longer the patient remains hypokalemic despite extra potassium and restricted sodium intake, proceed with the workup.

4. Document that *plasma renin activity* is low, most simply by obtaining a blood sample after 2 hours of upright posture immediately before beginning the saline suppression test of plasma aldosterone. A low-sodium diet or a diuretic may be used to demonstrate renin suppression (Fig. 13.4) but the extra trouble hardly seems necessary.

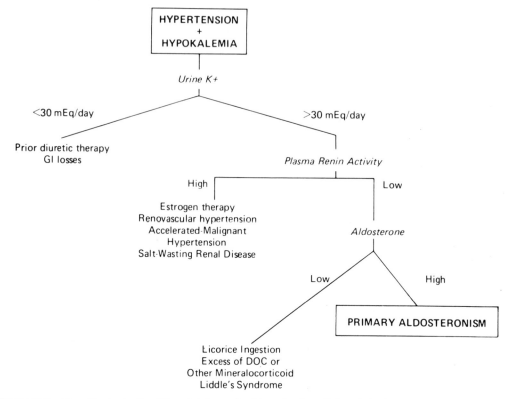

**Figure 13.6.** Flow diagram for the differential diagnosis of hypertension with hypokalemia.

5. Document that aldosterone levels are elevated and do not suppress normally. The use of a single plasma aldosterone measurement is not adequate since diurnal and episodic changes can occur (Kem et al, 1973) and such factors as posture and activity may have marked effects (Hoefnagels et al, 1980).

—Saline suppression test of plasma aldosterone:

The best approach utilizes a simple saline suppression test of plasma aldosterone (Kem et al, 1971). Plasma aldosterone is measured before and after the infusion of 2 L of normal saline over 4 hours. Patients with primary aldosteronism have higher basal levels but, more importantly, fail to suppress these levels after saline to below 10 ng/dl (Fig. 13.4). Some patients with adrenal hyperplasia may suppress to a level between 5 and 10 ng/dl after saline, so that the normal level may need to be set at 5 ng/dl when screening is done for hyperplasia (Holland et al, 1984).

—Captopril suppression test of plasma aldosterone:

Whereas plasma aldosterone levels were markedly suppressed 3 hours after oral intake of 1 mg of captopril per kilogram of body weight in patients with essential hypertension or renovascular hypertension, they remained elevated in those with primary hyperaldosteronism (Thibonnier et al, 1982). Although some have found the response to captopril to give valid data (Lyons et al, 1983), others have not (Muratani et al, 1986).

—24 hour urinary aldosterone assays:

An elevated level in a single 24-hour urine specimen collected with proper attention to sodium and potassium intake is strong evidence for the diagnosis of primary aldosteronism.

—Suppression tests of urinary aldosterone:

Since occult secondary forms of aldosteronism may mislead the clinician, various suppression tests measuring 24-hour urinary aldosterone have been advocated to confirm the presence of primary aldosterone excess, including the use of intravenous saline (Espiner et al, 1967), intramuscular deoxycorticosterone acetate

(DOCA) (Biglieri et al, 1967), or oral flu-drocortisone. In the Cleveland series, a urine aldosterone level above 14 $\mu g/24$ hour after 3 days of salt loading provided the best separation between primary aldosteronism and essential hypertension (Bravo et al, 1983).

6. Document a favorable blood pressure response to the aldosterone antagonist spironolactone (Aldactone). Spark and Melby (1968) showed that patients with primary aldosteronism had at least a 20-mm Hg fall in their diastolic blood pressure after 5 weeks of spironolactone, 100 mg 4 times a day for 5 weeks.

Since the majority of patients with low renin hypertension without aldosteronism also respond to spironolactone, many false-positives have been noted. Thus, the procedure seems no longer appropriate as a diagnostic test, but it may have prognostic value since the response to spironolactone in patients with an adenoma closely resembled their subsequent response to surgery (Ferriss et al, 1978a).

7. Rule out glucocorticoid-suppressible hyperplasia.

Although not used as a test for aldosteronism, a 7- to 10-day course of dexamethasone, 0.5 mg 4 times daily, has been advocated to recognize the rare patients with glucocorticoid-suppressible adrenal hyperplasia, whose hypertension and hyperaldosteronism should be completely relieved (Salti et al, 1969).

8. Measurement of other steroids.

The precursor of aldosterone, 18-hydroxycorticosterone (18-OHB), may be elevated even more than the aldosterone level, both in blood (Biglieri and Schambelan, 1979) and urine (Vecsei et al, 1982). Serum levels are useful both in establishing the diagnosis and separating the two major types of adrenal pathology as will be noted later in this chapter (see Fig. 13.7).

Another potent mineralocorticoid, 19-nor-deoxycorticosterone (19-nor-DOC), may be elevated in patients with primary aldosteronism (Griffing et al, 1983) along with a derivative of cortisol, 18-hydroxycortisol (Ulick and Chu, 1982).

## Excluding Other Diseases

The various causes of secondary aldosteronism listed in Table 13.1 are easily excluded by the presence of edema and high levels of peripheral blood PRA. In addition, there are a number of "pseudoaldosteronism" conditions that should be identified by history and by the presence of low levels of aldosterone.

### Conditions with High PRA

*Diuretic-Induced Hyperaldosteronism.* With the chronic use of these drugs in the treatment of hypertension, plasma volume remains shrunken, stimulating renin release and thereby a mild degree of secondary aldosteronism. Patients should not be put through urine electrolyte, renin, or aldosterone studies while on diuretics. At least 4 days should be allowed to overcome the effects of these agents, although potassium replenishment may take much longer.

*Surreptitious Gastrointestinal Losses.* Patients may either vomit or take laxatives surreptitiously. Profound hypokalemia, plasma volume depletion, and secondary aldosteronism may mimic primary aldosteronism—if by chance the patient is also hypertensive (Wolff et al, 1968).

*Hypertension During Pregnancy.* Normal pregnancy is a form of secondary aldosteronism with high PRA but with normal plasma electrolytes (Chapter 11). The occurrence of preeclampsia tends to lower the renin and aldosterone levels, although they are still above the nonpregnant range. Primary aldosteronism has been recognized during pregnancy in hypokalemic patients with even higher aldosterone levels than expected and, most importantly, suppressed PRA (Colton et al, 1984).

*Renovascular Hypertension.* Peripheral blood PRA levels may not be elevated but should not be suppressed, so the distinction should not be difficult. The degree of secondary aldosteronism is usually mild, although occasionally striking (Goldberg and McCurdy, 1963).

*Accelerated-Malignant Hypertension.* In about half of patients, hypokalemia is present as a consequence of the aldosteronism secondary to high PRA arising from the ischemic kidneys. A small number of patients having primary aldosteronism with malignant hypertension have been reported. In those in whom a PRA was measured, the level was suppressed (McAllister et al, 1971; Baxter and Wang, 1974; Aloia and Beutow, 1974). Renin measurements, therefore, should separate the few with primary aldosteronism from the many with the secondary form.

*Normotensive Patients with Pseudoaldosteronism.* Two other rare syndromes have been reported with hypokalemia but normal blood pressures: Bartter's and Gitelman's syndromes.

*Bartter's Syndrome.* Juxtaglomerular hyperplasia, hyperreninemia, and hyperaldosteronism with hypokalemic metabolic alkalosis and normotension (Bartter et al, 1962) appear to be caused by a defect in the transport of chloride in the thick ascending limb of the loop of Henle (Kurtzman and Gutierrez, 1975). A similar syndrome may result from renal sodium wasting (Cannon et al, 1968) or diuretic abuse (Ramos et al, 1980). The primary role of the kidney is further supported by the relief from hypokalemia noted in one patient after a renal transplant (Rubin, 1988).

*Gitelman's syndrome* is an even less common, familial disorder characterized by low serum potassium and magnesium levels due to their wastage into the urine by an unknown mechanism (Gitelman et al, 1966).

## Conditions with Low PRA

Unlike the previously discussed conditions with high PRA, there are some that simulate primary aldosteronism wherein PRA levels are low either because another mineralocorticoid is present or because abnormal renal salt retention occurs for unknown reasons. In all of these, aldosterone levels should also be low, whereas they are high in primary aldosteronism.

*Licorice or Carbenoxolone Ingestion.* As noted earlier, the glycyrrhetinic acid in licorice (and the ulcer drug carbenoxolone) inhibit the enzyme 11-beta-OHSD needed for conversion of the potent cortisol to the impotent cortisone in the kidney, thereby flooding the mineralocorticoid receptors with cortisol that exerts full mineralocorticoid action.

Relatively small amounts of confectionery licorice, 200 g daily for 10 days, produced sodium retention, kaliuresis, and suppression of PRA and aldosterone in normal people (Stewart et al, 1987). The metabolic changes were accompanied by a fall in cortisone and a rise in cortisol excretion. Patients who ingest large amounts of licorice may develop hypokalemia and hypertension. Since the syndrome results from excess mineralocorticoid activity, the similarity to primary aldosterone is striking, but endogenous aldosterone is suppressed. Licorice is added to some chewing tobacco, and, if the chewer swallows the saliva, pseudohyperaldosteronism may develop (Blachley and Knochel, 1980). A popular drink in France, pastis, contains liquorice extract and may also cause the syndrome (Cereda et al, 1983).

*Apparent Mineralocorticoid Excess.* The deficiency of 11-beta-OHSD may be congenital, leading to the syndrome of apparent mineralocorticoid excess, first reported in children (Werder et al, 1974) who were shown to have a defect in cortisol metabolism (Ulick et al, 1979). An adult with the same defect in the renal cortisol-cortisone shuttle has been reported with the expected hypertension, hypokalemia and suppression of renin-aldosterone (Stewart et al, 1988).

A variant has now been recognized with a normal cortisol-cortisone shuttle but another defect in cortisol clearance that apparently keeps the renal mineralocorticoid receptors flooded in the same manner (Ulick et al, 1989).

The possibility that partial defects in 11-beta-OHSD activity could be responsible for some "low-renin essential hypertension" is being actively explored (Lewicka et al, 1989).

*Excessive Secretion of Deoxycorticosterone.* Excess DOC may be produced in the following conditions:

—Cushing's syndrome, usually from ectopic ACTH-producing tumors;
—17-hydroxylase deficiency;
—21-hydroxylase deficiency;
—adrenal tumors, benign or malignant (Irony et al, 1987).

*Iatrogenic Mineralocorticoid Excess.* As with Cushing's syndrome induced by exogenous glucocorticoids, aldosteronism may be induced by exogenous mineralocorticoids, even when absorbed through the skin in an ointment for the treatment of dermatitis (Lauzurica et al, 1988). One miniepidemic was found to be caused by inadvertent use of a potent mineralocorticoid, 9-alpha-fluoroprednisone, in a nasal spray used for allergic rhinitis (Funder et al, 1979).

*Excessive Renal Sodium Conservation.* Liddle et al (1963) described members of a family with hypertension, hypokalemic alkalosis, and negligible aldosterone secretion apparently resulting from an unusual tendency of the kidneys to conserve sodium and excrete potassium even in the virtual absence of mineralocorticoids. These patients did not respond to aldosterone antagonists but did respond to triamterene (Dyrenium), which inhibits renal tubular sodium transport in the absence of aldosterone. Such patients appear to have a generalized defect in sodium transport (Gardner et al, 1971).

Another syndrome has been described with

increased renal sodium and chloride retention that causes hypertension and suppression of the renin-aldosterone mechanism, but with hyperkalemia (Gordon, 1986). The syndrome is familial and may be associated with short stature and poor dentition. Plasma levels of atrial natriuretic factor were not elevated as expected in the presence of volume expansion (Gordon et al, 1988).

This long listing of various diseases, most involving hypokalemia and many with hypertension, should not imply that the clinician must be concerned with a long and complicated differential diagnosis of primary aldosteronism. By following the diagnostic flow diagram shown in Figure 13.6, the correct diagnosis can usually be made with relative ease.

## ESTABLISHING THE TYPE OF ADRENAL PATHOLOGY

Once the diagnosis of primary aldosteronism is made, the type of adrenal pathology must be ascertained since the choice of therapy is different: surgery for an adenoma, medical for hyperplasia.

Various procedures are available for diagnosing the type of adrenal pathology (Table 13.5). The percentages given for six of the procedures are taken from Young and Klee's (1988) review of 47 published reports. The figure for dexamethasone scintigraphy is taken from Gross and Shapiro's (1989) review of 317 scans in 13 re-

ports. The large number of techniques recommended gives witness to the problems in making the differentiation and the importance of doing so. Fortunately, the resolution offered by nuclear imaging, particularly with computerized tomography (CT), is improving so rapidly that these noninvasive techniques will likely be the first, and the best, way to diagnose the type of adrenal pathology.

The currently available techniques can be divided into three groups: (1) measurement of plasma renin and aldosterone, which tend to be less abnormal in those with hyperplasia, reflecting their milder manifestations of aldosteronism; (2) attempts to suppress or stimulate aldosterone synthesis, assuming that adenomas are very responsive to ACTH but not to the renin-angiotensin system, whereas hyperplastic glands tend to be more responsive to manipulations of renin-angiotensin; and (3) direct confirmation by localizing the site of excess aldosterone secretion. The main problem with these procedures is the usually small size of aldosterone-producing adenomas, the smallest of the functional tumors rising from the adrenal.

### Individual Procedures

#### Aldosterone and Renin Levels

Although adenomas tend to be associated with higher blood pressure and aldosterone levels but

**Table 13.5.  Techniques to Differentiate Adrenal Adenoma (APA) from Bilateral Hyperplasia (IHA) in Patients with Primary Aldosteronism**

| Technique | Adenoma | Hyperplasia | Discriminatory Value |
|---|---|---|---|
| Basal aldosterone levels | High | Less high | Poor |
| Basal plasma 18-OHB | High (>50) | Less high | Excellent (82%) |
| Basal renin levels | Low | Less low | Poor |
| Multiple logistic analysis (PRA, aldosterone, K$^+$) | Greater degrees of abnormality | Lesser degrees of abnormality | Good |
| Upright posture: plasma aldosterone (PA) | Fall | Rise | Excellent (85%) |
| Suppression test (Change in PA) | | | |
|   DOC administration | None | Fall | Poor |
|   Florinef administration | None | Fall | Poor |
|   Response to spironolactone | None | Rise | Poor |
| Stimulation tests (change in PA) | | | |
|   ACTH | Rise | Less rise | Poor |
|   Saralasin | No change | Increase | Good (only one report) |
| Adrenal venography | Tumor | Bilateral enlargement | Good (66%) |
| Adrenal venous aldosterone | Increased on side of adenoma | Equal | Excellent (95%) |
| Adrenal scintiscan with | | | |
|   [131I]cholesterol | Unilateral update | Bilateral update | Good (72%) |
|   Plus dexamethasone | Persistent | Suppressed | Excellent (90%) |
| Adrenal computed tomography | Unilateral mass | Bilaterally enlarged | Good (73%) |

lower PRA and potassium levels than hyperplasia, these alone cannot make the differentiation.

### Suppression and Stimulation Tests

*Upright Posture.* This test depends upon changes in plasma aldosterone in response to variations in endogenous stimuli during 4 hours of upright posture (Ganguly et al, 1973). The premise is that adenomas are not responsive to postural increases in angiotensin (which stay suppressed anyway) but are exquisitely sensitive to diurnal changes in plasma ACTH, whereas hyperplasia is very responsive to postural changes in angiotensin (which should increase). Thus, patients with hyperplasia should have an even greater than normal *rise* in plasma aldosterone after 4 hours of standing, whereas patients with an adenoma show an anomalous *fall* in plasma aldosterone, in parallel with the falling plasma ACTH levels during the early morning hours.

These upright posture tests have provided fairly good, but not complete, discrimination. In the Indiana collection, 23 of 32 patients with adenoma had a postural fall in plasma aldosterone, but so did two of eight patients with hyperplasia (Weinberger et al, 1979). In the Cleveland series, only 20 of 33 patients with an adenoma had a postural fall as did one of 10 patients with hyperplasia (Bravo et al, 1983).

*Plasma 18-Hydroxycorticosterone.* Plasma 18-hydroxycorticosterone (18-OHB) levels have provided better separation, both in the basal (0800) and upright (1200) specimens (Biglieri and Schambelan, 1979) (Fig. 13.7).

*Suppression or Stimulation.* Other tests utilize ACTH or various mineralocorticoids to suppress or stimulate the adrenal (Table 13.5). Most have not worked well in part because some adenomas remain responsive to angiotensin II and therefore display the stimulation with upright posture or the suppression with saline or mineralocorticoids typical of hyperplasia (Gordon et al, 1987).

### Localizing Techniques

Until CT became available, invasive procedures—venography and sampling of adrenal venous blood—were usually needed because aldosterone-producing adenomas are often so small. But now, the accuracy provided by CT, magnetic resonance imaging, and scintigraphy promise to relegate the other procedures to infrequent use in the few cases not so identified.

*Adrenal Venography.* The procedure identifies most adenomas. However, the smaller size

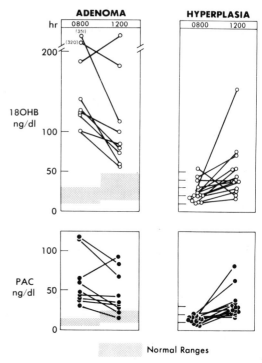

**Figure 13.7.** The 0800-hour recumbent and 1200-hour upright 18-hydroxycorticosterone (18-OHB) and plasma aldosterone concentration (*PAC*) levels in nine patients with adenoma and 14 patients with hyperplasia. (From EG, Biglieri, M, Schambelan: The significance of elevated levels of plasma 18-hydroxycorticosterone in patients with primary aldosteronism. *J Clin Endocrinol Metab* 49:87, 1979, Copyright, The Endocrine Society.)

and variation in the position of the right adrenal vein, which usually empties directly into the vena cava, may preclude its catheterization. Moreover, intraadrenal hemorrhage occurs in 10% or more of patients despite careful injection of dye.

*Adrenal Venous Plasma Aldosterone Assays.* Whereas venography may demonstrate adenomas with a diameter of 10 mm or more, assays of aldosterone from adrenal veins may lateralize adenomas as small as 3 mm (Davidson et al, 1975). In most series, patients with adenomas not only have a high aldosterone/cortisol ratio from the affected gland but also a lower ratio from the nonaffected gland than in the lower caval blood, indicative of contralateral suppression of aldosterone secretion. In the cases with hyperplasia, the ratio from both adrenals is higher than that found in the lower caval blood.

*Adrenal CT or MRI.* Most aldosterone-producing adenomas may be so identified, at least those down to 1.0 cm in diameter (Gross and

Shapiro, 1989 (Fig. 13.8). However, since some aldosterone-producing adenomas are smaller, some as small as 3 mm, the CT scan may miss them. MRI is less able to detect small aldosterone-producing tumors (Glazer et al, 1988), but improved technology may soon make it superior to CT scans (Council on Scientific Affairs, 1989).

*Adrenal Scintillation Scanning.* If the CT scan is not revealing, adrenal scintiscans offer as good discrimination and much less discomfort than adrenal vein catheterization. From 1971 to 1977, the procedure utilized [$^{131}$I]19-iodocholesterol as the tracer. Another isotope, 6-beta-[$^{131}$I]-iodomethyl-19-norcholesterol (NP-59), gives better adrenal uptake in much shorter time and superior images with less radiation exposure. Even better results have been achieved with suppression scintiscans using 0.5 or 1 mg of dexamethasone every 6 hours to discriminate between adenomas, which remain visible, and bilateral hyperplasia, which fades after a few days of dexamethasone. The NP-59 scintiscan shown in *D* of Figure 13.8 was obtained on the third day of dexamethasone, wherein the hyperplasia glands would still not be totally suppressed as would normal glands.

The published experiences with adrenal scintiscans have shown discrimination between adenoma and hyperplasia in 90% of cases (Gross and Shapiro, 1989).

Remember that those found to have hyperplasia should be considered for a trial of dexamethasone, looking for the rare glucocorticoid-suppressible syndrome. The problem of excluding adrenal hyperfunction in adrenal glands found incidentally to be enlarged by abdominal CT done for other reasons has been addressed in the first portion of Chapter 12.

## Overall Plan

The algorithm constructed by Young and Klee (1988) (Fig. 13.9) seems logical and well supported by data from various centers. The al-

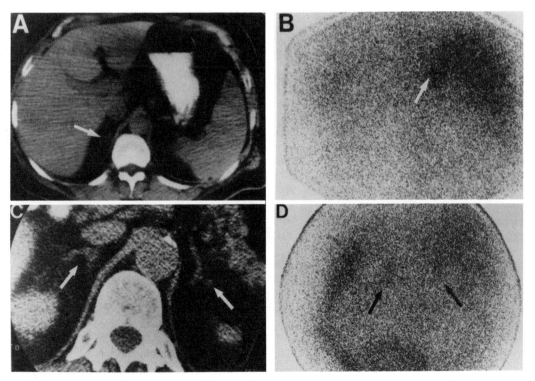

**Figure 13.8.** *A*, abdominal CT scan demonstrates a solitary adrenal mass (*arrow*). *B*, posterior abdominal NP-59 scintiscan [day 3 post NP-59 on dexamethasone suppression (DS)] identifies the abnormally functioning adrenal adenomas as a solitary focus of NP-59 update. The contralateral adrenal is not seen at this time interval. *C*, abdominal CT scan through the level of both adrenals (*arrows*) fails to demonstrate anatomic abnormalities in a case of PA due to bilateral adrenal hyperplasia. *D*, posterior abdominal NP-59 scintiscan (day 3 post NP-59 on DS) identifies faint, but definitely abnormal, bilateral NP-59 uptake (*arrows*). (From Gross MD, Shapiro B: *Semin Nuc Med* 19:122, 1989.)

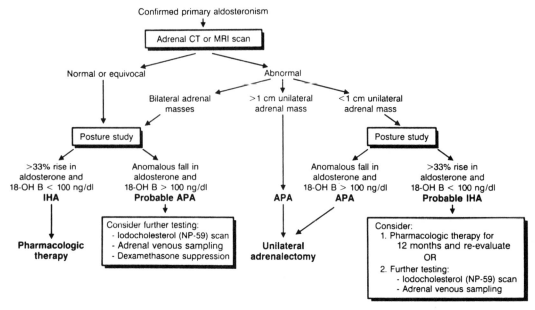

**Figure 13.9.** Algorithm for the diagnostic differentiation between adenoma (*APA*) and bilateral hyperplasia (*IHA*). The details are discussed in the text. *18-OH B*, 18-hydroxycorticosterone; *CT*, computed tomography; *MRI*, magnetic resonance imaging. (From Young WF Jr, Klee GG: *Endocrinol Metab Clin N Am* 17:367, 1988.)

gorithm starts with a CT or MRI scan of the adrenals. If a unilateral mass or two symmetrical glands are clearly seen, the diagnosis is established except for the rare occurrence of an incidental nonfunctioning tumor on one side and an adenoma on the other (Soma et al, 1989).

The algorithm next indicates a posture study, obtaining plasma aldosterone and 18-OHB levels before and after 4 hours of standing (0800 and 1200), which has been found to have better than an 80% accuracy in distinguishing the type of adrenal pathology (Young and Klee, 1988).

If the posture study is supportive of an adenoma but the CT or MRI scan does not show a unilateral mass, an adrenal scintiscan is the next procedure recommended, rarely to be followed by adrenal venous sampling.

## THERAPY

Having put the patient through as much of a workup as is needed, the type of adrenal pathology should be known with virtual certainty. If the diagnosis is *adenoma*, surgery should be done; if it is *bilateral hyperplasia*, medical therapy is indicated.

### Surgical Treatment

#### Preoperative Management

Once the diagnosis is made, a 3- to 5-week course of spironolactone therapy may be given,

both as an additional diagnostic study and as a guide to the probable response of the hypertension to removal of an adenoma if that is the lesion, or to chronic medical therapy if hyperplasia is the lesion (Ferriss et al, 1978a). Since most patients have an adenoma, additional advantage is gained with spironolactone therapy; not only should the hypertension be controlled, but the various disturbances of electrolyte composition and fluid volume should also be normalized, easing anesthetic, surgical, and postoperative management (Morimoto et al, 1970).

### Surgical Technique

Some surgeons use the lumbar approach, and others prefer the transabdominal one. With improved preoperative diagnosis of an adenoma, a unilateral extraperitoneal approach seems preferable (Auda et al, 1980).

If bilateral hyperplasia is found at surgery despite the preoperative diagnosis of an adenoma, only a left adrenalectomy should be done. In view of the poor overall results with bilateral adrenalectomy and its complications, one gland should be left intact.

### Postoperative Management

The patient, even if given spironolactone preoperatively, may develop hypoaldosteronism with an inability to conserve sodium and excrete potassium (Biglieri et al, 1966). The aldosterone deficiency may persist for some time after renin levels return to normal, analogous to the slowness of the return of cortisol production after prolonged ACTH suppression by exogenous glucocorticoids (Conn et al, 1964).

The aldosterone deficiency is usually not severe or prolonged and can be handled simply by providing adequate salt without the need for exogenous glucocorticoid or mineralocorticoid therapy. However, five of 33 patients who had unilateral adrenalectomy for an adenoma were symptomatically hypotensive 1 year later, some with low plasma cortisol, others with low plasma aldosterone and adrenaline levels (Gordon et al, 1989).

In most patients, the electrolyte abnormalities are corrected quickly and the renin-aldosterone system returns to normal within 6 months (Weinberger et al, 1982), but the hypertension may persist for some time, with a few patients requiring years for return of normal blood pressure. In 13 series published since 1978 involving 466 patients, 64% were cured of hypertension and 33% were improved (Shenker, 1989).

If the blood pressure fails to respond, hyperfunctioning adrenal tissue may have been left. More likely is the presence of coincidental essential hypertension or the occurrence of significant renal damage from the prolonged hypertension (O'Neal et al, 1970; Danforth et al, 1977). Few with bilateral hyperplasia respond to unilateral (Groth et al, 1985) or even to bilateral adrenalectomy (Ferriss et al, 1978a).

## Medical Treatment

Chronic medical therapy with spironolactone or amiloride with or without a thiazide diuretic is the treatment of choice for patients with hyperplasia, patients with an adenoma who are unable or unwilling to have surgery, those who remain hypertensive after surgery, and those with equivocal findings. Initial experience with a calcium antagonist, nifedipine, has shown excellent control of blood pressure and reduction of aldosterone levels in patients with hyperplasia (Nadler et al, 1985) but not in those with an adenoma (Bursztyn et al, 1988).

Therapy with spironolactone usually lowers the blood pressure and keeps it down (Ferriss et al, 1978a). After starting with doses of 100 to 200 mg a day, a satisfactory response may be maintained with as little as 50 mg a day. The combination of the spironolactone with a thiazide diuretic may provide even better control and allow for smaller doses of spironolactone (Bravo et al, 1972).

With these lower doses the various side effects were generally minor, and in only three of 95 cases were they severe enough to lead to withdrawal of the drug (Ferriss et al, 1978a). Aspirin should be avoided since it will antagonize the effects of spironolactone (Tweeddale and Ogilvie, 1973).

Patients with hyperplasia respond much better to medical therapy than to surgery. In half of the patients with hyperplasia, chronic spironolactone therapy kept the blood pressure normal for as long as 8 years (Ferriss et al, 1978a).

The rare patient who cannot tolerate spironolactone but still needs medical therapy can be controlled by a low salt intake plus another potassium-sparing diuretic such as triamterene (Ganguly and Weinberger, 1981) or amiloride (Griffing et al, 1982).

Various inhibitors of steroidogenesis may be useful, particularly in those with adrenal cancer. These include *trilostane*, a competitive inhibitor of adrenal 3-beta-hydroxysteroid dehydrogenase (Nomura et al, 1986); *ketoconazole*, an inhibitor of the P-450-dependent enzymes 11-beta- and 18-hydroxylase (Leal-Cerro et al, 1988), and, perhaps, CGS16949A, an inhibitor of aromatase (Demers et al, 1989). The only proven effective agent for adrenal carcinoma is o,p'-DDD (mitotane) (Shenker, 1989).

## CONCLUSION

Primary aldosteronism remains a fascinating disease that has probably generated as many publications as the number of patients found to have it as the cause of their hypertension. We turn from it to another adrenal endocrinopathy, also rare in its natural state but more often induced—Cushing's syndrome, and an even rarer group of congenital adrenal hyperplasias.

### References

Aloia JF, Beutow G: *Am J Med Sci* 268:241, 1974.

Andersen GS, Toftdahl DB, Lund OJ, et al: *J Hum Hypertens* 2:187, 1988.

Arriza JL, Weinberger C, Cerelli G, et al: *Science* (Wash DC) 237:268, 1987.

Arteaga E, Biglieri EG, Kater CE, et al: *Ann Intern Med* 101:316, 1984.

Auda SP, Brennan MF, Gill JR Jr: *Ann Surg* 191:1, 1980.

Baer L, Sommers SC, Krakoff KR, et al: *Circ Res* 26-27(Suppl 1):203, 1970.

Bartter FC, Pronove P, Gill JR Jr, et al: *Am J Med* 33:811, 1962.

Baxter RH, Wang I: *Scott Med J* 19:161, 1974.

Beevers DG, Nelson CS, Padfield PL, et al: *Acta Clin Belg* 29:276, 1974.

Beevers DG, Brown JJ, Ferriss JB, et al: *Q J Med* 45:401, 1976.

Berglund G, Andersson O, Wilhelmsen L: *Br Med J* 2:554, 1976.

Biglieri EG: *Am J Hypertens* 1:313, 1988.

Biglieri EG, Irony I, Kater CE: *J Steroid Biochem* 32:199, 1989.

Biglieri EG, McIlhoy MD: *Circulation* 33:78, 1966.

Biglieri EG, Schambelan M: *J Clin Endocrinol Metab* 49:87, 1979.

Biglieri EG, Schambelan M, Slaton PE, et al: *Circ Res* 26-27 (Suppl 1): *195, 1970.*

*Biglieri EG, Slaton PE Jr, Silen WS, et al: J Clin Endocrinol Metab* 26:553, 1966.

Biglieri EG, Slaton PE Jr, Kronfield SJ, et al: *JAMA* 201:510, 1967.

Blachley JD, Knochel JP: *N Engl J Med* 302:784, 1980.

Bravo EL, Tarazi RC, Dustan HP: *Circulation* 45-46 (Suppl 2):83, 1972 (abstract).

Bravo EL, Tarazi RC, Dustan HP, et al: *Am J Med* 74:641, 1983.

Bravo EL, Fouad-Tarazi FM, Tarazi RC, et al: *Hypertension* 11(Suppl I):I207, 1988.

Bursztyn M, Grossman E, Rosenthal T: *Am J Hypertens* 1:88S, 1988.

Cannon PJ, Leeming JM, Sommers SC, et al: *Medicine* (Baltimore)47:107, 1968.

Card WI, Mitchell W, Strong JA, et al: *Lancet* 1:63, 1953.

Cereda JM, Trono D, Schifferli J: *Lancet* 1:1442, 1983.

Colton R, Perez GO, Fishman LM: *Am J Obstet Gynecol* 150:892, 1984.

Conn JW, Rovner DR, Cohen EL, et al: *JAMA* 195:111, 1966.

Conn JW: *Harvey Lect* 62:257, 1968.

Conn JW, Cohen E, Rovner DR: *JAMA* 190:213, 1964.

Conn JW, Cohen ED, Rovner DR: *JAMA* 193:200, 1965.

Council on Scientific Affairs: *JAMA* 261:420, 1989.

Danforth DW, Orlando MM, Bartter FC, et al: *J Urol* 117:140, 1977.

Davidson JK, Morley P, Hurley GC, et al: *Br J Radiol* 48:435, 1975.

Demers LM, Melby J, Lipton A, Harvey H: Program 1989, Endocrine Society, June 21, 1989, Seattle, Abstract 414, pg. 126.

Dluhy RG, Williams GH: *J Clin Endocrinol* 29:1319, 1969.

Edwards CRW, Stewart PM, Burt D, et al: *Lancet* 2:986, 1988.

Espiner EA, Tucci JR, Jagger PI, et al: *N Engl J Med* 277:1, 1967.

Ferriss JB, Beevers DG, Boddy K, et al: *Am Heart J* 96:97, 1978a.

Ferriss JB, Beevers DG, Brown JJ, et al: *Am Heart J* 95:375, 1978b.

Ferriss JB, Brown JJ, Cumming AMM, et al: *Acta Endocrinol* 103:365, 1983a.

Ferris JB, Brown JJ, Fraser R, et al: *Handbook of Hypertension*, Robertson JIS (ed): *Clinical Aspects of Secondary Hypertension.* New York, Elsevier, 1983b, vol 2, p 132.

Flanagan MJ, McDonald JH: *J Urol* 98:133, 1967.

Fukuda K, Baba A, Kuchii M, et al: *J Hypertens* 6(Suppl 4):S261, 1988.

Funder JW, Adam WR, Mantero F, et al: *J Clin Endocrinol Metab* 49:841, 1979.

Ganguly A, Melada GA, Luetscher JA, et al: *J Clin Endocrinol Metab* 37:765, 1973.

Ganguly A, Weinberger MH: *Clin Pharmacol Ther* 30:246, 1981.

Ganguly A, Yum MN, Pratt JH, et al: *Clin Exp Hypertens* A5:1635, 1983.

Ganguly A, Weinberger MH, Guthrie GP, et al: *Hypertension* 6:305, 1984.

Gardner JD, Lapey A, Simopoulos AP, et al: *J Clin Invest* 50:2253, 1971.

Gardner JD, Simopoulos AP, Lapey A, et al: *J Clin Invest* 51:1565, 1972.

Gifford RW Jr: *Milbank Mem Fund Q* 47:170, 1969.

Gill JR Jr, Bartter FC: *J Clin Endocrinol Metab* 53:331, 1981.

Gitelman HJ, Graham JB, Welt LG: *Trans Assoc Am Phys* 79:221, 1966.

Glazer GM, Francis IR, Quint LE: *Invest Radiol* 23:3, 1988.

Goldberg M, McCurdy DK: *Ann Intern Med* 59:24, 1963.

Gomez-Sanchez CE, Gill JR Jr, Ganguly A, et al: *J Clin Endocrinol Metab* 67:444, 1988.

Gonzalez-Campoy JM, Romero JC, Knox FG: *Kidney Int* 35:767, 1989.

Gordon RD: *Hypertension* 8:93, 1986.

Gordon RD, Gomez-Sanchez CE, Hamlet SM, et al: *J Hypertens* 5(Suppl 5):S103, 1987.

Gordon RD, Hawkins PG, Hamlet SM, et al: *J Hypertens* 7(Suppl 6):S210, 1989.

Gordon RD, Ravenscroft PJ, Klemm SA, Tunny TJ, Hamlet SM: *J Hypertens* 6(Suppl 4):S323, 1988.

Griffing GT, Berelowitz B, Hudson M, et al: *J Clin Invest* 76:163, 1985.

Griffing GT, Cole AG, Aurecchia SA, et al: *Clin Pharmacol Ther* 31:56, 1982.

Griffing GT, Dale SL, Holbrook MM, et al: *J Clin Endocrinol Metab* 56:218, 1983.

Grim CE, Weinberger MH, Higgins JT, et al: *JAMA* 237:1331, 1977.

Gross MD, Shapiro B: *Semin Nuc Med* 19:122, 1989.

Groth H, Vetter W, Stimpel M, et al: *Cardiology* 72(Suppl 1):107, 1985.

Hamlet SM, Tunny TJ, Woodland E, et al: *Clin Exp Pharmacol Physiol* 12:249, 1985.

Hiramatsu K, Yamada T, Yukimura Y, et al: *Arch Intern Med* 141:1589, 1981.

Hoefnagels WHL, Drayer JIM, Smals AGH, et al: *J Clin Endocrinol Metab* 51:1330, 1980.

Holland OB, Brown H, Kuhnert L, et al: *Hypertension* 6:717, 1984.

Hyman D, Kaplan NM: *N Engl J Med* 313:642, 1985.

Irony I, Biglieri EG, Perloff D, Rubinoff H: *J Clin Endocrinol Metab* 65:836, 1987.

Jackson B, Valentine R, Wagner G: *Aust NZ J Med* 16:69, 1986.

Jeffries WB, Wang Y, Pettinger WA: *Am J Physiol* 254:F739, 1988.

Kageyama Y, Bravo EL: *Hypertension* 11:750, 1988.

Kaplan NM: *N Engl J Med* 269:1282, 1963.

Kaplan NM: *Ann Intern Med* 66:1079, 1967.

Kaplan NM: *Clinical Endocrinology*, Volume 2. New York: Grune & Stratton, 1968:468.

Dem DC, Weinberger MH, Mayes DM, et al: *Arch Intern Med* 128:380, 1971.

Kem DC, Weinberger MH, Gomez-Sanchez CE, et al: *J Clin Invest* 52:2272, 1973.

Kem DC, Tang K, Hanson CS, et al: *J Clin Endocrinol Metab* 60:67, 1985.

Kloppenborg PWC, Drayer JIM, Van Haelst AJG, et al: *Neth J Med* 17:239, 1974.

Kurtzman NA, Gutierrez LF: *JAMA* 234:758, 1975.

Lauzurica R, Bonal J, Bonet J, et al: *J Hum Hypertens* 2:183, 1988.

Leal-Cerro A, Garcia-Luna P, Villar J, et al: *N Engl J Med* 318:710, 1988.

Ledingham JGG, Bull MB, Laragh JH: *Circ Res* 20-21 (Suppl 2):177, 1967.

Lewicka S, Vecsei P, Abdelhamid S, et al: Program 1989, Endocrine Society, June 21, 1989, Seattle, Abstract 413, p 126.

Liddle GW, Bledsoe T, Coppage WS Jr: *Trans Assoc Am Phys* 76:199, 1963.

Lins P-E, Adamson U: *Acta Endocrinol (Copenh)* 113:564, 1986.

Lüscher T, Tenschert W, Salvetti A, et al: *Klin Wochenschr* 62:470, 1984.

Lyons DF, Kem DC, Brown RD, et al: *J Clin Endocrinol Metab* 57:892, 1983.

Mader IJ, Iseri LT: *Am J Med* 19:976, 1955.

Man in't Veld AJ, Wenting GJ, Schalekamp MADH: *J Cardiovasc Pharmacol* 6:S143, 1984.

Matsunaga M, Hara A, Song TS, et al: *Hypertension* 5:240, 1983.

McAllister RG Jr, Van Way CW, Dayani K, et al: *Circ Res* 28-29(Suppl 2):160, 1971.

Melby JC, Spark RF, Dale SL, et al: *N Engl J Med* 277:1050, 1967.

Menard MR, Friedman SM: *Hypertension* 7:873, 1985.

Morimoto S, Takeda R, Murakami M: *J Clin Endocrinol Metab* 31:659, 1970.

Moura A-M, Angeli M, Worcel M: *Kidney Int* 34(Suppl 26):S8, 1988.

Muratani H, Abe I, Tomita Y, et al: *Am Heart J* 112:361, 1986.

Neville AM, Symington T: *Cancer* (Phila) 19:1854, 1966.

Nomura K, Demura H, Horiba N, et al: *Acta Endocrinol* (Copenh) 113:104, 1986.

O'Neal LW, Kissane JM, Hartroft PM: *Arch Surg* 100:498, 1970.

Oberfield SE, Levine LS, Firpo A, et al: *Hypertension* 6:75, 1984.

Ramos E, Hall-Craggs M, Demers LM: *JAMA* 243:1070, 1980.

Reidbord H, Fisher ER: *Arch Pathol* 88:155, 1969.

Rubin A: *Acta Med Scand* 224:165, 1988.

Salti IS, Stiefel M, Ruse JL, et al: *Can Med Assoc J* 101:1, 1969.

Seldin DW, Rector JC Jr: *Kidney Int* 1:306, 1972.

Sen S, Bumpus FM, Oberfield S, et al: *Hypertension* 5(Suppl I):I-27, 1983.

Shenker Y: *Endocrin Metab Clin North Am* 18:415, 1989.

Soma R, Miyamori I, Nakagawa A, et al: *J Endocrinol Invest* 12:183, 1989.

Sonkodi S, Nicholls MG, Cumming AMM, et al: *Clin Endocrinol* 14:613, 1981.

Spark RF, Melby JC: *Ann Intern Med* 69:685, 1968.

Stewart PM, Wallace AM, Valentino R, et al: *Lancet* 2:821, 1987.

Stewart PM, Corrie JET, Shackleton CHL, et al: *J Clin Invest* 82:340, 1988.

Streeten DHP, Tomycz N, Anderson GH Jr: *Am J Med* 67:403, 1979.

Sutherland DA, Ruse JL, Laidlaw JC: *Can Med Assoc J* 95:1109, 1966.

Suzuki T, Abe H, Nagata S, et al: *Am J Cardiol* 62:1224, 1988.

Tarazi RC, Ibrahim MM, Bravo EL, et al: *N Engl J Med* 289:1330, 1973.

Thibonnier M, Sassano P, Joseph A, et al: *Cardiovasc Rev Rep* 3:1659, 1982.

Tunny TJ, Gordon RD: *Lancet* 1:272, 1986.

Tweeddale MG, Ogilvie RI: *N Engl J Med* 289:198, 1973.

Ulick S, Levine LS, Gunczler P, et al: *J Clin Endocrinol Metab* 49:757, 1979.

Ulick S, Chu MD: *Clin Exp Hypertens* A4:1771, 1982.

Ulick S, Chan CK, Rao KN, Edassery J, Mantero F: *J Steroid Biochem* 32:209, 1989.

Vaughan NJA, Slater JDH, Lightman SL, et al: *Lancet* 1:120, 1981.

Vecsei P, Abdelhamid S, Haack D, et al: *Clin Exp Hypertens* A4:1759, 1982.

Weinberger MH, Grim CE, Hollifield JW, et al: *Ann Intern Med* 90:386, 1979.

Weinberger MH, Grim CE, Kramer NJ, et al: *Clin Exp Hypertens* A4:1715, 1982.

Wenting GJ, Man in't Veld AJ, Derkx FHM, et al: *Clin Exp Hypertens* A4:1727, 1982.

Werder E, Zachmann M, VOllmin JA, et al: *Res Steroids* 6:385, 1974.

Williams ED, Boddy K, Brown JJ, et al: *J Hypertens* 2:171, 1984.

Wolff HP, Krück F, Brown JJ, et al: *Lancet* 1:257, 1968.

Young DB, Guyton AC: *Circ Res* 40:138, 1977.

Young WF JR, Klee GG: *Endocrinol Metab Clin N Am* 17:367, 1988.

# 14 Cushing's Syndrome and Congenital Adrenal Hyperplasia

In addition to aldosterone, an excess of other hormones secreted by the adrenal cortex may cause hypertension. The most common is cortisol excess, referred to as Cushing's syndrome. Less commonly involved are various other mineralocorticoids whose hypersecretion usually reflects inborn errors of cortisol synthesis.

## CUSHING'S SYNDROME

Cushing's syndrome is a serious disease with a mortality rate, even after successful therapy, 4 times above that of an age- sex-matched population (Ross and Linch, 1982). Much of the excess mortality is caused by cardiovascular disease. Hypertension, present in over 80% of patients with Cushing's syndrome, is a major risk factor for the development of premature cardiovascular disease.

### Etiology

The syndrome is caused by excess glucocorticoid, either cortisol with the idiopathic form or various exogenous steroids with the iatrogenic form. As shown in Figure 14.1, the idiopathic disease may be caused by:

—ACTH-dependent mechanisms with bilateral adrenal hyperplasia:
  —pituitary hypersecretion of adrenocorticotrophic hormone (ACTH), i.e., Cushing's *disease* (about 70% of all cases), or
  —ectopic ACTH from various tumors (about 12%) (Findling and Tyrrell, 1986)
—ACTH-independent mechanisms:
  —adrenal tumors, either benign or malignant (about 12%) or
  —primary adrenal hyperplasia (about 5%)

Some interesting variants have been reported, including these:

—bilateral adrenal adenomas (Mimou et al, 1985);
—unilateral nodular hyperplasia (Josse et al, 1980);
—spontaneously remitting disease (Kammer and Barter, 1979);
—cyclic or episodic disease (Atkinson et al, 1985);
—an association with overt hypothalamic disorders (Berlinger et al, 1977);
—transition from pituitary-dependent to pituitary-independent disease (Hermus et al, 1988);
—familial micronodular adrenocortical dysplasia (Hodge and Froesch, 1988);
—ACTH-independent bilateral macronodular hyperplasia (Malchoff et al, 1989).

### Hypertension in Cushing's Syndrome

Hypertension is present in about 80% of patients with Cushing's syndrome. It may be severe; in the series of Ross and Linch (1982), 10 of 70 patients had pressure exceeding 200/120 mm Hg, and all but one of these died despite treatment of the Cushing's syndrome. Among all 70, 55% had an abnormal electrocardiogram (ECG) and 28% had cardiomegaly.

Unlike what is seen in primary hypertension and some other secondary forms of hypertension, the elevated blood pressure (BP) in patients with Cushing's syndrome does not fall during sleep (Imai et al, 1988). Moreover, the normal nocturnal fall in BP can be eliminated with exogenous glucocorticoids.

#### Incidence with Exogenous Steroids

The high incidence of hypertension in naturally occurring Cushing's syndrome is in contrast to its relative rarity in patients who take exogenous glucocorticoids or ACTH (David et al, 1970). The incidence is thought to be so low

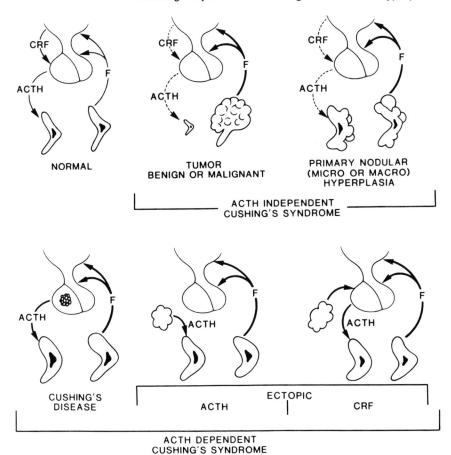

**Figure 14.1.** Etiologies of endogenous Cushing's syndrome. The lesions on the top arise within the adrenal. Those on the bottom arise within the pituitary (Cushing's disease) or from ectopic production of ACTH or CRF. (From Carpenter PC: *Endocrinol Metab Clin North Am* 17:445, 1988.)

because most patients are given steroid derivatives with less mineralocorticoid activity than cortisol. Even less trouble will be seen with alternate day therapy (Axelrod, 1976) or with low doses: Continuous therapy in the range of 10 mg/per day of prednisone did not induce hypertension (Jackson et al, 1981).

Even though hypertension is relatively infrequent with exogenous ACTH or nonmineralocorticoid glucocorticoids, significant rises of BP do occur within 5 days of their administration in fairly high doses to normal subjects (Whitworth et al, 1989). These rises in blood pressure developed in the absence of sodium retention or volume expansion. These findings suggest some direct "hypertensinogenic" effect of adrenal steroids beyond the mechanisms held responsible for the development of hypertension in endogenous Cushing's syndrome (Krakoff, 1988).

## Mechanisms for the Hypertension

Multiple mechanisms may be responsible for the hypertension so common in Cushing's disease. They are:

1. The salt-retaining action of the high levels of cortisol (Sudhir et al, 1989). Although only 1/300 as potent a mineralocorticoid as aldosterone, 200 times more cortisol is normally secreted, and this level is increased 2-fold or more in Cushing's disease.
2. Increased production of mineralocorticoids. Though usually noted in patients with adrenal tumors (Kater et al, 1986), increased levels of 19-nor-deoxycorticosterone (Ehlers et al, 1987), deoxycorticosterone (DOC), and, less commonly, aldosterone (Cassar et al, 1980) have been found in patients with all forms of the syndrome.
3. Increased levels and activity of renin-angio-

tensin. The levels of renin substrate are increased by exogenous cortisol and in patients with Cushing's syndrome (Saruta et al, 1986). A marked fall in blood pressure was noted with the angiotensin-converting enzyme inhibitor, captopril, in five of 10 patients with Cushing's syndrome (Greminger et al, 1984).

4. Increased sympathetic nervous system activity. Glucocorticoids induce the enzyme phenylethanolamine N-methyltransferase (PNMT), responsible for the conversion of norepinephrine to epinephrine, both in the adrenal gland and in the brain.

5. Increased vascular reactivity to catecholamines (Mendlowitz et al, 1958).

Other mechanisms may also be involved:

—an increased activity of the $Na^+$,$K^+$-ATPase pump in red blood cells (Wambach et al, 1984);
—an inhibition of the production of vasodilatory prostaglandins by glucocorticoids (Saruta et al, 1986);
—the hyperinsulinemia secondary to insulin resistance (Rebuffe'-Scrive et al, 1988), which is likely involved in the hypertension seen in other forms of upper body obesity (Kaplan, 1989).

## Clinical Features

Many more patients with cushingoid features are seen than the relatively few who have the syndrome. The differential can be made with fair reliability using the clinical features shown in the *top portion* of Table 14.1 (Ross and Linch, 1982). The index shows that the findings of bruising, myopathy, hypertension, plethora, edema, hirsutism, and red striae were of most power in discriminating patients with Cushing's syndrome from those with suggestive features who did not have the disease.

Various neuropsychiatric disturbances ranging from a mild decrease in energy to a severe depression were found in 62% of Ross and Linch's series. The depression common in Cushing's syndrome is in contrast to the euphoria frequently observed with glucocorticoid therapy. Non-Cushing's patients with endogenous depression may have hypercortisolism related to increased ACTH pulse frequency (Mortola et al, 1987), but their basal cortisol levels are usually normal and they do not hyperrespond to corticotrophin-releasing hormone (Gold et al, 1986).

Alcoholics often display numerous features suggestive of Cushing's syndrome, including

**Table 14.1. Discriminant Indices of Clinical Features in Cushing's Syndrome**[a]

| Clinical Features | Discriminant Index in Series | |
|---|---|---|
| | Present (70 Cases) | Collected (711 Cases) |
| Strong discrimatory value | | |
| Bruising | 10.3 | 10.5 |
| Myopathy | 8.0 | 7.1 |
| Hypertension | 4.4 | 5.1 |
| Plethora | 3.0 | 3.6 |
| Edema | 2.9 | 3.3 |
| Hirsutism in women | 2.8 | 2.7 |
| Red striae | 2.5 | 3.1 |
| Less discriminatory value | | |
| Menstrual irregularity | 1.6 | 1.6 |
| Truncal obesity | 1.6 | |
| Headaches | 1.3 | 1.1 |
| No discriminatory value | | |
| Acne | 0.9 | |
| Generalized obesity | 0.8 | |
| Impaired glucose tolerance | 0.7 | 0.7 |

[a]The index is obtained by dividing the prevalence of each feature in the separate series of patients with Cushing's syndrome, the authors' 70 cases, and the 711 cases collected from the literature by its prevalence in the series of Nugent et al (1964) of 159 mostly obese patients in whom the diagnosis of Cushing's syndrome was suspected but not biochemically substantiated.

From Ross EJ, Linch DC: *Lancet* 2:646, 1982.

hypertension and a failure to suppress plasma cortisol after overnight dexamethasone (Kapcala, 1987). Alcohol should be withdrawn for at least 2 weeks before studies are done.

## Laboratory Diagnosis*

The extent of the workup of patients suspected of having Cushing's varies with the clinical situation: A measurement of urine-free cortisol or an overnight 1-mg dexamethasone suppression test will be adequate for most with only minimally suggestive features; those with highly suggestive features should have both the low- and high-dose urinary suppression test (Fig. 14.2). The urine-free cortisol measurement is an excellent discriminator: Only 5% of patients with Cushing's but 95% of obese patients excrete less than 100 $\mu$g per day (Crapo, 1979). Random plasma cortisol levels provide much less discrimination because of the marked minute to minute variation, reflecting episodic secretion from the adrenals (Hellman et al, 1970). Though their plasma levels are almost always higher, patients with Cushing's syndrome also

*The data to be presented all use the traditional units of $\mu$g/dl or mg/d. To convert to SI units:
—Plasma cortisol from $\mu$g/dl to nmol/L: multiply by 27.6;
—Urine cortisol from $\mu$g/24 hour to nmol/d: multiply by 2.76;
—Urine 17-hydroxycorticoids from mg/d to $\mu$mol/d: multiply by 2.76;
—Plasma ACTH from pg/ml to pmol/L: multiply by 0.22.

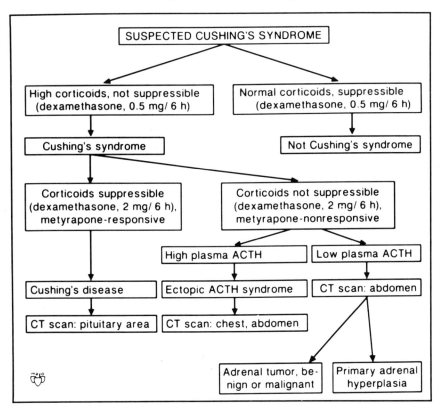

**Figure 14.2.** Evaluation of patients with suspected Cushing's syndrome. Because some medications alter ACTH production rate, patients should be medication free before initiation of assessment. *ACTH*, adrenocorticotropic hormone; *CT*, computed tomography. (From Carpenter PC: *Mayo Clin Proc* 61:49, 1986.)

secrete cortisol episodically (Liu et al, 1987). These variations show the need for some type of suppression test to assess adrenal hyperfunction adequately.

*Plasma Suppression.* For screening of patients with cushingoid features, the single bedtime 1-mg-dose dexamethasone suppression test, measuring the plasma cortisol at 8 a.m. the next morning, has worked very well with fewer than 2% false-negative results (Crapo, 1979).

False-positive results are seen in 10 to 20% of non-Cushing's patients (Crapo, 1979). One reason is too rapid inactivation of the exogenous dexamethasone to produce suppression of the pituitary-adrenal system in patients taking drugs that stimulate the hepatic drug-metabolizing enzymes such as dipheylhydantoin, barbiturates, tolbutamide, rifampin, and perhaps alcohol (Elias and Gwinup, 1980).

Another reason may be the overriding effect of stress or endogenous depression. Patients in a hospital frequently fail to suppress nearly as well as they do when restudied as outpatients (Connolly et al, 1968). Patients with endogenous depression may also fail to respond to dexamethasone (Carroll et al, 1980).

*Dexamethasone Suppression.* If the screening test is abnormal or the clinical evidence is very strong, the presence of hypercortisolism can be virtually assured by the finding that urine (and, perhaps, plasma) levels of cortisol cannot be normally suppressed by a "low dose" of 0.5 mg of dexamethasone every 6 hours for 2 days (Liddle, 1960). This amount of dexamethasone is equivalent to about 40 mg of cortisol, approximately twice the normal daily secretion rate. In Crapo's review, 240 of 241 controls without Cushing's syndrome suppressed below 4.0 mg/day of urine 17-hydroxycorticosteroid (17-OHCS) or 25 $\mu$g/day of urine-free cortisol, whereas only nine of 154 patients with Cushing's syndrome suppressed below those levels.

To circumvent the need for multiple 24-hour urine collections, plasma cortisol may be measured. When blood was obtained at 8 a.m. on the morning after the 2 days of low-dose dexamethasone, serum cortisol was below 2.2 $\mu$g/dl in 31 of 32 without Cushing's syndrome and above 9.1 $\mu$g/dl in 12 of 13 with Cushing's syndrome (Kennedy et al, 1984).

Dexamethasone suppression tests may give anomalous results because excessive hormone secretion may be cyclic (Atkinson et al, 1985) or variable, even from an adenoma (Green and Van't Hoff, 1975). One patient has been described whose hypothalamic-pituitary feedback mechanism failed to recognize dexamethasone but did suppress with cortisol (Carey, 1980).

## Establishing the Cause of the Syndrome

Once Cushing's syndrome has been diagnosed, the type of pathology needs to be accurately determined to guide therapy. The ability to visualize both the pituitary and adrenals with greater ease and accuracy by means of computed tomography (CT) and magnetic resonance imaging (MRI) will reduce the dependence upon functional tests.

### Laboratory Studies

The longest and largest experience has been with dexamethasone suppression, but other procedures, such as the metyrapone test (Sindler et al, 1983) or corticotropin-releasing hormone stimulation (Nieman et al, 1986), may be used.

*Dexamethasone Suppression* (Fig. 14.2). The "high-dose" test is an extension of the "low-dose" test, predicated on the resetting of the pituitary-cortisol feedback mechanism at a higher level in those with ACTH-dependent Cushing's disease arising in the pituitary: Whereas a low dose of dexamethasone, i.e., the equivalent of 40 mg of cortisol per day, will not suppress the hyperfunctioning pituitary, a high dose, i.e., the equivalent of 160 mg of cortisol per day, usually will. On the other hand, not even the high dose will usually suppress an adrenal tumor or an ectopic ACTH-producing tumor. With a 40% decrease from baseline urinary cortisol on the second day of 2.0 mg every 6 hours as indicative of suppression, 84 of 91 patients with pituitary Cushing's syndrome suppressed, whereas only one of 44 with an adrenal tumor and four of 20 with ectopic ACTH tumor suppressed (Crapo, 1979).

*Plasma ACTH.* Plasma ACTH levels should clearly separate the three major forms of Cushing's syndrome (Fig 14.1), with adrenal tumors having very low levels, pituitary hyperfunction having "normal" levels (which are abnormally high in the presence of elevated plasma cortisol), and ectopic Cushing's syndrome having very high levels. ACTH and lipotropins (LPH) are synthesized through a common precursor, proopiomelanocortin, in the pituitary. Kuhn et al (1989) have found that assays of plasma ACTH and LPH give excellent separation between the three forms of Cushing's syndrome, with even better results from the LPH assay, perhaps because LPH is more stable in blood. Rarely, sampling of inferior petrosal venous sinus blood will be needed to localize ACTH-secreting pituitary microadenomas (Oldfield et al, 1985).

*Corticotropin-Releasing Factor Test.* The availability of ovine or human corticotropin-releasing factor (CRF) provides another way to differentiate various forms of cortisol excess. A marked rise in plasma ACTH and cortisol occurs after an intravenous bolus of long-acting ovine CRF in patients with pituitary Cushing's, but no change is seen in either ACTH or cortisol in patients with ectopic ACTH secretion (Nieman et al, 1986).

### Radiological Studies

If the hormonal tests indicate ACTH-independent disease, the adrenal glands should be scanned by CT or MRI (Carpenter, 1988). [131]I-6-$\beta$-iodomethylnorcholesterol (NP-59) scintigraphy will identify some lesions that are too small to be seen on CT (Fig et al, 1988).

If the tests indicate ACTH-dependent disease, CT or MRI scans should look for a pituitary or ectopic tumor. The majority of CT scans of the pituitary are negative in patients with Cushing's disease. A positive scan actually diminishes the probability of clinical remission following transsphenoidal surgery: At the Mayo Clinic, 95% of those with negative pituitary CT scans had a postoperative remission, but only 68% of those with a positive preoperative scan had a remission (Carpenter, 1988).

CT scans of the lungs and abdomen should be performed in those suspected of ectopic ACTH production.

## Treatment of Cushing's Syndrome

### Treatment of the Hypertension

Until definitive therapy is provided, the hypertension that accompanies Cushing's syndrome can temporarily be treated with the usual antihypertensive agents described in Chapter 7. Since excess fluid volume is likely involved, a diuretic, perhaps in combination with the aldosterone antagonist spironolactone, is an appropriate initial choice. In view of the possible involvement of both renin-angiotensin and the sympathetic nervous system, a beta-blocker that will inhibit both of these may be an appropriate second drug.

## Treatment of Cushing's Syndrome

The choice of definitive therapy depends upon the cause of the syndrome, and many choices are available (Table 14.2). Benign adrenal tumors should be surgically removed (Välimäki et al, 1984). For adrenal cancers and ectopic ACTH tumors, removal of the adrenal may be helpful, but chemotherapy is usually needed (Schteingart, 1989). For the most common type of Cushing's syndrome, that due to pituitary ACTH hypersecretion, transsphenoidal microsurgical removal of pituitary tumors has become the treatment of choice in both adults (Jeffcoate, 1988; Mampalam et al, 1988) and children (Styne, et al, 1984). Pituitary irradiation may be given by alpha-particles from a cyclotron (Linfoot, 1981) or from yttrium-90 interstitial implants (Sandler et al, 1987).

In the future, drugs that selectively inhibit corticotropin-releasing factor may have a primary place. At present, such drugs are a secondary line of therapy (Schteingart, 1989), including bromocriptine (Lamberts et al, 1980) or cyproheptadine (Wiesen et al, 1983). Patients in whom pituitary surgery is inappropriate or who have adrenal tumors can be successfully treated with inhibitors of adrenal steroid synthesis, often combined with external irradiation. The largest experience has been with mitotane ($o,p'$-DDD) (Schteingart, 1989), but results with

**Table 14.2. Therapies for Cushing's Syndrome**

Surgery
  Pituitary: Transsphenoidal microresection
            Transfrontal hypophysectomy
  Adrenal: Unilateral adrenalectomy
           Bilateral adrenalectomy
Radiation
  External: High voltage x-ray (cobalt) ± mitotane, etc.
            alpha-particle, proton beam (cyclotron)
  Internal: Implants of yttrium-90, gold-198
Drugs
  Acting upon CNS neurotransmission
    Bromocriptine (Parlodel)
    Cyproheptadine (Periacten)
    Sodium valproate
  Acting upon adrenocortical steroid synthesis
    o,p'-DDD (mitotane, Lysodren)
    Metyrapone (Metopirone)
    Aminoglutethimide (Elipten)
    Trilostane (WIN 24,540)
    Ketoconazole (Nizoral)
  Acting as a competitive glucocorticoid antagonist (RU 486)

the inhibitor of cytochrome P-450-dependent adrenal enzymes, ketoconazole, for long-term therapy of ACTH-dependent disease have been generally excellent (Sonino, 1987). In the future, glucocorticoid antagonists such as RU-486 may be more widely used since they are so well tolerated (Nieman et al, 1985).

## Course of Hypertension

As with most secondary causes of hypertension, the blood pressure may remain elevated despite removal of the cause. In the series of O'Neal et al (1970), 26% of those with bilateral adrenal hyperplasia remained hypertensive after adrenal surgery. Many of these had arteriolar nephrosclerosis that the authors attribute to the long-standing hypertension and that they blame for the persistence of the hypertension. In some, the hypertension may not recede for as long as a year (Aso and Kinoshita, 1975). This delay could reflect the use of excessive steroid replacement therapy. Thus, hypertension is common with Cushing's syndrome; it may be severe and may persist unless the disease is cured quickly.

## CONGENITAL ADRENAL HYPERPLASIA

The two most common forms of adrenal cortical excess, primary aldosteronism (Chapter 13) and Cushing's syndrome, are almost always acquired and are often associated with benign tumors. The other type of adrenal cortical hormone excess is congenital and is associated with diffuse hyperplasia. Most instances of congenital adrenal hyperplasia (CAH) are manifested in early childhood by virilization, and the most common type, the 21-hydroxylase deficiency, responsible for perhaps 90% of all CAH, is not associated with hypertension. Late-onset or attenuated 21-hydroxylase deficiency usually manifests as hirsutism and may be accompanied by a mild defect of mineralocorticoid synthesis as well (Fiet et al, 1989).

Of the less common forms of CAH, two are associated with hypertension because of the presence of large amounts of mineralocorticoid hormones (Table 14.3). Though most of these are also seen among young children, some only become obvious during adolescence or adult life. Additionally, at least a few adult hypertensives have their hypertension as a result of partial defects in adrenal steroidogenesis, which may be clinically manifested only by hirsutism

**Table 14.3. Syndromes of Congenital Adrenal Hyperplasia**

| | Site of Defect | | Steroid Levels[a] | | | | Clinical Features | |
|---|---|---|---|---|---|---|---|---|
| | Increased Precursor | Decreased Product | 17-KS | 17-OH-P or P'triol | DOC | Aldo | Virili-zation | Hyper-tension |
| 21-hydroxylase | | | | | | | | |
| Nonsalt wasting | 17 hydroxypro-gesterone | 11-deoxycortisol, cortisol | ↑ | ↑ | N | ↑ | + + + + | No |
| Salt-wasting | Progesterone | 11-deoxycorti-costerone, cortisol | ↑ | ↑ | ↓ | ↓ | + + + + | No |
| 11-hydroxylase | 11-deoxycortisol 11-deoxycorti-costerone | Cortisol Cortisterone | ↑ | ↑ | ↑ | ↓ | + + + | Yes |
| 17-hydroxylase | Progesterone Pregnenolone | Cortisol 17-hydroxypreg-nenolone | ↓ | ↓ | ↑ | ↓ | 0 | Yes |
| 3β-ol-dehydrogenase | Pregnenolone | Progesterone, cortisol | ↑ | ↓ | ↓ | ↓ | + | No |

[a]17-KS, 17-ketosteroids; 17-OH-P, 17-hydroxyprogesterone; P'triol, pregnanetriol; DOC, deoxycorticosterone; Aldo, aldosterone, N, normal.

(Guthrie et al, 1982) or manifestations of hypokalemia (Zachmann et al, 1983). A pattern suggesting a partial deficiency of adrenal 11-hydroxylase with high levels of DOC and deoxycortisol, both basal and after ACTH stimulation, has been measured in 15 patients with what appears to be ordinary primary hypertension (de Simone et al, 1985). Whether such a partial CAH is involved in a significant number of hypertensives remains to be seen.

Defects in all of the enzymes involved in adrenal steroid synthesis shown in Figure 14.3 have been recognized. These defects are inherited in an autosomal recessive manner, and many are obvious at birth. Their manifestations result from inadequate levels of the end products of steroid synthesis, in particular, cortisol. The low levels of cortisol call forth increased secretion of ACTH, further increasing the accumulation of the precursor steroids proximal to the enzymatic block and stimulating steroidogenesis in those pathways that are not blocked.

The clinical manifestations vary with degree of enzymatic deficiency and the mix of steroids

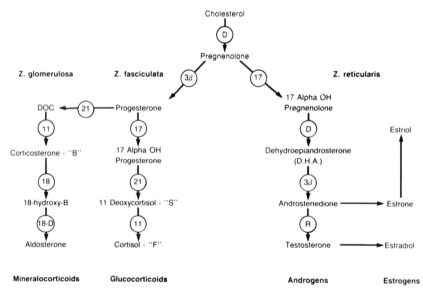

**Figure 14.3.** Major biosynthetic pathways in the three zones of the adrenal cortex. The enzymes involved are shown within the circles: *D*, desmolase; *3β*, 3-β-ol-dehydrogenase; *17*, 17-hydroxylase; *11*, 11-β-hydroxylase; *21*, 21-hydroxylase, *18*, 18-hydroxylase; *18-D*, 18-dehydrogenase; *R*, reductase.

secreted by the hyperplastic adrenal glands. Therapy is with glucocorticoid, usually cortisol, though dexamethasone may provide more prolonged ACTH suppression with fewer systemic side effects (Khalid et al, 1982).

The two forms of CAH that have hypertension as part of their syndrome are the 11-hydroxylase defect, wherein 11-deoxycorticosterone (DOC) is in excess along with adrenal androgens, and the 17-hydroxylase defect, which also has an excess of DOC but a deficiency of androgen production. Though these are rare causes of hypertension, recall that partial enzymatic deficiencies have been observed in hirsute women (Guthrie et al, 1982), so some hypertensive adults may have unrecognized, subtle forms of CAH.

## 11-Hydroxylase Deficiency

The 11-hydroxylase deficiency syndrome is usually recognized in infancy because, as shown in Figure 14.4, the defect sets off production of excessive androgens (Bongiovanni and Root, 1963; White et al, 1987). The enzyme deficiency prevents the hydroxylation of 11-deoxycortisol, resulting in cortisol deficiency. The defect also prevents the conversion of DOC to corticosterone and aldosterone. The high levels of DOC induce hypertension and hypokalemia, the expected features of mineralocorticoid excess. Thus, the syndrome features virilization of the infant, hypertension, and hypokalemia.

It is recognized by the high levels of 11-deoxycortisol and DOC in urine and plasma (Franks, 1972). By more detailed study, patients can be shown to have an 18-hydroxylase deficiency in the zona fasciculata as well (Levine et al, 1980). Patients have been described with the syndrome who can make cortisol and corticosterone, suggesting either a partial defect or the presence of two independent 11-beta-hydroxylating systems (Gregory and Gardner, 1976). The report of a pattern of steroids suggesting a partial 11-hydroxylase deficiency in patients with what appears to be ordinary primary hypertension (de Simone et al, 1985) remains to be documented.

Treatment, as for all of the syndromes of CAH, is with glucocorticoid, which should relieve the hypertension and hypokalemia and allow the child to develop normally. Since aldosterone synthesis is blocked with glucocorticoid therapy that successfully reduces DOC production, sodium wastage may become manifest after therapy is instituted (Zadik et al, 1984).

## 17-Hydroxylase Deficiency

Unlike the 21-hydroxylase and 11-hydroxylase deficiencies, CAH caused by a 17-hydroxylase deficiency is associated with an absence of sex hormones, leading to incomplete masculinization in males and primary amenorrhea in females. Since 17-hydroxylase activity is also lacking in the gonads, the defect prevents conversion of the precursor pregnenolone into androgens and estrogens (Fig. 14.5). Though most affected 46,XY males are phenotypically fe-

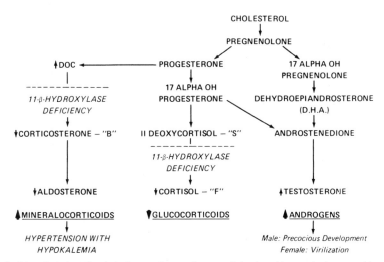

**Figure 14.4.** Defect in adrenal synthesis in the syndrome of congenital adrenal hyperplasia caused by a deficiency of the 11-hydroxylase enzyme.

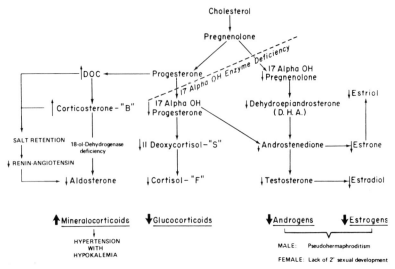

**Figure 14.5.** Defect in adrenal steroid synthesis in the syndrome of congenital adrenal hyperplasia caused by a deficiency of the 17-hydroxylase and, perhaps, the 18-ol-dehydrogenase enzymes.

males, some may appear as partially virilized males at birth, presumably because they have less severe enzyme deficiency (Dean et al, 1984). The syndrome usually is not recognized until after the age of puberty when sexual development does not progress in a normal manner in patients who are phenotypically female. Only a few cases have been recognized, but adolescents with hypertension and abnormal sexual development should be suspect (Winter et al, 1989).

Since the 17-hydroxylase deficiency interferes with cortisol synthesis, the resultant increase in ACTH stimulates the adrenal to do what it can—synthesize large amounts of the potent mineralocorticoid DOC, as well as 18-hydroxyDOC and 19-nor-DOC (Griffing et al, 1984). Hypertension and hypokalemia supervene. The hypertension can be very severe in nature (Fraser et al, 1987). The syndrome therefore includes hypertension; hypokalemia; hypogonadism; very low urinary 17-ketosteroids; and high levels of DOC, 18-OHDOC, and 19-norDOC.

Aldosterone synthesis would be expected to be increased in the presence of large amounts of its precursor corticosterone. However, low levels of aldosterone have been found in most cases (Biglieri et al, 1966). This could result from one or both of the mechanisms shown on the *left* in Figure 14.5. An additional deficiency of the 18-ol-dehydrogenase enzyme, needed to convert corticosterone to aldosterone, has been

suggested (Waldhäusl et al, 1978). On the other hand, the salt retention induced by the high levels of DOC produced by continuous ACTH stimulation would be expected to suppress the renin-angiotensin mechanism, the primary stimulus for aldosterone synthesis in the zona glomerulosa (Kater et al, 1982), so no additional biosynthetic defects other than the 17-hydroxylase deficiency need be evoked.

Regardless of the details, the entire syndrome can be corrected with glucocorticoid therapy—usually cortisol in doses of 10 to 30 mg/day.

## Other Forms of Mineralocorticoid Hypertension

In addition to the classic forms of CAH listed in Table 14.3, a rare form of congenital hyperaldosteronism associated with adrenal hyperplasia is described in Chapter 13 as having these characteristics: familial, inherited as an autosomal dominant, and glucocorticoid-suppressible.

Even rarer are two hypertensive syndromes associated with mineralocorticoid excess. One is a primary resistance to cortisol, likely resulting from a defect in the glucocorticoid receptor, that leads to an increased secretion of mineralocorticoids (Chrousos et al, 1983). The second, described in Chapter 13, is a deficiency of the 11-beta-hydroxysteroid dehydrogenase (11-beta-OHSD) enzyme in the kidney that allows high levels of cortisol to bind to mineralocorticoid receptors (Edwards et al, 1988). This syndrome of "apparent mineralocorticoid excess" is reproduced by inhibition of 11-beta-OHSD by licorice, and partial deficiencies may turn out to be more common than the few overt cases now recognized. Stewart et al (1988) find a loss of 11-beta-OHSD activity in patients with chronic renal disease, so this may be playing a role in the hypertension so common in this condition.

Now that the various renal and adrenal causes of hypertension have been covered, we shall turn to an even larger variety of less common forms.

## References

Armbruster H, Vetter W, Reck G, et al: *Int J Clin Pharmacol* 12:170, 1975.

Aso Y, Kinoshita K: *Urol Int* 30:386, 1975.

Atkinson AB, Kennedy AL, Carson DJ, et al: *Br Med J* 291:1453, 1985.

Axelrod L: *Medicine* (Baltimore) 55:39, 1976.

Bagshawe KD: *Lancet* 2:284, 1960.

Berlinger FG, Ruder HJ, Wilber JF: *J Clin Endocrinol Metab* 45:1205, 1977.

Biglieri EG, Herron MA, Brust N: *J Clin Invest* 45:1946, 1966.

Boggan JE, Tyrrell JB, Wilson CB: *J Neurosurg* 59:195, 1983.

Bongiovanni AM, Root AW: *N Engl J Med* 268:1283, 1342, 1391, 1963.

Carey RM: *N Engl J Med* 302:275, 1980.

Carpenter PC: *Mayo Clin Proc* 61:49, 1986.

Carpenter PC: *Endocrinol Metab Clin North Am* 17:445, 1988.

Carroll BJ, Schroeder K, Mukhopadhyay S, et al: *J Clin Endocrinol Metab* 51:433, 1980.

Cassar J, Loizou S, Kelly WF, et al: *Metabolism* 29:115, 1980.

Chrousos GP, Vingerhoeds ADM, Loriaux DL, et al: *J Clin Endocrinol Metab* 56:1243, 1983.

Connolly CK, Gore MBR, Stanley N, et al: *Br Med J* 2:665, 1968.

Crapo L: *Metabolism* 28:995, 1979.

David DS, Gieco MH, Cushman P Jr: *J Chronic Dis* 22:637, 1970.

Dean HJ, Shackleton CHL, Winter JSD: *J Clin Endocrinol Metab* 59:513, 1984.

de Simone G, Tommaselli AP, Rossi R, et al: *Hypertension* 7:204, 1985.

Edwards CRW, Stewart PM, Burt D, et al: *Lancet* 1:986, 1988.

Ehlers ME, Griffing GT, Wilson TE, et al: *J Clin Endocrinol Metab* 64:926, 1987.

Elias AN, Gwinup G: *Metabolism* 29:582, 1980.

Fiet J, Bueux B, Raux-Demay M-C, et al: *J Clin Endocrinol Metab* 68:542, 1989.

Findling JW, Tyrrell JB: *Arch Intern Med* 146:929, 1986.

Fig LM, Gross MD, Shapiro B, et al: *Ann Intern Med* 109:547, 1988.

Franks RC: *J Clin Endocrinol Metab* 35:831, 1972.

Fraser R, Brown JJ, Mason PA, et al: *J Hum Hypertens* 1:53, 1987.

Gold PW, Loriaux DL, Roy A, et al: *N Engl J Med* 314:1329, 1986.

Green JRB, Van't Hoff W: *J Clin Endocrinol Metab* 41:235, 1975.

Gregory T, Gardner LI: *J Clin Endocrinol Metab* 43:469, 1976.

Greminger P, Vetter W, Groth H, et al: *Klin Wochenschr* 62:855, 1984.

Griffing GT, Wilson TE, Holbrook MM, et al: *J Clin Endocrinol Metab* 59:1011, 1984.

Guthrie GP, Wilson EA, Quillen DL, et al: *Arch Intern Med* 142:729, 1982.

Hellman L, Weitzman ED, Roffward H, et al: *J Clin Endocrinol Metab* 30:686, 1970.

Hermus AR, Pieters GF, Smals AG, et al: *N Engl J Med* 318:966, 1988.

Hodge BO, Froesch TA: *Arch Intern Med* 148:1133, 1988.

Imai Y, Abe K, Sasaki S, et al: *Hypertension* 12:11, 1988.

Jackson SHD, Beevers DG, Myers K: *Clin Sci* 61:381, 1981.

Jeffcoate WJ: *Br Med J* 296:227, 1988.

Josse RG, Bear R, Kovacs K, et al: *Acta Endocrinol* 92:495, 1980.

Jubiz W, Meikle AW, Levinson RA, et al: *N Engl J Med* 283:11, 1970.

Kammer H, Barter M: *Am J Med* 67:519, 1979.

Kapcala LP: *Am J Med* 82:849, 1987.

Kaplan NM: *Arch Intern Med* 149:1514, 1989.

Kater CE, Biglieri EG, Brust N, et al: *J Clin Endocrinol Metab* 55:295, 1982.

Kater CE, Czepielewski MA, Biglieri EG, et al: *J Hypertension* 4(Suppl 6):S604, 1986.

Kennedy L, Atkinson AB, Johnston H, et al: *Br Med J* 289:1188, 1984.

Khalid BAK, Burke CW, Hurley DM, et al: *J Clin Endocrinol Metab* 55:551, 1982.

Krakoff LR: *Cardiol Clin* 6:537, 1988.

Kuhn JM, Proeschel MF, Seurin DJ, et al: *Am J Med* 86:678, 1989.

Lamberts SWJ, Klijn JGM, De Quijada M, et al: *J Clin Endocrinol Metab* 51:207, 1980.

Levine LS, Rauh W, Gottesdiener K, et al: *J Clin Endocrinol Metab* 50:258, 1980.

Liddle GW: *J Clin Endocrinol Metab* 20:1539, 1960.

Linfoot JA: *Clin Neurosurg* 27:83, 1981.

Liu JH, Rasmussen DD: *J Clin Endocrinol Metab* 64:1027, 1987.

Malchoff CD, Rosa J, DeBold CR, et al: *J Clin Endocrinol Metab* 68:855, 1989.

Mampalam TJ, Tyrell JB, Wilson CB: *Ann Intern Med* 109:487, 1988.

Mendlowitz M, Gitlow S, Naftchi N: *J Appl Physiol* 13:252, 1958.

Mimou N, Sakato S, Nakabayashi H, et al: *Acta Endocrinol* 108;245, 1985.

Mortola JF, Liu JH, Gillin JC, et al: *J Clin Endocrinol Metab* 65:962, 1987.

Nieman LK, Chrousos GP, Kellner C, et al: *J Clin Endocrinol Metab* 61:536, 1985.

Nieman LK, Chrousos GP, Oldfield EH, et al: *Ann Intern Med* 105:862, 1986.

Oldfield EH, Chrousos GP, Schulte HM, et al: *N Engl J Med* 312:100, 1985.

O'Neal LW, Kissane JM, Hartroft PM: *Arch Surg* 100:498, 1970.

Rebuffe'-Scrive M, Krotkiewski M, Elfverson J, et al: *J Clin Endocrinol Metab* 67:1122, 1988.

Ross EJ, Linch DC: *Lancet* 2:646, 1982.

Sandler LM, Richards NT, Carr DH, et al: *J Clin Endocrinol Metab* 65:441, 1987.

Saruta T, Suzuki H, Handa M, et al: *J Clin Endocrinol Metab* 62:275, 1986.

Schteingart DE: *Endocrniol Metab Clin North Am* 18:311, 1989.

Sindler BH, Griffing GT, Melby JC: *Am J Med* 74:657, 1983.

Sonino N: *N Engl J Med* 317:812, 1987.

Stewart PM, Whitworth JA, Burt D, et al: *J Hypertension* 6:947, 1988 (abst).

Styne DM, Grumbach MM, Kaplan SL, et al: *N Engl J Med* 310:889, 1984.

Sudhir K, Jennings GL, Esler MD, et al: *Hypertension* 13:416, 1989.

Välimäki M, Pelkonen R, Porkka L, et al: *Clin Endocrinol* 20:229, 1984.

Waldhäusl W, Herkner K, Nowotny P, et al: *J Clin Endocrinol Metab* 46:236, 1978.

Wambach G, Schmülling V, Kaufmann W: *J Hypertension* 2:96, 1984.

White PC, New MI, Dupont B: *N Engl J Med* 316:1580, 1987.

Whitworth JA, Gofdon D, Andrews J, et al: *J Hypertension* 7:537, 1989.

Wiesen M, Ross F, Krieger DT: *Acta Endocrinol* 102:436, 1983.

Winter JSD, Couch RM, Muller J, et al: *J Clin Endocrinol Metab* 68:309, 1989.

Zachmann M, Tassinari D, Prader A: *J Clin Endocrinol Metab* 56:222, 1983.

Zadik Z, Kahana L, Kaufman H, et al: *J Clin Endocrinol Metab* 58:384, 1984.

# 15 Other Forms of Secondary Hypertension

Coarctation of the Aorta
Hormonal Disturbances
  Hypothyroidism
  Hyperthyroidism
  Hyperparathyroidism
  Acromegaly

Carcinoid
Sleep Apnea
Neurological Disorders
Psychogenic Hyperventilation
Acute Stress

Medical Conditions
Surgical Conditions
Increased Intravascular Volume
Drugs and Other Substances That
  Cause Hypertension

The preceding chapters covered the major types of hypertensive diseases listed in Table 1.10, accounting for perhaps 98% of the total. Others that deserve consideration will be covered in this chapter. Coarctation, described in this chapter, and congenital adrenal hyperplasia, in Chapter 14, are seen mainly in children; additional coverage of hypertension in childhood follows in Chapter 16.

## COARCTATION OF THE AORTA

Constriction of the lumen of the aorta may occur anywhere along its length but most commonly just beyond the origin of the left subclavian artery, at or below the insertion of the ligamentum arteriosum. This lesion makes up about 7% of all congenital heart disease and presents either an infantile or adult form, differing in pathological and clinical features. Hypertension in the upper extremities with diminished or absent femoral pulses is the usual presentation (Fixler, 1988).

### Infantile Coarctation

The narrowing involves a larger segment of the aorta and is usually accompanied by serious cardiac anomalies. If the coarctation is proximal to the ductus arteriosus, pulmonary hypertension, congestive failure, and cyanosis of the lower half of the body occur early in life. From 45 to 84% of infants found to have coarctation die during their first year of life (Campbell, 1970), but better results with surgery are possible (Shinebourne et al, 1976).

### Adult Coarctation

Those born with less severe postductal lesions may have no difficulties during childhood. However, they almost always develop prema-

ture cardiovascular disease, and in the two largest series of autopsied cases seen prior to effective surgery the mean age of death was 34 years (Abbott, 1928; Reifenstein et al, 1947). The causes of death reflect the load upon the heart and the associated cardiac and cerebral lesions:

| | |
|---|---|
| Congestive heart failure | 25% |
| Rupture of the aorta | 21% |
| Bacterial endocarditis | 18% |
| Intracranial hemorrhage | 11% |

Coarctation may affect the abdominal aorta, either as a congenital lesion (Bergqvist et al, 1988) or as an acquired form of arterial fibroplasia (Keech et al, 1988).

### Mechanism of Hypertension

Beyond the obvious obstruction to blood flow, the coarctation may lead to a generalized increase in vascular resistance in tissues below the stenosis, suggesting a systemic vasoconstrictor mechanism (Liard and Spadone, 1985). In experimental models, the normotensive vessels below the aorta also thicken (Stacy and Prewitt, 1989), which could explain the occasional persistence of hypertension after repair of the lesion.

In experimental models, the renin-angiotensin system is inappropriately turned on in the presence of an expanded body fluid volume (Bagby and Mass, 1980). In patients, plasma renin levels may not be elevated under basal conditions (Sehested et al, 1983), but they may rise inordinately after diuretics or standing and exercise (Parker et al, 1982).

### Recognition of Coarctation (Table 15.1)

Hypertension in the arms with weak femoral pulses in a young person strongly suggests coarctation. With minimal constriction, symp-

**Table 15.1. Symptoms and Signs of Coarctation**

| Symptoms | Signs |
| --- | --- |
| Headache | Hypertension |
| | Hyperdynamic apical impulse |
| Cold feet | Murmurs in front or back of chest |
| Pain in legs with exercise | Pulsations in neck |
| | Weak femoral pulse |

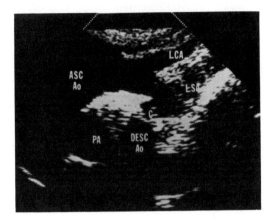

**Figure 15.1.** Two-dimensional echocardiogram showing aortic arch with discrete coarctation (*C*). *ASC Ao*, ascending aorta; *LCA*, left carotid artery; *LSA*, left subclavian artery; *Desc Ao*, descending aorta; *PA*, pulmonary artery. (From Sahn DJ, Anderson F: *An Atlas for Echocardiographers: Two-dimensional Anatomy of the Heart.* Copyright, New York, Wiley Medical Publications, 1982:454.)

toms may not appear until late in life. Often the heart is large and shows left ventricular strain on the electrocardiogram. The chest x-ray can be diagnostic, with the "3 sign" from dilation of the aorta above and below the constriction and notching of the ribs by enlarged collateral vessels (Smyth and Edwards, 1972). The diagnosis is now usually made by echocardiography (Fig 15.1). Color Doppler flow mapping will provide additional useful information (Simpson et al, 1988). Neither magnetic resonance imaging nor angiography is usually needed since echo usually confirms the diagnosis.

Atypical aortic coarctations in adults most likely represent aortitis (Lande, 1976). Takayasu's arteritis, or pulseless disease, usually affects the aortic arch and may also involve the descending aorta (Ishikawa, 1978). This large vessel vasculitis may be successfully treated with glucocorticoids, cytotoxins, and surgery (Shelhamer et al, 1985).

**Management of Coarctation**

*Severe Disease.* If the disease is associated with other cardiac defects and induces heart fail-

ure in the first few weeks of life, early repair is necessary. Although the surgical mortality for patients under 6 weeks is 45%, this is almost half the 86% mortality observed in those not operated on (Shinebourne et al, 1976). If the infant is less afflicted, the operation should be performed electively between 6 months and 1 year of age; if postponed, hypertension is more likely to persist despite relief of aortic obstruction.

*Mild Disease.* If the disease is milder and no troubles occur during infancy, surgery should be performed before age 9 (Cohen et al, 1989) and probably between the ages of 4 and 6 years (Fixler, 1988). Immediately after surgical repair, the blood pressure (BP) may paradoxically rise. In most patients, this is transient and likely represents both renin-angiotensin and sympathetic nervous hyperactivity (Benedict et al, 1978). It may persist, often associated with mesenteric arteritis, inducing severe abdominal pain and, occasionally, intestinal infarction (Sealy, 1953). Prophylactic use of beta-blockers has been shown to prevent the postoperative rises in both blood pressure and plasma renin activity (Leenen et al, 1987).

Even with early surgery, hypertension may persist (Murphy et al, 1989), but the prognosis is certainly improved. The prevalence of hypertension is closely related to the age at repair: In the Mayo Clinic series, the prevalence was 7% in those operated on as infants but 33% in those operated on after age 14 (Cohen et al, 1989). About 20% of those children who are normotensive after repair have an excessive BP rise during exercise and need to be followed more closely (Simsolo et al, 1988).

*Angioplasty.* Balloon dilation angioplasty has been increasingly used (Rao et al, 1988) and may become the treatment of choice, but concerns about subsequent aneurysm formation persist (Fixler, 1988).

**HORMONAL DISTURBANCES**

**Hypothyroidism**

Among 40 patients prospectively followed over the time they became hypothyroid after radioiodine therapy for thyrotoxicosis, 16 (40%) developed a diastolic blood pressure (DBP) above 90 mm Hg (Streeten et al, 1988). These investigators found hypothyroidism in 3.6% of 688 consecutively seen referred hypertensive patients and noted reversal of the hypertension in one-third of these patients given thyroid hormone replacement therapy.

### Mechanism of Hypertension

Hypothyroid patients tend to have a low cardiac output due to a fall both in heart rate and in stroke volume (Bing and Swales, 1983). To maintain tissue perfusion, they have a high peripheral resistance, from a combination of increased responsiveness of alpha-adrenergic receptors and an increased level of sympathetic nervous activity (Wennlund and Linde, 1984). These would tend to raise diastolic pressures more than systolic, the usual pattern seen in hypothyroidism.

### Hyperthyroidism

An elevated systolic but lowered diastolic blood pressure is usual in patients with hyperthyroidism, associated with a high cardiac output and reduced peripheral resistance.

### Hyperparathyroidism

Beyond a possible role for increased levels of parathyroid hormone in the pathogenesis of primary hypertension described in Chapter 3, the presence of autonomous hyperfunction of the parathyroid glands—primary hyperparathyroidism—is associated with about a doubling of the rate of hypertension (Salahudeen et al, 1989). From the other perspective, there is an increased prevalence of hyperparathyroidism, as high as 1%, among patients with hypertension (Rosenthal and Roy, 1972). Patients with previously unrecognized primary hyperparathyroidism may have a sharp rise in plasma calcium levels after start of thiazide therapy; if the calcium level is above 10.5 mg/dl on thiazides and if hypercalcemia persists after the thiazide is stopped, the diagnosis should be considered (Christensson et al, 1977).

### Mechanism

The mechanism for the hypertension is uncertain: Hypercalcemia raises the blood pressure, probably by a direct effect on peripheral resistance that may be caused by an increased vascular reactivity to sympathetic nervous stimulation (Vlachakis et al, 1982). The renin-aldosterone mechanism and whole-body exchangeable sodium were similar in those hyperparathyroid patients who were hypertensive as in those who were normotensive (Salahudeen et al, 1989). However, others find that plasma renin activity and cortisol levels are higher and

fall after parathyroidectomy (Richards et al, 1988).

### Postoperative Course

After successful correction of the hypercalcemia by removal of a parathyroid adenoma, most find that hypertension does *not* remit (Richards et al, 1988; Jespersen et al, 1989; Lafferty and Hubay, 1989; Salahudeen et al, 1989). Others find that it does in about half of patients (Horky' et al, 1986; Diamond et al, 1986). Moreover, BP was reduced by administration of vitamin D to a group with mild hyperparathyroidism (Lind et al, 1988). Obviously, the relations between parathyroid disease and BP are complicated.

### Pseudohypoparathyroidism

Half of a group of adults with pseudohypoparathyroidism type I, caused by target organ resistance to parathyroid hormone, were hypertensive (Brickman et al, 1988).

### Acromegaly

Hypertension is found in about 40% of patients with acromegaly (Thuesen et al, 1988) and may disappear when the disease is successfully treated (Davies et al, 1985). The blood pressure is elevated because of sodium retention caused by the high levels of growth hormone. The volume expansion, in turn, stimulates the secretion of the digitalis-like factor (Deray et al, 1987) postulated to be the natriuretic hormone (see Chapter 3). The heart is enlarged and cardiac output is increased by 50% (Thuesen et al, 1988).

The diagnosis of acromegaly is made by finding high and usually nonsuppressible levels of growth hormone and insulin-like growth factor I (Barreca et al, 1989).

Acromegaly remains difficult to cure: The best results are with transsphenoidal surgery (Thomas, 1983). The somatostatin analogue octreotide may provide long-term suppression of growth hormone secretion and clinical improvement (Tauber et al, 1989).

### Carcinoid Syndrome

Among 34 cases of carcinoid, nine had hypertension, and most of these had significant renal damage (Schwartz, 1970). Even in some without renal disease, severe hypertension has been reported (Rosenberg, 1968).

# SLEEP APNEA

Sleep apnea is a common aggravating factor for hypertension, particularly in obese middle-aged men. Despite a number of recent papers describing the association and documenting relief of hypertension after relief of sleep apnea, the syndrome is infrequently considered and diagnosed. Along with alcohol abuse, sleep apnea is one of the most frequent causes of reversible hypertension, far more common than the various adrenal hyperfunction states that have received so much more attention. Among habitual snorers, who frequently have sleep apnea (Hoffstein et al, 1988), hypertension is about 2 times more common than among nonsnorers (Waller and Bhopal, 1989).

## Definition

Sleep apnea is defined as the occurrence of at least 30 periods of respiratory cessation lasting 10 or more seconds in nonrapid eye movement (non-REM) sleep during a 7-hour period (Guilleminault et al, 1976). Three types have been defined: *central* sleep apnea, wherein no breathing efforts occur; *obstructive*, wherein breathing efforts continue but, because of upper airway obstruction, air movement ceases; and *mixed*, wherein both central and obstructive elements are present (Lavie et al, 1982).

## Clinical Features

The syndrome can only be diagnosed with certainty by an overnight sleep study involving continuous recordings of respiration, electroencephalogram (EEG), electromyograph (EMG), and eye movements along with electrocardiogram (ECG) and oxygen saturation.

The presence of the syndrome should be suspected in any patient who snores loudly, particularly overweight middle-aged men who have repetitive episodes of gasping, choking, or loud snorting during sleep (often only recognized by the patient's bed partner) that are often accompanied by excessive daytime sleepiness and morning headaches. The presence of repetitive bradycardia (during apnea) and tachycardia (when breathing restarts) on a nighttime continuous ECG monitor may be a tip-off to the diagnosis (Burack, 1984).

Hypertension is seen in 60 to 80% of patients with the full-blown syndrome, and as many as 30% of hypertensive patients have sleep apnea (Kales et al, 1984; Lavie et al, 1984; Williams et al, 1985) (Table 15.2). Of the 15 hypertensive

**Table 15.2. Sleep Apnea in a Hypertensive Population[a]**

| | 50 Normotensives | 50 Hypertensives on Therapy |
|---|---|---|
| Mean blood pressure | 131/80 | 154/88 |
| Sleep apnea > 30 apneic periods > 10 sec/night | 0 | 30% |
| Sleep apneic activity: 3–29 periods/night | 24% | 34% |

[a]Data from Kales A, Bixler EO, Cadieux RJ, et al: *Lancet* 1:1005, 1984.

patients in the study by Kales et al who had sleep apnea, six were within 20% of their ideal weight, so gross obesity is not a requisite for the syndrome. Unfortunately, the subjects in all three of these studies, though not selected because of features suggestive of sleep apnea, were all receiving antihypertensive medications, most of which are known to have central nervous system (CNS) side effects. Warley et al (1988) found no excessive arterial hypoxemia among 30 untreated hypertensives, so the syndrome may be less common than the series of treated patients would suggest.

## Mechanism of Hypertension

Whatever is responsible for the sleep apnea, when it occurs a series of hemodynamic changes are induced that may give rise to cyclic systemic hypertension (Schroeder et al, 1978) (Fig. 15.2). Sympathetic nervous hyperactivity (Hedner et al, 1988) and neuroendocrine dysfunction (Grunstein et al, 1989) are usually seen. The manner in which the cyclic periods may lead to permanent hypertension is uncertain, but there clearly may be prolonged periods of sustained daytime hypertension that disappear after relief of sleep apnea.

## Treatment

Those who are massively overweight or who have obvious obstructive defects in the upper airways may get relief from weight loss and nasal continuous positive airway pressure (nCPAP) with an accompanying decrease in blood pressure (Jennum et al, 1989). Tracheostomy may be needed for those with severe sleep apnea, and it may be followed by prompt and dramatic relief of hypertension (Burack, 1984).

## NEUROLOGICAL DISORDERS

A number of seemingly different disorders of the central and peripheral nervous system may

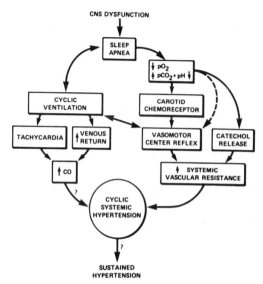

**Figure 15.2.** Proposed mechanism for cyclic systemic hypertension with sleep apnea that may lead to sustained hypertension. (From Schroeder JS, Motta J, Guilleminault C: *Sleep Apnea Syndromes.* New York: Alan R. Liss, 1978:191.)

cause hypertension. Many may do so by a common mechanism involving sympathetic nervous system discharge from the vasomotor centers in response to an increased intracranial pressure. The rise in systemic pressure is useful in restoring cerebral perfusion (Plets, 1989). However, the classical hypertensive response to brain ischemia (Cushing phenomenon) involves bradycardia rather than the expected tachycardia from catechol excess.

Unlike the situation in many neurological diseases, hypertension is *less* common in patients with Alzheimer's disease, apparently receding as the process worsens without an association with weight loss (Garbarino et al, 1989).

As noted in Chapters 4 and 7, patients with acute stroke may have transient marked elevations in BP. Rarely, episodic hypertension suggestive of a pheochromocytoma may occur after cerebral infarction (Funck-Brentano et al, 1987).

### Brain Tumors

Intracranial tumors, especially those arising in the posterior fossa, may cause hypertension. In some, paroxysmal hypertension and other features suggestive of catecholamine excess may point mistakenly to the diagnosis of pheochromocytoma (Bell and Doig, 1983). The problem may be confounded by the increased incidence of neuroectodermal tumors, some within the central nervous system in patients with pheochromocytoma. Unlike patients with a pheochromocytoma who always have high catechol levels, patients with a brain tumor may have increased catecholamines during a paroxysm of hypertension but normal levels at other times.

### Quadriplegia

Patients with transverse lesions of the cervical spinal cord above the origins of the thoracolumbar sympathetic neurons lose central control of their sympathetic outflow. Stimulation of nerves below the injury, as with bladder or bowel distension, may cause reflex sympathetic activity via the isolated spinal cord, inducing hypertension, sweating, flushing, piloerection, and headache, a syndrome described as autonomic hyperreflexia (Johnson et al, 1975).

The hypertension may be so severe and persistent as to cause cerebral vascular accidents and death. During hypertensive episodes in five patients whose mean arterial blood pressure rose from 95 to 154, the heart rate fell from 72 to 45, cardiac output was unchanged, and peripheral resistance rose markedly (Naftchi et al, 1978). Plasma volume was reduced by 10 to 15%, which may explain the propensity of these patients to develop hypotension when the hypertensive stimulus is removed.

### Severe Head Injury

Immediately after severe head injury, the blood pressure may rise because of a hyperdynamic state mediated by excessive sympathetic nervous activity (Simard and Bellefleur, 1989). If the hypertension is persistent and severe, a short-acting beta-blocker, e.g., esmolol, should be given. Caution is needed in the use of vasodilators such as hydralazine and nitroprusside, which may increase cerebral blood flow and intracranial pressure (Van Aken et al, 1989).

### Other Neurological Disorders

Hypertension related to high catechol levels may occur during Guillain-Barré syndrome (Ventura et al, 1986). Encephalitis and other acute neurological diseases may cause transient hypertension (Davies and Rowlatt, 1978). Paroxysmal hypertension may develop after sinoaortic baroreceptor denervation (Aksamit et al, 1987) or dysfunction (Kuchel et al, 1987).

### PSYCHOGENIC HYPERVENTILATION

During acute hyperventilation or panic attacks, the blood pressure may rise acutely and significantly (White and Baker, 1987). The recurrent spells, often associated with tremor, tachycardia, and headache, may suggest a pheochromocytoma. Even more commonly, hyperventilation is responsible for many of the symptoms noted by recently discovered hypertensives who are anxious over their diagnosis. Along with the symptoms, hyperventilation may cause myocardial and vascular contractions, leading to coronary spasm (Previtali et al, 1989), as well as a rise in systemic BP (Fig. 15.3).

## ACUTE STRESS

Hypertension may appear during various acute stresses, presumably reflecting an overshoot or an overreaction to sympathetic discharge. Problems related to anesthesia and surgery are covered in Chapter 7.

### Medical Conditions

#### Hypoglycemia

Hypertension may appear during hypoglycemia, particularly if it develops in diabetics receiving noncardioselective beta-blockers, wherein alpha-mediated vasoconstriction may be unopposed (Lloyd-Mostyn and Oram, 1975).

#### Acute Pancreatitis

Of 42 patients with acute pancreatitis 40 had transient hypertension that often was of a severe degree (Sankaran et al, 1974). Though this could reflect a flood of catecholamines, there may be a release of increased amounts of renin from the initial volume contraction and an increased conversion of inactive renin to the active form by proteolytic enzymes released from the inflamed pancreas (Greenstein et al, 1987).

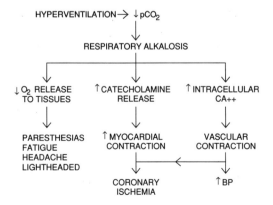

**Figure 15.3.** The mechanisms by which acute hyperventilation may induce various symptoms, coronary ischemia, and a rise in blood pressure.

#### Alcohol Withdrawal

Even without pancreatitis, transient hypertension often accompanies the withdrawal from alcohol in chronic alcoholics (Saunders et al, 1979). Additionally, even without withdrawal, hypertension is more common among those who consume more than an average of 2 ounces of alcohol per day, as covered in Chapter 3.

#### Sickle Cell Crisis

Hypertension may reflect pain or renal ischemia (Sellers, 1978). As with patients with other hematological disorders, severe hypertension may occur in sickle cell patients given multiple transfusions (Warth, 1984).

#### Porphyria

Attacks of acute intermittent porphyria often include hypertension and tachycardia, associated with increased levels of plasma catecholamines. Platelets from patients having acute porphyria take up and accumulate less norepinephrine, suggesting that the high levels of circulating catechols may result from blockade of reuptake into sympathetic neurons (Beal et al, 1977).

#### Cold Exposure

Hypertension subsequently developed in seven of 11 people who experienced pulmonary edema when scuba diving or surface swimming in cold water (Wilmshurst et al, 1989).

### Surgical Conditions

#### Burns

Hypertension appears in about 25% of patients with significant second and third degree burns (Brizio-Molteni et al, 1979). The blood pressure usually rises within 3 to 5 days, may last 2 weeks, and may, on occasion, induce encephalopathy (Lowrey, 1967). The mechanism may involve activation of either the sympathetic nerves or renin-angiotensin.

#### Perioperative

In addition to those mentioned in the coverage of anesthesia and hypertension in Chapter 7, there are numerous reasons why hypertension may be a problem during and soon after surgery. As an example, the application of a tourniquet during lower limb surgery was accompanied by hypertension in 11% of patients (Kaufman and Walts, 1982). Children who have surgery for leg lengthening and for correction of flexion contractures about the knee may develop hypertension (Harandi and Zahir, 1974), but this may also occur when traction is applied for the treatment of fractures (Linshaw et al, 1979) or during immobilization by casts (Turner et al, 1979).

Hypertension may appear in the immediate postoperative period for many reasons. Sixty of 1844 had readings in excess of 190/100 in the recovery room (Gal and Cooperman, 1975). Of these, 60% had a past history of hypertension. The elevated pressures usually appeared within 30 minutes after the end of surgery and lasted about 2 hours. The probable causes of this transient hypertension were: pain (36%), hypoxia and hypercarbia (19%), and physical and emotional excitement (32%).

### Cardiovascular Surgery

Hypertension may accompany various cardiovascular surgical procedures for various reasons (Estafanous and Tarazi, 1980) (Table 15.3).

*Coronary Bypass.* Since so many coronary artery bypass graft (CABG) procedures are being done, the hypertension seen after this procedure has received special attention. About one-third of patients will have hypertension after coronary bypass surgery, usually starting within the first 2 postoperative hours and lasting 4 to 6 hours (Colvin and Kenny, 1989). Those who have

**Table 15.3. Hypertension Associated with Cardiac Surgery[a]**

Preoperative
  Anxiety, angina, etc.
  Discontinuation of antihypertensive therapy
  "Rebound" from blocking agents in patients with
    coronary artery disease
Intraoperative
  Induction of anesthesia
    Specific drugs
    Hypertension due to tracheal intubation and
      nasopharyngeal, urethral, or rectal manipulation
  Precardiopulmonary bypass (during sternotomy and
    chest retraction)
  Cardiopulmonary bypass
  Postcardiopulmonary bypass (during surgery)
Postoperative
  Early—within 2 hours
    Obvious cause: hypoxia, hypercarbia, ventilatory
      difficulties, hypothermia, shivering, arousal from
      anesthesia
    With no obvious cause: after myocardial
      revascularization; less frequently after valve
      replacement; early (Sealy type I) hypertension
      after resection of aortic coarctation
  Intermediate—12 to 36 hours after surgery: Sealy
    type II after repair of aortic coarctation
  Late—weeks to months: after aortic valve
    replacement by homografts

[a]Data from Estafanous FG, Tarazi RC: *Am J Cardiol* 46:685, 1980.

been on beta-blockers preoperatively (Whelton et al, 1980) and those who have a Type A behavior pattern (Kahn et al, 1980) may be more prone to develop hypertension.

The hypertension appears to reflect an increase in peripheral resistance resulting from sympathetic overactivity (Fouad et al, 1978; Cooper et al, 1985) whereas the renin system does not appear to be involved (Weinstein et al, 1987). Immediate therapy may be important to prevent postoperative heart failure or myocardial infarction. Besides stellate ganglion blockade, various parenteral vasodilators have been found to work. These include nitroprusside, nitroglycerin (Colvin and Kenny, 1989), trimetaphan (Corr et al, 1986), and nifedipine (van Wezel et al, 1987). Preoperative labetalol has been found to reduce the frequency of hypertension during CABG surgery (Dubois et al, 1984) and it may be used postoperatively (Orlowski et al, 1989). An ultrashort-acting beta-blocker, esmolol, has worked very well (Gray et al, 1987).

*Other Cardiac Surgery.* Hypertension may also occur, though less frequently, after other operations on the heart, including closure of atrial septal defects (Cockburn et al, 1975), valve replacement (Estafanous et al, 1978), and cardiac transplantation (Carruthers et al, 1984). Closure of a peripheral arteriovenous shunt may precipitate acute hypertension by various mechanisms, including activation of the renin-angiotensin mechanism (Rocchini et al, 1978).

*Carotid Endarterectomy.* Postoperative hypertension may be particularly serious in patients with known cerebrovascular disease who have carotid endarterectomy, perhaps because of sudden exposure of the damaged intracerebral vessels to both high pressure and blood flow (Caplan et al, 1978). Treatment might be most logically with a short-acting beta-blocker (esmolol) or labetalol (Orlowski et al, 1988) rather than with a vasodilator that might further increase cerebral blood flow.

## INCREASED INTRAVASCULAR VOLUME

If vascular volume is raised a significant degree over a short period of time, the renal natriuretic response may not be able to excrete the load, particularly if renal function is also impaired. This is likely the mechanism for hypertension after resuscitation (Ledgerwood and Lucas, 1974) and in some postoperative situations.

**Table 15.4. Hypertension Induced by Chemical Agents[a]**

| Mechanism | Examples |
| --- | --- |
| Expansion of fluid volume | |
|   Increased sodium intake | Antacids, processed foods (Chapter 6) |
|   Mineralocorticoid effects | Licorice (Stewart et al, 1987), cortisone, anabolic steroids (Bretza et al, 1980) |
|   Stimulation of renin-angiotensin | Estrogens (oral contraceptives) (Chapter 11) |
|   Blockade of diuretic effects (inhibition of prostaglandins) | Nonsteroidal antiinflammatory agents (Patak et al, 1975) |
| Stimulation of sympathetic nervous activity | |
|   Sympathomimetic agents | Cocaine (Virmani et al, 1988) |
| | Nose drops: phenylephrine (Saken et al, 1979) |
| | Nasal decongestants: pseudoephedrine (Mariani, 1986) |
| | Appetite suppressants: phenylpropanolamine (Pentel, 1984) |
| | Methylphenidate (Ritalin) (Ballard et al, 1976) |
| | Phencyclidine (Sernulan) poisoning (Eastman and Cohen, 1975) |
|   Interactions with monamine oxidase inhibitors | Foods with high tyramine content (red wines, aged cheese, etc.) (Liu and Rustgi, 1987) |
| | Sympathomimetics (Blackwell, 1986) |
|   Anesthetics | Ketamine (Pipkin and Waldron, 1983) |
|   Narcotic antagonist | Naloxone (Levin et al, 1985) |
|   Ergot alkaloids | Ergometrine (Browning, 1974) |
|   Antidopaminergies | Bromocriptine (Parlodel) (ADR, 1983) |
| | Metoclopamide (Roche, 1985) |
| Interference with antihypertensive drugs | |
|   Inhibition of prostaglandin synthesis (diuretics, beta-blockers) | Nonsteroidal anti-inflammatory drugs (Durao et al, 1977) |
|   Inhibition of neuronal uptake (block guanethidine, clonidine, methyldopa) | Nontricyclic antidepressants (Briant et al, 1973) |
| Paradoxical response to antihypertensive drugs | |
|   Withdrawal, followed by increased catechols | Clonidine (Metz et al, 1987) |
|   Unopposed alpha-adrenergic vasoconstriction | Beta-blockers (Drayer et al, 1976) |
|   Intrinsic sympathomimetic activity | Pindolol (Collins and King, 1972) |
|   Combination of beta-blocker and alpha-agonist | Propranolol plus clonidine (Warren et al, 1979) or methyldopa (Nies and Shand, 1973) |
| Unknown mechanisms | |
|   Heavy metal poisoning | Lead (Bertel et al, 1978) |
| | Thallium (Bank et al, 1972) |
|   Chemicals | Ethylene glycol dinitrate (Carmichael and Lieben, 1963) |
| | Methyl chloride (Scharnweber et al, 1974) |
| | Polychlorinated biphenyl (Kreiss et al, 1981) |
|   Insecticides | Parathion (Tsachalinas et al, 1971) |
|   Insect bites | Spiders (Weitzman et al, 1977) |
| | Scorpion (Gueron and Yaron, 1970) |
|   Diagnostic agents | Indigo carmine (Wu and Johnson, 1969) |
| | Pentagastrin (Merguet et al, 1968) |
| | Thyrotropin-releasing hormone (Rosenthal et al, 1987) |
|   Therapeutic agents | Lithium (Michaeli et al, 1984) |
| | Digitalis (Cohn et al, 1969) |
| | Cyclosporine (Curtis et al, 1988) |
| | Disulfiram (Volicer and Nelson, 1984) |

[a]Modified from Messerli FH, Frohlich ED: *Arch Intern Med* 139:682, 1979, copyright 1979, American Medical Association.

## Erythropoietin Therapy

Recombinant human erythropoietin is now being widely used to correct the anemia of chronic renal failure. As the hematocrit rises, so do blood viscosity and blood pressure (Raine, 1988). There is a need to correct the anemia slowly so as not to induce severe hypertension (Tomson et al, 1988).

## Polycythemia

Patients with primary polycythemia are often hypertensive, and some hypertensives have a relative polycythemia that may go away when the blood pressure is lowered (Chrysant et al, 1976). With a high hematocrit, cerebral blood flow may be significantly reduced, putting the patient at additional risk (Hudak et al, 1986). With venesection and a fall in hematocrit, cerebral blood flow increases (Humphrey et al, 1979).

## Hyperviscosity

The hypertension seen in polycythemic states could also reflect increased blood viscosity that, by impairing renal perfusion, could stimulate renin release. One striking example of malignant hypertension has been reported in a patient with marked hyperviscosity caused by myeloma (Rubio-Garcia et al, 1989).

### After Transfusions

A syndrome of hypertension, convulsions, and cerebral hemorrhage has been reported in eight patients with thalassemia after they were given multiple blood transfusions (Wasi et al, 1978). Since the episodes often developed days after the transfusions, they were considered not to reflect volume overload, but rather the presence of unknown vasopressor substances. Similar episodes have been reported in others receiving multiple transfusions, particularly in the presence of renal insufficiency (Eggert and Stick, 1988).

### Inappropriate Antidiuretic Hormone

Hypertension has been reported in patients with inappropriate secretion of antidiuretic hormone, presumably related to an overexpanded vascular volume (Whitaker et al, 1979).

### DRUGS AND OTHER SUBSTANCES THAT CAUSE HYPERTENSION

A variety of drugs, a few foods, and poisons may cause hypertension in various ways (Oren et al, 1988) (Table 15.4). Some of these, such as sodium-containing antacids, alcohol, insulin, licorice, oral contraceptives, cyclosporine, and monoamine oxidase inhibitors, are covered elsewhere because of their frequency or special features.

Perhaps the most commonly encountered form of chemically induced hypertension is that related to the use of foods and drugs containing large amounts of sodium. More dramatic effects will be seen with the use of sympathomimetic agents. Large amounts of these drugs, available over-the-counter for use as nasal decongestants and appetite suppressants, may raise the blood pressure enough to induce, on rare occasions, hypertensive encephalopathy, strokes, and heart attacks (Pentel, 1984).

The multiple interferences with the effectiveness of various antihypertensive agents are covered in Chapter 7. With increasing use of prostaglandin inhibitors, the possibility of interference with the effects of both diuretics and beta-blockers (Durao et al, 1977) should be kept in mind. Tricyclic antidepressants may induce postural hypotension on the one hand and interfere with the antihypertensive effect of certain drugs on the other (Marshall and Forker, 1982).

Perhaps the safest way to prevent these various interactions and interferences is to advise hypertensives to avoid all over-the-counter drugs and to be sure to make those who prescribe medications aware of their antihypertensive drug regimens.

### Street Drugs

Marijuana or delta-9-tetrahydrocannabinol (THC) in moderate amounts will increase the heart rate but usually lowers the blood pressure (Hollister, 1986).

Heroin and other drugs taken intravenously may lead to severe renal damage, likely from an immunological response (Rao et al, 1974).

Cocaine and amphetamines may cause significant though transient hypertension and may interfere with action of adrenergic inhibitors. Most cocaine-related deaths are associated with myocardial injury similar to that seen from catecholamine excess and aggravated by acute hypertension (Virmani et al, 1988).

### References

Abbott M: *Am Heart J* 3:392, 1928.
ADR Highlight No. 83-12, FDA (HRN-730), 5600 Fishers La., Rockville, MD 20857, 1983.
Aksamit TR, Floras JS, Victor RG, et al: *Hypertension* 9:309, 1987.
Bagby SP, Mass RD: *Hypertension* 2:631, 1980.
Ballard JE, Boileau RA, Sleator EK, et al: *JAMA* 236:2870, 1976.
Bank WJ, Pleasure DE, Suzuki K, et al: *Arch Neurol* 26:456, 1972.
Barreca A, Ciccarelli E, Minuto F, et al: *Acta Endocrinologica* (Copeh) 120:629, 1989.
Beal MF, Atuk NO, Westfall TC, et al: *J Clin Invest* 60:1141, 1977.
Bell GM, Doig A: *Handbook of Hypertension, Clinical Aspects of Secondary Hypertension*, Vol 2. New York: Elsevier, 1983:291.

Benedict CR, Grahame-Smith DG, Fisher A: *Circulation* 57:598, 1978.
Bergqvist D, Bergentz S-E, Ekberg M, et al: *Acta Med Scand* 223:275, 1988.
Bertel O, Buhler FR, Ott J: *Br Med J* 1:551, 1978.
Bing RF, Swales JD: *Handbook of Hypertension, Clinical Aspects of Secondary Hypertension*, Vol 2. New York: Elsevier, 1983:276.
Blackwell B: *Br J Psychiatry* 148:216, 1986.
Bretza JA, Novey HS, Vaziri ND, et al: *Arch Intern Med* 140:1379, 1980.
Briant RH, Reid JL, Dollery CT: *Br Med J* 1:522, 1973.
Brickman AS, Stern N, Sowers JR: *Am J Med* 85:785, 1988.
Brizio-Molteni L, Molteni A, Cloutier LC, et al: *Scand J Plast Reconstr Surg* 13:21, 1979.

Browning DJ: *Med J Aust* 1:957, 1974.
Burack B: *Am Heart J* 107:543, 1984.
Campbell M: *Br Heart J* 32:633, 1970.
Caplan LR, Skillman J, Ojemann R, et al: *Stroke* 9:457, 1978.
Carmichael P, Lieben J: *Arch Environ Health* 7:424, 1963.
Carruthers SG, Webster EG, Kostuk WJ, et al: *Am J Cardiol* 53:334, 1984.
Christensson T, Hellstrom K, Wengle B: *Arch Intern Med* 137:1138, 1977.
Chrysant SG, Frohlich ED, Adamopoulos PN, et al: *Am J Cardiol* 37:1069, 1976.
Cockburn JS, Benjamin IS, Thomson RM, et al: *J Cardiovasc Surg* 16:1, 1975.
Cohen M, Fuster V, Steele PM, et al: *Circulation* 80:840, 1989.
Cohn JN, Tristani FE, Khatri IM: *Am Heart J* 78:318, 1969.

Collins IS, King IW: *Curr Ther Res* 14:185, 1972.

Colvin JR, Kenny GNC: *Anaesthesia* 44:37, 1989.

Cooper TJ, Clutton-Brock TH, Jones SN, et al: *Br Heart J* 54:91, 1985.

Corr L, Grounds RM, Brown MJ, et al: *Br Heart J* 56:89, 1986.

Curtis JJ, Luke RG, Jones P, et al: *Am J Med* 85:134, 1988.

Davies DL, Beastall GH, Connell JMC, et al: *J Hypertension* 3(Suppl 3):S413, 1985.

Davies J, Rowlatt RJ: *Br Med J* 2:1608, 1978.

Deray G, Rieu M, Devynck MA, et al: *N Engl J Med* 316:575, 1987.

Diamond TW, Botha JR, Wing J, et al: *Arch Intern Med* 146:1709, 1986.

Drayer JIM, Keim JH, Weber MA, et al: *Am J Med* 60:987, 1976.

Dubois C, Fischler M, Schlumberger S, et al: *J Hypertension* 2:432, 1984.

Durao V, Prata MM, Goncalves LMP: *Lancet* 3:1005, 1977.

Eastman JW, Cohen SN: *JAMA* 231:1270, 1975.

Eggert P, Stick C: *Lancet* 1:1344, 1988.

Estafanous FG, Tarazi RC: *Am J Cardiol* 46:685, 1980.

Estafanous FG, Tarazi RC, Buckley S, et al: *Br Heart J* 40:718, 1978.

Fixler DE: *Cardiol Clin* 6:561, 1988.

Fouad FM, Estafanous FG, Tarazi RC: *Am J Cardiol* 41:564, 1978.

Funck-Brentano C, Pagny J-Y, Menard J: *Br Heart J* 57:487, 1987.

Gal TJ, Cooperman LH: *Br J Anaesth* 47:70, 1975.

Garbarino KA, Levitt JR, Feinsod FM: *Am J Med* 86:734, 1989.

Gray RJ, Bateman TM, Czer LSC, et al: *Am J Cardiol* 59:887, 1987.

Greenstein RJ, Krakoff LR, Felton K: *Am J Med* 82:401, 1987.

Grunstein RR, Handelsman DJ, Lawrence SJ, et al: *J Clin Endocrinol Metab* 68:352, 1989.

Gueron M, Yaron R: *Chest* 57:156, 1970.

Guilleminault C, Tilkian A, Dement WC: *Annu Rev Med* 27:465, 1976.

Harandi BA, Zahir A: *J Bone Joint Surg* 56A:1733, 1974.

Hedner J, Ejnell H, Sellgren J, et al: *J Hypertension* 6(Suppl 4):S529, 1988.

Hoffstein V, Rubinstein I, Mateika S, et al: *Lancet* 2:992, 1988.

Hollister LE: *Pharmacol Reviews* 38:1, 1986.

Horky' K, Broulik P, Pacovsky' V: *J Hypertension* 4(Suppl 6):S585, 1986.

Hudak ML, Koehler RC, Rosenberg AA, et al: *Am J Physiol* 251:H63, 1986.

Humphrey PRD, Marshall J, Russell RWR, et al: *Lancet* 3:873, 1979.

Ishikawa K: *Circulation* 57:27, 1978.

Jennum P, Wildschiødtz G, Christensen NJ, et al: *Am J Hypertens* 2:847, 1989.

Jespersen B, Pedersen EB, Charles P, et al: *Acta Endocrinologica* (Copenh) 120:362, 1989.

Johnson B, Pallares V, Thomason R, et al: *Milit Med* 140:345, 1975.

Kahn JP, Kornfeld DS, Frank KA, et al: *Psychosom Med* 42:407, 1980.

Kales A, Bixler EO, Cadieux RJ, et al: *Lancet* 1:1005, 1984.

Kaufman RD, Walts LF: *Br J Anaesth* 54:333, 1982.

Keech AC, Westlake GW, Wallis PL, et al: *Am Heart J* 115:1328, 1988.

Kreiss K, Zack MM, Kimbrough RD, et al: *JAMA* 245:2505, 1981.

Kuchel O, Cusson JR, Larochelle P, et al: *J Hypertension* 5:277, 1987.

Lafferty F, Hubay CA: *Arch Intern Med* 149:789, 1989.

Lande A: *AJR* 127:227, 1976.

Lavie P, Alroy G, Halpern E: *Isr J Med Sci* 18:523, 1982.

Lavie P, Ben-Yosef R, Rubin AE: *Am Heart J* 108:373, 1984.

Ledgerwood AM, Lucas CE: *Arch Surg* 108:531, 1974.

Leenen FHH, Balfe JA, Pelech AN, et al: *Am Heart J* 113:1164, 1987.

Levin ER, Sharp B, Drayer JIM, et al: *Am J Med Sci* 290:70, 1985.

Liard J-F, Spadone J-C: *J Hypertension* 3:281, 1985.

Lind L, Wengle B, Wide L, et al: *Am J Hypertens* 1:397, 1988.

Linshaw MA, Stapleton FB, Gruskin AB, et al: *J Pediatr* 95:994, 1979.

Liu L, Rustgi AK: *Am J Med* 82:1060, 1987.

Lloyd-Mostyn RH, Oram S: *Lancet* 1:1213, 1975.

Lowrey GH: *J Trauma* 7:140, 1967.

Mariani PJ: *Am J Emerg Med* 4:141, 1986.

Marshall JB, Forker AD: *Am Heart J* 103:401, 1982.

Merguet P, Ewers HR, Brouwers HP: *Kongr Innere Med* 80:561, 1968.

Messerli FH, Frohlich ED: *Arch Intern Med* 139:682, 1979.

Metz S, Klein C, Morton N: *Am J Med* 82:17, 1987.

Michaeli J, Ben-Ishay D, Kidron R, et al: *JAMA* 251:1680, 1984.

Murphy AM, Blades M, Daniels S, et al: *Am Heart J* 117:1327, 1989.

Naftchi NE, Demeny M, Lowman EW, et al: *Circulation* 57:336, 1978.

Nanton MA, Olley PM: *Am J Cardiol* 37:769, 1976.

Nies AS, Shand DG: *Clin Pharmacol Ther* 14:823, 1973.

Oren A, Grossman E, Messerli FH, et al: *Cardiol Clin* 6:467, 1988.

Orlowski JP, Shiesley D, Vidt DG, et al: *Crit Care Med* 16:765, 1988.

Orlowski JP, Vidt DG, Walker S, et al: *Cleve Clin J Med* 56:29, 1989.

Parker FG Jr, Streeten DHP, Farrell B, et al: *Circulation* 66:513, 1982.

Patak RV, Mookerjee BK, Bentzel CJ, et al: *Prostaglandins* 10:649, 1975.

Pentel P: *JAMA* 252:1898, 1984.

Pipkin FB, Waldron BA: *Clin Exp Hypertens* 5:875, 1983.

Plets C: *Am J Cardiol* 63:40C, 1989.

Previtali M, Ardissino D, Barberis P, et al: *Am J Cardiol* 63:17, 1989.

Raine AEG: *Lancet* 1:97, 1988.

Rao PS, Najjar HN, Mardini MK, et al: *Am Heart J* 115:657, 1988.

Rao TKS, Nicastri AD, Friedman EA: *N Engl J Med* 190:19, 1974.

Reifenstein GH, Levine SA, Gross RE: *Am Heart J* 33:146, 1947.

Richards AM, Espiner EA, Nicholls MG, et al: *J Hypertension* 6:747, 1988.

Rocchini AP, Rosenthal A, Schuster S: *Am Heart J* 95:497, 1978.

Roche H: *N Engl J Med* 312:1125, 1985.

Rosenberg FB: *Arch Intern Med* 121:95, 1968.

Rosenthal E, Najm YC, Maisey MN, et al: *Br Med J* 294:806, 1987.

Rosenthal FB, Roy S: *Br Med J* 4:396, 1972.

Rubio-Garcia R, de Garcia-Diaz J, Ortiz MC, et al: *Am J Med* 87:119, 1989.

Sahn DJ, Anderson F: *An Atlas for Echocardiographers: Two-dimensional Anatomy of the Heart*. New York: Wiley Medical Publications, 1982:454.

Saken R, Kates GL, Miller K: *J Pediatr* 95:1077, 1979.

Salahudeen AK, Thomas TH, Sellars L, et al: *Clin Sci* 76:289, 1989.

Sankaran S, Lucas CE, Walt AJ: *Surg Gynecol Obstet* 138:235, 1974.

Saunders JB, Beevers DG, Paton A: *Clin Sci* 57:295s, 1979.

Scharnweber HC, Spears GN, Cowles SR: *JOM* 16:112, 1974.

Schroeder JS, Motta J, Guilleminault C: *Sleep Apnea Syndromes*. New York: Alan R. Liss, 1978:191.

Schwartz DT: *Angiology* 21:568, 1970.

Sealy WC: *Surg Gynecol Obeste* 97:301, 1953.

Sehested J, Kornerup HG, Pderesen EB, et al: *Cur Heart J* 4:52, 1983.

Sellers BB: *J Pediatr* 92:941, 1978.

Shelhamer JH, Volkman DJ, Parrillo JE, et al: *Ann Intern Med* 103:121, 1985.

Shinebourne EA, Tam ASY, Elseed AM, et al: *Br Heart J* 38:375, 1976.

Simard JM, Bellefleur M: *Am J Cardiol* 63:32C, 1989.

Simpson IA, Sahn DJ, Valdes-Cruz LM, et al: *Circulation* 77:736, 1988.

Simsolo R, Grunfeld B, Gimenez M, et al: *Am Heart J* 115:1268, 1988.

Smyth PT, Edwards JE: *Circulation* 46:1027, 1972.

Stacy DL, Prewitt RL: *Am J Physiol* 256:H213, 1989.

Stewart PM, Wallace AM, Valentino R, et al: *Lancet* 2:821, 1987.

Streeten DHP, Anderson GH Jr, Howland T, et al: *Hypertension* 11:78, 1988.

Tauber JP, Tauber BMT, Vigoni F, et al: *J Clin Endocrniol Metab* 68:917, 1989.

Thomas JP: *Br Med J* 286:330, 1983.

Thuesen L, Christensen SE, Weeke J, et al: *Acta Med Scand* 223:337, 1988.

Tomson CRV, Venning MC, Ward MK: *Lancet* 1:351, 1988.

Tsachalinas D, Logaras G, Paradelis A: *Eur J Toxicol Environ Hyg* 4:46, 1971.

Turner MC, Ruley EJ, Buckley KM, et al: *J Pediatr* 95:989, 1979.

Van Aken H, Cottrell JE, Anger C, et al: *Am J Cardiol* 63:43C, 1989.

van Wezel HB, Bovill JG, Koolen JJ, et al: *Am Heart J* 113:266, 1987.

Ventura HO, Messerli FH, Barron RE: *J Hypertension* 4:265, 1986.

Virmani R, Robinowitz M, Smialek JE, et al: *Am Heart J* 115:1068, 1988.

Vlachakis ND, Fredericks R, Velasquez M, et al: *Hypertension* 4:452, 1982.

Volicer L, Nelson KL: *Arch Intern Med* 144:1294, 1984.

Waller PC, Bhopal RS: *Lancet* 1:143, 1989.

Warley ARH, Mitchell JH, Stradling JR: *Q J Med* 68:637, 1988.

Warren SE, Ebert E, Swerdlin A-H, et al: *Arch Intern Med* 139:253, 1979.

Warth JA: *Ann Intern Med* 144:607, 1984.

Wasi P, Pootrakul P, Piankijagum A, et al: *Lancet* 2:602, 1978.

Weinstein GS, Zabetakis PM, Clavel A, et al. *Ann Thorac Surg* 43:74, 1987.

Weitzman S, Margulis G, Lehmann E: *Am Heart J* 93:89, 1977.

Wennlund A, Linde B: *J Clin Endocrniol Metab* 59:258, 1984.

Whelton PK, Flaherty JT, MacAllister NP, et al: *Hypertension* 2:291, 1980.

Whitaker MD, McArthur RG, Corenblum B, et al: *Am J Med* 67:511, 1979.

White WB, Baker LH: *Arch Intern Med* 147:1973, 1987.

Williams AJ, Houston D, Finberg S, et al: *Am J Cardiol* 55:1019, 1985.

Wilmshurst PT, Nuri M, Crowther A, et al: *Lancet* 1:62, 1989.

Wu CC, Johnson AF: *Henry Ford Hosp Med J* 17:131, 1969.

# 16 Hypertension in Childhood and Adolescence

Ellin Lieberman, M.D.

A separate discussion of pediatric hypertension is needed in a book focused primarily on the disease as seen in adults because: (1) Many physicians care for children and adults; (2) criteria for the diagnosis of hypertension in an individual less than 16 years of age are based on techniques and data that differ from those used in adults; (3) techniques for the evaluation and treatment of children and adolescents also differ; (4) the existence of primary (essential) hypertension in parents has important implications for their offspring; (5) primary hypertension may have its origins in infancy and childhood; and (6) attention to cardiovascular risk factors during the first two decades in life may prevent or retard the development of vascular complications associated with hypertension.

This chapter focuses on the problems of measurements and of interpretation of blood pressure levels in children, on the significance of elevated blood pressure levels, and on the special issues involving neonatal hypertension, reflux nephropathy, and hypertensive emergencies. Table 16.1 summarizes secondary causes encountered in pediatrics including some not listed in Table 1.10, which deals with patients of all ages. Special comments pertinent to a pediatric perspective are included. A discussion of major nonrenal causes has been excluded because they are covered elsewhere in this text: coarctation of the aorta in Chapter 15, adrenocortical disorders in Chapters 13 and 14, pheochromocytoma in Chapter 12.

Knowledge concerning childhood hypertension has expanded during the past two decades.

Attention has been focused on epidemiology, cardiovascular risk factors, clinical evaluation, and treatment. Clinicians now have an opportunity to apply information from field studies and clinical reports to their medical practice. Long-term data concerning outcome variables are still lacking and require extrapolation from experience with adults. Areas that remain controversial and uncertain are identified so that the reader can distinguish assumptions from facts.

## BLOOD PRESSURE MEASUREMENTS

Accurate recording and interpretation of blood pressure levels in infants, children, and adolescents require usage of appropriate equipment, agreement concerning which Korotkoff sounds are used for diastolic pressure, and, most importantly, the availability of adequate data from large numbers of normal children examined with similar techniques. The following is an adaptation for children of the portion of Chapter 2 that deals with blood pressure measurements in adults.

### Technique

The fewest errors result if the observer employs the technique outlined below, recording the levels, the position of the child, and the size of the cuff used. The mercury manometer should be in place at eye level to avoid errors introduced by parallax, and the child's arm should be placed at heart level.

### Cuff Size

The choice of blood pressure cuff depends on the size and not on the age of the child. The

**Table 16.1.  Causes of Hypertension in Children and Adolescents**

| Cause | Author's Comments |
|---|---|
| **Renal** | |
| Bilateral involvement | |
| Glomerulonephritis, acute or chronic | Children and adolescents with these renal disorders have a constellation of symptoms, signs, and laboratory findings such that their evaluation is focused; diagnostic studies should be expedited systematically and intervention should be prompt. |
| Previous infection (e.g., streptococcal) | |
| Henoch-Schönlein purpura | |
| Lupus erythematosus | |
| Hemolytic-uremic syndrome | |
| Hypersensitivity reactions | Not always associated with hypertension. |
| Acute renal failure (acute interstitial nephritis, acute shutdown, acute tubular necrosis) | Hypertension in this setting is most often due to volume overload. |
| End stage renal disease (ESRD) | Severe, chronic, resistant hypertension often present when glomerular filtration rate (GFR) is $< 5$ ml/min/1.73M$^2$ |
| Bilateral or unilateral involvement | |
| Asymmetric renal disease | A significant cause of **malignant** and life-threatening hypertension in pediatrics. This diagnosis has generally been underemphasized in the literature. |
| Malformations including bilateral polycystic kidneys, hypoplasia, ureteropelvic junction obstruction | This group of anomalies is readily documented by renal ultrasound ± nuclear scans in patients older than one month and with normal renal function. Patients with autosomal recessive polycystic renal disease often have life-threatening hypertension and congestive heart failure in the first months of life. |
| Pyelonephritis with or without hydronephrosis | **Reflux Nephropathy** with scarred, small kidneys is a prominent cause of **malignant** hypertension, especially in girls ages 7 to 18 years. |
| Tubulopathies: cystinosis, medullary cyst disease, nephronophthisis | Hypertension characteristically absent until severe decrease in GFR and volume overload supervene. |
| Renal arterial disorders | |
| Renal artery stenosis (unilateral, bilateral or segmental), Takayasu's disease (affecting renal arteries), neurofibromatosis | Usually associated with moderate to **malignant** hypertension in pediatric patients from $< 16$ months to 18 years. Atypically patient has milder fixed hypertension and requires evaluation. |
| Renal calculi | Unusual cause of hypertension unless due to pain, acute obstruction, or association with scarred kidneys. |
| Renal vein thrombosis ± vena caval thrombosis | May or may not have associated hypertension; usually mild, easy to recognize, and to treat. |
| Thrombosis, embolus | Especially important in neonates and young infants. Hypertension may resolve after 6 months or more of medical therapy. |
| Tumors (renal): Wilms', juxtaglomerular tumors | Wilms' has characteristic features and usually minimal if any hypertension; rarely associated with hyperreninemia and severe hypertension. Juxtaglomerular tumors: rare under 20 years of age; **malignant** hypertension with secondary aldosteronism; diagnosis may only be validated by surgery. |
| Trauma | Renal trauma acutely usually does not cause severe hypertension; but, long-term follow-up of severe trauma may be associated with moderate to severe hypertension. |
| **Cardiovascular** | |
| Coarctation of the aorta | May be difficult diagnosis in neonate, readily diagnosed in older pediatric patients. The second most common cause of secondary hypertension after all renal disorders. |
| Hypoplasia of abdominal aorta (coarctation of the abdominal aorta; mid-aortic arch syndrome) | Children and adolescents may present with markedly stunted growth; others may appear normal, and the severity of their hypertension is correlated with the magnitude of renal artery involvement. |
| **Endocrine** | |
| Adrenal | |
| Congenital adrenal hyperplasia | Usually diagnosed in early infancy. Salt-wasting, hyperkalemia and genital changes are characteristic features. |
| 11-hydroxylase deficiency | Very rare and associated with virilization and excessive growth. |
| 17-hydroxylase deficiency | Very rare, associated with hypogonadism. |
| Cushing's syndrome | Diagnosed by inspection. |
| Primary hyperaldosteronism | Extraordinarily rare cause of hypertension in pediatrics. |

**Table 16.1. Causes of Hypertension in Children and Adolescents—Continued**

| Cause | Author's Comments |
|---|---|
| **Endocrine** | |
| Adrenal—*continued* | |
| Dexamethasone-suppressible hyperaldosteronism | Rare; low PRA; autosomal dominant. |
| Pheochromocytoma | Patients have wide variety of complaints, including **malignant hypertension**; orthostatic hypotension, diaphoresis, weight loss, polyuria, visual complaints of varying degrees of severity. |
| Thyroid | |
| Hyperthyroidism | A very rare cause of hypertension and usually suspected from clinical findings. |
| Hyperparathyroidism/hypercalcemia | Hypercalcemia-induced hypertension should be considered in immobilized patients, patients on vitamin D therapy, with sarcoidosis (rare), and with tumors involving bone marrow. |
| Turner's syndrome (gonadal dysgenesis) | Hypertension may be due to coarctation, renal anomalies, or unknown etiology. |
| **Central nervous system** | |
| Infections, space-occupying lesions | Hypertension is component of altered central nervous system function. Usually not severe. |
| Dysautonomia (Riley Day syndrome) | Hypertension and hypotension characterize disorder. |
| **Burns** | **Severe**, typically transient hypertension may accompany extensive third degree burns, likely secondary to catecholamines. |
| **Orthopedic injuries and procedures** | Hypertension frequently accompanies transient trauma to long bones, leg lengthening, and placement of Harrington rods for scoliosis. |
| **Tumors (nonrenal): neuroblastoma, rhabdomyosarcoma, carcinomas** | Hypertension is usually mild and easy to treat. Cause is obvious. |
| **Drug ingestion and abuse** | |
| Sympathomimetics including amphetamines, ephedrine, polyephrine eye drops. | Patients may present with severe hypertension that readily resolves with drug withdrawal unless renal damage has occurred. |
| Glucocorticoids and mineralocorticoids | Mild hypertension unless agents being used as part of regimen for significant underlying renal disease. |
| Oral contraceptive agents | Mild hypertension that usually resolves with drug withdrawal. |
| Phencyclidine (PCP or "angel dust") | Severe hypertension that is responsive to emergency therapy. |
| Rebound hypertension with withdrawal of antihypertensive agents | Important in young children who develop acute gastroenteritis and vomit maintenance oral antihypertensive agents. |
| Poisonings (lead, mercury) | |

appropriate blood pressure cuff is one with a bladder that completely and comfortably encircles the girth of the arm, with or without overlap. At least three-fourths of the length of the child's upper arm should be covered by the bladder with adequate space in the antecubital fossa to allow proper placement of the head of the stethoscope. Available commercial cuffs have bladders with varying dimensions as shown in Table 16.2 (Report of the Second Task Force on Blood Pressure Control in Children, 1987).

If the ideal cuff and bladder are not available, use of a larger cuff is recommended to avoid spuriously high levels (Moss, 1981). The large adult cuff with large bladder dimensions is frequently required to obtain accurate measurements in a youngster with fat or muscular upper arms.

As with an adult with a large arm, inappropriate use of the regular adult cuff with such a child may provide falsely elevated blood pressure levels.

**Ultrasound**

Measurement of blood pressure in newborns and small infants is easy by the use of ultrasound by the Doppler method. The appropriate-sized cuff is wrapped around the upper arm with a transducer directly over the brachial artery. The systolic pressure is recorded when the intensity of reflected sound waves increases and the observer hears a sound. Continued deflation of the cuff results in a distinct muffling of the ultrasound signal that is interpreted as the diastolic pressure. This method provides data comparable to other noninvasive indirect procedures (Kirk-

**TABLE 16.2.  Dimensions of Bladders of Commercially Available Cuffs**

| | Range of Dimensions of Bladder (cm) | |
|---|---|---|
| | Width | Length |
| Newborn | 0.5–1.0 | 5.0–5.0 |
| Infant | 4.0–6.0 | 11.5–18.0 |
| Child | 7.5–9.0 | 17.0–19.0 |
| Adult | 11.5–13.0 | 22.0–26.0 |
| Large adult arm | 14.0–15.0 | 30.5–33.0 |
| Adult thigh | 18.0–19.0 | 36.0–38.0 |

land and Kirkland, 1972; Dweck et al, 1974) and direct intraarterial measurements (Moss, 1981), but accuracy of this method for diastolic levels remains undocumented (Weismann, 1988).

## Procedure

Children, especially in the toddler age group, are often anxious and restless. They require time to relax and to familiarize themselves with their surroundings and with the examiner. Younger children often respond favorably to a simple demonstration of the equipment and to realization that pain is not involved. Children often are more at ease in the sitting position than in a supine position. Even when these steps are taken and the child is quiet and cooperative, the Korotkoff sounds are often difficult to hear because they are softer in children than in adults.

When the child is ready and in a comfortable position, the arm is placed at heart level. By convention (Report of the Second Task Force, 1987), the right arm, sitting position, has been selected so that measurements can be compared over time. Inflation and deflation of the cuff are done in the same manner as with adults. The major difference is that the fourth Korotkoff phase (K4), i.e., point of muffling, has been selected as the best indirect measure of diastolic pressure in infants and children, up to 13 years of age (Kirkendall et al, 1981; Report of the Second Task Force, 1987). Use of the K4 phase is known to overestimate and use of the fifth phase (K5), i.e., disappearance of the sounds, to underestimate the diastolic pressure in children as compared with direct intraarterial recordings (Moss, 1981).

## Recording

To avoid confusion, the blood pressure measurement should be recorded as follows: right arm, sitting position, 9-cm cuff: 100/70/40 (i.e., K1, K4, and K5). Recording the measurement in this manner reduces the likelihood of extraneous variability in repeated measurements and allows comparisons of subsequent readings.

Nonetheless, the onset of the muffling sound (K4) may not be heard easily, and observer bias may cause repetitive recordings of the same numbers. Periodic quality control checks will assure that such errors are not introducing and perpetuating mistakes.

## Interpretation

The interpretation of blood pressure measurements in children has been impeded by the lack of well-designed epidemiological studies, by the variation in techniques, and by differences between recommendations for blood pressure measurement, guidelines endorsed by the American Heart Association from 1967 until 1981 (Kirkendall et al, 1981), guidelines from the Report of the Joint National Committee (1984), and the recent recommendations from the Second Task Force (1987). With these most recent recommendations, clinicians are now able to define what levels of blood pressures in the individual child clearly constitute an abnormality and what significance those levels have (Report of the Second Task Force, 1987).

Reference standards for the determination of percentiles for blood pressure levels are available from the Second Report of the Task Force, 1987. Figures 16.1 through 16.3 represent distribution curves for boys; similar curves for girls are available in the Report. Unfortunately only the first blood pressure reading was used to derive the blood pressure distribution curves, but they were obtained on over 70,000 white, black, and Mexican-American children from nine separate sources. The three sets of curves include systolic and diastolic pressure levels for boys and girls at birth to 12 months of age and from 1 to 13 years of age using the IV Korotkoff sound (K4) as the best indirect reflection of diastolic pressure and curves for both boys and girls from 13 to 18 years of age utilizing the V Korotkoff sound (K5). Data are supplied for integration of height and weight into the interpretation of the curves. If a child is taller and heavier than the 90th percentile and his/her blood pressure level falls into that decile, the child is *not* regarded as hypertensive. On the other hand, if the child is short and lean, the same blood pressure level is regarded as abnormal (Report of the Second Task Force, 1987).

## EPIDEMIOLOGICAL DATA AND SURVEYS

Since the report of Zinner et al, in 1974, surveys of blood pressure patterns in children

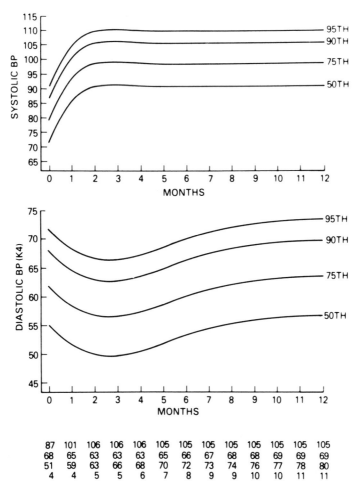

**Figure 16.1.** Age-specific percentiles of blood pressure measurements in boys—birth to 12 months of age; Korotkoff phase IV (K4) used for diastolic blood pressure. (From Report of the Second Task Force on Blood Pressure Control in Children—1987. *Pediatrics* 79:1, 1987.)

have sought to identify infants and children destined for hypertension in later life. These studies have provided cross-sectional and longitudinal data on neonates (deSwiet et al, 1984), on urban children and adolescents (Kotchen et al, 1974; Gillum et al, 1980; Hediger et al, 1984; Sinaiko et al, 1989), on Latin children (Kilcoyne 1974; Fixler et al, 1979; Gutgesell et al, 1981), black children, and adolescents (Kilcoyne 1974; Kotchen et al, 1974; Gutgesell et al, 1981; Sinaiko et al, 1989), on mature American children (Gillum et al, 1980), and on Japanese adolescents (Tochikubo et al, 1986). These studies did not identify significant abnormalities detectable early in childhood to explain why some racial groups are at increased risk from cardiovascular disease, but recent studies by Murphy et al (1988) demonstrated increased cardiovascular reactivity among black children as compared with white children, and McDonald et al (1987) reported that sodium-lithium countertransport was positively associated with systolic blood pressure in black children.

Consensus has been reached: Of all of the factors the most predictive one for sustained blood pressure elevation is an antecedent elevated blood pressure (Prineas et al, 1983; Hofman et al, 1985; Michels et al, 1987; Shear et al, 1986). However, Rames et al (1978), Fixler et al (1983) and Lauer et al (1984) have shown that children whose initial blood pressure levels fall within the highest quartile may on follow-up fall into a lower quartile. The converse was also true within each cohort. Lauer et al (1985) concluded that the significance of blood pressure levels could not be assessed without integrating data for height and weight.

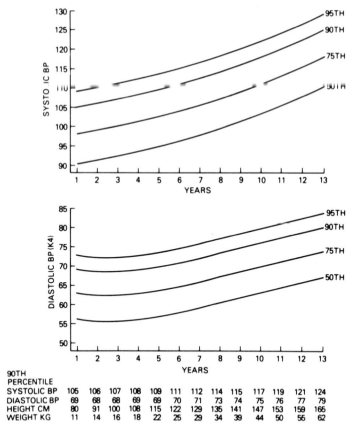

**Figure 16.2.** Age-specific percentiles of blood pressure measurements in boys—1 to 13 years of age; Korotkoff phase IV (K4) used for diastolic blood pressure. (From Report of the Second Task Force on Blood Pressure Control in Children—1987. *Pediatrics* 79:1, 1987.)

## Tracking

Table 16.3 summarizes results of five representative longitudinal studies of the extent to which children's blood pressure levels track. Zinner et al (1974) were the first investigators to study the tracking behavior of children. Follow-up of 365 of their original cohorts revealed increased evidence of tracking with rising correlation coefficients (Zinner et al, 1978). A 15-year prospective study of Welsh children confirmed long-term tracking with increasing correlation coefficients when the cohort was older at the examination (Rosner et al, 1977). The correlation coefficient between ages 3 years and 4 years was 0.47 for systolic blood pressure (deSwiet et al, 1980) after a 1-year follow-up. Data from Bogalusa were extended to 8 years using the mean of six blood pressure measurements (Shear et al, 1986). Furthermore, both prior systolic blood pressure levels and family history of hypertension independently predicted

the Year 9 systolic blood pressure group (Shear et al, 1986). When three prior serial blood pressure measurements were in the upper quartile, the Year 9 blood pressure remained in the same quartile in 68% of children for systolic pressure and in 62% for diastolic (Shear et al, 1986). Review of Table 16.3 reveals that correlation coefficients are higher for systolic than for diastolic pressures, are higher for older children than younger, and are higher when the mean of several measurements is used to derive the correlation coefficient.

Longitudinal studies of children with blood pressure patterns in the 95th percentile have revealed more consistent tracking when the study group is of adolescent age, obese, the offspring of hypertensive parents, or if echocardiographic changes exhibiting increased left ventricular wall mass are present. Current data indicate that an adolescent whose blood pressure has over time exceeded the 95th percentile and whose weight has also exceeded the 95th percentile is at greater

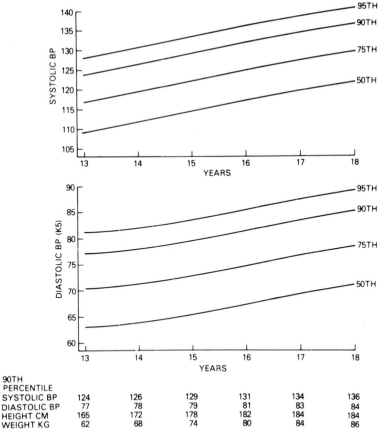

| 90TH PERCENTILE | | | | | | |
|---|---|---|---|---|---|---|
| SYSTOLIC BP | 124 | 126 | 129 | 131 | 134 | 136 |
| DIASTOLIC BP | 77 | 78 | 79 | 81 | 83 | 84 |
| HEIGHT CM | 165 | 172 | 178 | 182 | 184 | 184 |
| WEIGHT KG | 62 | 68 | 74 | 80 | 84 | 86 |

**Figure 16.3.** Age-specific percentiles of blood pressure measurements in boys—13 to 18 years of age; Korotkoff phase V (K5) used for diastolic blood pressure. (From Report of the Second Task Force on Blood Pressure Control in Children—1987. *Pediatrics* 79:1, 1987.)

**Table 16.3. Evidence for Tracking of Blood Pressure Levels in Children and Adolescents**

| Authors (yr) | Number | Initial Age Range (yr) | Follow-up Interval (yr) | R Values | |
|---|---|---|---|---|---|
| | | | | Systolic | Diastolic |
| Rosner et al (1977) | 56 | 15–19 | 15 | 0.51 | 0.32 |
| Zinner et al (1978) | 365 | 6–18 | 4[a] | 0.46 | 0.36 |
| | | 2–14 | 7–8[b] | 0.32 | 0.16 |
| deSwiet et al (1980) | 259 | 3 | 1 | 0.47 | |
| Shear et al (1986) | 1501 | 2–14 | 8 | 0.41 | 0.35 |
| Michels et al (1987) | 142 | 5.9–9.5 | 9 | 0.36 | 0.24[c] |

[a]Third survey versus second survey.
[b]Third survey versus first survey.
[c]Boys only.

risk than are his/her thinner peers with lower blood pressure levels (Fixler et al, 1983).

## Factors Determining Blood Pressure

Attempts to define the factors that determine blood pressure during childhood and adolescence have been summarized in a NHLBI symposium (Loggie et al, 1983). The importance of

the recognition of such factors lies in the generally accepted view that, if they were identified in childhood, then primary prevention of hypertension might become a realistic public health and clinical goal.

Multiple factors have been reported to correlate with blood pressure levels in children (Table 16.4). In addition to those listed, age (Zinner

**Table 16.4. Epidemiologic Factors Related to Blood Pressure Levels in Children and Adolescents**

Genetic
  Parental and sibling blood pressure levels—
    Mongeau, 1987
  Erythrocyte sodium flux—McDonald et al, 1987
  Urinary kallikrein level—Zinner et al 1976; Sinaiko et al 1982
  Haptoglobin phenotype 1-1—Weinberger et al, 1987
Environmental
  Socioeconomic status—Kotchen et al, 1974
  Rural versus urban residence—Kotchen and Kotchen, 1978
  Migration from developing area—Beaglehoe et al, 1978
  Pulse rate—Prineas et al, 1983
  Small for Gestational Age (S.G.A.)—Gennser et al, 1980; Barker et al, 1988
Mixed genetic and environmental
  Height—Lauer et al, 1985; Kahn and Bain, 1987
  Weight—Lauer et al, 1985
  Muscle mass—Wilson et al, 1985
  Sodium/potassium excretion—Prineas et al, 1983
  Stress—Parker et al, 1987
  Skinfold thickness—Aristimuno et al, 1984

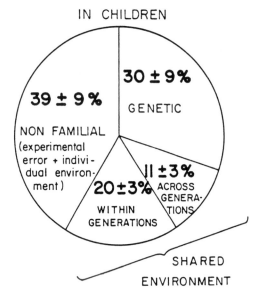

**IN CHILDREN**

**Figure 16.4.** Explanation of phenotypic variability for diastolic blood pressure in children (ISE). (From Mongeau J-G: Heredity and blood pressure in humans: An overview. *Pediatr Nephrol* 1:69, 1987.

et al, 1974; Lauer et al, 1984), sex (Goldring et al, 1977), and race (Goldring et al, 1977) have been shown to relate to blood pressure in children.

Analysis of these studies does not permit separation of genetic from nongenetic factors. Mongeau (1987) (Fig. 16.4) reviewed data from the Montreal adoption study, which led to a statistical assessment of the variability of blood pressure in children attributable to genetic (30

± 9%), nonfamilial (39 ± 9%), environmental (20 ± 3%), and shared environmental factors across generations (11 ± 3%). The specifics of genetic factors that are clearly separable from environmental influences or that overlap, e.g., body build, response to stress, or handling of a salt load, still require delineation.

The various factors listed in Table 16.4 are the major ones that have been found to correlate with blood pressure levels in young people. Most factors can be categorized as either genetic or environmental, but some have features of both. Height, body mass, and muscular development depend not only on genetic influences but also on nutrition and exercise. As noted in Chapter 3, salt intake may only exert its effect on blood pressure in those who are genetically predisposed to higher blood pressure levels and are salt sensitive. Blood pressure reactivity to some forms of stress varies with family history for hypertension (Falkner et al, 1979; Parker et al, 1987). Studies of children indicate that the single best correlate of elevated blood pressure is body mass.

**Genetic Factors**

The influence of genetic factors on blood pressure has been shown by the finding of a correlation of parental blood pressure levels with those of their natural offspring (Zinner et al, 1971, 1974; Lee et al, 1976; Kotchen et al, 1979; Higgins et al, 1980a and 1980b; Munger et al, 1988), the lack of correlation of parental blood pressure levels with those of their adopted children (Biron et al, 1976; Mongeau et al, 1987), and comparisons of siblings (Hennekens et al, 1976) and twins (monozygotic and dizygotic) and their families (Havlik et al, 1979; Rose et al, 1979). Overall the studies indicate that genetic factors play a strong but still ill-defined role (Mimura, 1973; Feinleib et al, 1975; Mongeau et al, 1987).

A number of potential differences between normotensive children with normotensive parents (FH −) and normotensive offspring of hypertensive parents (FH +) have been examined in an attempt to identify which child may be destined for future hypertension. These include:

—PRA was higher in FH + than in FH − although there was no difference in blood pressure levels (Shibutani et al, 1988).
—A 10-minute arithmetic test led to different blood pressure responses in adolescent controls, offspring of hypertensive parents, and

hypertensive adolescents, with the FH+ group responding more than the controls and less than their hypertensive peers (Falkner et al, 1979). When these studies were extended to include salt loading and then repeated mental stress testing on day 14, the FH+ group had greater diastolic and systolic levels after salt loading (Falkner et al, 1983).

—Increased forearm vascular resistance and decrease in forearm blood flow was demonstrated in FH+ but not in FH− in response to a short math test (Anderson et al, 1987).

—Diastolic blood pressure rose in response to stress tests in FH+ children (Parker et al, 1987).

—Diastolic blood pressure rose more and 24-hour urinary catecholamine excretion was higher in 11-year-old FH+ children than in age-matched FH− children (Ferrara et al, 1988).

—Exaggerated blood pressure responses were found with submaximal exercise on a bicycle ergometer in FH+ adolescents as compared with FH− adolescents (Molineax and Steptoe, 1988).

—Ambulatory blood pressure levels in FH+ adolescents had significantly higher mean diastolic levels during school hours (Wilson et al, 1988).

—Higher interventricular septum/posterior wall mass ratio on M mode echocardiograms was found in FH+ but not in FH− (deLeonardis et al, 1988).

—Although results of erythrocyte sodium relationships are conflicting, a difference in sodium-lithium countertransport was noted in FH+ adolescents as compared with their FH− peers (McDonald et al, 1987).

All of these observations suggest that physiological or pathophysiological changes may be at work long before clearcut hypertension emerges in children. The challenge is to select that test or combination of tests that has the greatest reliability in predicting the future blood pressure behavior of a given child.

As noted in Chapter 3, some studies of red blood cells from hypertensive individuals and their normotensive offspring reveal altered sodium fluxes as compared with normotensives and their offspring (Canessa et al., 1980; Garay et al., 1980). Trevisan et al (1988) did not find that a positive family history determined intracytic sodium or sodium-lithium countertransport in children. Abnormal whole-body and erythrocyte handling of $^{22}Na^+$ has been demonstrated in first degree relatives of hypertensives (Henningsen et al., 1979), but Prineas et al (1983) did not find the rate of $^{22}Na^+$ flux to be related to the blood pressure levels in children nor to parental blood pressure levels. Mongeau (1985) reported studies of erythrocyte sodium handling in FH+ offspring as follows: 9/15 had decreased cotransport, 5/11 had increased countertransport and 5/12 had a sodium leak. Trevisan et al (1988) observed that sodium-lithium countertransport was related to systolic and diastolic blood pressure in boys, but the associations lost significance when height and weight were considered. It, therefore, remains unclear whether the transmission of primary hypertension is related to the transmission of markers for sodium transport by red blood cell membranes in children. Similar uncertainty was noted in Chapter 3 concerning adults.

Longitudinal studies have demonstrated that urinary kallikrein levels are inversely correlated with blood pressure and cluster in families (Zinner et al, 1976; Zinner et al, 1978; Sinaiko et al, 1982). Lower levels of urinary kallikrein have also been found in cross-sectional studies of black children (Zinner et al., 1978). The significance of kallikrein excretion in relation to blood pressure patterns in children remains unclear.

### Environmental Factors

Of the environmental factors, increased body mass has increasingly been recognized as a major determinant of higher blood pressure levels throughout childhood and adolescence (Table 16.5). Studies that are either positively or negatively correlated with blood pressure levels are listed. In the United States, blood pressure rises with age in both sexes regardless of race (Report of the Second Task Force, 1987). Other factors that have been correlated to varying degrees with higher blood pressure levels in some studies include: lower socioeconomic status, lower family income, parental education, increased pulse rate, urban versus rural residence, and migration to a more industrialized area. The educational level attained by parents has not been correlated with blood pressure levels of their offspring. One study (Johnson et al, 1987) correlated suppressed anger in black adolescents with an increase in blood pressure, whereas Gillum et al (1985) did not find a correlation between blood pressure and personality. The trend toward increasing levels of blood pressure in childhood

**Table 16.5. Environmental Factors and Blood Pressure in Children**

| Factor | Positive Association Author, Year | No or Negative Association Author, Year |
|---|---|---|
| Increased body mass | Goldring et al, 1977<br>Londe et al, 1977<br>Voors et al, 1977<br>Harlan et al, 1979<br>Lyndes et al, 1980<br>Gutgesell et al, 1981<br>Lauer et al, 1984<br>Second Task Force, 1987<br>Feld and Springate, 1988 | |
| Increased height | Voors et al, 1977<br>Lauer et al, 1985<br>Kahn et al, 1986<br>Second Task Force, 1987 | |
| Lower socioeconomic status | Holland and Beresford, 1975<br>Kotchen and Kotchen, 1978 | Hunter et al, 1979<br>Gillum et al, 1985 |
| Low birth weight for gestational age | Simpson et al, 1981<br>Cater and Gill, 1984<br>Gennser et al, 1988<br>Barker et al, 1989 | |
| Hypertension during pregnancy | Kotchen et al, 1979 | Ounsted et al, 1985 |
| Increased pulse | Miller and Shekelle, 1976<br>Shekelle et al, 1978<br>Papa et al, 1983<br>Hediger et al, 1984<br>Barker et al, 1989 | Lee et al, 1976 (Newborn)<br>Voors et al, 1979<br>Hohn et al, 1983<br>Labarthe, 1986 |
| Urban versus rural | Kotchen and Kotchen, 1978 | |
| Parents educational level | Miller and Shekelle, 1976<br>Hunter et al, 1979<br>Gillum et al, 1985 | |
| Personality traits | Buck and Stenn, 1979<br>Gillum et al, 1985 | |
| Decreased urinary kallikrein | Zinner et al, 1976<br>Zinner et al, 1978<br>Sinaiko et al, 1982 | Hohn et al, 1983 |

and adolescence is not understood and cannot be attributed to the hormonal changes of puberty (Londe et al, 1975).

*Sodium Intake.* Sodium has increasingly been incriminated as a major factor in the emergence of primary hypertension as a disease of civilized societies (see Chapter 3). A short-term study of infants up to 6 months of age demonstrated that those fed a normal sodium diet had systolic pressure 2.1 mm Hg higher than those randomized to a low sodium diet (Hofman et al, 1983); however, when these babies were followed to 1 year of age the difference was only 1.0 mm Hg (Hofman et al, 1985). Whether excessive sodium ingestion during infancy (and often throughout childhood) sensitizes the vascular tree so that hypertension emerges at some later date in susceptible children is unknown.

A major problem that has precluded detailed investigations of the relation of sodium to blood pressure in childhood is the poor reliability of urinary collections for determination of sodium excretion. One study using random urine collections (Berenson et al, 1979) did not reveal any correlation between blood pressure levels and sodium excretion. Another study failed to find a correlation of blood pressure levels with overnight urinary sodium excretion nor with urinary sodium:potassium ratios (Prineas et al, 1983). On the other hand, a study of 73 children from the sixth to eighth grades of the Chicago school system, which included 7 days of 24-hour urine sodium measurements, showed a positive correlation (Liu et al, 1979). However, a subsequent publication from this group indicated that the findings were not reproducible and blood pressure levels did not correlate with urinary sodium excretion (Cooper et al, 1983).

The difficulty in defining a causal relationship between salt and blood pressure may, in part, result from the need to combine excessive sodium ingestion with a genetic predisposition to hypertension. Altschul and Grommet (1980) reviewed the evidence relating salt ingestion to blood pressure and suggested that all studies be examined in the light of positive or negative family histories for hypertension. The response of blood pressure to a mathematical stress was measured before and after a 2-week period on 10 g of extra salt in 40 individuals who had participated in longitudinal studies (Falkner et al, 1986). When blacks were grouped according to family history there was a significant difference in weight gain after sodium load. Before sodium loading there was no difference in the blood pressure response to mental stress. After sodium load, individuals displaying a $\geq 5$ mm Hg were regarded as sodium sensitive (SS) and had a greater blood pressure response to stress testing after the load. The greatest response occurred in SS individuals with a positive family history.

A recent study based on haptoglobin phenotypes revealed that those children with the 1-1 phenotype had higher blood pressures than those with other phenotypes (Weinberger et al, 1987), and those with the 1-1 phenotype were more likely to be salt sensitive (Luft et al, 1988). Salt sensitivity was much more frequent in blacks than whites.

Further investigation of the association of haptoglobin phenotypes and blood pressure responses to salt restriction in black and white children and adolescents is needed before extrapolating these observations to wide-scale public health measures aimed at prevention and treatment of primary hypertension. Appropriate studies are not yet available in children as to whether responses to sodium loading or alternatively to sodium restriction are interrelated to changes in potassium and/or calcium homeostasis. A study designed to answer questions related to sodium restriction as well as possible beneficial effects of potassium and calcium supplementation is under way in Minneapolis (Prineas et al, 1986).

## Cardiovascular Risk Factors

Hypertension alone or in combination with other risk factors has been shown to have a deleterious effect on the cardiovascular system beginning in childhood (Newman et al, 1986; Sinaiko et al, 1985; Seguro et al, 1986; Kwiterovich, 1986).

The relationship of hypertension and serum lipoprotein levels to early atherosclerosis in children and adolescents was assessed in an autopsy study of 35 persons who had, as children, been part of the Bogalusa Heart Study (Newman et al, 1986). Mean systolic blood pressure tended to be higher in the 4 subjects with coronary-artery fibrous plaques than in those without them. Aortic fatty streaks were strongly related to antemortem levels of total and low density lipoprotein (LDL) cholesterol and were universally correlated with the ratio of LDL cholesterol to LDL plus very low density lipoprotein (VLDL) cholesterol.

Many studies have sought changes on echocardiograms in children and adolescents whose blood pressures have tracked at the 90th percentile or above. An increase in cardiac performance was found by Sinaiko et al (1985). Increased left ventricular mass, increased wall thickness to radius ratio, and increased cardiac index were found by Seguro et al (1986). Left ventricular mass indexed for body surface area (LVMI) in children 12 to 15 years of age with blood pressure greater than or equal to 95th percentile was increased (Rokkedal-Nielsen et al, 1989) whereas in another study by the same investigators of children 8 to 10 years of age, LVMI did not increase (Rokkedal-Nielsen et al, 1989). Recently, Doppler ultrasound in normal adolescents revealed a direct relationship between diastolic blood pressure and the ratio of late to early peak diastolic filling that was independent of left ventricular hypertrophy (Graettinger et al, 1987).

Oral contraceptive use by female adolescents has been associated with hypertension, hypercholesterolemia, hypertriglyceridemia, and lower high density lipoprotein (HDL) cholesterol levels than in nonusers (Kwiterovich, 1986).

## Significance of Elevated Readings

The 1987 Second Task Force on Blood Pressure Control in Children focused attention on the problems of interpretation and evaluation of elevated blood pressure measurements in young people. The report reflects a conservative approach to labeling children as hypertensive and of investigating abnormal levels. Blood pressure recording and follow-up of abnormal levels are regarded as an essential component of the primary care of children. The definitions provided by the Task Force are shown in Table 16.6.

Based on data derived from single blood pressures obtained in over 70,000 infants, children, and adolescents, the Report also provided numbers signifying significant and severe hypertension by age group. In children younger than 13

**Table 16.6. Definitions from Second Task Force on Blood Pressure Control in Children**[a]

| Term | Definition |
|------|-----------|
| Normal BP | Systolic and diastolic BPs < 90th percentile for age and sex |
| High normal BP[b] | Average systolic and/or average diastolic BP between 90th and 95th percentiles for age and sex |
| High BP (hypertension) | Average systolic and/or average diastolic BPs ≥ 95th percentile for age and sex with measurements obtained on at least three occasions |

[a]Modified from the Report of the Second Task Force on Blood Pressure Control in Children—1987: *Pediatrics* 79:1, 1987.
[b]If the BP reading is high normal for age, but can be accounted for by excess height for age or excess lean body mass for age, such children are considered to have normal BP.

years of age, diastolic pressure was measured by K4 and in those older than 13 years of age by K5. Numbers that clearly exceed the 90th percentile for both systolic and diastolic pressures are illustrated in Figures 1 through 3. The report cautions, however, that weight must be taken into account when interpreting the data. Accordingly, a child whose blood pressure and height exceed the 90th percentile is regarded as normotensive. By use of these curves, children can be categorized as normotensive (i.e., less than the 90th percentile), high normal (between the 90th and 95th percentile), or hypertensive (three recorded blood pressures exceeding the 95th percentile) providing clear reference standards for the clinician to assess the blood pressure pattern of a specific child.

The choice of 90th and 95th percentiles for identification of a systolic or diastolic pressure as high-normal or abnormal is arbitrary as are the numbers presented for significant and severe hypertension (Table 16.7). Nevertheless, this approach provides a basis for clinical decision

making that heretofore was lacking. Practitioners previously depended on extrapolation from adult experience, data from earlier, often noncomparable surveys, or from the recognition that a child had symptomatic hypertension at any given set of numbers.

## EVALUATION OF CHILDREN AND ADOLESCENTS WITH ELEVATED BLOOD PRESSURE

### General Guidelines

Asymptomatic children and adolescents who have a single casual blood pressure recording that exceeds the 90th percentile for systolic or diastolic pressure according to the age-specific distributions of blood pressure for boys and girls should have the blood pressure remeasured within 3 months. A blood pressure value exceeding the 90th percentile but below the 95th may be regarded as normal if height is increased above the 90th percentile but abnormal if due to adiposity. According to data derived from screening programs (Kilcoyne et al, 1974; Fixler et al, 1979; Hediger et al, 1984) and epidemiological surveys (Rames et al, 1978), the likelihood of repeated measurements being elevated is small. The probability of the elevation being sustained is heightened if the child is obese or has a hypertensive parent. Furthermore, if an adolescent has been consistently overweight for height, the chances of his blood pressure remaining elevated and/or his becoming hypertensive are greatly increased.

One approach to the evaluation of abnormal blood pressure measurements in children and adolescents is to obtain ambulatory blood pressure levels. A study of 84 hypertensive children ages 6 to 23 years with ambulatory recordings revealed that application to pediatrics was limited because (1) the pressurometer only detected K5, (2) the Second Task Force 1987 recom-

**Table 16.7. Classification of Hypertension by Age Group**[a]

| Age (yr) | Significant Hypertension | | Severe Hypertension | |
|----------|--------------------------|----------|---------------------|----------|
| | Systolic | Diastolic | Systolic | Diastolic |
| | (BP Greater Than) (mm Hg) | | (BP Greater Than) (mm Hg) | |
| Infants (<2) | 112 | 74 | 118 | 82 |
| Children (3–5) | 116 | 76 | 124 | 84 |
| Children (6–9) | 122 | 78 | 130 | 86 |
| Children (10–12) | 126 | 82 | 134 | 90 |
| Adolescents (13–15) | 136 | 86 | 144 | 92 |
| Adolescents (16–18) | 142 | 92 | 150 | 98 |

[a]Modified from the Report of the Second Task Force on Blood Pressure Control in Children—1987: *Pediatrics* 79:1, 1987.

mended that blood pressure be measured in a sitting position, (3) the full range of cuff sizes needed for children is not available for the ambulatory blood pressure monitor, and (4) ambulatory standards for normal blood pressure measurements currently do not exist (Daniels et al, 1987). Until more data are available with improved technology, ambulatory recordings have little role in pediatric hypertension.

Echocardiographic abnormalities have been demonstrated by several investigators in adolescents with persistently elevated blood pressure levels including changes in left ventricular wall thickness (Laird and Fixler, 1981), left ventricular wall mass (Schieken et al, 1982), and indices reflecting ventricular performance (Johnson et al, 1983). The questions raised by these studies that remain unanswered include: Are these changes reflective of target organ damage or are they an integral part of the process that raised the blood pressure? do these findings signify that intervention should be initiated? and, are there preferred strategies or medications that would reverse the anatomical or hemodynamic abnormalities in a beneficial manner?

One study examined the impact of a combined nutritional-pharmacological intervention on the blood pressure of children in the highest decile to determine whether intervention could prevent hypertension (Berenson et al, 1983). Chlorthalidone and propranolol were used as therapeutic agents. Over a 6-month period 50 children initially in the highest decile lowered their pressure (systolic and diastolic levels) to below the 90th percentiles. The investigators concluded that their results supported community-wide intervention programs to prevent hypertension in individuals identified at risk. On the other hand, many caution against this approach because some teenagers with repeatedly elevated blood pressure levels have become normotensive without therapy on follow-up, which extended up to 8 years (Kilcoyne, 1974; Aschinberg et al, 1977; Rames et al, 1978).

## Evaluation

### History

Evaluation of children with persistently elevated blood pressure (i.e., over the 95th percentile on three occasions) includes ascertainment of these historical features: (1) primary or essential hypertension, or complications of uncontrolled hypertension, i.e., stroke, heart attack, and kidney failure of unknown origin in first degree relatives; (2) familial obesity; (3) familial hyperlipidemia; (4) blood pressure levels of siblings; and (5) past events or present occurrences that might influence blood pressure such as prior renal disease or urological surgery, use of pressor agents, i.e., sympathomimetics and, in some cases, oral contraceptives. Attention should be focused on drug abuse with emphasis on street drugs known to elevate blood pressure, such as amphetamines and phencyclidine.

### Physical Examination

The physical examination should include the patient's height and weight because of the association of obesity with elevated blood pressure levels in childhood and adolescence (Report of the Second Task Force, 1987). The pulse should be recorded because some reports indicate an association of an increased pulse rate with higher levels of pressure. The physical examination is oriented toward signs of secondary causes of hypertension such as decreased femoral pulses, abdominal bruits, and cushingoid stigmata. In children, in contrast to adults, retinal arteriolar tortuosity, arteriovenous crossing, and increased arterial light reflex more likely reflect long-standing hypertension than atherosclerosis.

### Laboratory Studies

The likelihood of an asymptomatic child with persistently elevated blood pressure having a recognizable cause for the blood pressure elevation is remote. The history and physical examination usually reveal evidence of secondary causes of hypertension. Therefore, detailed diagnostic studies of children without suggestive evidence of secondary hypertension are not warranted. The skewed emphasis in the medical literature on rare secondary causes of hypertension that require detailed and sophisticated investigative studies has led to a tendency to pursue an all-inclusive evaluation. Children with persistently elevated blood pressure are usually not sick and may not have fixed hypertension. Few laboratory studies are needed (Report of the Second Task Force, 1987); they include urinalysis and serum urea nitrogen, serum creatinine, and uric acid. Additional studies may be obtained if the child's condition changes. Echocardiography is the best means to detect increased left ventricular wall thickness or septal hypertrophy (Laird and Fixler, 1981). Our findings at Childrens Hospital of Los Angeles (CHLA) are in accord with their observations. The 1987 Second Task Force Report also recommends obtaining an echocardiogram, especially if pharmacological intervention is contemplated, so that reversal of abnormalities can be monitored and correlated with adequacy of blood pressure control.

## Preventive Measures

Because the natural course for children with persistently elevated blood pressure remains unknown, definite recommendations for prevention of fixed hypertension cannot be made. Extrapolation of data from epidemiological surveys in children and adults does, however, permit proposals for health maintenance. As noted earlier, sustained obesity is a definite risk factor for fixed hypertension in young people. Reduction of excess weight, moderation of salt intake, avoidance of smoking and pressor agents, plus an active dynamic sports program may prove beneficial. Sodium intake should be assessed and the total amount of sodium lowered in children with greatly excessive intakes and if salt-sensitive hypertension is suspected. It is premature to recommend supplemental potassium and calcium intakes, but these areas bear watching because prospective studies are being conducted (Prineas et al, 1986). All suggestions must be presented in a positive, nonthreatening manner to avoid an unnatural concern about hypertension and its sequelae and to prevent changes in life style that have an undesirable effect on the quality of life for the child and his/her family.

## OBESITY AND HYPERTENSION

Obesity-associated hypertension is separated from primary and secondary hypertension because observations in pediatrics suggest that this group represents a subtype among hypertensive populations (Report of the Second Task Force, 1987; Feld and Springate, 1988). The clinical definition of obesity is a weight that exceeds the average for a given height by 20% or more; for practical purposes such an approach is usually all that is needed. Refinements of the descriptions of body fat include Body Mass Index (BMI) or Quetelet index, defined as weight/height$^2$, triceps skinfold thickness (TSF) and circumference at the midpoint of the right upper arm (RAC). The problem of determining the contribution of excess body weight to sustained high blood pressure is complicated by the occurrence of increasing body weight and increasing blood pressure levels as children mature. In

the Minneapolis study, of 753 children who participated in nine screenings, TSF tracked high, i.e., remained in the upper tertile of the distribution at each of the screenings, in 66 (8.8%), BMI in 138 (18.3%) and for both in 58 (7.7%). Their data suggested a greater effect of high tracking indices on systolic pressure than on diastolic pressure (Prineas et al, 1985).

Well-designed clinical studies analyzing the effects of weight loss on blood pressure patterns are lacking among children. However, numerous clinical observations attest to the normalization of blood pressure after weight loss in children and adolescents and emphasize the importance of nonpharmacological intervention to achieve normalization of pressure (Court et al, 1974; Aschinberg et al, 1977; Rames et al, 1978). Few reports, however, provide long-term follow-up and therefore leave unanswered the question as to whether sustained weight loss and sustained normotension persist over a long term.

The management of obese hypertensive children requires involvement of a dietitian and the child's entire family. Court et al (1974) described 21 obese hypertensive children (2 to 14 years of age); three of six normalized their blood pressure with weight loss. In another study six of 10 obese children with persistently elevated blood pressure levels lowered their blood pressure to less than the 95th percentile with weight reduction (Rames et al, 1978). Frequently obesity occurs in a familial pattern, and without a dedicated approach to the entire family with sensitivity to the psychosocial aspects of eating, efforts at weight reduction are doomed to failure. Dietary modifications should also take into account changes in salt intake and the need to change the type and composition of fat intake.

## PRIMARY HYPERTENSION

As a result of epidemiological studies, screening programs, tracking studies, and heightened clinical awareness, an increasing number of young children and adolescents whose blood pressure has been persistently abnormal are being identified as having primary (essential) hypertension (Loggie, 1975; Londe and Goldring, 1976). This group is rarely symptomatic and rarely has secondary causes. Ogborn et al (1987) reported that 43 of 103 hypertensive children and adolescents had primary hypertension. Conclusive information as to the incidence and prevalence of primary hypertension in the United States is still lacking. This problem may be compounded by the immigration of different ethnic groups whose blood pressure patterns may have changed after entry into this country.

Controversy still persists as to the need for and extent of investigation to exclude secondary causes of hypertension. The point of contention between the author and other experts is focused on how many tests are appropriate as the *initial* step in evaluation (Table 16.8). Arguments favoring extensive workups are: Many physicians caring mainly for hypertensive adults believe that persistent hypertension in individuals less than 20 years of age is usually secondary; detailed diagnostic studies are indicated to avoid overlooking a secondary (and presumably remediable) cause of hypertension (Klein et al, 1981); and adolescents with primary hypertension are usually asymptomatic with mild hypertension, therefore all symptomatic children with moderate hypertension should be *extensively* investigated. An opposing view is that an all-inclusive approach for all hypertensive children is unnecessary, costly, and in some instances physically and psychologically damaging.

During the past 5 years working committees (the International Committee, Heidelberg, 1985 [Schärer et al, 1986] and the Second Task Force Report, 1987) and investigators (Dillon, 1987; Ogborn and Crocker, 1987; Feld and Springate, 1988) have published recommendations concerning the investigation of hypertensive children (Table 16.8). If a child is asymptomatic and has had a blood pressure that has tracked on several occasions or over years in the 95th percentile or greater in the absence of obesity, the child is regarded as hypertensive (Report of the Second Task Force, 1987). The initial evaluative steps include a thorough history and physical examination.

## Family History

Approximately 50% of children with primary hypertension come from families in whom the family history for primary hypertension or its complications in a first degree relative are positive (Londe et al, 1971). Although all children whose parents have primary hypertension are at greater risk than their peers, not all offspring are at the same risk. The likelihood of primary hypertension and its complications is suspected by blood pressure tracking in the highest percentiles. The monitoring of such high risk children includes serial blood pressure recordings, serial height/weight measurements, and, if feasible, assessments of dietary intake.

## Symptoms

Primary hypertension in childhood and adolescence is frequently asymptomatic although like adults many do develop symptoms. The most frequent symptom is headache. The hypertension-associated headache has no particular features that distinguish it from other pediatric conditions. In adolescent athletes, headaches often occur after strenuous exercise. An occasional child complains of severe, throbbing frontal headaches that may or may not be relieved by analgesics. Symptoms such as seizures, nosebleeds, dizziness, or syncope are rare. Their presence suggests that hypertension has been exacerbated by pressor agents, i.e., sympathomimetics, or by an emotional crisis, particularly in adolescents. Otherwise, these symptoms are more often a reflection of severe secondary hypertension.

## Physical Findings

Obesity is the most frequently detected abnormality and has been noted in as many as 50% (Londe et al, 1971), with the highest prevalence among black female adolescents. Careful physical examination is unlikely to reveal any other positive physical findings. An occasional child may have early changes of hypertensive retinopathy including arteriolar narrowing and mild tortuosity when hypertension is chronic in duration and moderate in severity. Clues to secondary causes of hypertension (Table 16.1) should be systematically sought and sequentially excluded by the absence of abnormalities.

## Laboratory Studies

If no secondary cause of hypertension has been identified by history and physical examination, routine recommended studies include: urinalysis, serum urea nitrogen, creatinine, uric acid, and echocardiogram. The latter study may have two uses: To help identify anatomical changes and to evaluate hemodynamic alterations. Roentgenograms of the chest and electrocardiograms should not be routinely obtained because they are not as sensitive as echocardiograms (Laird and Fixler, 1981). In asymptomatic adolescents whose blood pressure levels are distinctly elevated, e.g., diastolic levels consistently greater than 100 mm Hg, but who have unremarkable histories and physical examinations, additional tests are often obtained even though the yield is low (Aschinberg et al, 1977; Loggie, 1974; Silverberg et al, 1975). In a small group of adolescent patients with primary hy-

**Table 16.8. Recommendations for Initial Investigation of Sustained Hypertension**

| Test | Lieberman (CHLA) 1989 | TASK FORCE 1987 | Schärer et al, 1986 | Dillon, 1987 | Ogborn and Crocker, 1987 | Feld and Springate, 1988 |
|---|---|---|---|---|---|---|
| Urinalysis | X | X (+Culture) | X | X | X | X |
| Blood count | X | X | X | | | |
| BUN/creatinine | X | X | X | X | X | X |
| Uric acid | | X | | | | X |
| Electrolytes | | X | X | X | X | X |
| PRA | | | X | X | X | |
| P-Aldosterone | | | | X | X | |
| P-Catechol | | | | X | | |
| U-VMA/Metabolites | | | X | X | X | |
| 24-Hour U-Protein, creatinine | | | | | X | |
| P-Magnesium, calcium, phosphorus, alkaline phosphatase | | | | | X | |
| Thyroid function | | | | | X | |
| P-Cortisol | | | | | X | |
| Chest x-ray | | | X | X | X | X |
| Electrocardiogram | | | X | X | X | |
| Echocardiography | X | X | X | | | X |
| DMSA/DTPA | X | | X | X | X | X |
| Renal US | X | | X | X | | X (OR IVP) |

pertension at CHLA, there has been a tendency toward a high hemoglobin and hematocrit, as reported by Tochikubo et al (1986). Hyperuricemia (Gruskin et al, 1983) and a tendency toward slightly higher serum calcium and phosphorus levels (Perlman et al, 1983) have been reported, but their significance remains unclear. Secondary hypertension has been said to be more frequent among white female teenagers (Loggie, 1975), but our experience does not confirm this view.

The rationale for obtaining an all-inclusive diagnostic evaluation is the same as that for adults, based on the concept that an occult secondary cause may be detected. However, the data base on which to reach an opinion is much smaller among children. Review of experience at CHLA and elsewhere with hypertensive adolescent patients suggests that the number of occult cases of secondary hypertension is small (Loggie, 1974; Silverberg et al, 1975; Levine et al, 1976). In other words, the majority of secondary causes of hypertension reveal themselves with a careful history, methodical physical examination, and minimal laboratory screening studies. Recommendations in pedia-

tric patients also take into account the severity of hypertension and the age of the patient. The younger the patient and the higher the blood pressure, the more likely an underlying etiology will be found. At CHLA the initial laboratory evaluation includes urinalysis, blood count, blood urea nitrogen (BUN) and creatinine, renal scan (DTPA or DMSA), renal ultrasound, and echocardiogram (Table 16.8).

In adolescents with moderate hypertension, the performance of a rapid sequence or hypertensive intravenous pyelogram has been deleted from radiological evaluations because it is an insensitive study for renovascular disease (Korobkin et al, 1976) and because ultrasonography coupled with scans are more helpful in determining renal size, renal scars, and alteration in renal function. Nonetheless arteriography is still indicated whenever other evidence of renal involvement is noted.

### Prepubertal Children

Guidelines for the initial investigation of prepubertal children suspected of having primary hypertension are available (Report of the Second Task Force, 1987; Schärer et al, 1986). They differ from the author's approach in the number of first-ordered tests. Experience at CHLA indicates that a significant number of children with secondary forms of hypertension (often renal) can be identified using a selective approach (Fig. 16.5). Note that if initial findings are normal, the evaluation should proceed to rule out all reasonable possibilities. The higher the blood pressure and the more severe its manifestations, the more likely a secondary cause of hypertension will be detected (Table 16.9). Nevertheless, a significant proportion of prepubertal hypertensive children, up to 10 to 15%, will not have a recognizable secondary cause. In symptomatic prepubertal FH — children whose physical examination fails to reveal diagnostic clues, the same screening laboratory studies advocated for adolescents plus renal ultrasound and renal scans are recommended (Table 16.8). Even though subtle adrenal cortical abnormalities are extraordinarily rare in this age group, serum potassium and bicarbonate levels should be obtained to search for evidence of primary or secondary aldosteronism. Measurement of plasma renin activity (PRA) has been advocated in children suspected of having primary hypertension to determine their renin profile (Gruskin et al,

1986), but studies that base therapy on such profiles are lacking in pediatrics. PRA levels must be obtained under standardized conditions and interpreted by age (Kotchen et al, 1972; Stark et al, 1975). PRA levels are high in infancy and gradually reach adult levels by the age of 16 years (Hiner et al, 1976).

## Treatment

Treatment of primary hypertension in children and adolescents is still empirical because long-term studies of diet with or without drug therapy do not exist. Short-term observations suggest that weight reduction often leads to normalization of elevated pressures (Court et al, 1974; Rames et al, 1978). In the absence of adequate data on safety and effectiveness of drug therapy, the decision as to whether a specific child should receive medications must be individualized. The question has not been answered as to whether pharmacological therapy in an asymptomatic hypertensive prepubertal child will interfere with growth and development, but there are no data to suggest such deleterious effects.

The first step in young children with persistently elevated levels of pressure includes a dietary assessment of caloric and salt intake. This

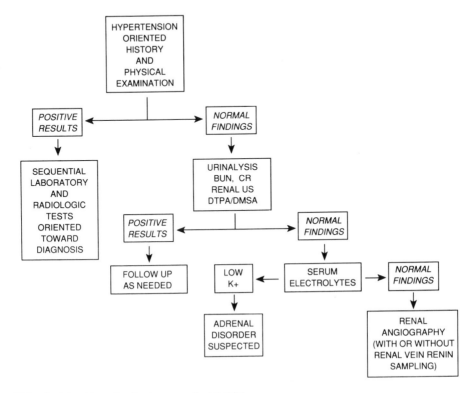

**Figure 16.5.** Sustained hypertension in a prepubertal child.

**Table 16.9. Causes of Hypertension in Children and Adolescents[a]**

| | Lieberman | | Uhari and Koskimies, 1979 | | Gill et al, 1976 | | Loirat et al, 1982 | | Still and Cottom, 1967 | |
|---|---|---|---|---|---|---|---|---|---|---|
| | No. | % | No. | % | No. | % | No. | % | No. | % |
| Number of cases | 256 | | 110 | | 100 | | 100 | | 55 | |
| Age range (yrs) | 0–21 | | 0–16 | | 0–15 | | 0–17 | | 0–14 | |
| **PRIMARY HYPERTENSION** | 55 | | 21 | | 2 | | 12 | | 3 | |
| *% of all causes* | *21* | | *20* | | *2* | | *12* | | *5* | |
| **SECONDARY HYPERTENSION** | 201 | (100) | 92 | (100) | 98 | (100) | 88 | (100) | 52 | (100) |
| *% of all causes* | *79* | | *80* | | *98* | | *88* | | *95* | |
| All renal causes | 151 | (75) | 45 | (49) | 76 | (78) | 78 | (89) | 38 | (73) |
| Renovascular disease | 17 | (9) | 4 | (4) | 6 | (6) | 9 | (10) | 5 | (10) |
| Coarctation | 9 | (4) | 37 | (40) | 15 | (15) | | | | |
| Adrenal causes or pheochromocytoma | 4 | (2) | 1 | (1) | 0 | | 1 | (1) | 2 | (4) |
| Nonrenal tumor | 7 | (3) | 0 | | 0 | | | | 0 | |
| Central nervous disorders | 4 | (2) | 0 | | 0 | | | | 0 | |
| Systemic disorders | 3 | (2) | 0 | | 0 | | | | 0 | |
| Others | 6 | (3) | 5 | (5) | 1 | (1) | | | 1 | (2) |

[a]Modifed from: deSwiet M: *B Med Bull*, 42:172, 1986.

evaluation should be undertaken in the context of the family's nutritional habits as well as their own cultural matrix. In pediatrics, even more than in adult medicine, food plays a central role in the nurturing process involving the child and his/her family. Primary hypertensives may be salt sensitive and this tendency may be greater in blacks than in other groups, and therefore attempts to reduce salt intake in black children may be more useful than indicated in the current pediatric literature. It is not known whether salt reduction should be accompanied by potassium supplementation, but enough evidence is available to suggest that a potassium-rich diet might be useful. Supplementation with calcium has not been evaluated.

Older children and adolescents often eat in places other than their own homes. The ubiquitous presence of sodium makes it very difficult for patients on a sodium-restricted intake to find easy ways of eating usual childhood foods with their friends. Many fast food chains now offer salad bars, but peer pressure may result in the selection of high sodium foods. An order of one superburger, french fries, and a chocolate shake adds up to about 1100 calories and at least 1 g of sodium without addition of salt at the table. The adolescent and his/her physician need to decide how to approach treatment and determine whether altering sodium intake will pose a significant psychological burden. If they decide to lower salt intake, dietary counseling coupled with self monitoring of urinary sodium may prove effective (Tochikubo et al, 1986).

## Drug Therapy

Treatment of asymptomatic, mildly hypertensive children and adolescents requires confronting a young person with the fact of illness, even though he/she does not feel sick. In particular, the adolescent who is seeking group acceptance, as well as a definition of personal identity, must cope with the notion of long-term, unremitting illness that may foreshorten one's life span if one does not comply. Treatment of adolescents requires sensitivity to the special problems of adolescents including their need to participate in the decisions that affect them. In hypertensive children and adolescents who cannot or will not reduce their salt and caloric intake or in children who do not respond to dietary changes, pharmacological therapy should be provided with the usual choice of diuretic or beta blocker. The 1987 Second Task Force recommends beginning with less than a full dose of thiazide-type diuretics or less than a full dose of adrenergic inhibitor. In children with mild elevations of blood pressure, thiazide therapy is often successful and has few side effects, although acute volume depletion represents an immediate adverse effect. Long-term metabolic changes in children and adolescents treated with diuretics have not been reported; nevertheless, it is prudent to monitor young people for changes in lipids, glucose, and uric acid (Perez-Stable and Carolis, 1983). If the child does not respond to thiazide diuretics, the addition of a beta-blocker is recommended for those without asthma. All children and adolescents receiving a beta-blocker should have their pulse rate recorded and should exercise for 1 to 2 minutes to ensure that they can raise their pulse adequately when they are stressed (i.e., 20 beats/minute or more). Children and parents should be cautioned about rebound hypertension if vomiting occurs or if the drug is abruptly stopped.

Unlike the situation among adults, concern about long-term adverse cardiovascular effects has not yet changed pediatric recommendations to consider starting with vasodilators or angiotensin-converting enzyme (ACE) inhibitors that do not alter cholesterol and triglycerides. If either diuretics or beta-blockers in sufficient dosage does not provide blood pressure control, an ACE inhibitor may be warranted. These agents have been used in children with renal hypertension but not with primary hypertension. If adequate control is still not achieved, the diagnosis may be incorrect, e.g., dexamethasone-suppressible hyperaldosteronism (note: positive family history in this condition may mimic family history of patient with primary hypertension). Accordingly, if a response is not achieved, reevaluation with or without consultation is required.

Sometimes drug therapy can be stopped to determine whether it is still needed. Little data about discontinuation of therapy exist in pediatrics. Experience at CHLA suggests that the greatest success, although uncommon, occurs with salt and/or weight reduction. Periodic blood pressure checks should be done to document the course of the child's blood pressure because many will still require treatment. Gill et al (1976) noted that propranolol induced excessive bradycardia in several children and cardiac failure in two; Kallen et al (1980) reported life-threatening hypoglycemia in children receiving propranolol.

Further discussion of treatment of hypertension appears in the sections on secondary causes (neonatal and renal) and on hypertensive emergencies in pediatrics.

### Recommendations About Athletics

A significant gap persists between the recommendations of health professionals (Strong, 1979; Report of the Second Task Force, 1987) and the attitudes of school coaches or others involved in clearing children and adolescents with elevated blood pressure for participation in sports. In the absence of definitive data, I believe that asymptomatic children and adolescents with mildly elevated blood pressures should be encouraged to participate in dynamic exer-

cises. If they become symptomatic, they should be evaluated. Participation in some sports, especially football, requires that team members undergo continuing weight lifting programs. In youngsters who are asymptomatic before, during, and after these exercises, it is difficult to prohibit their participation. However, the Second Task Force (1987) cautions that weight lifting may lead to increased muscle mass and a secondary increase in blood pressure. The Report of the Second Task Force (1987) recommends aerobic exercises and, in the absence of data on long-term effects of weight lifting and heart disease, it is suggested that isometric exercise be avoided. In all symptomatic individuals, in all youngsters on treatment, and in those with electrocardiographic or echocardiographic changes of left ventricular hypertrophy, isometric exercises are potentially hazardous, and aerobic exercises should be substituted.

### SECONDARY HYPERTENSION

In *prepubertal* hypertensive children, the largest number have a renal etiology of their disease. The results of several published series are presented in Table 16.9. Differences in the distribution of causes and the percentage of primary hypertension can be attributed to the source of the data. Those publications describing severely ill children (Gill et al, 1976; Still and Cottom, 1967) are skewed toward renal causes whereas Lieberman (1983) surveyed five Los Angeles hospitals for both inpatients and outpatients identified as hypertensive. Ogborn and Crocker (1987) studied children with sustained hypertension. It is of interest that in these five series, neither primary aldosteronism nor thyroid disease was reported. The need to include tests to diagnose primary aldosteronism and dexamethasone-suppressible hypertension during the initial evaluation phase is unclear although PRA and electrolytes are recommended by some (Schärer et al, 1986; Dillon, 1987; Ogborn and Crocker, 1987). In *postpubertal* children, the number with renal hypertension varies with the setting in which the adolescent is seen. Adolescents with severe hypertension referred to a hospital for evaluation and treatment are most likely to have a renal etiology, whereas those with mild hypertension are more likely to have primary hypertension. The number of pediatric patients with obscure etiologies for underlying hypertension is quite small. That fact should be kept in perspective so that expensive and often invasive tests are reserved for individuals with significant symptomatic hypertension of unclear cause.

## Neonatal Hypertension

Neonatal hypertension represents a special situation. Data are now available for determining whether given levels of blood pressure represent significant abnormalities for term infants (Table 16.10). With the advent of highly organized and well-equipped neonatal intensive care units, neonatal hypertension has been increasingly recognized since the 1970's.

### Etiology

Factors that increase the risk of neonatal hypertension are the use of umbilical artery catheters, extracorporeal membrane oxygenation (ECMO), bronchopulmonary dysplasia and asphyxia. Major causes of neonatal hypertension are presented in Table 16.11. Buchi and Siegler (1986) reported that 53 infants admitted with hypertension represented 0.7% of all neonatal tertiary care admissions. Of these, 23 had an identifiable etiology, of which all but two were renal in origin; these two had coarctation. Furthermore, these workers found that the results of urinalysis, BUN, serum creatinine and PRA tests were predictive of both etiology and outcome. In the entire group of 53, 81% were normotensive without therapy by 1 year of age (Buchi and Siegler, 1986). Another report described ophthalmological features resembling those of hypertensive retinopathy in adults in 11 hypertensive infants that resolved by 1 year of age (Fanaroff et al, 1985). In the Buchi and Siegler series (1986) four of 53 died, two of causes unrelated to hypertension, one of hypertension-related heart failure, and one of hypertensive encephalopathy. These authors concluded that the diagnostic workup including urinalysis, BUN, serum creatinine, and PRA would detect the majority of neonates with an identifiable renal

**Table 16.10. Definition of Hypertension in Term Infants[a]**

| Age Group | 95th Percentile Value (mm Hg) | | |
|---|---|---|---|
| | Systolic | Diastolic | Mean |
| Birth | 90 | 60 | 70 |
| 7 Days | 92 | 69 | 77 |
| 8 Days to 1 Month | 106 | 74 | 85 |

[a]From Feld LG, Springate JE: Hypertension in Children. *Curr Prob in Pediatr* 18(6):317, 1988, Year Book Publishers, reproduced with permission.

**Table 16.11. Causes of Neonatal Hypertension**

Renal
  Malformations: cystic renal diseases, renal hypoplasia or dysplasia, obstructive uropathy secondary to congenital anomalies
  Renovascular: renal artery stenosis/thrombosis, renal vein thrombosis (de novo, 2° to umbilical artery catheter, ECMO, idiopathic arterial calcification)
  Renal tumors: Wilms' tumor, neuroblastoma
  Renal failure

Cardiovascular
  Coarctation of the aorta

Pulmonary
  Bronchopulmonary dysplasia
  Pneumothorax

Medications
  Corticosteroids/ACTH/mineralocorticoids
  Ocular phenylephrine
  Narcotic-addicted mother (heroin, methadone)

Endocrine/metabolic
  Congenital adrenal hyperplasia
  Turner's syndrome
  Urea cycle abnormalities

Abdominal wall defect(s)
  Closure

cause. If these tests are abnormal, renal ultrasound and pyelography are advised. Nuclear scans are not mentioned although Adelman (1987) recommends them. Angiography was not performed. The authors recommend pharmacological therapy and careful follow-up. If the response to treatment is unsatisfactory, additional diagnostic tests are advised.

*Renal Artery Disease.* Before the introduction of umbilical artery catheters, acquired renal arterial abnormalities were usually associated with extension of neonatal renal vein thrombosis or with embolization from patent ductus arteriosus (Durante et al, 1976). With the advent of neonatal intensive care units, the use of umbilical artery catheters has become commonplace. Complications of their use include renal artery thrombosis and stenosis with associated hypertension (Adelman, 1987). Initial experience with early nephrectomy for renal artery thrombosis was associated with a high death rate (Plumer et al, 1976). Subsequent use of aggressive medical therapy resulted in improved survival and decreased the need for nephrectomy (Adelman, 1978). Hypertensive neonates require prompt and appropriate antihypertensive therapy (Table 16.12). Adelman in 1978 reported survival in 15 of 17 neonates treated medically and provided follow-up of 12 of these for up to 8.8 years (with a mean of 5.7 years) (Adelman, 1987). Of the 12 survivors with follow-up information, all were normotensive. Two had died

**Table 16.12.  Treatment of Neonatal Hypertension**

| Name of Drug | Drug Dose[a] | Route | Comment |
|---|---|---|---|
| Furosemide | 0.5–2.0 mg/kg/q 6–8 hours | i.v. or p.o. | Hypokalemia and alkalosis can be anticipated along with volume depletion; chronic usage is associated with **hypercalciuria**, may lead to **nephrocalcinosis** and fractures. |
| Hydralazine | 0.1–0.2 mg/kg/q 6 hours | i.v. or p.o. | Tachycardia may require adrenergic blockage. |
| Methyldopa | 5–10 mg/kg/q 6 hours | i.v. or p.o. | Well tolerated; effective agent; monitor renal function so that dose can be lowered if glomerular filtration rate is reduced. |
| Propranolol | 0.5–2 mg/kg/q 6 hours | p.o. | Usually not first line agent; studies in neonates not available; use with caution because of bradycardia. |
| Diazoxide | 1–3 mg/kg/dose (no more than 4 times/24 hours) | i.v. | Useful emergency agent; caution needed because of danger of extravasation and sloughing. |
| Nitroprusside | 0.5–5.0 mcgm/kg/min | i.v. | Useful agent but must be administered continuously; requires intensive care unit and monitoring of BP; thiocyanate levels must be obtained at least every 24 hours to avoid toxic drug levels. |
| Captopril | 0.05–0.25 mg/kg/dose/q 8 hours | p.o. | Careful initiating of low dose captopril may avoid renal failure. Dose increases should be initiated at defined intervals only if control is clearly inadequate, and renal function is normal. Drug appears more potent with a longer duration of action than in older children. |
| Nifedipine | Dose not established. | | |

[a]Lowest starting dose is given.

of nonrenal, nonhypertensive causes. Two remained below the 3rd percentile for height and weight. Mean calculated creatinine clearance for the 10 survivors was 99.8 ml/minute/1.73m². In Adelman's view, vigorous medical management is effective in achieving blood pressure control, and surgical intervention is unwarranted unless uncontrolled hypertension persists. If surgery is deemed necessary, it may be safely postponed throughout the first year of life if blood pressure control is adequate, if the infant is growing appropriately, and if renal function is normal.

**Evaluation**

The major difference in the approach advocated by Adelman (1983), by Vailas et al (1986), and by the author is the need for diagnostic studies during the neonatal period. If the diagnosis of neonatal renovascular hypertension is suspected, renal scans and pyelograms are not essential. However, scintigraphy comparing baseline studies with single-dose captopril scans may be useful in predicting which neonate may develop renal failure with captopril treatment (Sfakianakis et al, 1988). Data from scans are often included in discussions of neonatal hypertension (Adelman, 1987; Vailas et al, 1986). Portable renal ultrasound may assist in excluding other etiologies for renal hypertension. If the index of suspicion is high that renal arterial disease is the etiology for hypertension, therapy takes priority over diagnosis. These neonates may be safely managed without confirmation of the diagnosis by angiography. Peripheral and renal vein renin studies are of no diagnostic value because renin levels are elevated in sick and stressed neonates. In the author's opinion the risk of invasive studies, especially angiography outweighs potential benefits. These infants respond to pharmacological therapy. Captopril is especially useful but also potent; its dose should be lower than for older children (Sinaiko et al, 1986) (Table 16.12). Its use must be monitored very carefully; fatal neonatal renal failure has been reported (Bifano et al, 1982). Echocardiography has been advocated as a useful means of monitoring improved cardiac function in response to captopril therapy in a hypertensive infant (McGonigle et al, 1987). Invasive diagnostic studies can be postponed until the infant is stable, normotensive, and larger. As these infants approach 6 months of age, antihypertensive therapy may be discontinued without adverse effects; only a small percentage have persistent and drug-resistant hypertension. At that time, if renal ultrasound or scintigrams demonstrate a nonfunctioning unilateral and contracted kidney, nephrectomy may be curative.

## Reflux Nephropathy

Vesicoureteric reflux is the term used to describe the retrograde flow of urine from the bladder into the ureter(s) and kidney(s). The more severe the reflux, the higher the grade. With severe reflux the ureters become dilated and tortuous; the pelvocalycine outline becomes distorted by pelvic dilatation, and often renal scarring coexists. This constellation of features now known as reflux nephropathy was previously called chronic atrophic pyelonephritis.

Reflux nephropathy is a well-recognized antecedent of hypertension that is often severe and most often progresses to end stage renal disease regardless of medical and surgical intervention. Although its incidence and prevalence are unknown, reflux nephropathy is more common in girls. The diagnosis should be considered in any child with urinary tract infection; children with uncomplicated infections have urinalyses that are protein free unless they have high fever. If proteinuria is detected in a hypertensive child with a history of urinary tract infections and in the absence of fever, the child should be evaluated for reflux nephropathy. Noninvasive screening for upper tract abnormalities can now easily be accomplished with renal ultrasound. If any suspicious findings are encountered, voiding cystourethrography (VCUG) under standardized conditions should be done when the child is not infected.

The decision as to the optimal management plan rests on the clinical judgment of the physician, the severity of reflux, analysis of renal function, assessment of the family's ability to carry out long-term medical therapy, and cost considerations. Two important studies comparing medical and surgical treatment of vesicour-

eteric reflux are under way (International Reflux Study Committee, 1981; Birmingham Reflux Study Group, 1984). A symposium that reviews the subject in depth is available (Hodson et al., 1984). Braren et al (1988) described growth failure in hypertensive children with reflux. Catchup growth did not occur after successful antireflux surgery. Clearly this area of pediatrics requires in-depth study. Hopefully the results of the ongoing Birmingham and International studies may provide answers.

## Management of Sustained Hypertension

Clinicians responsible for the management of children with disorders not amenable to surgery are handicapped by the absence of long-term studies of treatment, including the follow-up of children and adolescents through periods of normal growth. Moreover, in the past, articles describing therapy could not separate the impact of each drug from that of polypharmacy (Pennisi et al., 1977; Potter et al., 1977; Boerth, 1980; Sinaiko et al., 1980; Green et al., 1981). Among those agents used in children, the long-term effectiveness of minoxidil has been described in 11 pediatric patients treated for a minimum of 6 months (Sinaiko et al, 1980). The major adverse reactions are salt and water retention and hypertrichosis that remits with discontinuation but is often severely disfiguring for both boys and girls. Rebound hypertension after minoxidil withdrawal has been reported (Makker and Moorthy, 1980). Methyldopa was used in 22 hypertensive children of whom 13 had impaired renal function (O'Dea and Mirkin, 1980). All children were receiving other antihypertensive agents, and therefore the hypotensive actions of methyldopa could not be assessed. However, these authors found an increase in methyldopa metabolites in those patients with altered renal function. They speculated that the increased sensitivity of azotemic hypertensive children to methyldopa might be explained by the accumulation of metabolites.

Captopril has been shown to be as effective in children as in adults (Oberfield et al, 1979; Sinaiko et al, 1983; Friedman and Chesney, 1983; Callis et al, 1986; O'Dea et al, 1988). Recent reports have emphasized the development of hyperkalemia as an acute event and proteinuria associated with immune complex nephropathy as a long term problem (Mirkin and Newman, 1985). Other problems include cough, ageusia, and renal failure. Bouissou et al, (1986) reported on 25 children (ages 1.5 to 18 years) with renal hypertension who received 29 courses of captopril ther-

**Table 16.13.** Treatment of Chronic Hypertension

| Name of Drug | ORAL DOSE[a] | COMMENT |
|---|---|---|
| **Diuretics** | | |
| Chlorothiazide or | 10 mg/kg/q 12 hours | Not effective in patients with decreased glomerular filtration rate (GFR). Observe for **acute volume depletion**, decreased $K_s$, decreased $Na_s$ long-term effects for children unknown. |
| Hydrochlorothiazide | 1 mg/kg/q 12 hours | |
| Furosemide | 1 mg/kg/dose q 6 hours | Especially valuable in patients with decreased GFR. Causes hypercalciuria, **nephrocalcinosis**, and bone demineralization. |
| **Vasodilators** | | |
| Hydralazine | 0.5–1 mg/kg/dose q 8 hours | Frequently causes reflex tachycardia, abdominal discomfort, headache. especially i.v. **Lupus-like syndrome is rare in pediatrics.** |
| Minoxidil | 0.025–0.05 mg/kg/q 12 hours | Salt and water retention can be modulated or prevented by concomitant diuretics. **Hypertrichosis** is important problem in pediatrics; resolves with discontinuation of drug. **Rebound** hypertension occurs with abrupt discontinuation. (Dose lower than Second Task Force, 1987). |
| Prazosin | 20–25 mcg/kg/dose q 8 hours | No studies of drug in pediatrics; clinical experience indicates that drug is well tolerated. First dose effect dictates that patient receives initial dose supine; some children have **hair loss** with chronic use. |
| Nifedipine | 0.25–0.5 mg/kg/dose 10 mg–Adolescents | Evidence suggests useful drug for severe, symptomatic hypertension. Well tolerated except for tachycardia. Headache, flushing, dizziness occur. |
| **Beta-adrenergic antagonists** | | |
| Propranolol | 0.5–2.0 mg/kg/q 12 hours | Avoid in asthma and heart failure; may have problem with bradycardia, bronchospasm; hypoglycemia reported, especially in patients with inadequate oral intake; **rebound** hypertension with drug interruption. May impair mental performance and adversely affect lipids. |
| Atenolol | 1–2 mg/kg/q 24 hours | No published experience in pediatrics; may be associated with some bronchospasm or mild bradycardia. Advantage over other adrenergic agents is lack of central nervous system effects, once only daily dosage, fewer side effects than other adrenergic blockers. |
| Labetalol | 100 mg bid Adolescents | Has alpha- and beta-adrenergic actions; does not affect exercise or alter lipids. |
| **Central nervous system alpha-adrenergic agonists** | | |
| Methyldopa | 10 mg/kg/q 6 hours | Dose adjustment required with decreased GFR. Interferes with mental concentration; sedation is common. May cause Coombs+ test. **Rebound** hypertension reported on interrupting drug. |
| Clonidine | 0.1–0.2 mg/24 hours | May be effective once daily; initial drowsiness; **rebound** hypertension occurs with abrupt discontinuation. Experience with use of weekly patch in children/adolescents—not published. |
| **Angiotensin-converting (ACE) inhibitors** | | |
| Captopril Infants: Older: | 0.01–0.25 mg/kg q 12 hours 0.25–0.5 mg/kg/q 8 hours | Modification of dose needed in neonates, decreased GFR and renal artery stenosis. In these 3, monitor blood pressure and creatinine carefully. May cause increased $K_s$, thrombocytopenia, neutropenia, nephropathy with secondary proteinuria, ageusia, cough, immune complex. |
| Enalapril | mg/kg/dose not established Start at 2.5 mg/kg/day and monitor need to increase to bid, and then to larger dose. | No skin rashes, ageusia, taste loss, dry cough as with captopril. Currently being studied in pediatrics. Initial experience suggest agent is superior to captopril in terms of side effects, tolerance, and effectiveness. Monitor for neutropenia in lupus and other connective diseases. No adverse lipid effects. |

[a]Lowest starting dose is given.

**Table 16.14. Hypertensive Emergencies in Pediatrics**

Symptoms
  Headache
  Blurred vision, scotoma, transient blindness
  Lethargy, coma, seizures
  Abdominal pain
Signs
  Height and/or weight < 3rd percentile
  Evidence of cerebrovascular accident
  Periorbital edema
  Facial palsy
  Hypertensive retinopathy
  Congestive heart failure
  Abdominal bruit

**Table 16.15. Causes of Hypertensive Emergencies in Pediatrics**

Renal
  Acute glomerulonephritis
  Chronic renal failure/end stage renal disease
  Hemolytic uremic syndrome
  Reflux nephropathy
  Renal artery stenosis
  Systemic lupus erythematosus
  Transplant rejection
Nonrenal
  Coarctation of the aorta
  Drug ingestion
  Pheochromocytoma
  Volume overload

apy during a mean period of 14.8 months. Effective blood pressure control occurred in all but 13%; the latter improved with addition of a beta-blocker. Miller et al (1986) studied 14 children with renal hypertension treated with enalapril for 3½ months to 1 year. The drug was well tolerated; however, two children had an increase in proteinuria. The major advantage of ACE inhibitors are their beneficial effect on renal hemodynamics in children with altered renal function.

Children with chronic renal hypertension may require one or more agents shown in Table 16.13. Titration of dosages up to desirable effects with avoidance of unpleasant side effects is a formidable task. Affected children, their families, and responsible physicians all face a time-consuming often tedious process of controlling blood pressure without precipitating renal dysfunction.

Despite the limitations in knowledge concerning the treatment of children with chronic renal hypertension, therapeutic goals can be reached. Blood pressure levels should be reduced over weeks to months to the safest tolerable levels. Although lowering of blood pressure levels more quickly may alleviate both physician and patient anxiety, the shorter time span does not permit the child adequate time to equilibrate. In general, unless the child has signif-

icant symptomatic hypertension, there is no urgency to lower levels rapidly. The child's vasculature is less vulnerable to the ravages of hypertension so that the known complications of stroke, myocardial infarction, and progressive kidney failure seen in the adult are unlikely.

## Hypertensive Emergencies

An emergency exists when the blood pressure becomes markedly elevated for age and symptoms or signs directly attributable to uncontrolled high blood pressure develop (Table 16.14).

The major causes of hypertensive emergencies in pediatrics are relatively few and are easily diagnosed (Table 16.15).

Treatment of hypertensive emergencies in young individuals has been made safer, easier, and more effective with the availability of agents listed in Table 16.16. The goal of treatment is a safe reduction of elevated pressure by decreasing both the systolic and diastolic levels by approximately 33% within the first 6 hours. The remainder of blood pressure reduction to a preset goal should take place within 36 to 72 hours. Sublingual nifedipine has been studied in infants and children (Rascher et al, 1986; Siegler and Brewer, 1988; Evans et al, 1988); the majority of patients respond and the majority do not experience side effects. Use of this agent provides a safe reliable means of blood pressure reduction (Rascher et al, 1986; Siegler and Brewer, 1988; Evans et al, 1988). The duration of response, however, is highly variable. Intravenous labetolol frequently appears in the European literature as a useful agent (Dillon, 1987; Dillon, 1988), but it has not been studied or used extensively in the United States for children with hypertensive emergencies. Once the blood pressure is lowered to a level at which the patient becomes asymptomatic, oral agents (chosen by the diagnosis and action of each medication) can be introduced so that the patient can be gradually weaned from parenteral therapy (if used) or become less dependent on drugs used for hypertensive crises.

## CONCLUSION

Hypertension in children and adolescents is now recognized as an important pediatric problem, and guidelines for the evaluation of single measurements as well as multiple recordings are available. The determinants of blood pressure are becoming better understood. The diagnosis, evaluation, and therapy are now based on a solid

**Table 16.16. Treatment of Hypertensive Emergencies**

| Drug | Onset of Action | Dose and Route | Comments |
|---|---|---|---|
| Nifedipine | Minutes | 0.25–0.5 mg/kg/dose Sublingual | Avoids acute drops in BP |
| Captopril | Minutes | Infants: 0.05–0.25 mg/kg/dose Children: 0.1–0.2 mg/kg/dose p.o. | May acutely drop BP and cause acute renal failure |
| Hydralazine | Minutes | 0.1–0.2 mg/kg i.v. | Tachycardia, headache 2° to cerebral vasodilation |
| Diazoxide | Minutes | 3–5 mg i.v. bolus | Usually requires furosemide because of salt and $H_2O$ retention. Do not repeat within 1 hour |
| Labetolol | Minutes | 1–3 mg/kg i.v. | May drop BP acutely |
| Nitroprusside | Seconds | 1–8 mcgm/kg/min i.v. | Drug of choice, requires intensive care unit because of difficulty in drug delivery. |
| Phentolamine | Seconds | 0.1–0.2 mg/kg i.v. | Alpha-blocker. For Rx of pheochromocytoma. |

foundation. Recommendations described in this chapter, although based on limited experience, should serve the clinician in the management of most hypertensive children and adolescents.

**Acknowledgment**

The author wishes to acknowledge the invaluable secretarial assistance of Cari Adams in the preparation of this chapter.

**References**

Adelman RD: *Pediatr Clin North Am* 25:99, 1978.

Adelman RD: In Loggie JMH, Horan MJ, Gruskin AB, et al (eds): *NHLBI Workshop on Juvenile Hypertension*, p. 267. New York, Biomedical Information Corporation, 1983.

Adelman RD: *Pediatr Nephrol* 1:35, 1987.

Altschul AM, Grommet JK: *Nutr Rev* 38:393, 1980.

Anderson EA, Mahoney LT, Lauer RM, et al: *Hypertension* 10:544, 1987.

Aristimuno GG, Foster TA, Voors AW, et al: *Circulation* 69:895, 1984.

Aschinberg LC, Zeis PM, Miller RA, et al: *JAMA* 238:322, 1977.

Barker DJP, Osmond C, Golding J, et al: *Br Med J* 298:564, 1989.

Beaglehoe R, Eyles E, Salmond C, et al: *Am J Epidemiol* 108:283, 1978.

Berenson GS, Voors AW, Dalferes ER Jr, et al: *J Lab Clin Med* 93:535, 1979.

Berenson GS, Voors AW, Webber LS, et al: *Hypertension* 5:41, 1983.

Bifano E, Post EM, Springer J, et al: *J Pediatr* 100:143, 1982.

Birmingham Reflux Study Group: In Hodson CT, Heptinstall RH, Winberg J (eds): *Reflux Nephropathy Update: 1983*, Basel, Karger, 1984, p 169.

Biron P, Mongeau J-G, Bertrand D: *Can Med Assoc J* 115:773, 1976.

Boerth RC: In Onesti G, Kim KE (eds): *Hypertension in the Young and the Old*, p. 211. New York, Grune & Stratton, 1980.

Bouissou F, Meguira B, Rostin M, et al: *Clin Exp Hypertens* A8:841, 1986.

Braren V, West JC Jr, Boerth RC, et al: *Urology* 32:228, 1988.

Buchi KF and Siegler RL: *J Hypertens* 4:525, 1986.

Buck C, Stenn PG: *J Psychosom Res* 23:13, 1979.

Callis L, Vila A, Catalá J, et al: *Clin Exp Hypertens* A8:847, 1986.

Canessa M, Adragna N, Solomon HS, et al: *N Engl J Med* 302:772, 1980.

Cater J, Gill M: In Illslev R, Mitchell RG (eds): *Low Birth Weight, a Medical Psychological and Social Study*, p. 191. Chichester, John Wiley, 1984.

Cooper R, Liu K, Trevisan M, et al: *Hypertension* 5:135, 1983.

Court JM, Hill GJ, Dunlop M, et al: *Austr Paediatr J* 10:296, 1974.

Daniels SR, Loggie JMH, Burton T, et al: *J Pediatr* 111:397, 1987.

deLeonardis V, DeScalzi M, Falchetti A, et al: *Am J Hypertens* 1:305, 1988.

deSwiet M: *Br Med Bull* 42:172, 1986.

deSwiet M, Fayers PM, Shinebourne EA: *Br Med J* 1:1567, 1980.

deSwiet M, Fayers PM, Shinebourne EA: *J Hypertens* 2:501, 1984.

Dillon MJ: *Pediatr Nephrol* 1:59, 1987.

Dillon MJ: *Arch Dis Childh* 63:347, 1988.

Durante D, Jones D, Spitzer R: *J Pediatr* 89:978, 1976.

Dweck HS, Reynolds DW, Cassady G: *Am J Dis Child* 127:492, 1974.

Evans JHC, Shaw NJ, Brocklebank: *Arch Dis Childh* 63:975, 1988.

Falkner B, Kushner H, Hkalsa DK, et al: *J Hypertens* 4:(Suppl 5)S381, 1986.

Falkner B, Lowenthal DT, Affrime MB, et al: *Am J Cardiol* 51:459, 1983.

Falkner B, Onesti G, Angelakos ET, et al: *Hypertension* 1:23, 1979.

Fanaroff AA, Stork EK, Carlo W, et al: *In Children's Blood Pressure, 85th Ross Conference*, 1985.

Feinleib M, Garrison R, Borhani N, et al: In Paul O (ed): *Epidemiology and Control of Hypertension*, p. 3. Miami, Symposia Specialists, 1975.

Feld LG and Springate JF: *Curr Prob Pediatr* 18:317, 1988.

Ferrara LA, Moscato TS, Pisanti N, et al: *Cardiology* 75:200, 1988.

Fixler DE, Baron A, Laird WB, et al: In Loggie JMH, Horan MJ, Gruskin AB, et al (eds): *NHLBI Workshop on Hypertension*, p. 37. New York, Biomedical Information Corporation, 1983.

Fixler DE, Laird WP, Fitzgerald V, et al: *Pediatrics* 63:32, 1979.

Friedman AL, Chesney RW: *J Pediatr* 103:806, 1983.

Garay RP, Elghozi J-L, Dagher G, et al: *N Engl J Med* 302:769, 1980.

Gennser G, Rymark P and Isberg BM: *Br Med J* 296:1498, 1988.

Gill DG, Mendes da Costa B, Cameron JS, et al: *Arch Dis Childh* 51:951, 1976.

Gillum RF, Prineas RJ, Gomez-Marin O, et al: *J Chron Dis* 38:187, 1985.

Gillum RF, Prineas RJ, Palta M, et al: *Hypertension* 2:744, 1980.

Goldring D, Londe S, Sivakoff M, et al: *J Pediatr* 91:884, 1977.

Graettinger WF, Weber MA and Gardin JM: *J Am Coll Cardiol* 10:1280, 1987.

Green TP, Nevins TE, Houser MT, et al: *Pediatrics* 67:850, 1981.

Gruskin AB, Perlman SA, Baluarte JH, et al: In Loggie JMH, Horan MJ, Gruskin AB, et al (eds): *NHLBI Workshop on Juvenile Hypertension*, p. 305, New York, Biomedical Information Corporation, 1983.

Gruskin AB, Perlman SA, Baluarte JH, et al: *Clin Exp Hypertens* A8:741, 1986.

Gutgesell M, Terrell G, Labarthe D: *Hypertension* 3:39, 1981.

Harlan WR, Cornoni-Huntley J, Leaverton PE: *Hypertension* 1:559, 1979.

Havlik RJ, Garrison RJ, Katz SH, et al: *Am J Epidemiol* 109:512, 1979.

Hediger ML, Schall JI, Katz SH, et al: *Pediatrics* 74:1016, 1984.

Hennekens CH, Jesse MJ, Klein BE, et al: *Prev Med* 5:60, 1976.

Henningsen NC, Mattsson S, Nosslin B, et al: *Clin Sci* 57:321s, 1979.

Higgins M, Keller JB, Moore F, et al: *Am J Epidemiol* 111:142, 1980a.

Higgins M, Keller JB, Metzner HL, et al: *Hypertension* 2 (Suppl I)I-117, 1980b.

Hiner LB, Gruskin AB, Baluarte HJ, et al: *J Pediatr* 89:258, 1976.

Hobson CJ, Heptinstall RH, Winberg J (eds): *Reflux Nephropathy Update: 1983*, Basel, Karger, 1984.

Hofman A, Hazebroek A, Valkenburg HA: *JAMA* 250:370, 1983.

Hofman A, Valkenburg HA, Maas J, et al: *Int J Epidemiol* 14:91, 1985.

Hohn AR, Riopel DA, Keil JE, et al: *Hypertension* 5:56, 1983.

Holland WW, Beresford SAA: In Paul O (ed): *Epidemiology and Control of Hypertension*, p. 375. Miami, Symposia Specialists, 1975.

Hunter SM, Frerichs RR, Webber LS, et al: *J Chron Dis* 32:441, 1979.

International Reflux Study Commission: *Pediatrics* 67:392, 1981.

Johnson EH, Spielbarger CD, Worden TJ, et al: *J Psychosomat Res* 31:287, 1987.

Johnson GL, Kotchen JM, McKean HE, et al: *Am Heart J* 105:113, 1983.

Kahn HS, Bain RP: *Hypertension* 9:390, 1987.

Kahn HS, Bain RP, Pullen-Smith B: *J Chron Dis* 39:521, 1986.

Kallen RJ, Mohler JH, Lin HL: *Clin Pediatr* 19:567, 1980.

Kilcoyne MM: *Circulation* 50:1014, 1974.

Kilcoyne MM, Richter RW, Alsup PA: *Circulation* 50:758, 1974.

Kirkendall WM, Feinleib M, Freis ED, et al: *Hypertension* 3:509A, 1981.

Kirkland RT, Kirkland JL: *J Pediatr* 80:52, 1972.

Klein AA, McCrory WW, Engle MA: *Cardiovasc Clin* 11:11, 1981.

Korobkin M, Perloff DL, Palubinskas AJ: *J Pediatr* 88:388, 1976.

Kotchen JM, Kotchen TA: *J Chronic Dis* 31:581, 1978.

Kotchen JM, Kotchen TA, Cottrell CM, et al: *J Chronic Dis* 32:653, 1979.

Kotchen JM, Kotchen TA, Schwertman NC, et al: *Am J Epidemiol* 99:315, 1974.

Kotchen TA, Strickland AL, Rice TW, et al: *J Pediatr* 80:938, 1972.

Kwiterovich PO: *Pediatrics* 78:349, 1986.

Labarthe DR: *Clin Exp Hypertens* A8:495, 1986.

Laird WB, Fixler DE: *Pediatrics* 67:255, 1981.

Lauer RM, Anderson AR, Beaglehoe R, et al: *Hypertension* 6:307, 1984.

Lauer RM, Burns TH, Clarke WR: *Pediatrics* 75:1081, 1985.

Lee Y-H, Rosner B, Gould JB, et al: *Pediatrics* 58:722, 1976.

Levine LS, Lewy JE, New MI: *NY State J Med* 76:40, 1976.

Lieberman E, In Kotchen TA, Kotchen JM (eds): *Clinical Approaches to High Blood Pressure in the Young*, p 237. Boston, John Wright, 1983.

Liu K, Cooper R, Soltero I, et al: *Hypertension* 1:631, 1979.

Loggie JMH: *Postgrad Med* 56:133, 1974.

Loggie JMH: *Hosp Pract* 10:81, 1975.

Loggie JMH, Horan MJ, Gruskin AB, et al(eds): *NHLBI Workshop on Juvenile Hypertension*. New York, Biomedical Information Corporation, 1983.

Loirat C, Pillion G, Blum C: *Adv Nephrol* 11:65, 1982.

Londe S, Goldring D: *Am J Cardiol* 37:650, 1976.

Londe S, Goldring D, Gollub SW, et al: In New MI, Levine LS (eds): *Juvenile Hypertension*, p. 13. New York, Raven Press, 1977.

Londe S, Bourgoignie JJ, Robson AM, et al: *J Pediatr* 78:569, 1971.

Londe S, Johanson A, Kronemer NS, et al: *J Pediatr* 87:896, 1975.

Luft FC, Miller JZ, Cohen ST, et al: *Am J Cardiol* 61:1H, 1988.

Lynds BG, Seyler SK, Morgan BM: *Am J Pub Health* 70:171, 1980.

Makker SP, Moorthy B: *J Pediatr* 96:762, 1980.

McDonald A, Treviasan M, Cooper R, et al: *Hypertension* 10[Suppl I]:I-42, 1987.

McGonigle LF, Beaudry MA, Coe JY: *Arch Dis Childh* 62:614, 1987.

Michels VV, Bergstrath EJ, Hoverman VR, et al: *Mayo Clin Proc* 62:875, 1987.

Miller K, Atkin B, Rodel PV, et al: *J Hypertens* 4(Suppl 5):S413, 1986.

Miller RA, Shekelle RB: *Circulation* 54:993, 1976.

Mimura G: *Singapore Med J* 14:278, 1973.

Mirkin BL, Newman TJ: *Pediatrics* 75:1091, 1985.

Molineux and Steptoe A: *J Hypertens* 6:361, 1988.

Mongeau JG: *Int J Pediatr Nephrol* 6:41, 1985.

Mongeau JG: *Pediatr Nephrol* 1:69, 1987.

Moss AJ: *West J Med* 134:296, 1981.

Munger RG, Prineas RJ, Gomez-Marin O: *J Hypertens* 6:647, 1988.

Murphy JK, Alpert BS, Walker SS, et al: *Hypertension* 11:308, 1988.

Newman WP III, Freedman DS, Voors AW, et al: *New Engl J Med* 314:138, 1986.

Oberfield SE, Case DB, Levine LS, et al: *J Pediatr* 95:641, 1979.

O'Dea RF, Mirkin BL: *Clin Pharmacol Ther* 27:37, 1980.

O'Dea RF, Mirkin BL, Alward CT, et al: *J Pediatr* 113:403, 1988.

Ogborn MR, Crocker JFS: *Am J Dis Child* 141:1205, 1987.

Ounsted MK, Cockburn JM, Moar VA, et al: *Arch Dis Childh* 60:631, 1985.

Papa A, Dal Canton A, Capuno, et al: *Proc EDTA* 20:551, 1983.

Parker FC, Croft JB, Cresanta JL, et al: *Am Heart J* 113:1174, 1987.

Pennisi AJ, Takahashi M, Bernstein BH, et al: *J Pediatr* 90:813, 1977.

Perez-Stable E, Carolis PV: *Am Heart J* 106:245, 1983.

Perlman SA, Prebis JW, Gruskin AB, et al: *Semin Nephrol* 3:149, 1983.

Plumer LB, Kaplan GW, Mendoza SA: *J Pediatr* 89:802, 1976.

Potter DE, Schambelan M, Salvatierra O Jr, et al: *J Pediatr* 90:307, 1977.

Prineas RJ, Gillum RF, Gomez-Marin O: In Loggie JMH, Horan MJ, Gruskin AB, et al (eds): *NHLBI Workshop on Juvenile Hypertension*, p. 21. New York, Biomedical Information Corporation, 1983.

Prineas RJ, Gomez-Marin O, Gillum RF: In *Report of the 85th Ross Conference on Pediatric Research*, 120, 1985.

Prineas RH, Gomez-Marin O, Sinaiko A: *Clin Exp Hypertens* A8:583, 1986.

Rames LK, Clarke WR, Connor WE, et al: *Pediatrics* 61:245, 1978.

Rascher W, Bonzel KE, Ruder H, et al: *Clin Exp Hypertens* 8A:859, 1986.

Report of the Joint National Commission on Detection, Evaluation and Treatment of High Blood Pressure: *Arch Int Med* 144:1045, 1984.

Report of the Second Task Force on Blood Pressure Control in Children—1987: *Pediatrics* 79:1, 1987.

Rokkedal-Nielsen J, Hansen HS, Froberg K, et al: *Scand J Clin Lab Inv* 49:32, 1989.

Rose RJ, Miller JZ, Grim CE, et al: *Am J Epidemiol* 109:503, 1979.

Rosner B, Hennekens CH, Kass EH, et al: *Am J Epidemiol* 106:306, 1977.

Schärer K, Rascher W, Ganten D, et al (eds): Proceedings of the Second International Symposium on Hypertension in Children and Adolescents, Heidelberg (FRG): *Clin Exp Hypertens* A8:495, 1986.

Schieken RM, Clarke WR, Prineas R, et al: *Circulation* 66:428, 1982.

Seguro C, Sau F, Rusazio M, et al: *J Hypertens* 4:(Suppl 6)S34, 1986.

Sfakianakis GN, Sfakianaki E, Paredes A, et al: *Biol Neonate* 54:246, 1988.

Shear CL, Burke GL, Freedman DS, et al: *Pediatrics* 77:862, 1986.

Shekelle RB, Liu S, Raynor WJ: *Pediatrics* 61:121, 1978.

Shibutani Y, Sakamoto K, Katsuno S, et al: *J Hypertens* 6:489, 1988.

Siegler RL, Brewer ED: *J Pediatr* 112:811, 1988.

Silverberg DS, Van Nostrand C, Juchli B, et al: *Can Med Assoc J* 113:103, 1975.

Simpson G, Mortimer JG, Silva PA, et al. In: Onesti G, Kim KE (eds). *Hypertension in the Young and Old*, p 153. New York, Grune and Stratton, 1981.

Sinaiko AR, Bass J, Gomez-Marin O, et al: *J Hypertens* 4(Suppl 5):S378, 1985.

Sinaiko AR, Glasser RJ, Gillum RF, et al: *J Pediatr* 100:938, 1982.

Sinaiko AR, Gomez-Marin O, Prineas RJ: *J Pediatr* 114:664, 1989.

Sinaiko AR, Kashtan CE, Mirkin BL: *Clin Exp Hypertens* A8:829, 1986.

Sinaiko AR, Mirkin BL, Hendrich DA, et al: *J Pediatr* 103:799, 1983.

Sinaiko AR, O'Dea RF, Mirkin BL: *J Cardiovasc Pharmacol* 2(Suppl 2):S181, 1980.

Stark P, Beckerhoff R, Leumann EP, et al: *Helv Paediatr Acta* 30:349, 1975.

Still JL, Cottom D: *Arch Dis Childh* 42:34, 1967.

Strong WB: *Pediatrics* 64:693, 1979.

Tochikubo O, Sasaki O, Umemura S, et al: *Hypertension* 8:1164, 1986.

Trevisan M, Strazzullo P, Cappuccio FP: *J Hypertens* 6:227, 1988.

Uhari M, Koskimies O: *Acta Paediatr Scand* 68:193, 1979.

Vailas GN, Brouillette RT, Scott JP, et al: *J Pediatr* 109:101, 1986.

Voors AW, Berenson GS, Dalferes ER, et al: *Science* (Wash DC) 204:1091, 1979.

Voors AW, Webber LS, Frerichs RR: *Am J Epidemiol* 106:101, 1977.

Weinberger MH, Miller JZ, Fineberg NS, et al: *Hypertension* 10:443. 1987.

Weismann DN: *Pediatrics* 82:112, 1988.

Wilson PD, Ferencz C, Dischinger PC, et al: *Am J Epidemiol* 127:946, 1988.

Wilson SL, Gaffney FA, Laird WP, et al: *Hypertension* 7:417, 1985.

Zinner SH, Levy PS, Kass EH: *N Engl J Med* 284:401, 1971.

Zinner SH, Margolius HS, Rosner B, et al: *Am J Epidemiol* 104:124, 1976.

Zinner SH, Margolius HS, Rosner B, et al: *Circulation* 58:908, 1978.

Zinner SH, Martin LF, Sacks F, et al: *Am J Epidemiol* 100:437, 1974.

# Index

Page numbers followed by *t* denote tables; those followed by *f* denote figures.